Histology from a Clinical Perspective

SECOND EDITION

Histology from a Clinical Perspective

SECOND EDITION

Dongmei Cui, M.D. (Hon.), Ph.D.
Associate Professor
Medical Histology and Cell Biology and Dental Histology
Division of Clinical Anatomy
Department of Neurobiology and Anatomical Sciences
University of Mississippi Medical Center
Guest Lecture
Kunming Medical University
Visiting Professor
St. George's University School of Medicine

William P. Daley, M.D.
Professor
Department of Pathology
University of Mississippi Medical Center

Gongchao Yang, M.D.
Professor
Department of Academic Information Services
Department of Neurobiology and Anatomical Sciences
University of Mississippi Medical Center

Edgar R. Meyer, M.A.T., Ph.D.
Assistant Professor
Department of Neurobiology and Anatomical Sciences
School of Medicine
Assistant Director
Master of Science in Biomedical Sciences Program
School of Graduate Studies in the Health Sciences
University of Mississippi Medical Center

James C. Lynch, Ph.D.
Emeritus Professor
Department of Neurobiology and Anatomical Sciences
University of Mississippi Medical Center

Expert Consultants and Contributors:

John P. Naftel, Ph.D.
Emeritus Professor
Department of Neurobiology and Anatomical Sciences
University of Mississippi Medical Center

Duane E. Haines, Ph.D.
Emeritus Professor
Department of Neurobiology and Anatomical Sciences
University of Mississippi Medical Center

Jonathan D. Fratkin, M.D.
Former Professor
Medical Pathology
Department of Pathology
University of Mississippi Medical Center

Illustrators

Michael P. Schenk, B.S., M.S.M.I., C.M.I., F.A.M.I.
Walter Kyle Cunningham, B.A., M.S.M.I.
Tong Yang, D.M.D.
Dongmei Cui, M.D. (Hon.), Ph.D.
James C. Lynch, Ph.D.
John P. Naftel, Ph.D.
Holly R. Fischer, M.F.A.

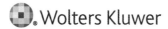. Wolters Kluwer

Philadelphia • Baltimore • New York • London
Buenos Aires • Hong Kong • Sydney • Tokyo

Senior Acquisitions Editor: Crystal Taylor
Development Editors: Kelly Horvath (freelance), Amy Millholen
Editorial Coordinator: Oliver Raj
Editorial Assistant: Parisa Saranj
Marketing Manager: Phyllis Hitner
Production Project Manager: Catherine Ott
Design Coordinator: Stephen Druding
Art Director: Jennifer Clements
Manufacturing Coordinator: Margie Orzech
Prepress Vendor: Straive

Second Edition

9 8 7 6 5 4 3 2 1

Printed in Mexico

Cataloging-in-Publication Data available on request from the Publisher

ISBN: 978-1-9751-5244-4

---

shop.lww.com

QUADM0522

Dedication

To my mentor, Dr. Duane E. Haines, for his wonderful mentoring
and guidance during my early academic career, who has supported
and inspired me to embark on this book.

To my mentors, Drs. John P. Naftel, James C. Lynch, Michael N. Lehman,
and Paul J. May for their understanding and constant support
during my academic journey.

To my students, my colleagues, and friends who have encouraged, supported,
and helped me bring this project to fruition.

—*Dongmei Cui*

Preface

Histology from a Clinical Perspective is based on the first edition of *Atlas of Histology with Functional and Clinical Correlations*. In this new edition, we recognize fundamental shifts in the educational paradigm for professional students. A modest reduction in hours available for basic science instruction, a clear shift to integrate clinically relevant information within the structure of basic science courses, and the packaging of basic science and clinical concepts in a way that is most advantageous to the educational goals of the student pursuing a career in medicine, dentistry, or the allied health professions. We continue to emphasize the importance of the correlation between histology and pathology and relevant examples of clinical cases, and we enhance the linkage of function of histology material to clinical scenarios. The following improvements have been made in this new edition.

First, more clinical correlations have been added. Photographs of some common pathologic conditions were chosen to enhance understanding of how normal tissues are modified by a disease process. Reviewers unanimously liked the inclusion of pathologic examples and the format with normal images (photograph and/or drawing) and a pathologic example appearing on the same page. We continued with this approach and added new examples. We believe that it is not only a major strength of this project but also specifically differentiates this book from others.

Second, a new feature *From Histology to Pathology* has been added to this new edition. Histology and pathology photos are arranged side by side, showing how the basic features of the normal tissue are modified by a pathologic process; this allows easy comparison of the difference between the normal and abnormal tissues and structures and reinforces concepts of basic tissue structure and how it may change under certain conditions. This insight perfectly integrates histology and pathologic concepts in a very simple way. It provides a bridge for medical students to prepare for their clinical years.

Third, clinical vignette questions have been added at the end of each chapter, and their answers can be found at the end of the book. Most questions in the USMLE are clinical vignette questions. Instructors are encouraged by the Association of American Medical Colleges (AAMC) and Institution Curriculum Committee to write clinical-type questions to prepare students for the national board examination. However, many instructors who teach basic science courses do not have clinical experience and face great challenges writing clinical vignettes. We provide clinical vignette questions written by authors having clinical experience and reviewed by both basic science educators and clinical faculty members.

Fourth, we recognize the value of cell structure and function and have included more details in the cell chapter in the new edition. We also added new content in multiple chapters to make the information readily available to the users.

Fifth, computed tomography (CT) images, computed tomography angiography (CTA) images, and, in some cases, stereoscopic 3D images were added in multiple chapters to address anatomic knowledge of organs at the beginning of the organ chapters or associated locations to help integrate and enhance understanding of the relationship between microanatomy and gross anatomy.

Sixth, the quality of the electron micrographs (EMs) has been greatly improved in the new edition. Also, we have some EM images with partially colored structures that emphasize the important features of microstructure and cells. We increased the number of new illustrations and photographs to help students understand the basic concept of the histology materials and associated functions.

Seventh, we have modified and added content to some tables. Clinical correlations have been added in some tables to help summarize the materials and associated clinical correlations.

Eighth, we have added anatomy knowledge for some organs at the beginning or associated locations of the organ chapters. The purpose of this approach is to integrate gross anatomy and microscopic anatomy knowledge to help and make it convenient for students who use integrated curricula.

The goal of *Histology from a Clinical Perspective* is not only to provide a practical and useful source of fundamental information concerning basic histology but also to use an innovative approach to show how tissues can be modified by a pathologic process. This integrated approach emphasizes learning of both normal structure *and* how the same tissues would appear in an abnormal state. We believe that this approach will provide a bridge for students between knowledge of basic histology and clinical concepts as well as enhance information that will directly contribute to their understanding of important medical concepts.

Acknowledgments

The authors express their sincere appreciation to Dr. John P. Naftel, Dr. Duane E. Haines, and Dr. Jonathan D. Fratkin for their excellent contributions to the first edition of the book, which served as a foundation, enabling us to continue building the second edition of this book. We are grateful for the Expert Consultants and Reviewers who contributed to the first and second editions of this project through their insightful review of chapters, many constructive suggestions, and providing tissue samples, slides, or other images. Our special thanks to Dr. Timothy Allen, Chair of the Pathology Department, University of Mississippi Medical Center, for his generous support during this project. We have also benefitted greatly from our pathology colleagues who offered generous support, gave feedback, and, in some cases, contributed images to this project. We express our sincerest appreciation to Dr. Steven Bigler, Dr. Jonathan D. Fratkin, Dr. Kay Allen, Dr. Alexandra Brown, Dr. Michael F. Flessner, Dr. Roland F. Garretson, Dr. J. Mark Reed, Dr. Gary W. Reeves, Dr. Jennifer Schulmeier, Dr. Billy Walker, Dr. Sigurds O. Krolls, Dr. Niping Wang, Dr. Bob Wineman, Dr. Melanie Casey, and Dr. Martin Bohlen.

The inclusion of CT and CTA images in this edition is made possible by the outstanding cooperation of our clinical and basic science colleagues. We express our sincere thanks to the following individuals: Dr. Andrew D. Smith, Dr. Tracy C. Marchant, Dr. John T. McCarty, Dr. Anson L. Thaggard, Dr. Judd Storrs, and Dr. Majid A. Khan. In addition, a number of individuals have contributed to and were involved in creating the 3D stereoscopic images in this book. We greatly appreciate the assistance of Dr. Jian Chen, Dr. Alexis N. Griffith, and Dr. Andrew W. Garza. We also greatly appreciate the support from Dr. Michael N. Lehman, Dr. Timothy D. Wilson, Dr. Allan R. Sinning, and Dr. Marianne L. Conway. Numerous individuals generously provided images or permission to use images. Their names appear in the Figure Credits. We greatly appreciate their professional courtesy. Our sincerest thanks to Dr. Chun Y. Seow, Dr. Peter D. Paré, Mr. Michale Schenk, Dr. Marc Lenoir, Dr. Remy Pujol, Dr. Karen Steel, Dr. David J. Lim, Dr. Timothy C. Hain, Dr. David J. Dickman, Dr. Mark J. Reed, Dr. Paul M. Knechtges, and Dr. Andrew P. Klein. We also express our appreciation to the Anatomical Record, Canadian Journal of Physiology and Pharmacology, the Web site Journey into the World of Hearing, and the Web site: www.dizziness-and-balance.com (please see detailed citations in the figure credits).

We express our special thanks to Ms. Varie Lynch for her careful and excellent editing, reviewing, and proofreading of each chapter on the first edition. We are grateful to Dr. John P. Naftel and Mr. Glenn Hoskins, who were the main source of electron micrographs (TEM and SEM). Histology slides were scanned by Mr. Marcus Williams. Tissue prepared by Ms. Dianne Holmes and Ms. Betty Chen was used in this project. We also thank Dr. Tong Yang, who created many original line drawings and helped with the preparation of the computer files for first edition submission to the publisher. Mr. Jerome Allison provided invaluable advice and assistance in computer-related matters. In addition, helpful comments were provided by Mr. David Lynch and Dr. Eddie Perkins, who offered a number of suggestions on various phases of the project.

Many line drawings were created for this work. These were largely the work of Mr. Michael Schenk and Mr. Walter Kyle Cunningham (Medical Illustrators) and Ms. Holly R. Fischer (MFA). We are enormously appreciative of their time, energy, and dedication to creating the best possible artwork for this book.

The completion of this work would not have been possible without the interest and support of the publisher, Wolters Kluwer/Lippincott Williams & Wilkins. We would like to thank Ms. Crystal Taylor (Senior Acquisitions Editor), Ms. Kelly Horvath (Development Editor), Mr. Oliver Raj (Editorial Coordinator), and Jennifer Clements (Art Director).

Figure Credits

Figure 2-5A,B: © D. Cui. Used with permission.

Figures 4-5A,B and 4-9: © D. Cui. Used with permission.

Figures 5-2A, 5-11A, and 5-12A: © D. Cui. Used with permission.

Figure 6-15: From Seow C.Y. and Paré P.D. "Ultrastructural Basis of Airway Smooth Muscle Contraction." *Can J Physiol Pharmacol*, 85:659-665, 2007. © NRC Canada or its licensors.

Figures 6-3A,B, 6-4B, and 6-7A,B: © D. Cui. Used with permission.

Figures 8-1A,B and 8-14B: © D. Cui. Used with permission.

Figures 10-6 and 10-7: © M. Schenk. Modified with permission.

Figure 13-8A: © D. Cui. Used with permission.

Figures 15-2 and 15-3: © M. Schenk. Modified with permission.

Figure 21-5A: Modified from Hardy M. "Observation on the innervation of the macula sacculi in man." *Anatomical Record*, 59:403-418, 1934, with permission.

Figure 21-9A: Image courtesy of M. Lenoir and R. Pujol from "Journey into the World of Hearing," http://www.cochlea.eu/en/by; R. Pujol et al., NeurOreille, Montpellier, with permission.

Figure 21-9B: © D. Cui. Used with permission.

Figures 21-9C and 21-15: Images courtesy of D.J. Lim, House Ear Institute, Los Angeles.

Figure 21-11C: Image courtesy of T.C. Hain, Northwestern University Medical School, www.dizziness-and-balance.com.

Figure 21-12C: Image courtesy of J.D. Dickman, Baylor College of Medicine.

Figure 21-13C: Image courtesy of J.M. Reed, University of Mississippi Medical Center.

Figure 21-14B: Image courtesy of P.M. Knechtges and A.P. Klein, Medical College of Wisconsin.

Expert Consultants and Reviewers (Second Edition)

March D. Ard, Ph.D.
Emeritus Professor
Department of Neurobiology and Anatomical
 Sciences
University of Mississippi Medical Center

Michele Barbeau, Ph.D.
Assistant Professor
Department of Anatomy and Cell Biology
Schulich School of Medicine and Dentistry
University of Western Ontario, Canada

Kimberly Bibb, M.D.
Assistant Professor
Department of Family Medicine
University of Mississippi Medical Center

Martin Bohlen, Ph.D.
Postdoctoral Fellow
Biomedical Engineering
Duke University

Jian Chen, M.D., Ph.D.
Physician
Pain Management
NEA Baptist Memorial Hospital

Marianne L. Conway, M.D.
Assistant Professor
Department of Neurobiology and Anatomical
 Sciences
University of Mississippi Medical Center

Edward R. Friedlander, M.D.
Professor of Pathology
William Carey University

Andrew W. Garza, M.D.
Emergency Medicine Resident
Graduate Medical Education
University of Mississippi Medical
 Center

Robert S. Gatewood, D.M.D.
Professor
School of Dentistry
University of Mississippi Medical Center

Vasavi R. Gorantla, Ph.D.
Associate Professor
Department of Anatomical sciences
St. George's University, Grenada

Sahar Hafeez, M.D., M.Sc., M.Phil. (Anat)
Associate Professor
Preclinical Sciences, Anatomy and Embryology
College of Osteopathic Medicine
William Carey University

Robert Hage, M.D., Ph.D., D.L.D., M.B.A.
Professor
Department of Anatomical sciences
St. George's University, Grenada

Béla Kanyicska, Ph.D.
Scientist-Educator
Associate Professor (Retired)
Department of Neurobiology and Anatomical
 Sciences
University of Mississippi Medical Center

Barbie Klein, Ph.D.
Assistant Professor
Department of Anatomy
University of California

Jessica B. Perkins, M.D.
Assistant Professor
Division of Allergy and Clinical Immunology
Department of Pediatrics
University of Mississippi Medical Center

Martin Sandig, Ph.D.
Associate Professor
Department of Anatomy and Cell Biology
Schulich School of Medicine and Dentistry
University of Western Ontario, Canada

Audra Schaefer, Ph.D.
Assistant Professor
Department of Neurobiology and Anatomical
 Sciences
University of Mississippi Medical Center

Erica Simmon, M.S.N.
Nurse Practitioner
Advanced Practice Registered Nurse
Women's Health Nurse Practitioner
University of Mississippi Medical Center

Allan R. Sinning, Ph.D.
Professor
Department of Neurobiology and Anatomical
 Sciences
University of Mississippi Medical Center

Niping Wang, D.M.D., Ph.D.
Associate Professor
School of Dentistry
University of Mississippi Medical Center

Jian Yang, M.D., Ph.D.
Senior Lecturer
School of Biomedical Sciences
LKS Faculty of Medicine
The University of Hong Kong

Tong Yang, D.M.D.
Dentist
Private Practice

Kathleen T. Yee, Ph.D.
Assistant Professor
Department of Neurobiology and Anatomical
  Sciences
University of Mississippi Medical Center

Guiyun Zhang, M.D., Ph.D.
Associate Professor
Department of Pathology, Anatomy & Cell
  Biology
Sidney Kimmel Medical College
Thomas Jefferson University

Expert Consultants (First Edition)

March D. Ard, Ph.D.
Emeritus Professor
Department of Neurobiology and Anatomical
  Sciences
University of Mississippi Medical Center

Ben R. Clower, Ph.D.
Former Professor
Department of Neurobiology and Anatomical
  Sciences
University of Mississippi Medical Center

Sigurds O. Krolls, D.D.S.
Former Professor
Department of Maxillofacial Surgery and Oral
  Pathology
School of Dentistry
University of Mississippi Medical Center

Robert E. Lynch, M.D., Ph.D.
Former Chief
Division of Pediatric Critical Care
St. John's Mercy Medical Center
St. Louis, Missouri

Paul J. May, Ph.D.
Professor
Department of Neurobiology and Anatomical
  Sciences
University of Mississippi Medical Center

Norman A. Moore, Ph.D.
Former Professor
Department of Neurobiology and Anatomical
  Sciences
University of Mississippi Medical Center

Allan R. Sinning, Ph.D.
Professor
Department of Neurobiology and Anatomical
  Sciences
University of Mississippi Medical Center

Susan Warren, Ph.D.
Professor
Department of Neurobiology and Anatomical
  Sciences
University of Mississippi Medical Center

Faculty Reviewers

Dr. Stanley A. Baldwin
Dr. Ranjan Batra
Dr. Hamed A. Benghuzzi
Dr. Carson J. Cornbrooks
Dr. Tamira Elul
Dr. John R. Hoffman
Dr. Roger B. Johnson
Dr. Kenneth R. Kao

Dr. Masatoshi Kida
Dr. Rebecca Lynn Pratt
Dr. Timothy Smith
Dr. J. Mattew Velkey
Dr. Peter J. Ward
Dr. Ellen Wood
Dr. Angela Wu

Student Reviewers (Medical, Dental, and Graduate Students)

Joseph D. Boone
Cassandra Bradby
J. Kevin Bridges
Melanie R. Casey
Laura Franklin
Christopher A. Harris
Christine Hsieh
Susan Huang
Jennifer Lau
Margaret Mioduszewski
Ryan C. Morrison
Arash Mozayan-Isfahani

Elizabeth S. Piazza
Raymond Reiser
R. Andrew Rice
Jonathan B. Steadman
Amanda G. Vick
Ryckie Wade
Niping Wang
Griffin West
Israel Wojnowich
Mary Allyson Young
Junlin Zhang

Contents

1 Illustrated Glossary of Histologic and Pathologic Terms

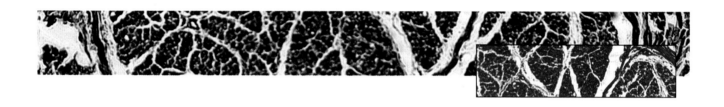

Descriptive Terms for Normal Cells
Cell Shape
Cytoplasm Features
Nucleus Features
Cell Size

Descriptive Terms for Abnormal Cells and Tissues
Acute Inflammation
Apoptosis
Atrophy
Calcification
Chronic Inflammation
Cellular Accumulations
Granulomatous Inflammation
Hyperplasia
Hypertrophy
Hydropic Change
Karyorrhexis
Metaplasia
Monomorphism
Multinucleation
Pleomorphism
Pyknosis
Scar
Necrosis
Pigments
Ulcer

Descriptive Terms for Normal Cells

Cell Shape

Squamous: This is an epithelial cell that has a flattened, "squamous" shape. Usually, the squamous cells we see in sections are cut edgewise so that they appear very thin, and about all we see is the flattened nucleus. The example here shows nuclei of three endothelial cells lining a vein full of erythrocytes.

Cuboidal: This is an epithelial cell with equal height and width. The example here is a layer of cuboidal epithelial cells lining a small duct in the pancreas.

Columnar: This is an epithelial cell with the height distinctly greater than the width. The example here is a layer of columnar cells lining a large duct in the pancreas.

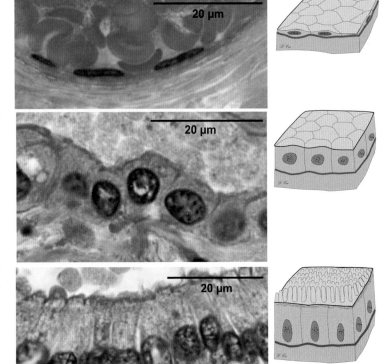

Spherical or ovoid: These terms describe ball-shaped or egg-shaped cells, respectively. The examples here are two spherical cells, a mast cell on the left and a plasma cell on the right. These residents of connective tissue can assume other shapes depending on pressures from neighboring structures.

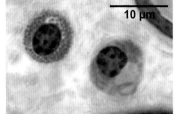

Fusiform: These cells are elongated and tapering at the two ends. The examples here are smooth muscle cells packed together in parallel. The elongated nucleus of each cell is easy to see, but the boundaries of the long spindle-shaped cells are difficult to distinguish.

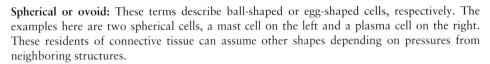

Polyhedral: Multiple flattened surfaces give the appearance of a pentagon, hexagon, and so on. The hepatocyte shown displays six sides.

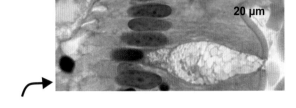

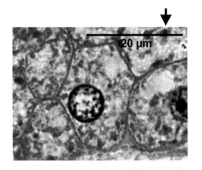

Polarized: These cells have a distinct orientation with one end of the cell being different from the other. Each columnar cell in the above example of intestinal epithelium has an apical end on the right that is different than the basal end on the left. The apical ends are exposed to the lumen. Most of the cells are absorptive cells that have a brush border and a dense row of microvilli extending from their apical surfaces. The cell that appears to have vacuoles filling the apical two thirds of its cytoplasm is a goblet cell, a mucus-secreting cell. What appear to be vacuoles are actually secretory vesicles that lost their contents during tissue processing.

Cytoplasm Features

Basophilia versus acidophilia (eosinophilia): In a hematoxylin and eosin (H&E)–stained section, basophilic components stain blue-purple; acidophilic components stain pink-red. The *arrow* indicates the basal part of the cytoplasm of a cell of a salivary gland duct. The acidophilic (*pink*) staining results from a concentration of mitochondria in this part of the cell. The *arrowhead* indicates the cytoplasm of a plasma cell. The basophilic (*bluish*) staining results from a concentration of rough endoplasmic reticulum.

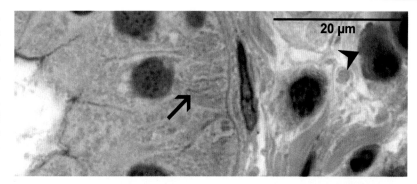

Granules: These vesicles stain because they retained at least some of their contents during tissue preparation. The *arrow* indicates small acidophilic granules filling the cytoplasm of an eosinophil. The *arrowhead* indicates large acidophilic secretory granules in the apical cytoplasm of a Paneth cell. Note that the basal cytoplasm surrounding the nucleus of the Paneth cell stains basophilic, indicating large amounts of rough endoplasmic reticulum in this region of the cell.

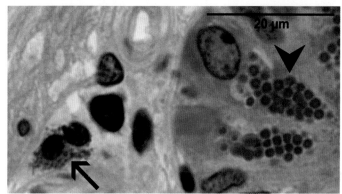

Vacuolated cytoplasm: This type of cytoplasm contains what appear to be empty holes. Usually, these represent either lipid droplets or vesicles whose contents were washed out during tissue processing. What appear to be empty spaces in the cells from the adrenal cortex shown here were actually occupied, in the living state, by droplets of lipid (cholesterol) that were extracted during tissue preparation.

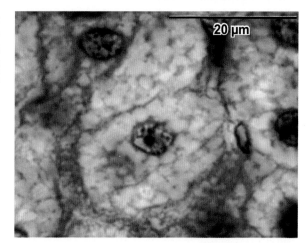

Abundant versus scant: This pair of terms describes a substantial amount (volume) of cytoplasm (*cell 1*) or a slight amount of cytoplasm (*cell 2*) surrounding the nucleus. These are inexact terms but are sometimes useful in describing a cell.

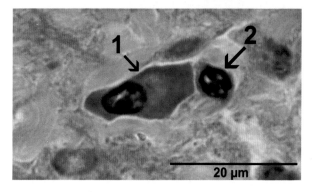

Nucleus Features

Large versus small: This is another imprecise set of terms, but useful when it is possible to make comparisons with nuclei of other cells in the field of view. *Label 1* indicates a relatively *large* nucleus; *labels 3, 4,* and *6* indicate *small* nuclei.

Euchromatic versus heterochromatic: Nuclei of most cells show us a mixture of *euchromatin* (dispersed, lightly stained, accessible to transcription) and *heterochromatin* (condensed, darkly stained, inactive). However, there is a wide variability in the relative proportions of the two forms. *Nucleus 1* has mostly euchromatin. *Nucleus 6* is highly heterochromatic. *Nuclei 3* and *4* have mixes of heterochromatin and euchromatin. Notice that the size of a nucleus is roughly proportional to its content of euchromatin.

Nucleoli prominent: The presence of an obvious nucleolus (*nucleus 1*) or nucleoli indicates that the cell is actively synthesizing ribosomes and, therefore, proteins.

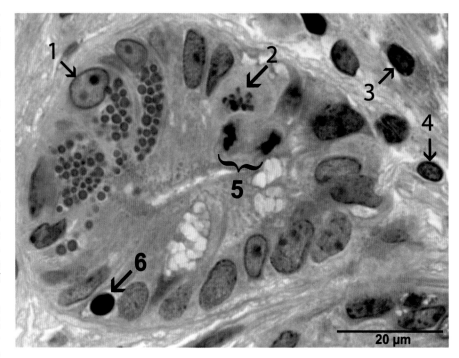

Typically, nucleoli are present in a nucleus that has most of its chromatin in the form of euchromatin, but there are exceptions (e.g., some malignant tumor cells).

Mitotic nucleus: When a cell divides, the nuclear envelope dissolves, and the chromosomes are dark, condensed particles. *Label 2* indicates the chromosomes of a metaphase cell. Label 5 indicates two clusters of chromosomes in an anaphase cell.

Simple versus segmented: A *simple* nucleus appears as a single structure that can have a variety of shapes (round, oval, indented, fusiform, irregular). All the nuclei in this photomicrograph are simple nuclei. A *segmented* nucleus, which is typical of some types of white blood cells, appears in sections as two or more distinct parts (lobes), as seen in the cell in the center of this small panel.

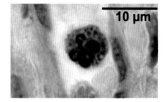

Inferences from nucleus appearance: The appearance of the nucleus provides some clues about the state of the cell's activity. Cells that are active in protein synthesis will usually have fairly large nuclei, prominent nucleoli, and a preponderance of euchromatin. Examples of such cells are rapidly dividing cells (which are busy duplicating cell constituents to be divided among daughter cells), cells that secrete proteins, and cells that have a very large area of membrane and a large volume of cytoplasm to maintain (e.g., neurons).

Cell Size

Large versus small: Although many cell types have diameters falling in the range of 10 to 20 μm, the total spectrum of cell sizes is much broader. There are cells much smaller (e.g., inactive lymphocyte is ~6 μm) or much larger (e.g., megakaryocyte is ~100 μm). If cell volume and surface area are considered, things can get more complicated, because many cells are not compact spheres or simple geometric shapes but have other shapes that can be extremely complex.

Descriptive Terms for Abnormal Cells and Tissues

Acute inflammation. H&E, ×388

Acute inflammation is an immediate response by the immune system due to tissue injury from many causes including infection, necrosis, and trauma. It results in a local increase in blood flow, tissue edema due to increased vascular permeability, and an increased number of acute inflammatory cells (chiefly polymorphonuclear leukocytes or neutrophils). A confluent collection of neutrophils is an **abscess**.

Image: Acute appendicitis showing an infiltration of neutrophils within layers of smooth muscle in the appendiceal wall is shown.

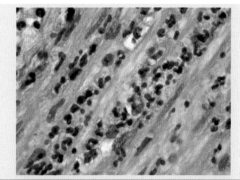

Apoptosis. H&E, ×155

Apoptosis is the process of cell death initiated by either physiologic or pathologic causes. Pathologic apoptosis may be seen in malignant neoplasms, cells damaged by radiation or chemicals, tissues infected by viruses, and immunologic damage as seen in graft versus host disease.

Image: Colonic mucosa demonstrating marked apoptosis of the crypt epithelial cells is shown in a patient with graft versus host disease following a bone marrow transplant.

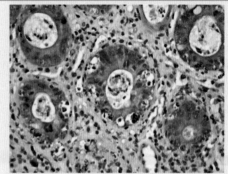

Atrophy. H&E, ×99

Pathologic **atrophy** refers to a decrease in cell size from various factors including denervation, decreased use, aging, decreased blood supply and nutrients, and pressure.

Image: Skeletal muscle showing denervation atrophy is pictured here. Note the larger, normal myocytes in the *right portion* of the image, and the smaller, atrophic myocytes in the *left portion* of the image. In this case, damage to a motor neuron or axon caused atrophy of a group of muscle fibers it served.

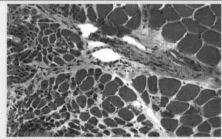

Calcification. H&E, ×199

Tissue **calcification** is abnormal and is broadly divided into **metastatic calcification** and **dystrophic calcification**. *Metastatic calcification* occurs in normal, healthy tissues in patients who are hypercalcemic due to vitamin D intoxication, renal failure, or increased parathyroid hormone or in patients with bone destruction. *Dystrophic calcification* occurs in dying or necrotic tissues in patients with normal serum calcium.

Image: Dystrophic calcification in an intraductal papilloma of the breast is shown. Tissues that assume a papillary morphology tend to develop calcifications at the tips of degenerating papillae. Other examples include papillary thyroid carcinoma and serous papillary neoplasms of the ovaries. Round, lamellated calcifications are called **psammoma bodies**.

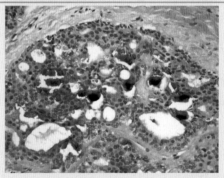

Chronic inflammation. H&E, ×199

Chronic inflammation is an ongoing inflammatory process, typically weeks to months in duration. It may be seen in infectious processes, like viral hepatitis, autoimmune disease, and toxic exposures. **Acute** and **chronic inflammations** commonly coexist, as in active chronic gastritis due to infection of the gastric mucosa by the bacteria *Helicobacter pylori*. The inflammatory cells participating in chronic inflammation include lymphocytes, plasma cells, mast cells, and eosinophils.

Image: This stomach biopsy shows chronic gastritis; note the plasma cells within the lamina propria. No neutrophils are seen, which would indicate a concomitant active, acute inflammatory process.

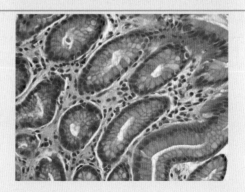

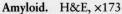

Alpha 1-antitrypsin. PASD (periodic acid-Schiff with diastase digestion), ×173
Alpha 1-antitrypsin deficiency is an autosomal recessive disorder characterized by low serum concentrations of the enzyme *alpha 1-antitrypsin*, which
inhibits or inactivates proteases and elastases. Alpha 1-antitrypsin deficiency
may cause neonatal hepatitis with later cirrhosis and pulmonary panacinar
emphysema.
Image: A liver biopsy in a patient with alpha 1-antitrypsin deficiency shows
accumulated alpha 1-antitrypsin as hyaline globules in this PAS stain. The globules remain after the tissue has been treated with diastase (diastase resistant).

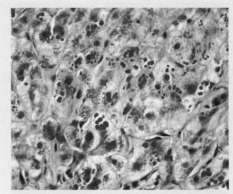

Amyloid. H&E, ×173
Amyloid is an abnormal protein caused by many pathological conditions, the
most common of which include **AL amyloid**, caused by light chains secreted by
plasma cells in plasma cell myeloma or monoclonal B-cell neoplasms; **AA amyloid**, seen in chronic inflammatory conditions; and **Aβ amyloid** in Alzheimer
disease. Many other types of amyloids exist.
Image: A lymph node containing AL amyloid in a patient with small lymphocytic lymphoma is shown. In H&E-stained preparations, amyloid is
amorphous and eosinophilic. Amyloid stained with Congo red shows a characteristic green birefringence when viewed with polarized light.

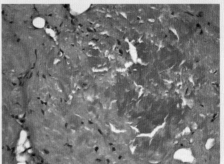

Fatty change. H&E, ×173
Fatty change, or **steatosis**, is the abnormal intracellular accumulation of lipid.
Although it can occur in many organs, it is most commonly seen in the liver
because of a variety of causes including alcohol abuse, hepatitis C, genetic predisposition, medications, toxins, and diabetes mellitus.
Image: This liver biopsy shows marked steatosis with intracellular lipid vacuoles.

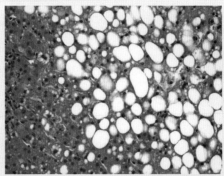

Lewy body. Immunohistochemistry for alpha-synuclein, ×431
A *Lewy body* is an intracytoplasmic oval with a halo, formed in neuromelanin-containing neurons in patients with idiopathic Parkinson disease.
Image: In this immunoperoxidase preparation, brown pigment indicates the
presence of alpha synuclein (*arrow*), the main protein in the inclusion.

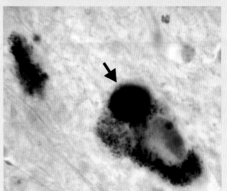

Neurofibrillary tangles. Silver stain, ×173
In patients with Alzheimer disease, microtubule-associated protein tau and
abnormally phosphorylated neurofilaments form *neurofibrillary tangles* within
neurons.
Image: This silver-stained slide shows a twisted, black helix (*arrows*) in the
cytoplasm of a neuron from a patient with Alzheimer disease.

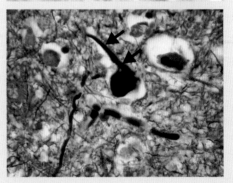

Granulomatous inflammation. H&E, ×99

Granulomatous inflammation is a type of chronic inflammation characterized by localized aggregates of macrophages called **epithelioid histiocytes**. Collectively, these collections of histiocytes are termed **granulomas**. Granulomatous inflammation is characteristic of certain bacterial infections, particularly *Mycobacterium tuberculosis*, fungal infections with organisms like *Histoplasma capsulatum*, and many other disease processes. Granulomatous inflammation may contain areas of necrosis, as in mycobacterial or fungal infections (caseous necrosis), or may be noncaseating as in the granulomatous disease sarcoidosis.

Image: This lymph node biopsy contains abundant noncaseating granulomas in a patient with sarcoidosis.

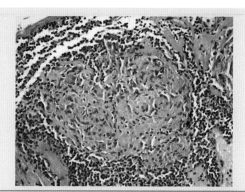

Hyperplasia. H&E, ×99

Hyperplasia represents the increase in the *number*, not size, of cells within an organ or a tissue. Contrast this to **hypertrophy** below in which the cell *size*, not number, increases. Hyperplasia and hypertrophy both may result in a larger organ or tissue. Hyperplasia can be the result of hormonal stimulation, as seen in hyperplasia of the endometrial cells of the uterus in response to estrogen stimulation.

Image: This is an endometrial biopsy showing hyperplasia of the glandular endometrium. The glands are increased in number and are abnormally close together. Endometrial hyperplasia is a risk factor for the development of adenocarcinoma of the endometrium.

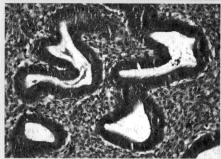

Hypertrophy. H&E, ×497

Hypertrophy is a compensatory mechanism by which the size of cells increases because of various stimuli, resulting in the increase in the size of the corresponding organ. Cardiac myocytes hypertrophy in response to increased workload because of hypertension or valvular dysfunction. In systemic hypertension, as the cardiac myocytes enlarge, the heart itself enlarges, producing left ventricular hypertrophy with a thickened muscular wall.

Image: This image of a hypertrophied cardiac myocyte in a patient with hypertension shows an enlarged, hyperchromatic (deeply staining) nucleus, referred to as a **"boxcar" nucleus**.

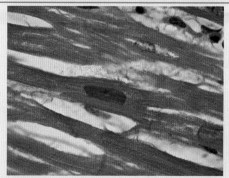

Hydropic change. H&E, ×155

Hydropic change is an early reversible cell injury characterized by cellular swelling due to perturbations in cellular membrane ion-pump function.

Image: This kidney biopsy shows swollen tubular epithelial cells with cytoplasmic clearing due to edema.

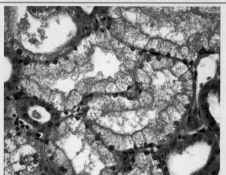

Karyorrhexis. H&E, ×747

Karyorrhexis refers to a pattern of nuclear change seen in irreversibly damaged cells, like pyknosis (below), in which the nucleus breaks apart and fragments.

Image: This image shows a nucleus undergoing karyorrhexis (*arrow*) in a malignant neoplasm.

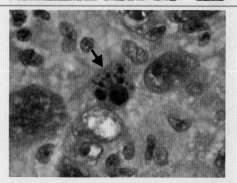

Metaplasia. H&E, ×199

Metaplasia is the reversible change of one mature cell type to another from an environmental stimulus. Examples of metaplasia include squamous metaplasia of the endocervical glandular epithelium of the cervix, squamous metaplasia of ciliated respiratory epithelium in smokers, and intestinal metaplasia of gastric mucosa from chronic gastritis.
Image: A section of stomach shows chronic gastritis with intestinal metaplasia. Note the presence of goblet cells (*arrow*) not normally present in the gastric mucosa.

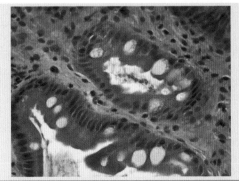

Monomorphism. H&E, ×155

Monomorphism is a term describing cell populations that show little difference in size and shape of the cell itself, the nucleus, or both. Benign neoplasms and well-differentiated malignant neoplasms may be monomorphic.
Image: This image shows a monomorphic population of cells in a duodenal gastrinoma. The cells are relatively uniform in size and shape, as are the nuclei.

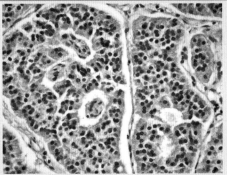

Multinucleation. H&E, ×155

Most normal cells contain a single nucleus, except for the osteoclast, which is **multinucleated**. Multinucleated cells can be seen in a variety of conditions including reactive bone conditions, malignant bone and soft tissue tumors, granulomatous inflammation, and foreign body giant cell reactions.
Images: The first image (*left*) shows a giant cell (*arrow*) in a granuloma of sarcoidosis. The second image (*right*) shows an extensive foreign body giant cell reaction (*dashed line*) to suture material (*arrow*).

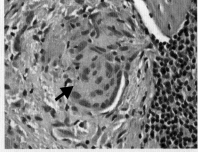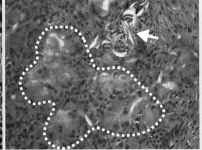

Pleomorphism. H&E, ×199

Pleomorphism is a term describing cell populations that show differences in the size and shape of the cell itself, the nucleus, or both. It is typically used to describe neoplasms. In general, poorly differentiated malignant neoplasms may have a pleomorphic appearance.
Image: This image shows extreme cellular and nuclear pleomorphism in this case of malignant fibrous histiocytoma, pleomorphic type. Compare this image to that of the monomorphic gastrinoma above.

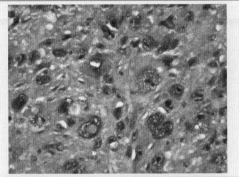

Pyknosis. H&E, ×747

Pyknosis is a morphologic change in the nucleus of an irreversibly damaged cell characterized by condensation and increased basophilia.
Image: This image shows pyknosis (*arrow*) in a dying cell in a malignant neoplasm.

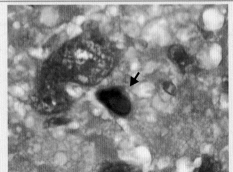

Scar. H&E, ×16

A **scar**, or **cicatrix**, is the result of a complex healing process involving an initial inflammatory response followed by the formation of new blood vessels, tissue remodeling, and wound contraction. Abnormal healing processes include keloid formation and hypertrophic scars.

Image: This image shows a dermal scar characterized by horizontal collagenous bands and an absence of skin adnexa-like hair follicles.

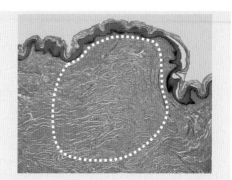

Necrosis

Necrosis represents the death of living cells due to irreversible cell injury. Depending on the tissue involved, necrosis will assume one of several morphologic patterns associated with the processes involved in cell death.

Caseous necrosis. H&E, ×97

Caseous necrosis is a form of necrosis characterized by obliteration of the underlying tissue architecture and the formation of amorphous granular necrotic debris, which grossly appears "cheesy," hence the name *caseous*. Caseous necrosis is highly characteristic of infection with *M. tuberculosis* and certain fungi and is a type of granulomatous inflammation.

Image: This image shows a lymph node biopsy with granulomatous inflammation and necrosis (*to the right of the dashed line*) in a patient with *H. capsulatum* infection.

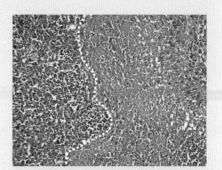

Coagulative necrosis. H&E, ×97

Coagulative necrosis is a form of necrosis characterized by preservation of cellular outlines. Examples include necrosis of cardiac myocytes in myocardial infarction and renal necrosis.

Image: This image shows global coagulative necrosis in a transplanted kidney due to compromised perfusion after the transplant. Note the preserved architecture with the glomerulus in the center surrounded by renal tubules. Note also the pale eosinophilic staining with lack of nuclear staining.

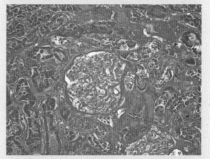

Fat necrosis. H&E, ×193

Fat necrosis is a specific type of necrosis seen in **fatty**, or **adipose, tissue**. Damage to adipocytes causes release of lipids and cell death followed by aggregates of foamy macrophages containing the released lipids. Fat necrosis is seen in damage to fatty tissue by trauma as well as enzymatic digestion as seen in acute pancreatitis.

Image: This image shows fat necrosis in subcutaneous adipose tissue after previous surgery. Note the abundant foamy macrophages containing lipid droplets (*arrow*).

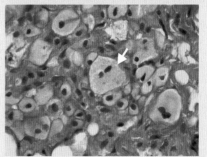

Liquefactive necrosis. H&E, ×48

Liquefactive necrosis may be seen after bacterial infections or infarcts involving the central nervous system.

Image: This image shows liquefactive necrosis in an infarcted area of the brain. Note the intact white matter in the *lower portion* of the image and the granular liquefactive necrosis in the *upper portion* of the image.

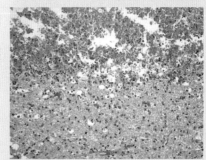

Pigments

Pigments are colored substances found within tissue macrophages or parenchymal cells. Pigments may be **endogenous**, those produced by the body, or **exogenous**, those originating outside of the body. **Melanin, lipofuscin,** and **hemosiderin** are the most common *endogenous* pigments. The most common *exogenous* pigment is **carbon.**

Anthracosis. H&E, × 155

Anthracosis is an exogenous pigment composed of carbonaceous material from smoking and air pollution. Inhaled carbon is taken up by alveolar macrophages and transported to lymph nodes. Anthracotic tissues are black in gross appearance.
Image: This lymph node from the hilar region of the lung shows abundant macrophages containing black carbonaceous material.

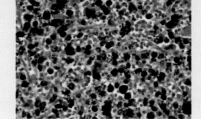

Melanin. H&E, ×388

Melanin pigment, a product of melanocytes, can normally be seen in the basal keratinocytes of the skin. In some chronic inflammatory skin conditions, melanin is released into the dermis and taken up by dermal macrophages, or **melanophages**.
Image: Black-brown melanin pigment is present within the papillary dermal macrophages.

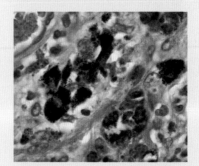

Lipofuscin. H&E, ×388

Also known as **lipochrome**, *lipofuscin* is a yellow-brown pigment related to tissue aging. Lipofuscin is insoluble and composed of phospholipids and lipids from lipid peroxidation. It is commonly seen in the liver and heart.
Image: This hypertrophic cardiac myocyte from an older individual contains lipofuscin granules adjacent to the nucleus.

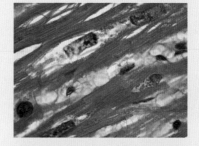

Hemosiderin. H&E, ×155 (left); Prussian blue, 3155 (right)

Hemosiderin is the tissue storage form of iron, which appears as granular, coarse, golden-brown pigment. Hemosiderin is formed from the breakdown of red blood cells and is taken up into tissue macrophages. It may be seen in tissues in which remote bleeding has occurred or in any condition in which excess iron is present.
Images: The first image (*left*) shows abundant hemosiderin-laden macrophages in soft tissue where past bleeding has occurred. The second image (*right*) is a Prussian blue preparation of the same tissue, showing the deep blue staining of hemosiderin.

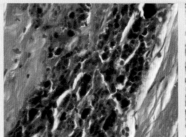 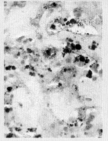

Ulcer. H&E, ×25

An **ulcer** represents the discontinuity of an epithelial surface, which may involve skin or mucous membranes. Ulcers may be caused by infectious processes, chemical exposures, prolonged pressure, or vascular compromise. They typically form crater-shaped lesions with a superficial fibrinopurulent layer and an underlying vascular and fibroblastic proliferation called **granulation tissue**.
Image: This is an image of a gastric ulcer. Note the intact mucosa transitioning to the ulcer with a fibrinopurulent surface. The formation of gastric ulcers is closely associated with infection with *H. pylori*. Gastric ulcers may be benign or malignant, representing gastric adenocarcinoma.

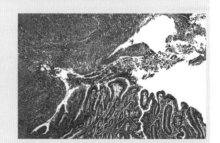

2 Cell Structure and Function

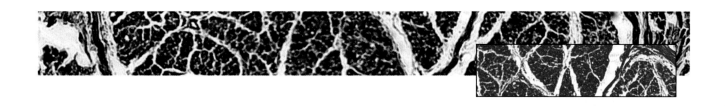

Introduction and Key Concepts for Cell Components
Nucleus
Cytoplasm
Cell Surface

Clinical Vignette Questions

Introduction and Key Concepts for Cell Components

The **cell** is the basic structural and functional unit of the body, and variations in **cell structure** account for the remarkable diversity in the morphology and function of the body's basic tissues and organs. The cell's repertoire of constituents is limited, but the possible combinations of quantities and arrangements of these constituents are numerous.

Nucleus

Nuclear envelope: This is a double-membrane structure consisting of a perinuclear cistern sandwiched between the inner and the outer nuclear membranes. The nuclear envelope protects the genetic material and separates it from the diverse molecules and structures of the cytoplasm. The nuclear envelope is continuous with the rough endoplasmic reticulum.

Nuclear pore: These gaps in the nuclear envelope are bridged by a pore complex of numerous proteins. This structure controls the traffic of molecules and particles between the nucleus and the cytoplasm.

Heterochromatin: This tightly coiled chromatin is inaccessible for transcription, and it appears as basophilic clumps in specimens prepared for light microscopy.

Euchromatin: This is chromatin in a more extended form, accessible to transcription. In the light microscope, it appears as less densely stained, basophilic regions of the nucleus.

Nucleolus: One or more of these spherical, basophilic structures develop in the nucleus if the cell is generating ribosomes.

Cytoplasm

Ribosome: This is an egg-shaped particle (~20 × 30 nm) that attaches to a messenger RNA (mRNA) molecule and generates a polypeptide according to the code provided by the nucleotide sequence of the mRNA strand.

Polyribosome: This is formed by the alignment of several ribosomes along the length of an mRNA molecule. When an mRNA for a cytosolic or mitochondrial protein is being translated, the polyribosome is not associated with endoplasmic reticulum, but rather it is suspended in the cytosol as a free polyribosome.

Rough endoplasmic reticulum (RER): This typically consists of flattened membrane-delimited cisternae that are studded with ribosomes. As polypeptides are synthesized by the ribosomes, they are sequestered by insertion into the cisternae. Small shuttle vesicles (transport vesicles) move the newly synthesized polypeptides from the RER to the Golgi complex.

Golgi complex: This consists of a stack of flattened membranous saccules (cisternae). The Golgi complex receives polypeptides from the RER, modifies them (e.g., by sulfation, glycosylation), and sorts and packages them according to their destination as constituents of lysosomes, secretory granules (e.g., pancreatic acinar cell), or cytoplasmic granules (e.g., neutrophilic leukocyte).

Secretory vesicle: Also called **secretory granules**, these are membrane-delimited packages of secretory products that can be either stored in the cytoplasm or immediately secreted by exocytosis of the vesicle at the cell surface.

Lysosome: This is a membrane-delimited vesicle characterized by its low pH and the content of a variety of hydrolases that can digest proteins, lipids, and polysaccharides. Lysosomes function both in the turnover of intrinsic cellular components and in the breakdown of the material ingested by endocytosis.

Other types of membrane-delimited vesicles: Substances other than the secretory products of secretory granules and the hydrolytic enzymes of lysosomes may be sequestered within vesicles. Examples are proteases within proteasomes, unfinished polypeptides in transfer vesicles, and oxidases and catalase in peroxisomes.

Smooth endoplasmic reticulum (SER): This is a membrane-delimited labyrinth, usually in the form of tubules rather than flattened cisternae. Its multiple functions include synthesis of membrane phospholipids, degradation of some hormones and toxic substances (liver), synthesis of steroid hormones, and sequestration of calcium stores (striated muscle).

Mitochondrion: This is a double-membrane organelle (like the nucleus) that generates adenosine triphosphate (ATP) to fuel energy-requiring activities of the cell. It also functions in some specialized synthetic pathways such as that for steroid hormones.

Cell Surface

Cilia: These are cylindrical extensions about 200 nm thick and 5 to 10 μm long. They are usually motile, with a whipping motion that consists of a power stroke and a recovery stroke. An axoneme of microtubules in a nine-doublet, two-singlet arrangement provides the stiffness and movement of cilia.

Microvilli: These are cylindrical, nonmotile extensions, typically about 80 nm in diameter and 1 μm long. In some cells, they are several micrometers long, in which case, they are called **stereocilia**. Actin filaments form the cores of microvilli.

Zonula occludens: Also called **tight junctions**, these are sites of fusion between plasmalemmas of adjacent epithelial cells that separate the lumen from the underlying connective tissue. Tight junctions prevent materials from passing from one compartment to another by diffusing through the space between adjacent epithelial cells.

Zonula adherens: These are sites of mechanical adhesion between adjacent epithelial cells. They are generally associated with and parallel to tight junctions. Actin filaments of the terminal web are anchored by proteins at the cytoplasmic faces of the membranes of the two cells.

Macula adherens: Also called **desmosomes**, these, like zonula adherens, are sites of mechanical adhesion between cells, but they are configured as spots rather than bands. Intermediate filaments are anchored to proteins at the cytoplasmic surfaces of the membranes of the two cells.

Gap junctions: Also called **nexus junctions**, these are sites of close (~2 nm) apposition between plasmalemmas of adjacent cells. The small space between the membranes is bridged by connexons, each of which is a cylindrical complex of proteins forming a pore. Gap junctions allow free flow of small ions between cells, so that the cells are electrically coupled.

Basolateral folds: Infoldings of the plasmalemma at the basal surface of an epithelial cell provide greatly increased surface area in support of extensive traffic of substances between the cytosol and the underlying interstitial compartment. Such folds are particularly prominent in epithelial cells that function in removing water and ions from a lumen. Lateral folds can have an additional function of contributing mechanical strength to a layer of cells by interlacing with complementary folds of an adjacent cell.

Basal lamina: This is an extracellular layer at the interface of a cell and the adjacent connective tissue. Basal laminae are characteristic of the basal surfaces of epithelia, but they are not restricted to epithelia. Examples of other cells with basal laminae are muscle cells and the Schwann cells that enshroud the axons of peripheral nerves.

Cytoskeleton

Actin filaments: These are thin (6 nm) filaments that form a feltwork (cortex) beneath the plasmalemma of many cells. They form a skeletal core of microvilli, and they also function in the movement of motile cells. In contractile cells, actin filaments interact with myosin (thick) filaments.

Intermediate filaments: These are relatively stable 10 nm to 12 nm filaments that provide structural support for the cell. Different specific proteins that form these filaments are characteristic of particular groups of cell types.

Microtubules: These are hollow tubes ~25 nm in diameter. In conjunction with other proteins, particularly kinesin and dynein, they serve as tracks for movement of materials within the cytoplasm. Microtubules also form centrioles and the basal bodies and axonemes (cores) of cilia.

SYNOPSIS 2-1 Functions of Major Cell Components

Nucleus
- *Nucleus*: Synthesizes all types of RNA; replicates its DNA.
- *Heterochromatin*: Condenses inactive DNA.
- *Euchromatin*: Renders DNA accessible to transcription.
- *Nucleolus*: Produces ribosomal RNA; assembles ribosome particles.
- *Nuclear envelope*: Segregates DNA from cytoplasmic constituents.
- *Nuclear pore*: Controls access of molecules that move between the nucleus and the cytoplasm.

Cytoplasm
- *Mitochondria*: Generate ATP and contribute to synthesis of some molecules.
- *Ribosome*: Translates mRNA to polypeptides.
- *Rough endoplasmic reticulum (RER)*: Synthesizes proteins to be confined by or associated with membranes.
- *Smooth endoplasmic reticulum (SER)*: Contributes to lipid metabolism, drug detoxification, and calcium regulation.
- *Golgi complex*: Modifies, packages, and traffics proteins.
- *Lysosome*: Degrades extraneous material.
- *Vesicles*: Segregate molecules from cytosol.

Cell Surface
- *Microvillus*: Increases the area of plasmalemma at a free (apical) surface of an epithelial cell.
- *Basal or basolateral fold*: Increases the area of plasmalemma at the basolateral surface of an epithelial cell.
- *Cilium*: Moves the material along the apical surface of an epithelial cell.
- *Basal lamina*: Contributes to the boundary between a cell and its surrounding interstitium.

Cytoskeleton
- *Actin filament*: Contributes to contraction, cell motility, and cell stiffness.
- *Myosin filament*: Interacts with actin to produce contraction.
- *Intermediate filament*: Contributes to structural (mechanical) strength of a cell.
- *Microtubule*: Provides tracks for intracellular movement of molecules and particles; generates movement of cilia and movement of chromosomes during cell division.

Centrosome: This is composed of a pair of centrioles embedded in amorphous material. The two centrioles are oriented at right

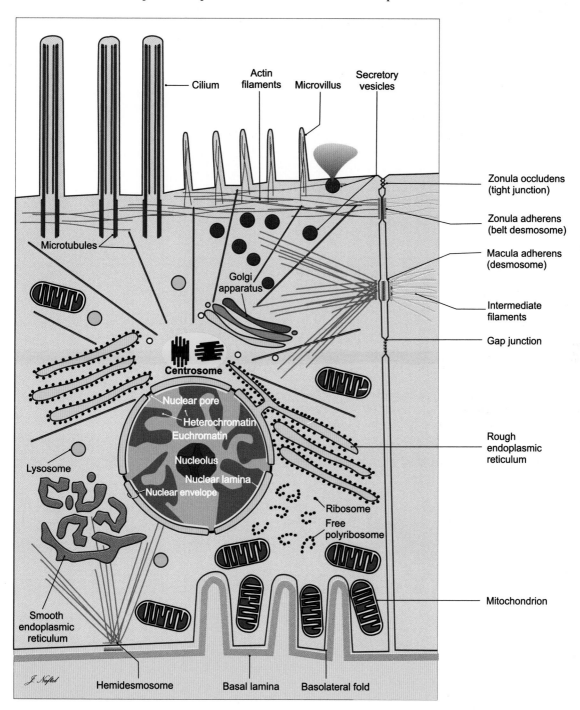

Figure 2-1. Overview of the cell.

The cell is the basic structural and functional unit of the human body. The human body contains a wide variety of cells, and the cells that share similar characteristics collectively form different tissues of the body with unique structures and functions. In general, each cell is composed of a **nucleus, cytoplasm,** and **plasma membrane (plasmalemma)**, also known as **cell membrane.** Some cells have more than one nucleus, and, although most cells have a round or an oval-shaped nucleus, some have an elongated, column-shaped nucleus. An active cell often has a **nucleolus** or multiple **nucleoli** within its nucleus. The **cytoplasm** is a gel-like solution with suspended organelles and other components enclosed inside of the cell membrane. The **cytosol** is the fluid part of the cytoplasm. It contains mainly water, salts, carbohydrates, and proteins, etc., which provide structure and support to the cell and allow movement of materials within the cell. The structural components of cytoplasm include **organelles, inclusions,** and elements of **cytoskeleton.** The **cell membrane** is a double-layer, selectively permeable membrane. It surrounds the entire cell to protect and confine cell contents, and its main function is to control and regulate the movements of materials in and out of the cell.

angles to each other, and each is composed of nine triplet sets of microtubules. The centrosome functions in organizing the array of

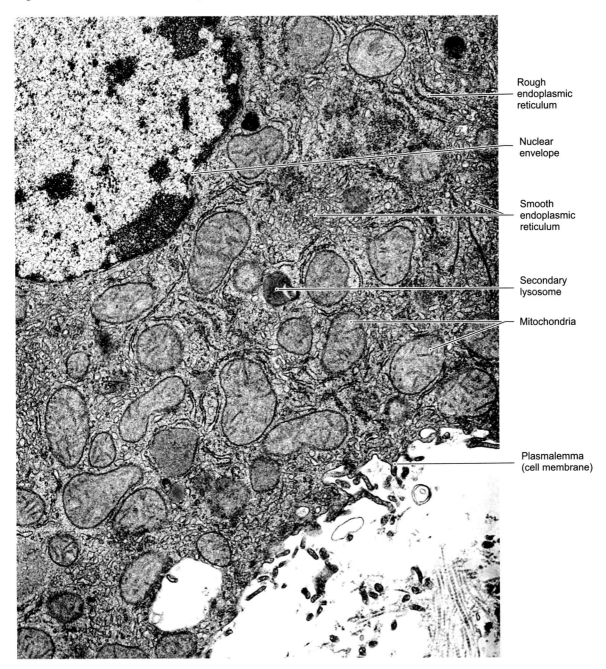

Figure 2-2. Membranes define the major components and compartments of the cell. EM, ×19,000

All **ultrastructural features** of cells can be viewed with electron microscopy under optimum conditions of specimen preparation, orientation, and magnification. The **unit membrane** that delimits the cell and many of its major components is seen as a thin, electron-dense line in transmission electron micrographs. Segments of membrane that are oriented vertically to the plane of section are most sharply defined, whereas membrane segments that are oriented at or nearly parallel to the plane of section cannot be readily discerned. Identification of the major organelles relies, to a great extent, on the characteristic arrangements of the membranes that define them. Two major structures, the **nucleus** and the **mitochondria**, are bounded by **double membranes**. Identification of mitochondria is aided by the infoldings of the **inner mitochondrial membrane** that form shelflike or tubular cristae, extending through the interior of the organelle. The **inner nuclear membrane** typically has heterochromatin apposed to it, and the **outer nuclear membrane** is often studded with ribosomes. The membrane that forms the **RER** encloses a cisternal space in the shape of either disks or tubules, and identification is confirmed by the presence of polyribosomes on the outer surface of the membrane. **SER** typically has a branching tubular form, so that, in sections, patches of circular, ovoid, and Y-shaped profiles of membrane are seen.

microtubules in the cell's cytoplasm and in developing the spindle apparatus during cell division.

A

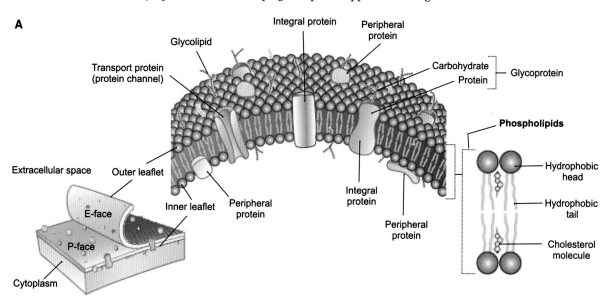

Figure 2-3A. Overview of the cell membrane (plasmalemma).

The cell membrane is also known as **plasma membrane (plasmalemma)**. It is composed of a double layer of phospholipids (forming outer leaflet and inner leaflet lipid bilayers) and membrane proteins. The prime function of cell membrane is to provide protection to the intracellular elements as well as giving shape to the cell. It also allows the transport of materials between the intra and extracellular environments through the process of **endocytosis** and **exocytosis**, respectively. **Membrane lipids** include **phospholipids, cholesterol,** and **glycolipids**. **Phospholipids** are composed of both polar parts (hydrophilic heads) and nonpolar parts (hydrophobic tails). **Cholesterols** connect phospholipids together and prevent them from drifting apart, also help to restrict movement of membrane proteins, and maintain the structural integrity of the membrane. **Glycolipids** are lipids with an attached carbohydrate and are located on the extracellular aspect of the outer membrane. They facilitate cellular recognition while also acting as membrane receptors. **Membrane proteins** include **integral proteins** and **peripheral proteins**. The **integral proteins** are embedded in the lipid bilayer of the cellular membrane. Examples of **integral proteins** include **transmembrane proteins**, such as **sodium channels**, and **glycoproteins**, such as **integrins**. The **peripheral proteins** are attached to the surface of cell membranes. Peripheral proteins are often attached to integral membrane proteins or located in the peripheral regions of the lipid bilayer, and they act as electron carriers. Examples of peripheral proteins include **cytochrome c, annexins, synapsin I,** and **spectrin**.

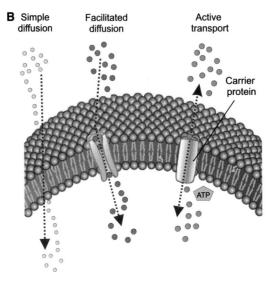

B Simple diffusion   Facilitated diffusion   Active transport

Carrier protein

ATP

Figure 2-3B. Cell membrane transport roles.

The **cell membrane** plays an important role in controlling the movement of substances in and out of cells via **passive transport** and **active transport**. **Passive transport** is a process in which the substances transfer across a cell membrane through a concentration gradient. Examples of passive transport include **osmosis, simple diffusion, facilitated diffusion,** and **filtration. Osmosis** involves the transfer of water from an area of lower concentration to an area of higher concentration via a semipermeable membrane. On the other hand, **diffusion** transfers molecules across the cell membrane from a higher concentration area to a lower concentration area. **Simple diffusion** transports small, uncharged molecules directly through the cell membrane without assistance. **Facilitated diffusion** transfers large and polar molecules through the cell membrane with assistance from **transmembrane proteins,** such as **channel proteins, aquaporins,** and **carrier proteins. Carrier proteins** have both passive and active transport functions. **Filtration** is a process of separating solid substance from a fluid, during the process a medium stops the passing of the substance. Fluid flows from an area of high pressure to an area of low pressure, such as in the production of urine, a constant pressure in the glomerular capillaries will filtrate plasma into the Bowman capsule. **Active transport** is an energy-dependent process that utilizes cellular energy and also requires the assistance of carrier proteins to transfer molecules across the cell membrane against an electrochemical gradient from areas of lower concentration to areas of higher concentration. Examples of active transport include the transfer of vesicle contents across cell membranes via **exocytosis** and **endocytosis. Exocytosis** refers to the process in which vesicles transfer their contents from the inside to the outside of the cell (substances leave the cell). **Endocytosis** refers to the process in which vesicles transfer materials from the outside to the inside of the cell (substances enter the cell).

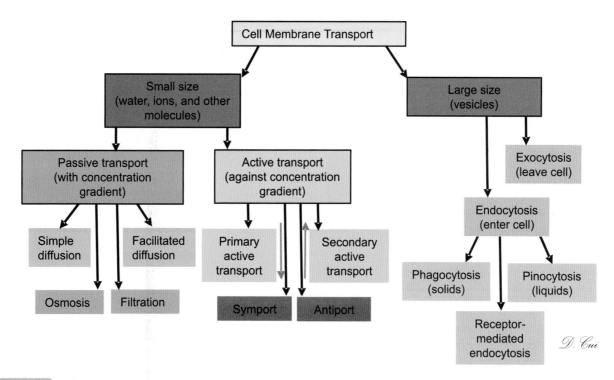

Figure 2-4. Cell membrane transport.

The **cell membrane** is semipermeable because it selectively allows the movement of fluid and certain molecules across it to maintain the internal environment of the cell. Small materials, such as water, ions, and other biological molecules, cross the cell membrane via both **passive transport** and **active transport**. The molecules moving from high concentration to low concentration across the membrane by passive transport use either **simple diffusion** or **facilitated diffusion**. Transport of oxygen (O_2), carbon dioxide (CO_2), and ethanol are examples of **simple diffusion**. Transport of glucose and amino acids are examples of **facilitated diffusion**, which requires the assistance of **carrier proteins** during the process of diffusion. Facilitated diffusion is faster than simple diffusion. Water moves from a region of lower solute concentration across the cell membrane into the region of higher solute concentration through a process known as **osmosis**. Under normal conditions, this movement of water is from the extracellular space into the intracellular space. Glomerular filtration of urine in the kidney is an example of **filtration**, which requires pressure to assist material transport. **Active transport** requires energy and additional help from **carrier proteins** when molecules move from a lower concentration environment into a higher concentration environment or when molecules move against a concentration gradient across the cell membrane. It includes **primary active transport** and **secondary active transport**. The movement of sodium ions (Na^+), potassium ions (K^+), calcium ions (Ca^{2+}), and hydrogen ions (H^+) across the cell membrane are examples of primary active transport, in which energy is derived directly from hydrolysis of ATP. Transportation of glucose and amino acids are examples of secondary active transport, in which transportation is indirectly linked to the hydrolysis of ATP. A transportation system that carries two molecules in the same direction across the cell membrane is called **symport**, such as a sodium-glucose transport protein. The transportation of one molecule in one direction, while another molecule is transported in the other direction, is called **antiport**, such as a sodium-potassium pump. **Vesicle transport** occurs via special types of active transport, including endocytosis, exocytosis, phagocytosis, and pinocytosis. **Exocytosis** is the movement of vesicle contents from the inside of the cell across the cell membrane to the outside of the cell (export), and examples include moving secretory vesicles (enzymes and hormones) from the cytoplasm of the cell to the outside environment. **Endocytosis** is the transportation of vesicles from extracellular fluid across the cell membrane into the cytoplasm of the cell (import). **Phagocytosis** (solid), **pinocytosis** (fluid), and **receptor-mediated endocytosis** are three types of endocytosis. **Phagocytosis** (cell eating) refers to the movement of solid particles via vesicles from the outside of the cell to the inside of the cell. For example, neutrophils use phagocytosis to engulf bacteria from the outside of the cell to the inside of the cell to digest them in the cytoplasm. **Pinocytosis** (cell drinking) refers to the process of moving fluid within vesicles from extracellular space across the cell membrane into the cell. **Receptor-mediated endocytosis**, also called clathrin-mediated endocytosis, is a type of endocytosis with the aid of a receptor for a specific molecule outside the cell. When that molecule, called the ligand, binds to the receptor on the external cell membrane, the protein clathrin forms a coat under the receptor on the internal side of the cell membrane. Clathrin causes the coated area of membrane to form into a vesicle that carries the ligand (and receptor) into the interior of the cell.

SYNOPSIS 2-2 Cell Membrane (Plasmalemma)

Membrane receptors are cell surface proteins that are embedded in the plasma membrane. They act as receptors for specific extracellular molecules. The binding of extracellular molecules to their receptors is a signal that triggers a series of events inside the cell.

Carrier proteins are membrane proteins that bind and transport specific molecules or ions across cell membranes. For example, calcium-binding carrier proteins transport calcium ions into the cell.

Channel proteins are membrane proteins that control the passage of ions or molecules into and out of the cell along the concentration gradient. Channels open to facilitate diffusion of ions across the membrane, and they close to inhibit diffusion, which maintains a difference in concentration inside and outside the cell.

Ligand-gated ion channels are a subclass of ion channels that open or close in response to the binding of specific ligands to membrane receptors. For example, ligand-gated sodium channels open when acetylcholine binds to nicotinic acetylcholine receptors on muscle cells.

Endocytosis and *exocytosis* transport materials contained in vesicles into and out of the cell. In endocytosis, a portion of the cell membrane forms an indentation and then a vesicle enclosing a small amount of extracellular fluid, which is transported into the cell. In exocytosis, an intracellular vesicle fuses with the cell membrane, emptying its contents into the extracellular space.

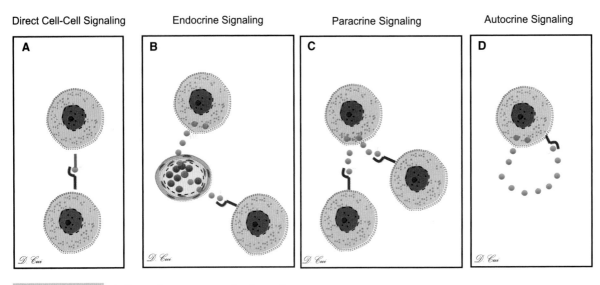

Direct Cell-Cell Signaling   Endocrine Signaling   Paracrine Signaling   Autocrine Signaling

Figure 2-5A–D. Cell membrane communication roles.

Cell-to-cell communication occurs via signaling molecules and membrane receptors. The signaling molecules are secreted by signaling cells. Signaling molecules can bind with membrane receptor proteins to promote cell-to-cell interactions and communications. (A) Cell signaling can occur from direct interaction between two neighboring cells (cell to cell). Synaptic signaling that occurs between two neurons via the actions of neurotransmitters at synapses is also an example of direct cell-to-cell communication. (B) Cell signaling can also occur through secreted and released signaling molecules that act on distant target cells. The signaling molecules, hormones, released by endocrine cells are carried through the bloodstream and act on distant target cells, which have specific receptors for the hormone. (C) In **paracrine signaling**, signaling molecules or hormones are released into the intercellular space and act on nearby cells. (D) **Autocrine signaling** is a special case in which the signaling molecules are secreted into the extracellular space, then bind to receptors on the secreting cell itself, so that the same cell is both the signaling and target cell. There are two types of signaling molecules: (1) **Hydrophobic (lipid-soluble) signaling molecules**, such as steroid and thyroid hormones, cross the cell membrane and bind to receptors inside the cell (cytoplasm or nucleus), and (2) **hydrophilic signaling molecules**, such as neurotransmitters and most hormones, bind to and activate cell surface receptors. **Membrane receptors** are mainly transmembrane proteins, such as glycoproteins, which are types of integral membrane proteins embedded in the lipid bilayer. **Membrane receptors** include **channel-linked receptors, enzyme-linked receptors,** and **G protein–coupled receptors (GPCRs)**. **Channel-linked receptors**, such as nicotinic acetylcholine (ACh) receptors, bind a signaling molecule, an event that opens or closes a channel to allow or block ions to pass through the cell membrane. **Enzyme-linked receptors**, such as insulin receptors, are membrane receptors that are associated with enzymes. **GPCRs**, also called **seven-transmembrane receptors**, pass on the signals with the help of G protein (guanine nucleotide–binding protein). When a signal molecule (ligand) binds with GPCR, the G protein on the cell membrane is activated. The G protein makes a conformational change resulting in exchange of guanosine diphosphate (GDP) for guanosine triphosphate (GTP) and the regulation of target proteins to generate intracellular second messengers that initiate cellular responses.

CLINICAL CORRELATION

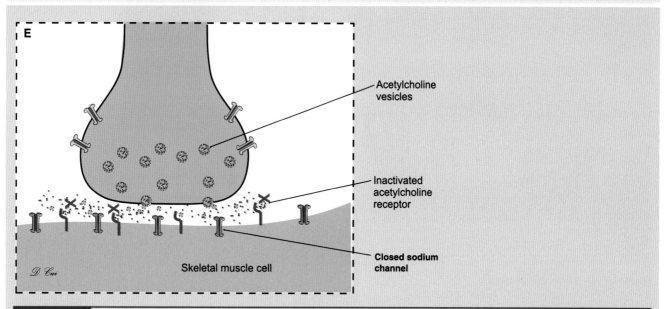

Acetylcholine
vesicles

Inactivated
acetylcholine
receptor

Closed sodium
channel

Skeletal muscle cell

D. Cui

Figure 2-5E. **Inactivated Acetylcholine Receptors (Snakebite).**

Snakebites cause over 100,000 human deaths worldwide annually. Snake venoms, produced by the parotid salivary glands of the poisonous snakes, are complex mixtures of proteins. Snake venoms exert a wide range of toxic actions, responsible for various clinical manifestations, ranging from local tissue damage to potentially life-threatening systemic effects. The neurotoxic effects of venom can inhibit presynaptic terminals from releasing ACh. Venom can also bind to the ACh receptors to prevent the opening of the **sodium channels**. The toxic effects can be generally categorized into neurotoxic, vasculotoxic, and myotoxic. Some snakes, like elapids, may have more neurotoxic effects, acting on the neuromuscular junction. The venom competes with **acetylcholine** at nicotinic receptors, **inactivating** the **acetylcholine receptor**, leading to muscular weakness and paralysis. Some venoms cause vasculotoxic effects, destroying endothelial cell membranes, leading to coagulation disorders and the lysis of red blood cells. Myotoxins cause muscle weakness and may lead to heart and respiratory muscle failure. Intravenous administration of antivenom is the only specific treatment to counteract the snake venom. Analgesics, ventilator support, fluid therapy, hemodialysis, and antibiotic therapy may also benefit.

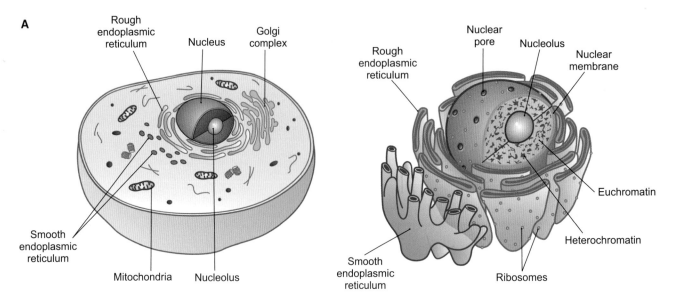

Figure 2-6A. Overview of nucleus.

The **cell nucleus** is located within the cell, stores genetic material, and regulates the activities of the cell. The cell nucleus is enclosed by a **nuclear envelope**, and it contains **heterochromatin**, **euchromatin**, and a nucleolus. The **nuclear envelope** is a double-layered structure constituting an **inner nuclear membrane** and an **outer nuclear membrane** as well as numerous **nuclear pores**. Heterochromatin is an inactive form of DNA that appears dark and electron dense. **Euchromatin** is active DNA that appears light and electron lucent. The **nucleolus** is a spherical structure inside the nucleus. It is the site of **ribosome** production, and it produces **ribosomal RNA** and plays an important role in the assistance of protein synthesis. More than one nucleolus can be found in the nucleus of a cell that is actively synthesizing proteins.

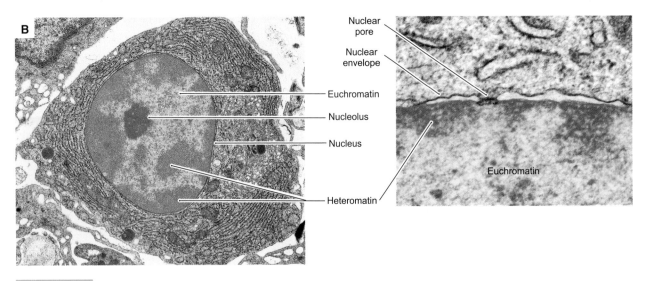

Figure 2-6B. **Cell nucleus.** EM, left ×17,000; right ×65,900

This is a transmission electron micrograph of a **cell nucleus** suspended in the cytoplasm of a protein-secreting cell (*A*). A small black condensed nucleolus is visible inside the nucleus. The **heterochromatin** appears relatively dark and dense and is distributed toward the periphery of the nucleus. The **euchromatin** appears light and surrounds the nucleolus. The **nuclear envelope** contains two layers of membranes (inner and outer), and it is interrupted by a nuclear pore (*B*). There are many nuclear pores in each nucleus, providing transport pathways between the nucleus and the cytoplasm.

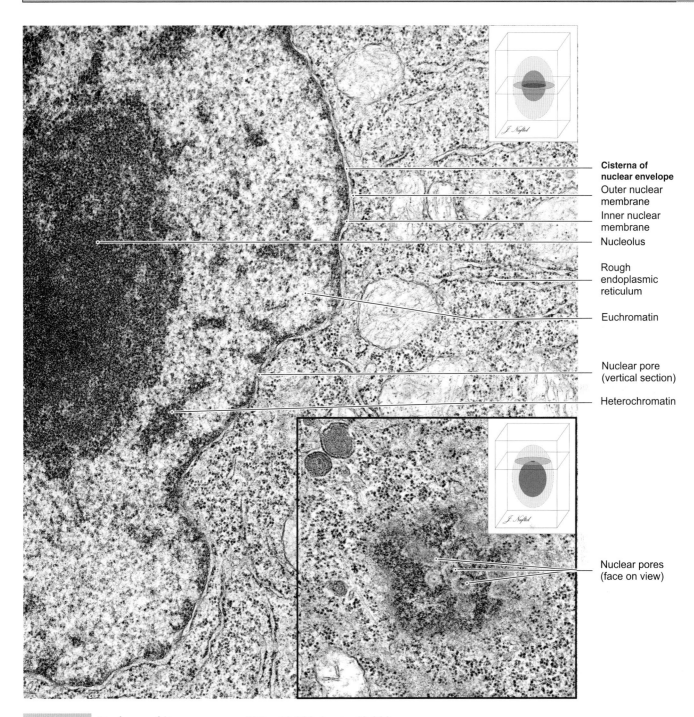

Cisterna of
nuclear envelope
Outer nuclear
membrane
Inner nuclear
membrane
Nucleolus

Rough
endoplasmic
reticulum

Euchromatin

Nuclear pore
(vertical section)

Heterochromatin

Nuclear pores
(face on view)

Figure 2-7. **Nucleus and its components.** EM, ×43,000; inset ×42,000

The **outer** and **inner nuclear membranes** and the **perinuclear cisternae** are readily identified in electron micrographs if there is adequate magnification and a favorable plane of section. In some cells, the outer nuclear membrane is studded with ribosomes, and the perinuclear cisternae are continuous with the cisternae of **RER**. In a cell that is actively synthesizing proteins, the **nuclear envelope** has numerous **nuclear pores** that can be identified in electron micrographs as interruptions in the double-membrane arrangement of the nuclear envelope. Some face-on views of nuclear pores can be seen in the *inset*. Note that the pores are not simply openings, but rather each has a diaphragm. Chromatin that is highly condensed, or **heterochromatin**, is much more electron dense than chromatin that is accessible to transcription, or **euchromatin**. Clumps of heterochromatin tend to be located adjacent to the inner nuclear membrane, with gaps that correspond to sites of nuclear pores. **Nucleoli** resemble heterochromatin but can usually be distinguished by a more complex substructure of granular, fibrous, and nucleolar organizer components.

Cell

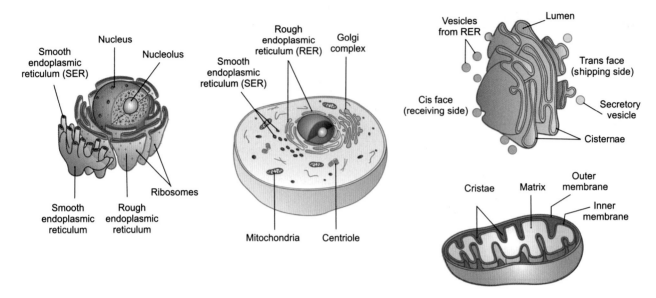

Figure 2-8. Overview of cytoplasm and organelles.

The **cytoplasm** contains cytosol, **cellular organelles, inclusions,** and **cytoskeleton. Cytosol** is a cellular fluid, a gel-like solution that provides support and maintains **organelles** in suspension within the cytoplasm. **Cellular organelles** are functional units located within the cytoplasm, and each organelle has its unique structure and function. The main organelles found in the cytoplasm include **mitochondria, rough endoplasmic reticulum (RER), smooth endoplasmic reticulum (SER),** the **Golgi complex, ribosomes, lysosomes,** and **vesicles. Cytoplasmic inclusions** are temporarily present in the cytosol and not able to carry out metabolic activities. Inclusions include stored nutrients, secretory products, and granules, such as glycogen, lipid droplets, lipofuscin, and the centrosome. The **cytoskeleton** is the skeleton of the cell, providing structural support and maintaining cell shape. The **actin filaments (microfilaments), myosin filaments, intermediate filaments,** and **microtubules** are the major elements of the cytoskeleton.

Mitochondria: elongated organelles, composed of a double-layered membrane (an outer and inner membrane). The outer mitochondrial membrane is smooth, while the inner membrane shows winding folds, the **cristae.** The fluid within the inner membrane is called the **matrix.** The main function of mitochondria is the production of energy (for cellular use) through the generation of ATP. They also contribute to the synthesis of some molecules.

Ribosomes: small granular particles where all protein synthesis occurs. Ribosomes are found attached to the surface of the **rough endoplasmic reticulum (RER)** and floating freely in the cytosol. A group of ribosomes aggregated to form a cluster structure known as **polyribosome,** which is attached to a single mRNA molecule and is commonly found in the cytosol.

Rough endoplasmic reticulum (RER): an organelle with a series of membranous folds with an inner lumen (**cisterna**) and an outer surface, which numerous mature **ribosomes** are attached. It is the primary site of protein synthesis and is closely associated with the **nucleus** and the **Golgi complex.** The main functions of this organelle include modifying, storing, and transporting proteins made by **ribosomes.** The proteins produced by the RER are utilized by both cytoplasm and cell membranes.

Golgi apparatus (Golgi complex): an organelle resembling a flattened stack of membranous. The Golgi complex is composed of multiple **cisternae** (saccules) with several regions: **cis Golgi network (CGN), medial Golgi network,** and **trans Golgi network (TGN).** The main functions of the Golgi complex include sorting, modifying, and packaging of proteins and lipids.

Smooth endoplasmic reticulum (SER): an organelle resembling a membranous tubular network without ribosomes on its outer surfaces. Although the SER connects to the RER, it has a different function, which does not relate to the protein synthesis. The main functions of SER include the synthesis and transport of **lipids** and **steroids.** Another function is **detoxification.** Therefore, the hepatocytes (liver cells) contain abundant SER, which is involved in the metabolism and ingestion of toxins.

Lysosome: a vesicle-like, membrane-bound organelle. It contains a variety of hydrolytic enzymes (**nucleases, proteases, glycosidases, phosphatases, lipases,** and **sulfatases**) that can degrade material and digest proteins. Lysosomes are commonly found in the cytoplasm of phagocytes. Lysosomes can be classified as primary lysosomes (early, small, before fusing with the phagosome) and secondary lysosomes (late, large, fused with a phagosome). **Secondary lysosomes,** also known as **heterolysosomes,** are relatively large and contain active enzymes. Digested materials are stored inside a membrane-bound vacuole called a **residual body.** For example, the **lipofuscin granules** in long-lived neurons are residual bodies. Lysosomal digestion can be divided into **heterophagy** (ingestion via phagocytosis/pinocytosis), **autophagy** (self-digestion of materials or organelles from within the cells itself), and **crinophagy** (ingestion of extra secretory granules) based on how and where the material is degraded.

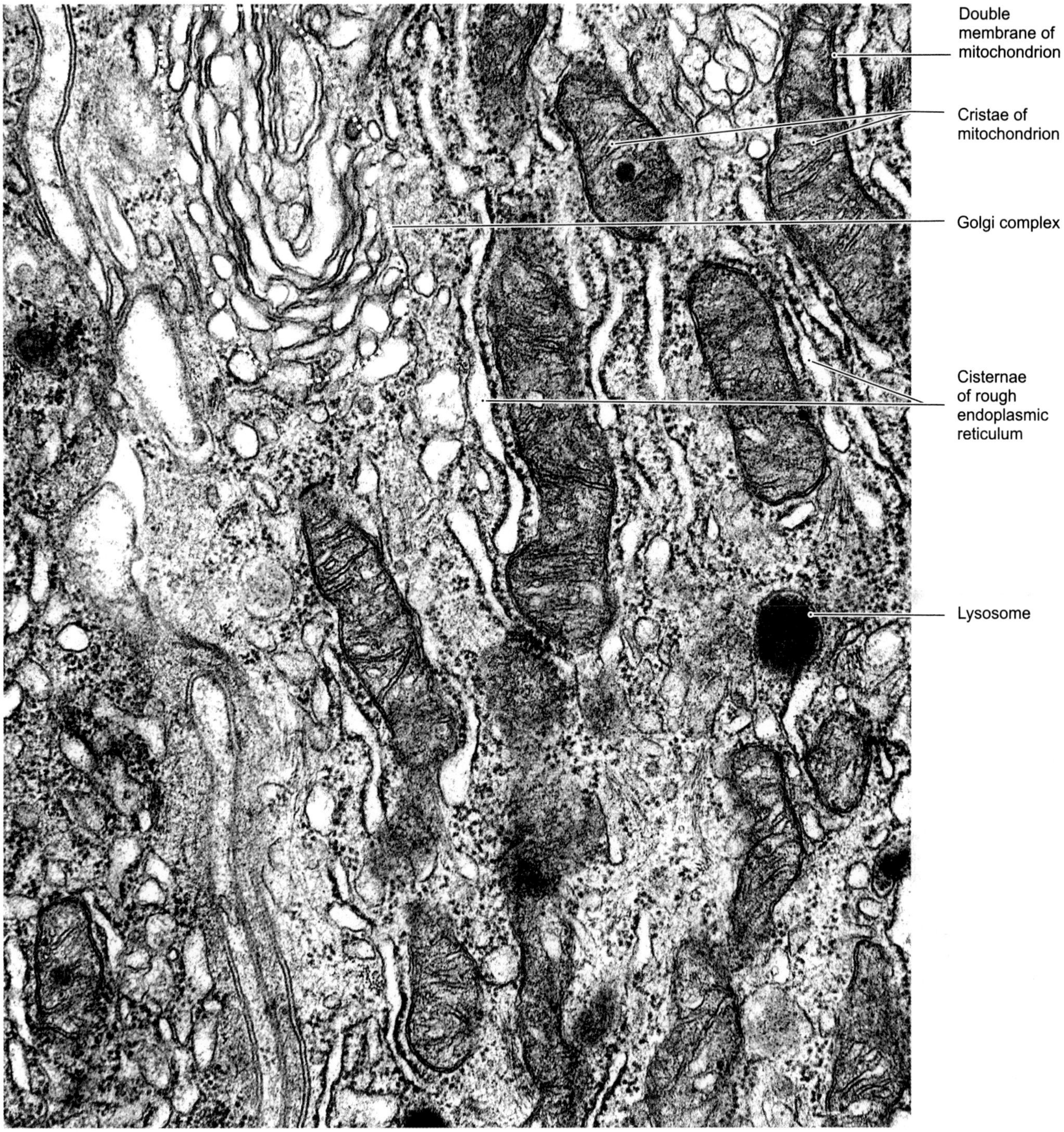
Double membrane of mitochondrion
Cristae of mitochondrion
Golgi complex
Cisternae of rough endoplasmic reticulum
Lysosome

Figure 2-9. **Cytoplasmic organelles.** EM, ×66,000

Mitochondria vary both in size and shape and in the appearance of their **cristae**, yet they are generally the easiest organelles to identify in transmission electron micrographs. The striking features are the **double membrane** and the **cristae**, which are inwardly directed extensions of the inner mitochondrial membrane. The **RER** typically consists of flattened, membrane-delimited sacs. The distinguishing feature of RER is the presence of ribosomes (polyribosomes) attached to the outer surface of the membrane. **SER** also consists of membrane-delimited spaces, but these are usually in the form of a labyrinth of branching tubules. The surface of the membrane of SER is smooth, with no attached ribosomes. **Golgi complexes** are composed of stacks of flattened, membrane-delimited sacs along with associated vesicles. Shapes of the sacs can vary, but often they are bowl shaped, so that there is a convex face (the forming face) and a concave face (the maturing face).

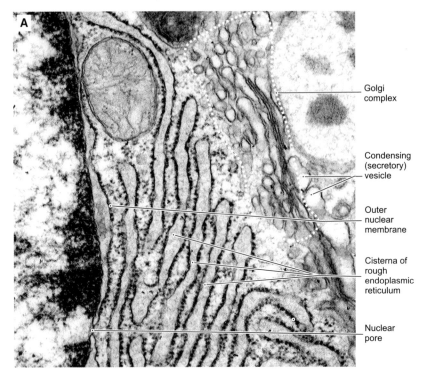

Figure 2-10A. Cytoplasmic organelles: Rough endoplasmic reticulum and the Golgi complex. EM, ×49,000

This view includes only a small area at the edge of the **nucleus** of a cell that is actively synthesizing proteins for secretion. Both euchromatin and heterochromatin can be seen, but the nucleolus, although present in the cell, is not in view here. The **nuclear pore** is the gateway for materials leaving the nucleus, for example, mRNA, tRNA (transfer RNA), and preribosomal particles. Entering the nucleus through nuclear pores are histones and other proteins of chromatin, DNA polymerases and RNA polymerases, and ribosomal proteins. The **outer nuclear membrane** is studded with ribosomes, an indication that the nuclear envelope is continuous with the **RER**, which is abundant in this cell. A part of the **Golgi complex** is identifiable as a stack of flattened membranous sacs with smooth surfaces. The small **vesicles** associated with the Golgi complex include transport vesicles that convey polypeptides from the RER.

Labels for Figure 2-10A:
- Golgi complex
- Condensing (secretory) vesicle
- Outer nuclear membrane
- Cisterna of rough endoplasmic reticulum
- Nuclear pore

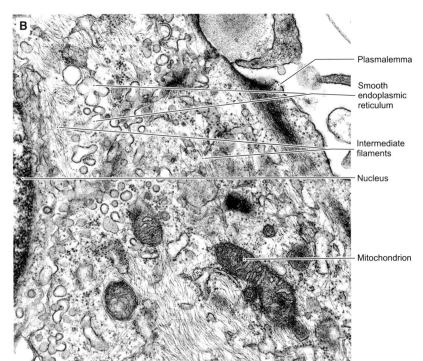

Figure 2-10B. Cytoplasmic organelles: Smooth endoplasmic reticulum. EM, ×33,000

Smooth endoplasmic reticulum is considerably less conspicuous in appearance than RER with its broad, flattened cisternae and arrays of attached ribosomes. The usual configuration of SER is a labyrinth of branching tubules with swellings. Thus, it presents in sections as profiles of smooth-surfaced circular or oval membranes, much the same as slices through spherical vesicles. The true distinctive structure of the SER is revealed by the occasional profiles that have a Y-shaped or branching lumen, as can be seen in this image. The cytoplasm in this view also contains some **mitochondria** and numerous **intermediate filaments** coursing through the cytosol. Some of the filaments near the **plasmalemma** of the cell are more likely actin filaments, which are concentrated in the **cortex** (outer layer) of many cells.

Labels for Figure 2-10B:
- Plasmalemma
- Smooth endoplasmic reticulum
- Intermediate filaments
- Nucleus
- Mitochondrion

A

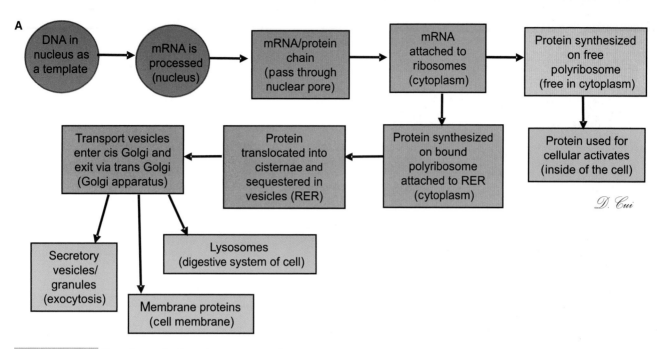

Figure 2-11A. Protein synthesis and transport pathway.

Protein synthesis is initiated in the **nucleus. Nucleoli** within the nucleus are the sites of ribosomal RNA production. DNA in the nucleus serves as a template from which mRNA is transcribed and processed and then released via **nuclear pores** from the nucleus into the cytoplasm. A single **mRNA** attaches to multiple ribosomes to form a functional group called a **polyribosome** in the cytoplasm and to initiate protein synthesis. Proteins are synthesized on **polyribosomes** found floating freely in the cytoplasm. These proteins are mainly used for cellular activities within the cell, such as cytoplasmic filament, mitochondria, and peroxisome formation. Proteins are also synthesized on the **bound polyribosomes** (polysomes) attached to **rough endoplasmic reticulum (RER)**. These proteins are translated into the cisternae of RER, and they undergo a series of processes of modification and sequestration. These processes include folding of proteins, modification of membrane proteins, covalent modification (such as phosphorylation and methylation), **cleavage** (reduction of a large initial protein to a smaller final structure for enzymes and secreted proteins), and **glycosylation** (formation of glycoproteins). Proteins are sequestered in vesicles in the RER and transferred via transport vesicles into the **Golgi apparatus** via the **cis face** (toward the RER) and exit the Golgi apparatus via the **trans face** (away from the RER). Proteins in transport vesicles are sorted, modified, and packaged in the Golgi apparatus. These proteins are used for **secretory granules, lysosomes**, and **membrane proteins**.

CLINICAL CORRELATION

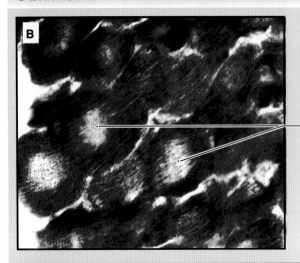

Absence of mitochondria
in the muscle fibers
with central core

| Figure 2-11B | Mitochondrial Disease (Central Core Myopathy). NADH, ×600 |

Central core disease is a mitochondrion-associated disease. It causes predominantly proximal **skeletal muscle weakness** in infants. The muscle weakness may cause delays in developmental milestones such as the initiation of walking. Often children with the disease have an abnormal gait and may appear to waddle. This weakness generally extends into adulthood, but it is not considered a severely progressive disease. Exercise and physical therapy can be of benefit. Muscle biopsies in affected patients reveal a **central clearing (central core)** of a portion or all the **myocytes** under routine and special histologic stains. Ultrastructural examination· of the central clearing reveals a marked **reduction** to a complete **absence of mitochondria**, the organelles responsible for **cellular respiration**, and **energy production**. The disease is due to a mutation in the **ryanodine receptor gene (RYR1)**. Some patients with central core myopathy are at risk for **malignant hyperthermia**, a severe reaction to certain anesthetics and depolarizing muscle relaxants.

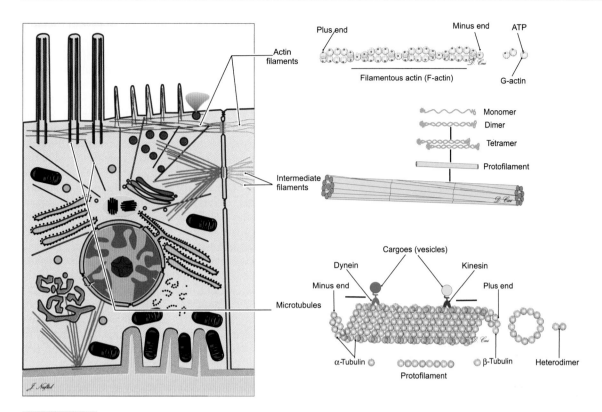

Figure 2-12. Overview of cytoskeleton.

The cytoskeleton is the network of filaments and tubules that provides a structural framework supporting the cell and serves as avenues for vesicle and organelle transport. It includes **actin filaments**, **intermediate filaments**, and **microtubules**.

Actin filaments are 5 to 7 nm in diameter and composed of numbers of globular **G-actin monomers** (**G actin**) that form a long two-helix structure known as **F actin**. Each **actin filament** has a **minus end** and a **plus end** with the polarity of polymerization and depolymerization. The functions of actin filaments include structural support to the cell (cell stiffness), cell motility, and cell contraction, such as the sliding of myosin filaments along actin filaments in the muscle cell during muscle contraction. Movement along microfilaments is mediated by motor proteins such as **myosin**.

Intermediate filaments are thicker than actin filaments and about 10 to 12 nm in diameter. They have no polarity and no motor proteins. The production of intermediate filament begins with assembling two **monomers** into a **dimer**, and two dimers form a **tetramer**. Tetramers join end to end to form a **protofilament**, and finally an intermediate filament is formed by approximately eight protofilaments. Intermediate filaments are composed of a large family of proteins and can be classified into five classes: (1) **type I acidic keratins** and **type II neutral-basic keratins**. Both classes are found in epithelial cells, such as cells in the epidermis of skin, hair, nails, and corneas. Types I and II provide structural support to and prevent the fracture of epithelial cells under tension. (2) **Type III** has four groups: **desmin, vimentin, glial fibrillary acidic protein (GFAP)**, and **peripherin**. Desmin is found in muscle cells, and **vimentin** is found in mesenchymal cells and mesenchymal-derived cells, such as fibroblasts and white blood cells. **Vimentin** can be used as a marker for mesenchymal derived tumor cells. GFAP is mainly found in glial cells (supporting cells) of the central nervous system, such as astrocytes and ependymal cells. **Peripherin** is mainly found in ganglion cells of the peripheral nervous system, and it also can be found in the neurons that have projections toward peripheral structures, such as spinal motor neurons. Type III intermediate–associated proteins (desmin, vimentin, GFAP, and peripherin) provide structural support and shape to nonepithelial cells. (3) **Type IV neurofilaments** are mainly found in the neurons of the central nervous system. Neurofilaments provide structural support and shape to the neuron cell body and help stabilize the extended axons of neurons. (4) **Type V lamins** are associated with the nucleus and are collectively known as the nuclear lamina. Lamins are found in the inner region of the nuclear envelope, and they interact with inner nuclear membrane proteins. The primary function of lamins is to help protect the DNA of the cell. (5) **Type VI nestin** is associated with radial growth of the axon and found in stem cells of the central nervous system. It can be used as a protein marker for the stem cells of the neurons.

Microtubules are hollow tubular structures of the cytoskeleton and measure about 25 nm in diameter. Each microtubule is composed of various fibrous proteins, including α-tubulin and β-tubulin. The α-tubulin and β-tubulin bind together to form a **heterodimer**, and then heterodimers form a **protofilament**. About 13 **protofilaments** assemble into a **microtubule**. Microtubules have a **minus end** and a **plus end**, with high polarity of polymerization and depolymerization. The motor proteins **kinesin** and **dynein** are associated with microtubules and assist with the movement of vesicles and other materials along microtubules. **Kinesin** bears **anterograde cargo**, helping move it toward the **plus end** (carrying materials to the periphery of the cell/cell surface); **dynein** bears **retrograde cargo**, helping move it toward the **minus end** of microtubules (carrying materials to the center of the cell). The functions of microtubules include structural support to the cell and directed movement of vesicles and other materials within the cytoplasm.

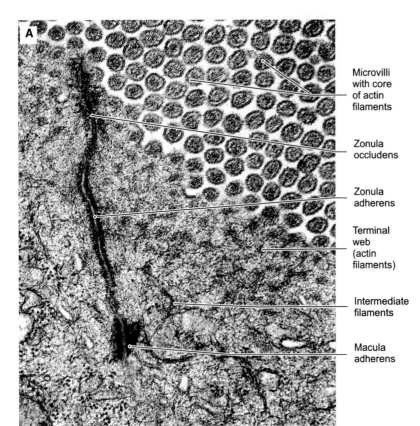

Microvilli with core of actin filaments

Zonula occludens

Zonula adherens

Terminal web (actin filaments)

Intermediate filaments

Macula adherens

Figure 2-13A. Cell surface and cytoskeleton, intestinal absorptive cells. EM, ×73,000

This image is restricted to a very small part of the surfaces of two **absorptive cells** (enterocytes) in the wall of the small intestine. The plane of section is tangential to the plane of the surface, so that the *right side* of the image shows numerous microvilli that project into the lumen and function to greatly increase the surface area exposed to the contents of the intestine. The electron-dense dots in the **cores** of the **microvilli** are **actin filaments**, which, in this case, provide stiffness rather than motility. These actin filaments extend from the microvilli into the cytoplasm as part of the **terminal web** of actin filaments near the cell surface. Components of a **junctional complex** provide a seal (**zonula occludens**) and adhesion (**zonula adherens** and **macula adherens**) between neighboring enterocytes. Beneath the terminal web of actin filaments are thicker filaments, **intermediate filaments**, which provide mechanical strength to the cell. Some of the intermediate filaments are anchored in the **macula adherens**.

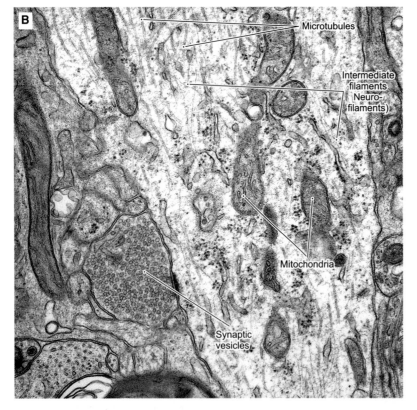

Microtubules

Intermediate filaments Neuro-filaments)

Mitochondria

Synaptic vesicles

Figure 2-13B. Cytoskeleton, the dendrite of a neuron. EM, ×20,000

The central structure in this view is a **dendrite of a neuron**. It is a process extending from the cell body of the cell. Dendrites and **axons**, the other type of neural process, require **cytoskeletal elements** both for mechanical support and for conveying essential molecules, particles, and organelles over distances that can be quite extensive. The structural support is provided mainly by the **intermediate filaments**, which are termed **neurofilaments** in neurons because of their specialized molecular structure. Intermediate filaments appear in electron micrographs as electron-dense single lines when they course within the plane of the section or as electron-dense dots when their orientation is vertical to the plane of the section. The movement of molecules and particles along the lengths of dendrites and axons requires **microtubules** as tracks and **motor molecules** (dyneins and kinesins) to transport the cargo structures and molecules along the microtubules. Because of their tubular structure, microtubules appear as a closely paired set of parallel lines when they course within the plane of the section or as circles when their orientation is vertical to the plane of the section.

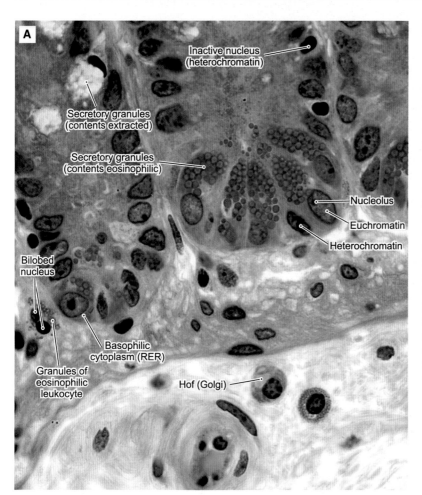

Figure 2-14A. Cell components in light microscopy. H&E, ×1,075

Only the larger **cell components** can be distinguished individually by light microscopy. Examples of such readily identifiable components include the **nucleus, nucleoli**, blocks of **heterochromatin** and **euchromatin**, larger **secretory vesicles**, and larger **secondary lysosomes**. Because of its limited resolution of about 0.2 μm, light microscopy cannot distinguish smaller cellular components, such as **ribosomes, centrioles, cytoskeletal elements**, and most **primary lysosomes** and **mitochondria**, although the presence of some of these structures can be inferred by their influence on staining reactions when they are present in abundance. For example, ribosomes, whether free or associated with endoplasmic reticulum, impart **basophilic** staining to a region of **cytoplasm** where they are concentrated. By contrast, mitochondria impart **acidophilic (eosinophilic)** staining to regions of cytoplasm where they are concentrated. In cells with a large **Golgi complex**, its presence can sometimes be distinguished as an unstained region adjacent to the nucleus.

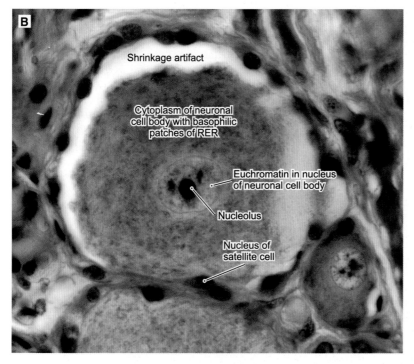

Figure 2-14B. Wide range of cell sizes, spinal ganglion sensory neuron. H&E, ×780

Human cells have a wide range of sizes and shapes. Some of the largest cell types, such as **oocytes** and **megakaryocytes**, can be as much as 100 μm in diameter. Similar diameters can be seen in cell bodies of neurons with long axons such as the sensory neurons in this illustration. The enormity of the cell body in the center of the image can be appreciated if its size is compared with that of the satellite cells that surround it. The **nucleolus** in the nucleus of the neuron is equal in size to the entire nucleus of the **satellite cell**. The large volume of cytoplasm that surrounds the nucleus of the neuron contains large expanses of **RER** and **Golgi complexes**. As large as the cell body is, it amounts to less than 1% of the total cell volume because the axon may be over a meter in length. Cell types with the smallest volumes include **spermatozoa, lymphocytes** (spherical cells with diameters as little as 5 μm), and **endothelial** and **alveolar cells** (extremely thin cells that allow exchange of gases and other materials between compartments).

Cell Ultrastructure

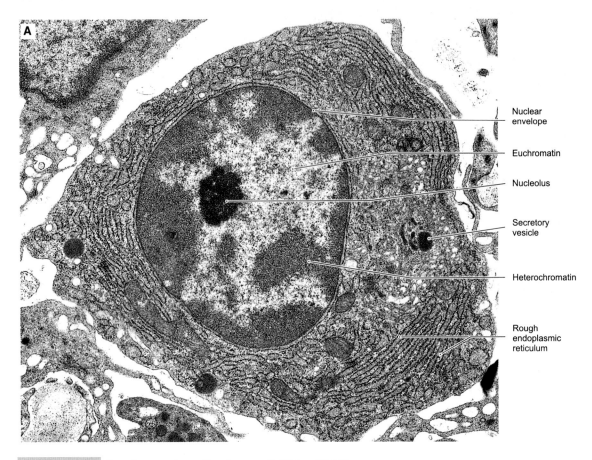

Figure 2-15A.   Protein-secreting cells, plasma cell. EM, ×17,000

Plasma cells function to synthesize and secrete **immunoglobulin**, a **glycoprotein**. Once these cells have differentiated from stimulated B lymphocytes, they secrete the antibodies as fast as they are generated for 1 to 2 weeks before they die. The major structures required for this process are **RER**, the **Golgi complex**, and **secretory vesicles**. The RER is the site of synthesis and sequestering of the polypeptides of the antibody. Posttranslational modification and packaging occur in the Golgi complex, and the secretory vesicles convey the product to the cell surface. Because plasma cells do not store the immunoglobulin, few, if any, secretory vesicles are seen in the cytoplasm. Rather, the cytoplasm is packed with RER, and there is a large Golgi complex (*not visible in this section*) located adjacent to the nucleus. The nucleus has one or more well-developed **nucleoli**, but there is a considerable amount of **heterochromatin**, considering that this is an active protein-secreting cell. The explanation may be that only one protein, an antibody molecule, is secreted, and the cell is terminally differentiated, so it will never divide. The immunoglobulin is secreted into the surrounding **interstitial compartment**, from which it can enter circulation through walls of small blood or lymph vessels. Even though the cell is not sharply polarized, the nucleus tends to occupy an eccentric position, with the Golgi complex near the center of the cell.

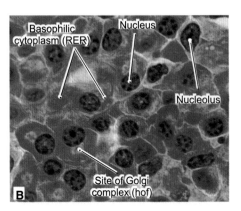

Figure 2-15B.   Light microscopic appearance of plasma cells. H&E, ×1,200

The appearance of **plasma cells** in light microscopy is consistent with the ultrastructure of these antibody-secreting cells. The nucleus has a mixture of **heterochromatin** and **euchromatin** in an arrangement that is variously described as a "clock face" or checkerboard pattern. A large **nucleolus** or two occupy the center of the nucleus. The **cytoplasm** is **basophilic** as a result of the ribonucleic acid associated with the extensive RER. Depending upon the orientation of the cell in the section, a pale area, called the **hof**, can be seen adjacent to the nucleus. This unstained area is the location of the **Golgi complex**.

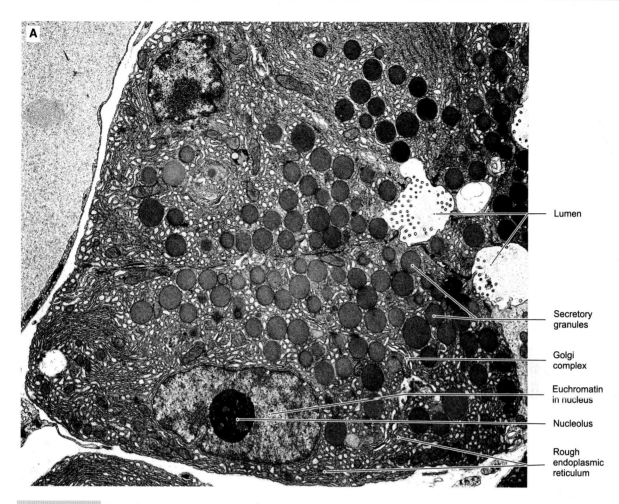

Figure 2-16A. Exocrine protein–secreting cells, pancreatic acinar cell. EM, ×7,000

There are many examples of glandular epithelial cells that function to **synthesize** and **secrete proteins** and **glycoproteins** into a **lumen**. All cells have in common the equipment needed for this function, and all cells are distinctly polarized, with a typical arrangement of cellular constituents. The necessary organelles are the **RER, Golgi complex,** and **secretory vesicles** (often called **secretory granules**). The RER functions to synthesize polypeptides, sequester them, and initiate posttranslational modifications such as glycosylation. The polypeptides are then shunted by small transport vesicles to the Golgi complex for further modification and packaging into secretory vesicles, which convey the products to the part of the cell's plasmalemma that borders a lumen or free surface. The nucleus of an **exocrine protein–secreting cell** can vary in shape and position, but it will typically have **nucleoli** evident and a substantial proportion of its **chromatin** in the **euchromatin** (transcription-capable) form.

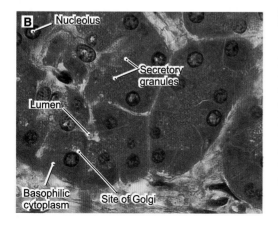

Figure 2-16B. Light microscopic appearance of an exocrine protein–secreting cell. H&E, ×750

Light microscopic views of **exocrine secretory cells** in sections are consistent with the structures that can be discerned in electron micrographs. The **nucleus** usually exhibits **nucleoli** and a considerable amount of **euchromatin**. The **cytoplasm** at the basal end of the cell is **basophilic** owing to the concentration of **RER** at this location. The position of the **Golgi apparatus** may be evident as a pale, unstained area of cytoplasm at the apical-facing edge of the nucleus. The sizes and staining characteristics of the **secretory granules** vary according to the type of cell and secretory product. In this example, the secretory granules are **acidophilic (eosinophilic)**.

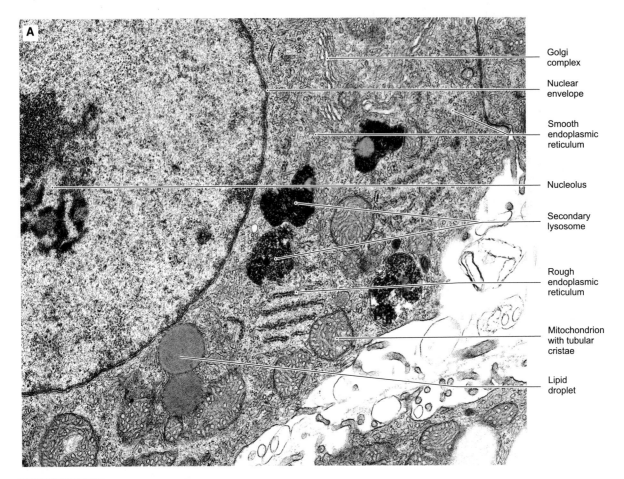

Figure 2-17A. Steroid hormone–secreting cells, adrenal cortex. EM, ×21,000

Adrenal cortical cells, testicular interstitial cells, and **ovarian follicular cells** are examples of cell types that function to **synthesize** and **secrete steroid hormones.** Each of these cells have in common the equipment needed for synthesis of steroid hormones. The necessary components include **lipid droplets** containing cholesterol esters as substrates, **SER,** and **mitochondria** that function together in the synthesis of hormones. The mitochondria characteristically have **cristae** that are **tubular** rather than shelflike.

Cell Membrane

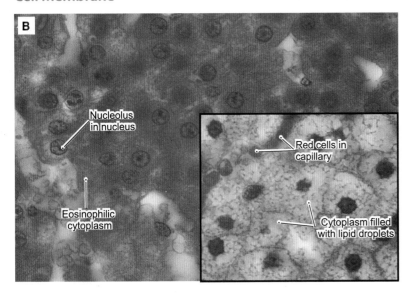

Figure 2-17B. **Light microscopic appearance of steroid hormone–secreting cells.** H&E, ×800 main panel and inset

Light microscopic views of **steroid hormone–synthesizing cells** reveal only a hint of the distinctive set of structures that characterize the cytoplasm of these cells. The **eosinophilia (acidophilia)** of the **cytoplasm** is largely attributable to the abundance of mitochondria. Steroid hormone–secreting cells vary in the amount of cholesterol stored in the form of **lipid droplets,** which appear in most preparations as empty vacuoles because their contents are extracted during specimen preparation. The cells in the *main panel* are in the **zona reticularis** and have few droplets, similar to the cell in the electron micrograph (Fig. 2-10A). The cells in the *inset* are from the **zona fasciculata** and have numerous lipid droplets.

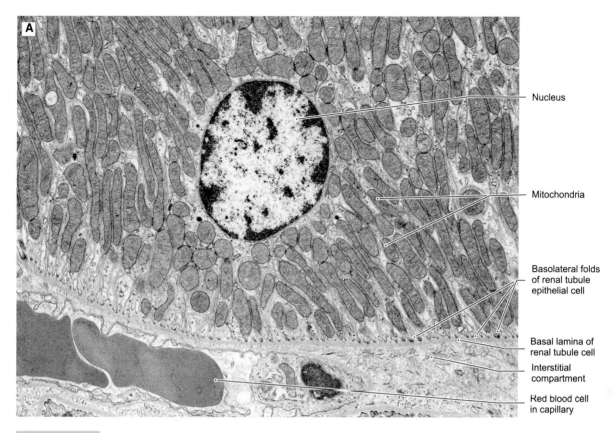

Nucleus

Mitochondria

Basolateral folds
of renal tubule
epithelial cell

Basal lamina of
renal tubule cell

Interstitial
compartment

Red blood cell
in capillary

Figure 2-18A. Ion-pumping cells, renal tubule. EM, ×9,060

Examples of **epithelial cells** that function primarily to **move ions** from a lumen to the **interstitial compartment** form the walls of some **renal tubules** and of some **ducts of salivary glands**. Perhaps surprisingly, the molecular pumps are located not in the apical cell membrane but rather in the **plasmalemma** of the basal and lateral surfaces of the cells. These **ATP-requiring** pumps transfer **sodium ions** from the cytosol of the cell into the interstitial compartment. Sodium ions are pulled from the lumen at the apex of the cell by the gradient created by the basolateral pumps. The surface area of the membrane containing the pumps is greatly increased by numerous, deep **basolateral folds**. The energy required to pump ions against a concentration gradient is supplied by numerous **mitochondria** packed into the cytoplasm of the basolateral folds.

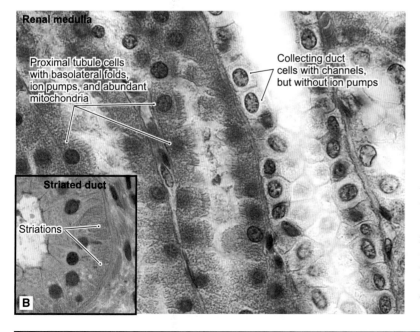

Renal medulla

Proximal tubule cells
with basolateral folds,
ion pumps, and abundant
mitochondria

Collecting duct
cells with channels,
but without ion pumps

Striated duct

Striations

B

Figure 2-18B. **Light microscopic appearance of ion-pumping cells.** H&E, ×770 main panel; ×710 inset

Light microscopic views of **cells that pump ions** from one compartment to another are consistent with the ultrastructural features of these cells. The **cytoplasm** is distinctly **acidophilic** (eosinophilic in an H&E-stained specimen) owing to the abundance of **mitochondria**, particularly in the basal portions of the cells. In paraffin sections such as the *main panel* view of the renal medulla, the **basolateral folds** are usually difficult to discern. The *inset* shows a plastic-embedded, 1-μm thick section of a duct from a **submandibular salivary gland**. Evidence of the basolateral folds can be seen here as vertical stripes in the basal cytoplasm of these cells, which function to retrieve ions from the secretion (saliva). This appearance is the basis of the term **striated duct** for this structure.

From Histology to Pathology

Normal neuron

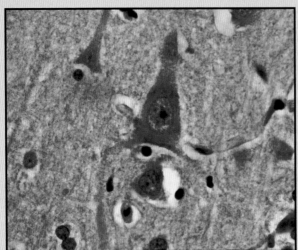

Neuromelanin-containing neurons

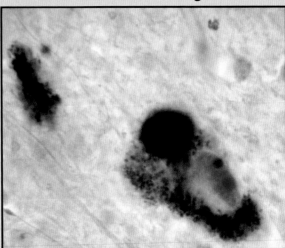

Figure 2-19. Normal neuron and neuromelanin-containing neurons. Left, H&E, ×600; right, immunohistochemistry for alpha-synuclein, ×431

Normal neuron on the *left*. **Neuromelanin-containing neurons** on the *right*, which is an intracytoplasmic oval with a halo (**Lewy body**), formed in neuromelanin-containing neurons in patients with idiopathic Parkinson disease. Brown pigment indicates the presence of alpha synuclein, the main protein in the inclusion.

Clinical Vignette Questions

1. A 13-year-old boy was hunting with his father and bitten by a snake. Shortly afterward, he collapsed and was sent to the emergency department. On arrival, he was drowsy but rousable. Several bite marks were noticed on his right leg. His blood tested positive for coral snake venom (elapid family). Elapid snakes mainly produce neurotoxins, leading to neurotoxicity. Which of the following is the correct mechanism by which this neurotoxin causes muscular weakness and paralysis?

A. Competition with a platelet activation receptor
B. Competition with acetylcholine at nicotinic receptors
C. Destruction of endothelial cell membranes
D. Blockade of calcium-sensing receptors

2. The mother of a 15-month-old boy is becoming concerned that her son is not walking as well as other children of his age. He has not attempted to walk frequently, and, when he does, he demonstrates a wide, waddling gait. The child's father has a history of delayed motor development and proximal muscle weakness into adulthood. In addition, the paternal grandfather had a history of malignant hyperthermia during an operation for appendicitis when a halothane anesthetic was used. The child's pediatrician refers the family to a child development physician who performs a muscle biopsy. The biopsy reveals abnormal myocytes with a conspicuous clearing in the middle of most muscle fibers examined. Based on the information provided, the patient's condition is associated with which of the following structures?

A. Golgi apparatus
B. Mitochondria
C. Lysosomes
D. Rough endoplasmic reticulum
E. Smooth endoplasmic reticulum

3 Epithelium and Glands

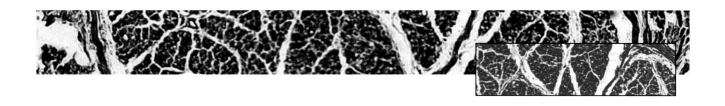

Classification of Epithelial Tissue

Simple Squamous Epithelium

Simple Cuboidal Epithelium

Simple Columnar Epithelium

Pseudostratified Columnar Epithelium

Stratified Squamous Epithelium (Keratinized)

Stratified Squamous Epithelium (Nonkeratinized)

Stratified Cuboidal Epithelium

Stratified Columnar Epithelium

Transitional Epithelium (Stratified Epithelium)

Specially Named Epithelial Tissue

From Histology to Pathology

Clinical Vignette Questions

Glands
Introduction and Key Concepts for Glands
Exocrine Glands Classified by Product
Exocrine Glands Classified by Mechanisms of Secretion
Exocrine Glands Classified by Morphology
Duct System

Exocrine Glands Classified by Product

Serous Gland

Mucous Gland

Mixed (Seromucous) Gland

Sebaceous Gland

Exocrine Glands Classified by Morphology

Unicellular Glands

Exocrine Glands Classified by Morphology

Multicellular Glands

Duct System of Exocrine Glands

From Histology to Pathology

Epithelium

Introduction and Key Concepts for Epithelium

Epithelium covers nearly all body surfaces. The basic functions of epithelial tissue are (1) protection of the body from abrasion and injury (e.g., skin and esophagus); (2) absorption of material from a lumen (e.g., tubules in kidney, small and large intestines); (3) transportation of material along a surface (e.g., cilia-mediated transport in the trachea); (4) secretion of mucus, hormones, and proteins (e.g., glands); (5) gas exchange (e.g., alveoli in the lung); and (6) lubrication between two surfaces (e.g., mesothelium of pleural cavity). Epithelium is an **avascular** tissue, which lacks a direct blood supply. Nutrients are delivered by diffusion from blood vessels in the neighboring connective tissue. Most epithelial tissues are renewed continuously.

Classification of Epithelial Tissues

Epithelium can be classified as **simple** or **stratified** based on the number of layers of cells. If there is a single layer of cells, it is referred to as *simple* epithelium. If there are two or more layers of cells, it is considered *stratified* epithelium. Epithelium is also classified according to the shape of the cells in the most superficial layer. If the surface cells are flattened in shape, it is called **squamous epithelium**. If surface cells are cuboidal in shape, it is called **cuboidal epithelium**. If the surface cells are tall, with their height much greater than their width, it is called **columnar epithelium**. If the surface cells change shape in response to stretching and relaxing, it is called **transitional epithelium (urothelium)**. As described below, these terms may be variously combined to designate layers of cells and shapes forming the superficial layer of the epithelium. In some cases, the height of an epithelial cell represents the level of metabolic activity. For example, epithelial cells lining the thyroid follicle usually exhibit as simple cuboidal epithelium. However, when the follicle cells are in a high metabolic state, they form a simple columnar epithelium. By contrast, when the follicle cells are in a low metabolic state, they form a simple squamous epithelium.

SIMPLE SQUAMOUS EPITHELIUM is composed of one layer of uniform flat cells, which rest on the **basement membrane**. Apical surfaces are smooth, and the width of the cells is greater than their height. The nuclei appear flattened and can easily be recognized following **hematoxylin** and **eosin staining (H&E)** because of the **basophilia** (affinity for blue stains) of the nucleic acids in the nuclei. This type of epithelium is found lining the posterior surface of the cornea; lining blood vessels and lymphatic vessels (where it is called **endothelium**); lining the surface of the body cavities, including the pericardial, pleural, and peritoneal cavities (where it is called **mesothelium**); and lining the alveoli of the lungs.

SIMPLE CUBOIDAL EPITHELIUM is composed of one layer of uniform cuboidal cells, which rest on the **basement membrane**. The cell's height, width, and depth are roughly equal. Nuclei are centrally placed and spherical in shape. Some cuboidal cells have long and abundant **microvilli**, which form a **brush border** on their apical surfaces. Such cells are found in the proximal tubules of the kidney. Other cuboidal cells have few, short microvilli which do not form a brush border; these cells can be found in the distal and collecting tubules of the kidney. Simple cuboidal epithelium is mainly found lining most of the tubules in the kidney and in some excretory ducts of glands.

SIMPLE COLUMNAR EPITHELIUM is composed of one layer of columnar cells resting on the **basement membrane**. The cell's height is greater than the width. The elongated ovoid nucleus is most often located in the basal region of the cell. The apical surface of this epithelium may reveal **microvilli**. Microvilli are often densely packed to form a **brush border** and function to increase the apical surface area of the cell to aid in absorption of fluid and other material from a lumen. Simple columnar epithelium can be found in the digestive tract, oviducts (fallopian tubes) in the female reproductive system, and ductuli efferentes testis of the male reproductive system.

PSEUDOSTRATIFIED COLUMNAR EPITHELIUM is composed of one layer of nonuniform cells that vary in shape and height. Cells resemble stratified cells, but all cells are in contact with the **basement membrane**. In general, most cells are tall columnar cells, but there are also some short **basal cells**, some of which are stem cells. The most widespread type of pseudostratified columnar epithelium is found in the respiratory tract and has long fingerlike, motile structures called **cilia** on the apical surface of the cells. Cilia aid in the transport of material across the surface of epithelial cells. Pseudostratified columnar epithelium is often referred to as **respiratory epithelium** because it is found in the linings of the respiratory tract, including the nasal cavity, trachea, and primary bronchi.

STRATIFIED SQUAMOUS EPITHELIUM contains several layers of cells, with cells in the superficial layer being flattened. Only the deepest layer of cells is in contact with the basement membrane. This type of epithelium protects the body against injury, abrasion, dehydration, and infection. This epithelium may be **keratinized** or **nonkeratinized**, depending on functional demands. *Keratinized stratified squamous epithelium* is found in the skin. The top layers consist of either thick or thin keratinized cells (flattened, nonnucleated dead cells) that are filled with tonofilaments. The thickness of the stratified squamous epithelium varies from region to region. *Nonkeratinized stratified squamous epithelium* is like keratinized squamous epithelium except that surface cells are nucleated instead of nonnucleated. This type of epithelium often covers wet surfaces and is found lining the oral cavity (soft palate, cheeks, and floor of the mouth), esophagus, vagina, and true vocal cords.

STRATIFIED CUBOIDAL EPITHELIUM is composed of two or three layers of cuboidal cells with the basal layer of cells often appearing nonuniform in distribution. It is mainly found lining large ducts of exocrine glands. The cells often have smooth apical surfaces and form barriers and ducts.

STRATIFIED COLUMNAR EPITHELIUM is also composed of two or three layers of cells. The top layer is columnar in shape, and the basal layer is usually cuboidal in shape. This is not a common type of epithelium and has a very limited distribution. Occasionally, it can be found in the conjunctiva of the eye and in some large ducts of the exocrine glands.

TRANSITIONAL EPITHELIUM is stratified epithelium, often referred to as **urothelium**, which lines the excretory channels leading from the kidney (renal calyces, ureters, bladder, and proximal segment of the urethra). It may contain four to six cell layers in the relaxed state. However, the histological appearance of the epithelium can change when stretched. In the empty bladder, the basal cells are mostly cuboidal, and the middle layer is polygonal, although surface cells bulge into the lumen. Surface cells are often described as "dome shaped" and are called **dome cells** or **umbrella cells**; they contain extra cell membrane material near the superficial (apical) surface. The dome cells may contain two nuclei. In the stretched bladder, the thickness of the epithelium is much reduced, and surface cells, as well as the intermediate cells, are extremely flattened.

Specializations of the Apical Surface (Apical Domain)

Apical surfaces of the epithelium may reveal **cilia, microvilli,** and **stereocilia**, depending on their function and location. (1) *Cilia* are elongated, motile structures that have a greater diameter and length than microvilli. The core of a cilium is composed of **microtubules** arranged in a consistent array of two central microtubules surrounded by a circle of nine peripheral pairs of microtubules. Cilia arise from electron-dense, cylindrical structures, called **basal bodies**, in the apical cytoplasm just below the cell membrane. There are many mitochondria at the apical surface of cells with motile cilia. The function of cilia is to aid in the transport of material along the surface of epithelial cells. Cilia are present in the pseudostratified ciliated columnar epithelium in the respiratory tract and ciliated simple columnar epithelium in the oviduct (fallopian tube). (2) *Microvilli* are smaller than cilia; each has a core that is composed of **actin microfilaments**. Microvilli are anchored to a network structure called the **terminal web**, which contains actin filaments to stabilize the microvillus. These specialized structures increase apical surface area to aid in absorption. Microvilli are commonly seen in simple columnar epithelium lining the small intestine and simple cuboidal epithelium lining the proximal tubules in the kidney. (3) *Stereocilia* are long microvilli, which consist of **actin microfilaments** and help with absorption. They can be found in the pseudostratified columnar epithelium in the epididymis and vas deferens of the male reproductive system.

Specializations of the Lateral Surface (Lateral Domain)

The **lateral surface** of epithelial cells contains cell junctions and cell adhesion molecules that are responsible for the cohesive nature of epithelial tissue. Intercellular connections of the epithelial cells include (1) **tight junctions (zonula occludens)**, that completely surround the apical cell borders to seal the underlying intercellular clefts from the outside environment; (2) **adherens junctions (zonula adherens/belt desmosome)**, found just beneath the tight junction, also forming a bandlike junction surrounding the entire cell and serving to attach adjacent cells; (3) **desmosomes (macula adherens)**, located beneath the adhering junctions, also assist in cell-to-cell attachment (the **junctional complex** is composed of tight junction, adherens junction, and desmosome); and (4) **gap junctions**, which are **communicating junctions**, provide a low-resistance channel to permit passage of ions and small molecules between adjacent cells. Gap junctions are present not only in epithelial tissues, but they can also be found in many other tissues (smooth muscle, cardiac muscle, and nerve tissues) in the body. However, gap junctions are not present in skeletal muscle, blood cells, and spermatozoa.

Specializations of the Basal Surface (Basal Domain)

Epithelial cells rest on a **basement membrane**, consisting of a **basal lamina** and a **reticular lamina**, which provide an underlying foundation for the cells. The term "basement membrane" is used in light microscopy observation, although the basement membrane is often difficult to visualize with the light microscope. The terms "basal lamina" and "reticular lamina" are ultrastructural terms and refer to features that require electron microscopy to be seen. Epithelial cells produce their own basement membrane. Cells are anchored to the basement membrane by **hemidesmosomes**, junctions that connect the cells to the underlying basement membrane. **Basal plasma membrane enfolding** may also be present in some epithelial cells (e.g., salivary gland excretory duct epithelium). This is a corrugation of the cell membrane in the basal (and sometimes lateral) regions of the cell, which increases cell surface area and is involved in ion and fluid transport. There are many **mitochondria** in the vicinity of the plasma membrane enfolding. These produce adenosine triphosphate (ATP) for active transport. The combination of the plasma membrane enfolding and the concentration of mitochondria results in a striated appearance in some of the epithelial cells.

SYNOPSIS 3-1 Functions of Epithelial Tissue

■ Promotes gliding between two surfaces (mesothelium of pleural cavity).
■ Senses changes in blood pressure, oxygen tension, and blood flow and controls blood coagulation (endothelium of blood vessels).
■ Pumps the excess fluid out of the stroma and keeps the cornea clear (simple squamous epithelium in cornea).
■ Mediates gas exchange (type 1 pneumocytes and simple squamous epithelium in the alveoli of the lung).
■ Absorbs material from a lumen (simple cuboidal epithelium in kidney and simple columnar epithelium in small and large intestines).
■ Transports material along a surface (pseudostratified ciliated columnar epithelium in the respiratory tract).
■ Provides conduit for fluid (simple and stratified cuboidal and columnar epithelia forming ducts of some large exocrine glands).
■ Protects the body from abrasion and injury (stratified squamous epithelium in the skin and esophagus).
■ Becomes highly distensible when the bladder is filled with urine and the tissue is stretched (transitional epithelium in bladder).
■ Secretes mucus, hormones, and proteins (secretory epithelium, glands).

Features of Epithelial Cells

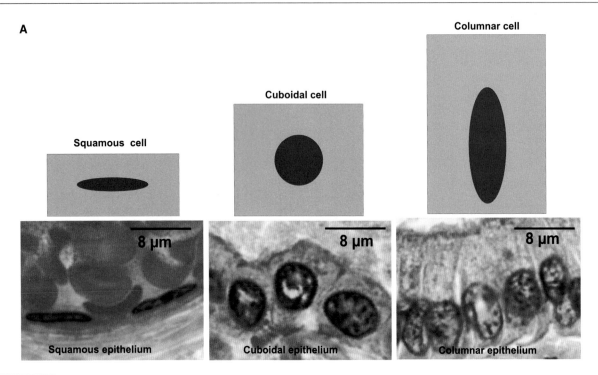

Figure 3-1A. Shapes of epithelial cells.

Epithelial cells are the basic units of epithelium. Epithelial cells come in various shapes, the most common shapes include squamous, cuboidal, and columnar. Squamous epithelial cells have a flattened "**squamous**" shape, and their nuclei often appear flattened. The width of squamous epithelial cells is much greater than their height. The cuboidal epithelial cells have a "**cuboidal**" shape, with their width and height relatively equal, like a box. Cuboidal epithelial cell nuclei often appear round and are frequently located in the center of the cell. The columnar epithelial cells have a cylindrical "**columnar**" shape because their height is greater than their width. Columnar epithelial cells are elongated, with an ovoid nucleus that is often located in the basal region of the cell. In addition to having different shapes, epithelial cells within epithelium are organized into layers. An epithelium with only one layer of epithelial cells is called **simple epithelium,** while an epithelium with two or more layers of cells is called **stratified epithelium.** The shapes of epithelial cells and the number of layers into which they are organized aid an individual in classifying the type of epithelium in which they reside. The classification of the epithelium is determined by the shape of its outermost layer of cells and by the number of layers it comprises. The shape of epithelial cells and the number of layers of these cells within an epithelium are correlated with their function. For example, **simple squamous epithelium** forms the lining of blood vessels, and its single layer of flattened cells provides a smooth surface that enables expedient blood flow, oxygen and nutrient exchange, and blood coagulation control. **Stratified squamous epithelium,** for instance, forms the epidermis of skin, which provides the body with a strong protection against abrasion, dehydration, and infection. Epithelial cells also have a unique, characteristic **apical surface (apical domain), lateral surface (lateral domain),** and **basal surface (basal domain).**

Basal Surface (Basal Domain)

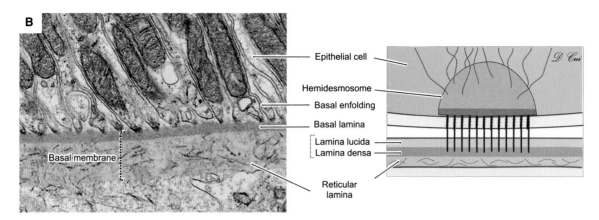

Figure 3-1B. **Specializations of the basal domain.** EM, ×18,360

Epithelial cells rest on a **basement membrane** to which they are anchored via junctions, **hemidesmosomes. The basement membrane** consists of the **basal lamina** and the **reticular lamina.** The **basal lamina** is also composed of two thin layers of structures: the **lamina lucida** and the **lamina densa.** Overall, the **basement membrane** provides an underlying foundation for the overlying epithelial cells. **Basal plasma membrane enfolding (basal enfolding)** or basolateral folds can also be found in some epithelial cells. These folds of the plasma membrane penetrate the cytoplasm and increase the surface area of the basal region of the epithelial cell's plasma membrane. This enhanced surface area increases the epithelial cell's ion and fluid transport. These folds also contain numerous mitochondria that provide the ATP energy necessary to power the active transport of ions and fluid.

Apical Surface (Apical Domain)
CILIA

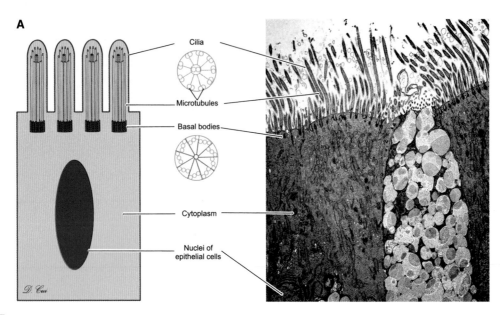

Figure 3-2A.   Cilia of epithelial cells. EM, ×6,300

The specialization of apical surface (apical domain) of the epithelial cells may reveal **cilia, microvilli,** and **stereocilia,** depending on their location and function. There are two types of **cilia:** motile cilia and non-motile cilia. (1) **Motile cilia** are elongated structures that have the ability to move. They can be found in the respiratory epithelium (ciliated pseudostratified columnar epithelium). In this EM, **cilia** rise from **basal bodies** and form the apical surface of a columnar epithelial cell adjacent to a mucus-producing goblet cell. Each cilium is composed of **microtubules** in a **9+2 arrangement** (nine pairs, or doublets, of microtubules on the periphery and two separate microtubules in the center). Each **basal body** is also composed of microtubules, but they are arranged in a pattern of nine peripheral triplets and no central microtubules. Each basal body supports its associated cilium and serves as a growth site for microtubules. Motile cilia produce a wavelike motion and help to remove mucus containing microorganisms and debris out of the respiratory tract. Motile cilia also can be found in the epithelial lining of the fallopian tube, where they help to move oocytes toward the uterus. (2) **Nonmotile cilia** are also called **primary cilia,** and they have no movable function. There is usually only one primary cilium per cell. Specialized primary cilia mainly serve as sensory antennae for cells, including such examples as hair cells and olfactory epithelial cells.

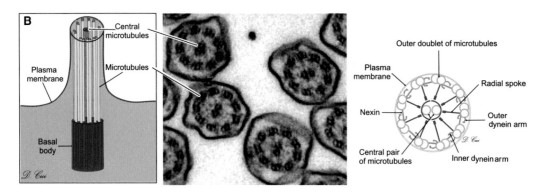

Figure 3-2B.   Internal structure of cilia. EM, ×74,000

Microtubules form the inner core of cilia, and they are anchored in the basal body. The structure of the axoneme (core) of a cilium can be readily appreciated from a high-magnification cross-sectional view. The microtubules have an extremely orderly, consistent arrangement into two separate, central microtubules surrounded by nine sets of doublet microtubules. This configuration is often termed the 9+2 arrangement. The proteins associated with microtubules include **dynein, nexin,** and **radial spoke**—all of which are found in the distal part of a cilium. **Axonemal dyneins** (inner and outer dynein) are motor proteins that form cross-bridges between two adjacent microtubules, allowing movement from one to the other. Nexin is the inter-doublet link protein that helps to both maintain the space along the microtubules and hold them together. Radial spoke is a multiunit protein, and it plays an essential role in the mechanical movement of the cilium and in transmitting signals that regulate the activity of dynein.

MICROVILLI AND STEREOCILIA

A

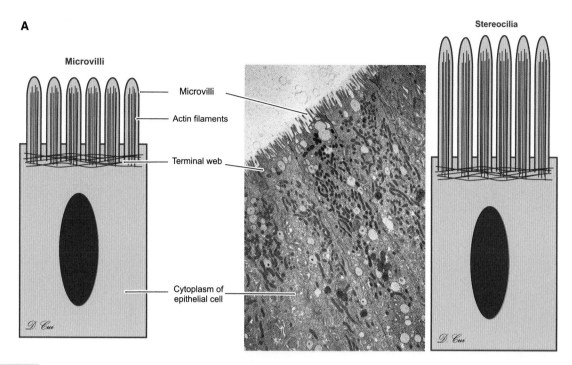

Figure 3-3A. Microvilli and stereocilia of epithelial cells. EM, ×6,300

Microvilli and **stereocilia** are two other forms of specialization of the apical surfaces (apical domains) of epithelial cells. (1) Smaller than cilia, **microvilli** are about **0.08 μm** in diameter and **1 μm** in length. Each microvillus has a core composed of 20 to 30 **actin filaments** known as **microfilaments**. **Microvilli** are anchored to the network structure **terminal web**, which contains mainly **actin filaments** (**microfilaments**) and associated proteins. Many examples of columnar and cuboidal epithelia comprise cells that bear **microvilli**, but absorptive cells lining the **small intestine** provide the premier example of tightly packed microvilli that provide a pronounced increase in surface area of the plasma membrane. (2) **Stereocilia** are **long microvilli**, and they have an internal structure like that of microvilli. They are less than **0.1 μm** in diameter and **10 μm** or **more** in length. Stereocilia, sometimes called **stereovilli**, can be found in the epithelium lining the **epididymis** and the **vas deferens** of the male reproductive system. Both microvilli and stereocilia are nonmotile, but they both largely increase the surface area of epithelial cells and aid in absorption.

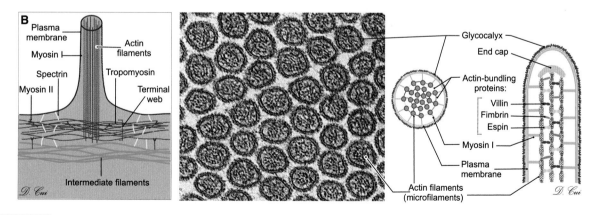

Figure 3-3B. Internal structure of microvilli. EM, ×74,000

Actin filaments (**microfilaments**) form the inner core of microvilli, and they extend from the **terminal web** into the **microvilli**. The cytoskeletal protein **spectrin** provides stability to the actin filaments within the **terminal web** and to the **plasma membrane**. **Myosin I** is a protein found in the peripheral region of microvilli, while the proteins **myosin II** and **tropomyosin** are found in the terminal web. The interaction of myosin I, myosin II, and tropomyosin with the **actin filaments** in the microvillus core that is anchored into the **terminal web** allows for the slight contraction of these actin filaments. Actin filaments within each **microvillus** are cross-linked by **actin-bundling proteins**, examples of which include **villin, fimbrin**, and **espin**. Villin also can be found at the tip (end cap) of the microvillus. In cross section, numbers of actin filaments appear as a cluster of small dots, and the fuzzy coating on the membranes of the microvilli is the **glycocalyx**.

Three Apical Specializations of Epithelium

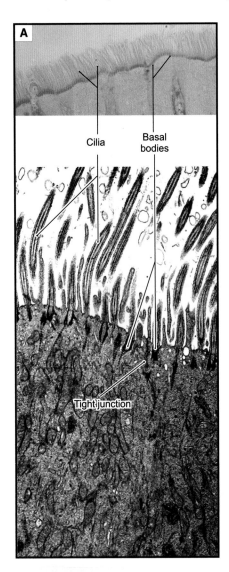

Figure 3-4A. Cilia, basal body, and junctional complex. EM, ×9,500; inset color photomicrograph ×724

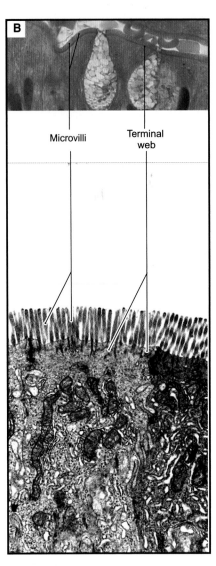

Figure 3-4B. Microvilli, terminal web, and junctional complex. EM, ×9,500; inset color photomicrograph ×723

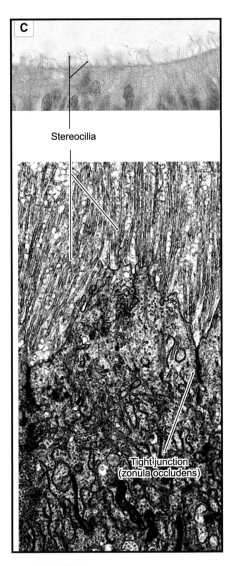

Figure 3-4C. Stereocilia and junctional complex. EM, ×9,500; inset color photomicrograph ×565

Cilia are 0.2 μm in diameter and 5 to 10 μm long, so they can be seen as individual structures with the light microscope. The core (**axoneme**) of each cilium is composed of **microtubules** and associated proteins, most notably the molecular motor **dynein**. The microtubules are arranged as nine peripheral doublets with two central singlets. Each cilium extends from a **basal body** just beneath the apical surface of the epithelial cell. Basal bodies also have microtubules as a major component. These form an orderly array of nine peripheral triplets with no central microtubules, an arrangement seen also in **centrioles**.

Microvilli of the intestinal epithelium are about 0.08 μm in diameter and 1 μm long, so they cannot be distinguished as individual structures with the light microscope, but the row of tightly packed microvilli can be seen as a **brush border**. The core of each microvillus contains a bundle of 6-nm **actin filaments**, which extend from the actin filaments that form the **terminal web** just beneath the apical surface of the cell.

Stereocilia are extremely long **microvilli**. Like ordinary microvilli, stereocilia are less than 0.1 μm in diameter, but they can attain lengths of 10 μm or more. Stereocilia are characteristic of the pseudostratified columnar epithelium of the ductus epididymis, which is the site of absorption of the large volumes of testicular fluid produced by the **seminiferous tubules**. The greatly expanded surface area afforded by the stereocilia probably contributes to this function.

Lateral Surface (Lateral Domain)

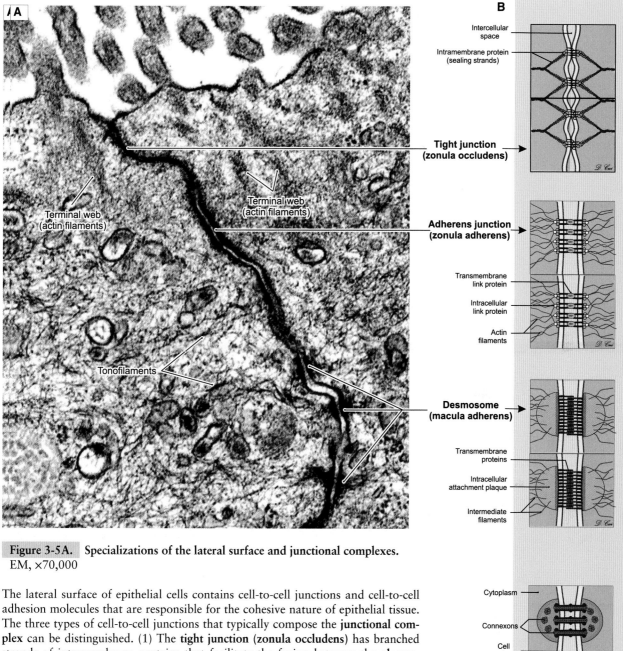

Figure 3-5A. Specializations of the lateral surface and junctional complexes. EM, ×70,000

The lateral surface of epithelial cells contains cell-to-cell junctions and cell-to-cell adhesion molecules that are responsible for the cohesive nature of epithelial tissue. The three types of cell-to-cell junctions that typically compose the **junctional complex** can be distinguished. (1) The **tight junction (zonula occludens)** has branched strands of intermembrane proteins that facilitate the fusion between the **plasmalemma** of two adjacent cells. This fusion effectively prevents materials in the extracellular space from crossing the epithelium through the passage between adjacent cells. (2) The **zonula adherens (adhering junction/belt desmosome) junction** composed of transmembrane and intracellular proteins provides a collar of mechanical adhesion between neighboring cells. The cytoskeleton of each cell at the level of the **zonula adherens** consists predominantly of **actin filaments** in a network termed the **terminal web**. (3) The **desmosome (macula adherens)** is one structure of an array of scattered junctions that provide spot-like mechanical adhesion between adjacent cells. **Cytokeratin filaments (tonofilaments)** of the **cytoskeleton** are anchored in the attachment plaques on the two cytoplasmic surfaces of each **desmosome**.

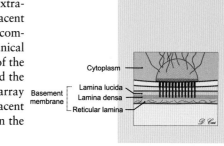

Figure 3-5B. Simplified representation of the components of the junctional complex.

Intercellular (cell-to-cell) connections of epithelial cells include (1) **tight junctions (zonulae occludentes)**, (2) **adherens junctions (zonulae adherentes)**, (3) **desmosomes (maculae adherentes)**, (4) **gap junctions**, and (5) **hemidesmosomes**. A junctional complex is composed of a tight junction, an adherens junction, and a desmosome. See Synopsis 3-1 for detailed information.

SYNOPSIS 3-2 Specialized Structures of the Epithelial Cell

- **Apical surface (domain):** Exposed to a luminal or external environment; site of primary function (absorption, protection, etc.).
  - *Cilia,* composed of microtubules in a 2+9 doublet arrangement, arise from basal bodies (which contain microtubules in an arrangement of nine peripheral triplets). Motile cilia have the ability to move, and they aid in the transport of material across the surface of the epithelium. Nonmotile cilia (primary cilia) which do not have the ability to move, mainly serve as sensory antennae (e.g., found in hair cells of the inner ears and olfactory epithelial cells). Microtubule-associated proteins include **dynein, nexin,** and **radial spoke.**
  - *Microvilli* are composed of actin filaments (microfilaments) anchored to a **terminal web.** The **actin-bundling proteins** include **villin, fimbrin,** and **espin.** Spectrin is a cytoskeletal protein which provides stability. Other actin-associated proteins which include myosin I, myosin II, and tropomyosin have contractile activity. Microvilli are coated with a glycocalyx, and they increase apical surface area of an epithelial cell to augment its absorption (e.g., found in internal lining of the small intestine).
  - *Stereocilia* are composed of **actin filaments (microfilaments).** They are especially long microvilli that have an internal structure similar to that of microvilli and that aid in absorption (e.g., found in the epithelial cells lining the epididymis and vas deferens).
- **Lateral surface (domain):** cell surface juxtaposed to the lateral surface of another cell and associated with junctional complexes.
- **Junctional complexes:** intercellular connections of the epithelial cells or between a cell and extracellular matrix.
  - *Tight junctions (zonula occludens),* specialized membrane proteins between the apical and lateral surface of the cell. Surround the apical borders and serve as impermeable barriers. Main transmembrane link proteins include **occludins, claudins,** and **ZO proteins. Actin filaments (microfilaments)** serve as cytoskeletal support for the tight junction.
  - *Adherens junctions (belt desmosome/zonula adherens),* beneath the tight junctions, form band-like junctions, and link the cytoskeleton of one cell to neighboring cells. They provide mechanical stability of the cells. Main transmembrane link proteins include **E-cadherin** and **catenin complexes. Actin filaments (microfilaments)** also serve as cytoskeletal support for the adherens junction.
  - *Desmosomes (macula adherens),* spot-like junctions which assist in cell-to-cell attachment. Main transmembrane link proteins include **desmogleins** and **desmocollin (cadherins). Intermediate filaments** serve as cytoskeletal support for the desmosomes.
  - *Hemidesmosomes* are junctions that anchor basal regions of epithelial cells to the basal lamina of the basement membrane. **Integrins** serve as main link proteins, and **intermediate filaments** serve as cytoskeletal support for the hemidesmosomes.
  - *Gap junctions,* also known as **communicating junctions,** permit passage of ions and small molecules between neighboring cells. **Connexin** serves as main link proteins for the gap junctions.
- **Basal surface (domain):** cell surface associated with hemidesmosomes and a basement membrane. Basolateral folds may also be present. Basolateral folds may also be present.
  - *Hemidesmosome,* a junction (one half of a desmosome) connecting cells to the underlying basement membrane.
  - *Basement membrane* consists of **basal lamina (lamina lucida and lamina dense)** and **reticular lamina,** which provide an underlying sheet for epithelial cells.
  - *Basolateral folds,* corrugations of the cell membrane in the lateral and basal regions of the cell, which increase cell surface area and are involved with ion and fluid transport.

Classification of Epithelial Tissue

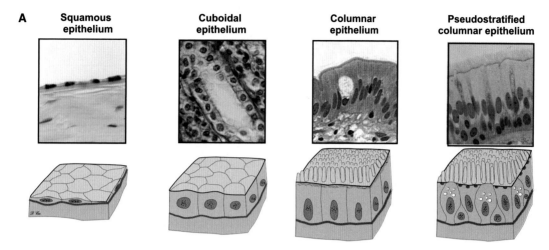

Figure 3-6A. Overview of types of simple epithelia (one layer of epithelial cells).

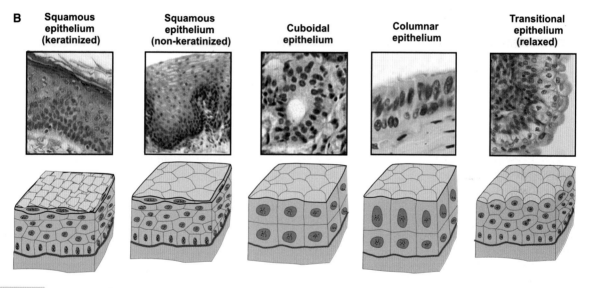

Figure 3-6B. Overview of types of stratified epithelia (two or more layers of epithelial cells).

Epithelium can be classified as **simple** or **stratified** based on the number of layers of cells. Epithelium is also classified according to the shape of the cells in the most superficial layer (Table 3-1).

TABLE 3-1 Classification of Epithelium

Shape of the Surface Cells	Simple Epithelium (Single Cell Layer)	Stratified Epithelium (Multiple Cell Layers)
Flat	Simple squamous epithelium	Stratified squamous epithelium (keratinized) Stratified squamous epithelium (nonkeratinized)
Cuboidal	Simple cuboidal epithelium	Stratified cuboidal epithelium
Columnar	Simple columnar epithelium Pseudostratified columnar epithelium	Stratified columnar epithelium
Dome From dome to flat		Transitional epithelium (relaxed) Transitional epithelium (distended)

Simple Squamous Epithelium
MESOTHELIUM

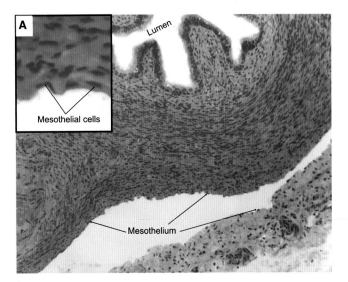

Figure 3-7A. Simple squamous epithelium, mesothelium of oviduct. H&E, ×155; inset ×310

Mesothelium is a term for the epithelial layer of the serous membranes (**peritoneum, pleura,** and **pericardium**) that line the body cavities and cover the organs that project into the cavities. The other component of these membranes is the loose connective tissue layer beneath the mesothelium. The membrane that lines the cavity wall constitutes the **parietal layer,** and the **visceral layer (serosa)** covers the organs located within the cavity.

The mesothelium secretes a slippery **lubricating fluid** that allows organs to easily slide against and over each other or against the cavity wall (e.g., beating heart, expanding or contracting lungs, peristaltic activity of the intestine) without damage to the mesothelium.

Excessive fluid in a mesothelial-lined cavity is called an "effusion," for example, a **pleural effusion.** Inflammation of the pleura is called **pleurisy;** of the peritoneum, it is called **peritonitis;** and of the pericardium, it is called **pericarditis.** These may exist in conjunction with a variety of clinical conditions or diseases.

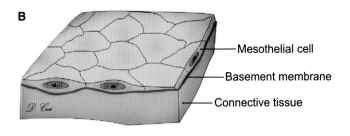

Figure 3-7B. Representation of a simple squamous epithelium lining a body cavity.

Mesothelial cells are flattened, generally pentagonal in shape, and form irregular borders with one another. The **basement membrane** is immediately adjacent to the mesothelium, which is barely visible with the light microscope. The basement membrane includes the **basal lamina** and an additional layer, the **reticular lamina.** The term "basal lamina" is used at the electron microscope level and includes the **lamina densa** and **lamina lucida. Connective tissue** is found beneath the basement membrane. The loose connective tissue beneath the basement membranes of mesothelia is the second component of the serous membranes lining the **peritoneal, pleural,** and **pericardial** cavities.

CLINICAL CORRELATION

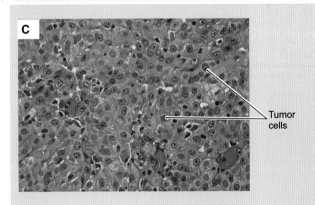

Figure 3-7C. Mesothelioma.

Mesothelioma (cancer of the mesothelium) is a neoplasm that arises from the surfaces of the **pleural** and **peritoneal** cavities. It is only occasionally found in the **pericardial** mesothelium. This type of tumor is more commonly seen in individuals who either were exposed to asbestos or who smoke. Mesothelioma cells develop long, slender, and curved microvilli. These tumors may invade nearby tissues and organs. In general, cancer cells are those that can **metastasize** (spread) from their original site to distant parts of the body, and mesotheliomas are no exception. The lymphatic system is a common route through which metastasis may occur.

A

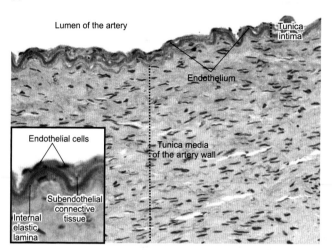

Lumen of the artery

Tunica intima

Endothelium

Tunica media of the artery wall

Endothelial cells

Subendothelial connective tissue

Internal elastic lamina

Figure 3-8A. **Simple squamous epithelium, endothelium of blood vessels.** H&E, ×219; inset ×310

Simple squamous epithelium lining the lumen surface of all types of blood vessels and lymphatic vessels is called an **endothelium** (sometimes a **vascular endothelium**). In this example, a single layer of squamous cells lines the inner layer, the **tunica intima**, of a medium artery. The endothelial cells are flattened and elongated, and they always rest on a thin **basement membrane**. Electron microscopy is required to see the ultrastructural features of the basement membrane. Endothelial cells of vessels sense changes in blood pressure, oxygen tension, and blood flow and respond to these changes by secreting substances, which have effects on the tone of vascular smooth muscle. Endothelial cells are also important in the control of blood coagulation; the endothelium produces von Willebrand factor that mediates platelet adhesion to collagen in subendothelial connective tissues at an injury site to stop bleeding. They also produce anticoagulant substances that prevent blood clotting and allow unobstructed flow of blood in normal conditions.

B

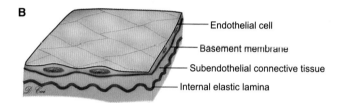

Endothelial cell

Basement membrane

Subendothelial connective tissue

Internal elastic lamina

Figure 3-8B. **Representation of simple squamous epithelium, artery endothelium.**

These **endothelial cells** are flattened and elongated, oriented parallel to the direction of blood flow, and rest on a **basement membrane**. The cells and basement membrane are linked by junctions called **hemidesmosomes**. Beneath the basement membrane is a **subendothelial layer of connective tissue**. The wavy structure is called the **internal elastic lamina**. The endothelium, subendothelial connective tissue, and the internal elastic lamina comprise the **tunica intima**.

CLINICAL CORRELATION

C

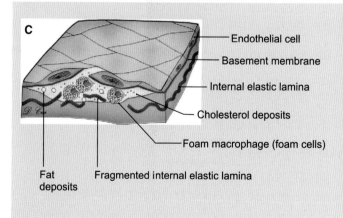

Endothelial cell

Basement membrane

Internal elastic lamina

Cholesterol deposits

Foam macrophage (foam cells)

Fat deposits

Fragmented internal elastic lamina

Figure 3-8C. **Atherosclerosis.**

Atherosclerosis is the formation of deposits of yellowish plaques that contain cholesterol, lipoid material, and **lipophages (macrophages)**. These deposits form the innermost layers of large- and medium-sized arteries. Of particular clinical significance are those plaques that form at the bifurcation of the common carotid artery into the internal and external carotid arteries and in the cerebral vessels. Although there are many possible causes of plaques, the more common are **endothelial dysfunction, dyslipidemia**, inflammatory and immunologic factors, and **hypertension**. As shown in this image, deposits of **cholesterol** and **fatty material** accumulate in the inner layers of the vessel resulting in damage to the vessel wall, including disruption of the **endothelium**. These deposits, when hardened, may occlude blood flow to distant tissues, and blood clots may form on exposed collagen in subendothelial connective tissue. Clot formation or dislodged pieces of plaque may result in vascular occlusion and **stroke**.

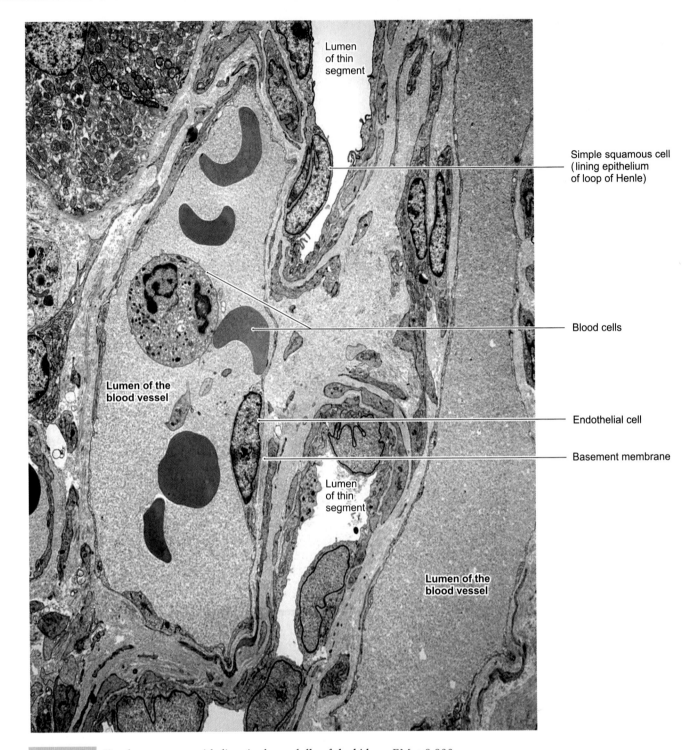

Lumen
of thin
segment

Simple squamous cell
(lining epithelium
of loop of Henle)

Blood cells

Lumen of the
blood vessel

Endothelial cell

Basement membrane

Lumen
of thin
segment

Lumen of the
blood vessel

Figure 3-9. **Simple squamous epithelium in the medulla of the kidney.** EM, ×8,900

This view of the medulla of the kidney provides two examples of **simple squamous epithelium**. The **endothelial cells** of the vessels (vasa recta) are extremely thin except at the nucleus. Red blood cells, a neutrophil, and a platelet can be seen in the **lumen of the blood vessel**. The cells that form the renal tubules shown here are squamous, but they are not as thin as the endothelial cells. These tubules are thin segments of the **loop of Henle**. There is considerable diffusion of water between the vasa recta vessels and the renal tubules in the medulla.

Simple Cuboidal Epithelium

THYROID GLAND

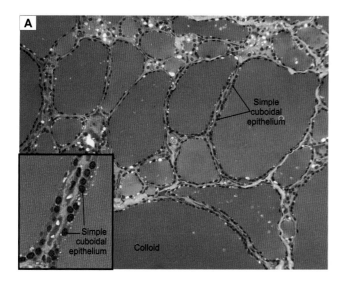

Figure 3-10A. Simple cuboidal epithelium, thyroid gland. H&E, ×155; inset ×537

Simple cuboidal epithelial cells that line the thyroid follicles of the thyroid gland are called **follicular cells**. Adjacent follicles are separated by a thin layer of connective tissue, containing occasional fibroblasts. Follicular cells are normally **cuboidal** in shape but become columnar when stimulated or in a state of hyperfunction (**hyperthyroidism**—excessively high levels of thyroid hormone secretion). At the other extreme, these cells may become flattened and squamous—like when they are inactive or in a state of hypofunction (**hypothyroidism**—excessively low levels of thyroid hormone secretion).

Follicular cells synthesize and release a precursor (**thyroglobulin**) of thyroid hormones (**T3** and **T4**) into the lumen of the follicle where it forms the colloid. Thyroid hormones are essential for normal brain and body development in infants and for the regulation of the metabolic rate in adults, and they affect the function of every organ system.

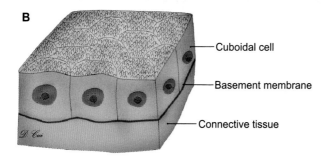

Figure 3-10B. Representation of simple cuboidal epithelium lining the thyroid follicle.

A layer of **cuboidal cells** rests on a thin **basement membrane**. The nuclei are round and located in the center of the cell. These cells have a large amount of **rough endoplasmic reticulum (RER)** and an elaborate **Golgi complex** in the cytoplasm, which reflects their high metabolic activity and production of secretory granules containing thyroglobulin. The thyroglobulin is secreted via **exocytosis** into the follicular lumen, where it is stored as a **colloid**. The apical (luminal) surface of these cuboidal cells is characterized by numerous short microvilli.

CLINICAL CORRELATION

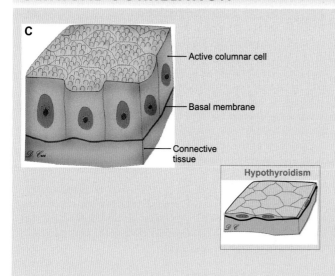

Figure 3-10C. Hyperthyroidism.

Hyperthyroidism is a condition characterized by the overproduction of thyroid hormone. In this condition, the follicular cells have changed from cuboidal cells to become **columnar cells** as a result of their high activity. Symptoms include nervousness, irritability, increased heart rate (**tachycardia**), increased perspiration, difficulty sleeping, muscle weakness, warm moist skin, trembling hands, and hair loss. This disorder is seen most often in women age 20 to 40 years. **Graves disease**, the most common form of hyperthyroidism, results from antibodies in the blood that mimic thyroid-stimulating hormone, stimulating the thyroid to grow and secrete excessive thyroid hormone. Symptoms of thyroid hyperfunction also can be induced by excessive thyroid hormone medication. At the other extreme, in **hypothyroidism**, there are very low levels of thyroid hormone secretion and follicular cells become flat, squamous cells; the patient may experience weight gain, somnolence, fatigue, and depression.

KIDNEY TUBULES

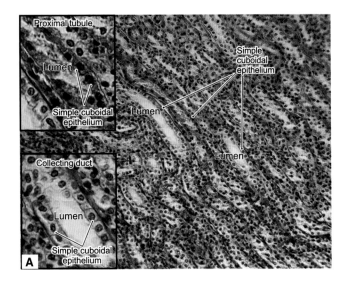

Figure 3-11A. Simple cuboidal epithelium, tubules of kidney. H&E, ×155; inset ×410

The appearance of this epithelium varies in different segments of the uriniferous tubules. For example, in the proximal tubules, the cuboidal cells have pink-stained cytoplasm and display numerous long **microvilli** on the apical surface. The microvilli generally fill the lumen and may appear disrupted in histological specimens, but this is an artifact of postmortem deterioration. The acidophilia of the cytoplasm of **proximal tubule cells** results partly from the numerous mitochondria that provide the ATP necessary to power the ion pumps in the basolateral membranes of these cells. The **cuboidal cells** of distal tubules have short and scanty microvilli. They display less acidophilia than the proximal tubules, although they do have mitochondria that support ion pumps. The cuboidal cells forming **collecting tubules** and **ducts** have few microvilli, and the cytoplasm is less stained. A defect in renal tubules can result in renal tubular **acidosis** (acidosis and electrolyte disturbance). (L, lumen.)

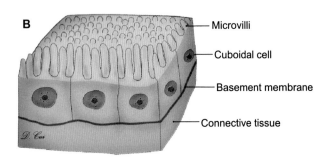

Figure 3-11B. Representation of simple cuboidal epithelium of the proximal tubule in the kidney.

These simple **cuboidal epithelial cells** have round nuclei that are in the center of the cells. The apical surface of the cell exhibits abundant long **microvilli**, indicating absorption and secretion functions. Most of the water, sodium, chloride, amino acids, proteins, and glucose in the glomerular filtrate are reabsorbed by the cuboidal cells of the proximal tubules and transported into the underlying **connective tissue**.

CLINICAL CORRELATION

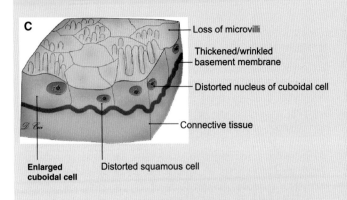

Figure 3-11C. Renal Fanconi Syndrome.
Renal Fanconi syndrome is mainly an impairment of proximal tubular function in the kidney resulting from an abnormality in the epithelial lining. The alteration of the epithelium can be caused by a variety of genetic defects (mostly in children) and by certain environmental factors. The result is that some substances that should be reabsorbed into the bloodstream are instead excreted in the urine. These substances include glucose, amino acids, phosphate, bicarbonate, and calcium. Their loss into the urine may lead to failure to thrive in children and decreased bone mineralization (**rickets** in children, **osteomalacia** in adults).

Some histological features typical of renal Fanconi syndrome are illustrated here. Epithelial cells become more **squamous** rather than cuboidal, **nuclei** are **distorted**, the **basement membrane** becomes **wrinkled** and **thickened**, and **microvilli** are **reduced** in number and length.

Simple Columnar Epithelium

SMALL INTESTINE

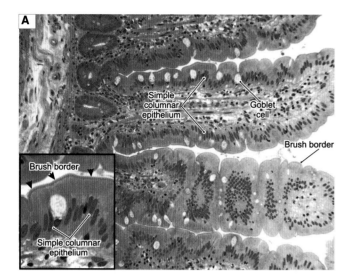

Figure 3-12A. Simple columnar epithelium, small intestine. H&E, ×155; inset ×408

This is a section taken from the ileum of the small intestine. The apical surface of the **columnar epithelium** reveals a **brush border**, consisting of **microvilli** with a **glycocalyx** coating. Microvilli are fingerlike structures that increase the surface area of the apical membrane where absorption of nutrients occurs. The cells with seemingly empty cytoplasm are **goblet cells**, which are mucus-secreting cells interspersed among the simple columnar absorptive cells (**enterocytes**). The nuclei of the epithelial cells are elongated, "hot-dog" shaped, and located toward the basal end of the cells. Sometimes, the simple columnar epithelium appears to be multilayered because of the cutting angle, but only a single layer of cells actually attaches to the basement membrane. **Simple columnar epithelium** is typical of the lining of the digestive tract, and it is also found in the oviducts, ductuli efferentes, and the ducts of some exocrine glands.

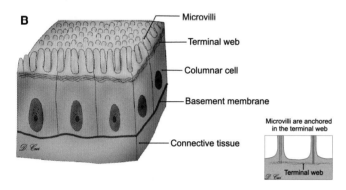

Figure 3-12B. Representation of simple columnar epithelium in the small intestine.

In the small intestine, **microvilli** enhance digestive and absorptive functions by increasing the area of the surface membrane of each **columnar epithelial cell**. This provides an expanded area of interface between the cell surface and the nutrients in the lumen. Each microvillus has a core that is composed of **actin microfilaments** anchored in a **terminal web** to stabilize the microvillus. Tall and slender columnar cells and the relationship of the terminal web are illustrated here. Individual microvilli, actin microfilaments, and actin filaments of the terminal web cannot be seen under light microscope.

CLINICAL CORRELATION

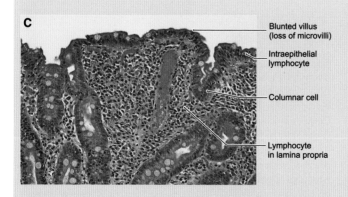

Figure 3-12C. Celiac (Coeliac) Disease.
Celiac (coeliac) disease is a disorder of the small intestine. **Gluten**, a substance found in wheat and barley, reacts with the lining of the small intestine (small bowel), leading to an attack by the immune system and damage to the microvilli and villi. If left untreated, celiac disease can lead to malabsorption; anemia; bone disease; and, rarely, some forms of cancer. The most important treatment is avoidance of all foods that contain gluten. Histologic features include blunting of villi, presence of lymphocytes among the epithelial cells (**intraepithelial lymphocytes**), and **increased lymphocytes** within the **lamina propria** (connective tissue).

Pseudostratified Columnar Epithelium

TRACHEA

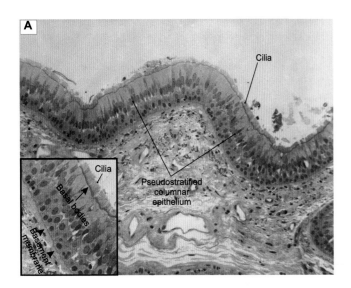

Figure 3-13A. Pseudostratified ciliated columnar epithelium, trachea. H&E, ×155; inset ×247

The cells of **pseudostratified ciliated columnar epithelium** vary in shape and height, and their nuclei are staggered, giving the false impression of being arranged in two or three layers of cells. However, the basal aspect of each cell is in contact with the **basement membrane**. Most cells are tall and columnar, but there are also short basal cells, some of which are **stem cells**. The most widespread type of pseudostratified columnar epithelium is **ciliated** and is found lining the trachea and primary bronchi, the auditory tube, and part of the tympanic cavity. **Nonciliated** pseudostratified columnar epithelium is found throughout the epididymis and vas deferens in the male reproductive tract. Cilia on the apical surfaces of some cells are closely packed like bristles of a brush. The pink line indicated by the *arrow (inset)* is formed by the **basal bodies**, from which the cilia arise. The arrangement of the nuclei in pseudostratified columnar epithelium is more irregular than in stratified columnar epithelium.

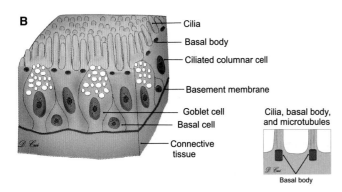

Figure 3-13B. Representation of the pseudostratified ciliated columnar epithelium of the trachea.

Secretory goblet cells are interspersed among the **ciliated columnar cells**. Cilia are elongated, motile structures that are about 5 to 10 times longer than microvilli. The core of a cilium is composed of **microtubules**, which are inserted into **basal bodies**, electron-dense structures in the apical cytoplasm just below the cell membrane. The function of cilia is to aid in the transport of material along the surface of the cells, such as moving mucus and particulate matter out of the respiratory tract. **Basal cells** are short, located in the basal portion of the epithelium, and do not reach the lumen. The epithelium may appear to have more than one layer; in fact, all its cells are in contact with the **basement membrane**.

CLINICAL CORRELATION

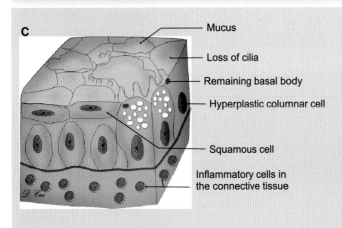

Figure 3-13C. Bronchitis.

Bronchitis is a disease marked by acute or chronic inflammation of the bronchial tubes (bronchi). The inflammation may be caused by **infection** (virus, bacteria) or by **exposure to irritants** (smoking or inhalation of chemical pollutants or dust). Cigarette smoking is the leading cause of chronic bronchitis. The inflammatory process inhibits the characteristic activity of **cilia**, which is to trap and eliminate pollutants. Inflammation also increases the secretion of **mucus**. The inflamed area of the bronchial wall becomes swollen, and excess mucus may obstruct the airway. In **chronic bronchitis**, the surface epithelium may undergo **hyperplasia** and **loss of cilia**; the pseudostratified epithelium is often replaced by squamous epithelium. This process is called **squamous metaplasia**.

RESPIRATORY EPITHELIUM

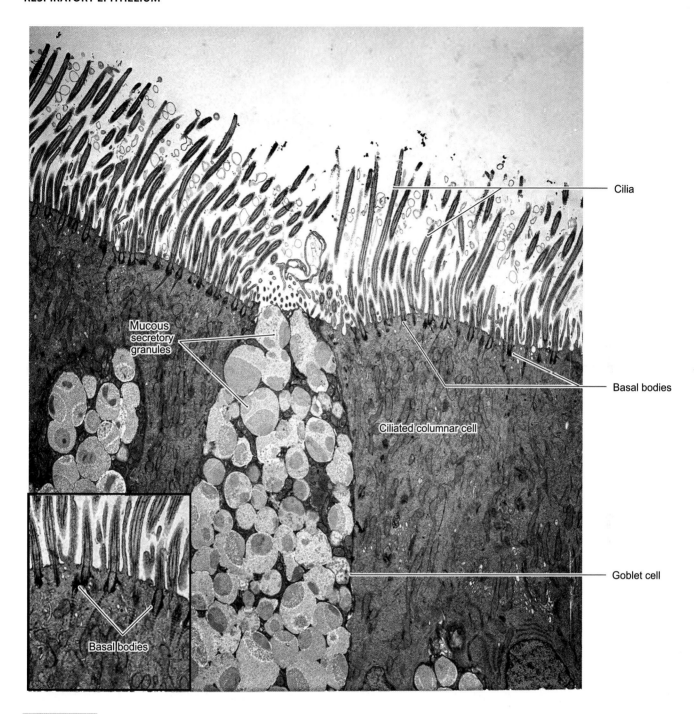

Figure 3-14. **Respiratory epithelium, example of ciliated pseudostratified columnar epithelium. EM, ×6,300; inset ×11,500**

This view of the respiratory epithelium includes only the apical half of the thickness of this **pseudostratified columnar epithelium.** Shown here are **goblet cells** and **ciliated cells,** the two most common of the approximately five cell types composing the respiratory epithelium. The *goblet cells* secrete **mucus** onto the surface of the epithelium. This mucus serves to trap airborne particles that have not been trapped by the nasal cavities. The *ciliated cells* convey the mucus with any captured material toward the larynx and the pharynx. **Mucociliary escalator** is the term sometimes used to refer to this system that protects the delicate respiratory structures of the lung from airborne microorganisms and foreign particulate matter.

Stratified Squamous Epithelium (Keratinized)

THICK AND THIN SKIN

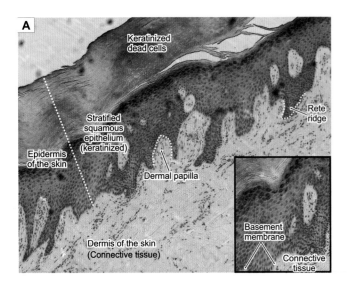

Figure 3-15A. Stratified squamous epithelium, palm of the hand (thick skin). H&E, ×78; inset ×96

Thick skin (palms and soles) and **thin skin** (most other body surfaces) are covered by **keratinized stratified squamous epithelium.** Skin includes epidermis (stratified squamous epithelium) and dermis (connective tissue). The top layer of the keratinized stratified squamous epithelium consists of dead cells (corneocytes), which lack nuclei. This tough **keratinized layer** resists friction and is impermeable to water. The cells of outer layers of the epithelium are flattened, and the middle and most basal layers of cells are more polyhedral or cuboidal. Only the cells in the deepest layer are in contact with the basement membrane. Note that the interface between the epithelium and the underlying connective tissue is expanded by unique features, such as dermal papillae and rete ridges throughout most of the stratified squamous epithelium. The *white dashed line* indicates the depth of the epithelial layer (epidermis) and the boundaries of the dermal papilla and rete ridge.

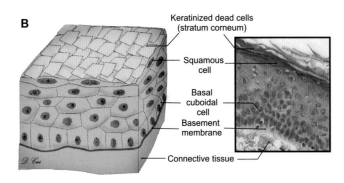

Figure 3-15B. Stratified squamous epithelium in thin skin. H&E, ×207

Stratified squamous epithelium that covers thin skin is like that of thick skin, although its **superficial keratinized layer (stratum corneum)** is much thinner than in thick skin. Keratinized stratified squamous epithelium is composed of several layers of cells. The superficial layers are formed by dead cells whose nuclei and cytoplasm have been replaced with **keratin.** Under the keratinized layer is the **squamous cell layer;** these cells are flat. The intermediate layers contain cells that are polyhedral. The cells close to the **basement membrane** are **cuboidal** in shape and are called **basal cells;** they are **stem cells** that are continuously dividing and migrating from the basal layer toward the surface as they differentiate.

CLINICAL CORRELATION

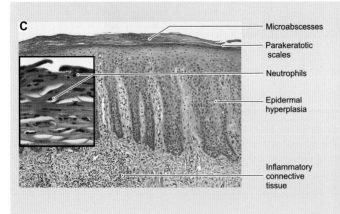

Figure 3-15C.   Psoriasis.
Psoriasis is a common chronic inflammatory skin disease typically characterized by pink- to salmon-colored plaques with silver scales and sharp margins. **T lymphocyte–mediated immunologic reactions** are believed to cause the clinical features. Symptoms and signs include itching, joint pain, nail pitting, and nail discoloration. Pathologic examinations reveal a thickened epidermis caused by increased epidermal cell turnover and extensive overlying **parakeratotic scales.** Neutrophils may migrate into the epidermis from dilated capillaries to form **microabscesses** (within the parakeratotic area of the **stratum corneum layer** of the epidermis) and **micropustules** (within the **stratum granulosum** and **spinosum layers** of the epidermis) as shown in this figure.

Stratified Squamous Epithelium (Nonkeratinized)
ESOPHAGUS

A

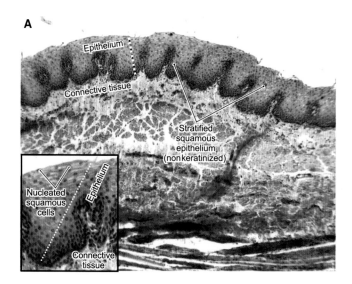

Figure 3-16A. Stratified squamous epithelium, esophagus. H&E, ×78; inset ×175

Stratified squamous epithelium (nonkeratinized) is usually wet on its surface and is found lining the mouth, oral pharynx, esophagus, true vocal cords, and vagina. Nonkeratinized stratified squamous epithelium is similar to keratinized squamous epithelium, but the flattened surface cells retain their nuclei, and there is no keratinization of these cells.

In some patients with long histories of **gastroesophageal reflux** and **heartburn**, the stratified squamous epithelium in the esophageal-stomach junction may be replaced by metaplastic columnar epithelium. The *dashed lines* illustrate the depth of the **epithelial layer.**

B

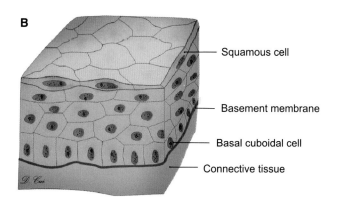

Figure 3-16B. Representation of nonkeratinized stratified squamous epithelium.

This type of epithelium is formed by multiple layers of cells. The top surface layers are composed of **flattened** and **nucleated** live cells, which do not form keratin. Other general features of **nonkeratinized stratified squamous epithelium** are similar to keratinized squamous epithelium: The basal layer has **cuboidal** or low column-shaped cells in contact with a **basement membrane**, intermediate layer cells are polyhedral in shape, and nuclei become progressively flatter as the cells move toward the surface.

CLINICAL CORRELATION

C

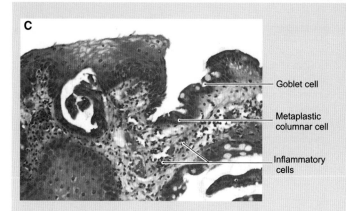

Figure 3-16C. Barrett Syndrome (Barrett Esophagus).
Barrett syndrome (Barrett esophagus) is a complication of chronic gastroesophageal reflux disease (GERD) marked by metaplasia of the stratified squamous epithelium of the distal esophagus into a simple columnar epithelium as a response to prolonged reflux-induced injury. Patients with Barrett syndrome have a high risk of developing adenocarcinoma (cancer of the esophagus). This image shows the metaplastic columnar cells and goblet cells that have replaced the normal squamous epithelium and the inflammatory cells (mainly lymphocytes and plasma cells) infiltrating the connective tissue.

Stratified Cuboidal Epithelium
SALIVARY GLAND

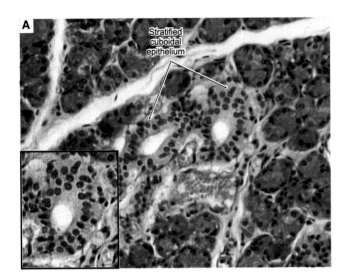

Figure 3-17A. Stratified cuboidal epithelium, salivary gland. H&E, ×175; inset ×234

Stratified cuboidal epithelium lines the ducts of the salivary glands. This uncommon type of epithelium has a very limited distribution. It may be found forming the ducts of some large exocrine glands and sweat glands. It functions to form a conduit for the secretory products of the gland. This type of epithelium is composed usually of only two layers of cuboidal cells, with the basal layer of cells often appearing incomplete.

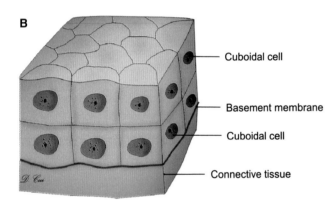

Figure 3-17B. Representation of stratified cuboidal epithelium in the duct of a salivary gland.

Stratified cuboidal epithelium usually has only two, occasionally three, layers of cuboidal cells. The top layer is composed of **uniform cuboidal cells**, whereas the basal cells sometimes appear to form an incomplete layer. Cells in stratified cuboidal epithelium often have smooth apical surfaces, and nuclei are centrally located.

CLINICAL CORRELATION

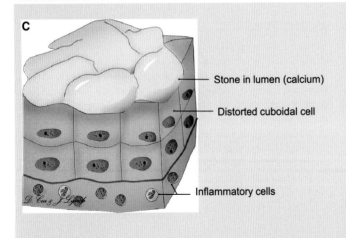

Figure 3-17C. Salivary Gland Swelling.

Salivary gland swelling with inflammation (**sialadenitis**) is a clinical condition that can result from blockage of a duct or ducts, so that saliva is not able to exit into the mouth. This causes the saliva to back up inside the duct, resulting in gland swelling. The patient will feel pain when chewing food. The most common cause of blockage is a **salivary stone (calculus)**, which forms from salts contained in the saliva. A blocked duct and gland filled with stagnant saliva may become infected with bacteria. A typical symptom of a blocked salivary duct is swelling that worsens just before mealtime. Sometimes, a small stone may be ejected into the mouth without medical intervention. A dentist may be able to push the stone out by pressing on the side of the obstructed duct. Removal of a stone may require surgery or lithotripsy treatment by focused, high-intensity acoustic pulses.

Stratified Columnar Epithelium
CONJUNCTIVA OF EYELID

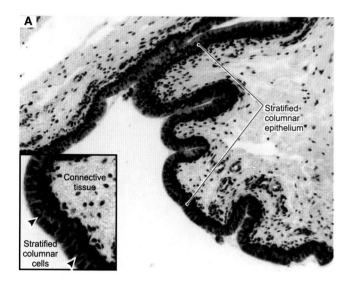

Figure 3-18A. Stratified columnar epithelium, conjunctiva of eyelid. H&E, ×155; inset ×295

Stratified columnar epithelium can be found lining the palpebral conjunctiva of the eyelid. The anterior surface of the eyelid is covered by keratinized stratified squamous epithelium (epidermis of thin skin); the posterior surface of the eyelid, which is in contact with the surface of the eyeball, is lined by stratified columnar epithelium as demonstrated here. The **basal cells** are cuboidal in shape, and the **surface layer cells** are low columnar in shape (only slightly taller than wide). The conjunctiva has a smooth surface that is kept moist and lubricated by tears and a mucinous substance in the normal condition. The *arrowheads* point to **columnar cells** of the surface layer of the epithelium (*inset*).

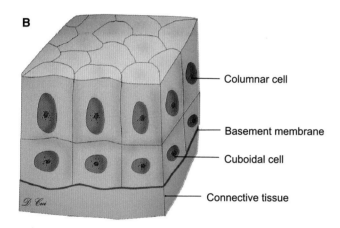

Figure 3-18B. Representation of the stratified columnar epithelium lining the conjunctiva of the eye.

Stratified columnar epithelium usually has two or three layers; the top layer is made up of **columnar cells,** and the basal layer normally consists of **cuboidal cells.** Stratified columnar epithelium is not a common type of epithelium and is found in only a few places in the body, for example, the larger ducts of some exocrine glands and the lining of the palpebral conjunctiva of the eyelid.

CLINICAL CORRELATION

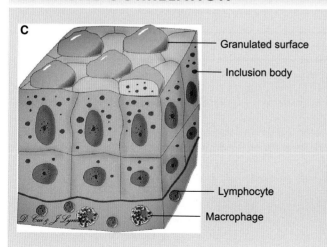

Figure 3-18C. Trachoma.

Trachoma is a chronic contagious conjunctivitis (eye disease) characterized by inflammatory granulation on the conjunctival epithelium surface caused by the bacteria *Chlamydia trachomatis.* This form of **"pink eye"** often presents with bilateral **keratoconjunctivitis** with symptoms of tearing, discharge, photophobia, pain, and swelling of the eyelids. It can cause eyelid deformities and turned-in eyelashes that scrape against the cornea. If left untreated, ulceration and infection of the cornea may occur. Trachoma can even cause loss of vision if scarring occurs on the central part of the cornea. **Lymphocytes** and **macrophages** invade underlying connective tissue as part of the inflammatory response. The epithelial **hyperplasia** and **inclusion bodies** in the epithelial cells are illustrated here.

Transitional Epithelium (Stratified Epithelium)

URINARY BLADDER

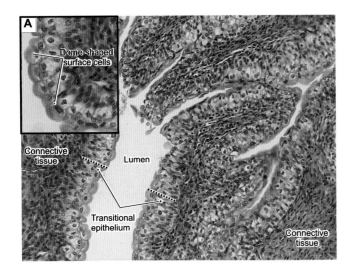

Figure 3-19A. Transitional epithelium, urinary bladder. H&E, ×155; inset ×250

Transitional epithelium has the special characteristic of being able to change shape to accommodate a volume change in the organ it lines. In the relaxed state, transitional epithelium contains four to six cell layers, and each surface cell appears dome shaped, often containing two nuclei (these cells are "binucleate"). This picture illustrates transitional epithelium in a relaxed state (in most slides, this tissue is unstretched and the surface cells appear dome shaped). The **lumen** of the bladder appears as a white space. The transitional epithelium lining the urinary tract including the bladder, ureter, and major calyces of the kidney is also referred to as **urothelium**. The *black dashed line* indicates the thickness of the epithelium.

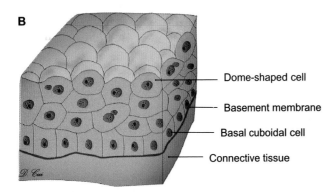

Figure 3-19B. Transitional epithelium (relaxed).

The **relaxed**, normal **transitional epithelium** is composed of four to six layers of cells. The cells located basally are smaller, low columnar or cuboidal cells. By contrast, the cells located in the most superficial layer are larger and exhibit a rounded, **dome shape** that bulges into the lumen.

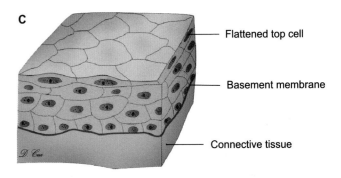

Figure 3-19C. Transitional epithelium (distended).

A presentation of **transitional epithelium** in the **distended state** is shown. These cells change shape according to the degree of distention of the bladder. When the transitional epithelium is stretched, the top dome-shaped cells become **flattened squamous cells** and the epithelium becomes thinner.

SYNOPSIS 3-3 Pathologic Terms for Epithelial Tissue

■ Metastasis: The spread of a malignant neoplasm from its site of origin to a remote site, usually through blood and lymphatic vessels.
■ Dyslipidemia: A general term describing a disorder of lipoprotein metabolism causing abnormal amounts of lipids and lipoproteins in the blood; certain dyslipidemias constitute a major risk factor for the development of atherosclerosis, such as hypercholesterolemia.
■ Osteomalacia: Abnormal bone mineralization producing weak, soft bones; may be caused by vitamin D deficiency or kidney disorders, including renal Fanconi syndrome.
■ Metaplasia: The reversible process by which one mature cell type changes into another mature cell type, as in squamous metaplasia of respiratory or glandular epithelia.
■ Microabscess: Collection of neutrophils and neutrophil debris within the parakeratotic scale in the skin disease psoriasis.
■ Micropustule: Collection of neutrophils within the epidermis, abutting the parakeratotic scale in the skin disease psoriasis.
■ Parakeratosis: Persistence of the nuclei of keratinocytes into the stratum corneum of the skin or mucous membranes; parakeratotic scales containing neutrophils are seen in the skin disease psoriasis.

Specially Named Epithelial Tissue

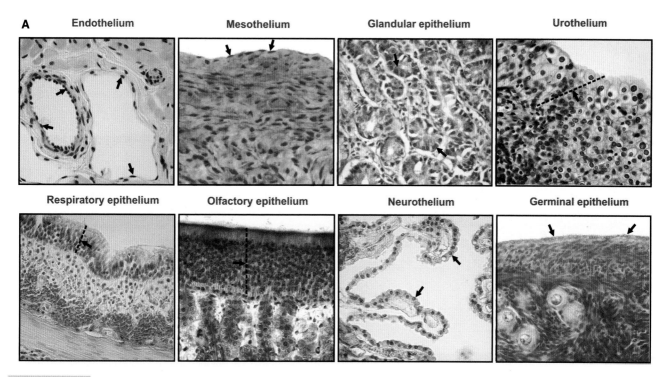

Figure 3-20A. Overview of specially named epithelial tissue. H&E, ×65,900

Epithelial tissues line the internal or external surface of many organs. These epithelia are often provided a special name, or identity, due to their specific location and unique function related to where they can be found. Here are some examples: (1) **Endothelium** is a type of simple squamous epithelium lining the inner luminal surface of blood vessels and lymph vessels. Endothelia provide a nonfriction lining for these vessels and allow smooth transport of blood and lymphatic fluid. (2) **Mesothelium** is also a simple squamous epithelium lining the outer surface of internal organs that project into body cavities and lining the surface of the body cavities. Mesothelia provide a protective layer and allow smooth movements, such as heart beats, lung contractions, and bowel peristaltic movements. (3) **Glandular epithelium** can be found in exocrine glands, which are associated with secretion and absorption. (4) **Urothelium** is a type of transitional epithelium that lines the urinary tract and allows expansion and distension of the bladder and ureters. (5) **Respiratory epithelium** is a ciliated pseudostratified columnar epithelium that lines the respiratory tract and provides protection and surface transport of mucus and debris. (6) **Olfactory epithelium** is a special type of pseudostratified columnar epithelium that lines the roof of the nose and which is composed of olfactory neurons able to detect the smell of odorants. (7) **Neurothelium** is a special simple cuboidal epithelium composed of cells derived from the neuroectoderm. Neurothelia are associated with the nervous system, and examples include ependymal cells lining the internal surfaces of the ventricles and spinal canal and epithelial cells lining the choroid plexus. (8) **Germinal epithelium** is a single layer of simple squamous-to-simple cuboidal epithelial cells lining the external ovarian surface. (*Not pictured:* Germinal epithelium also lines the seminiferous tubules of the testes).

CLINICAL CORRELATION

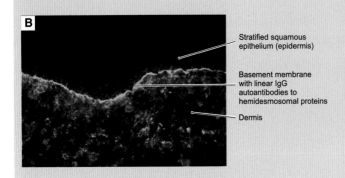

B
- Stratified squamous epithelium (epidermis)
- Basement membrane with linear IgG autoantibodies to hemidesmosomal proteins
- Dermis

Figure 3-20B **Bullous Pemphigoid.** Immunofluorescence for IgG, ×200

Bullous pemphigoid (BP) is a rare, autoimmune skin condition characterized by fluid-filled **blisters** (**bullae**), typically affecting older individuals. Clinically, BP may initially manifest as **pruritic** (itchy) scaly lesions in the nonbullous phase. In the bullous phase, tense fluid-filled blisters form, preferentially on the flexor forearms, inner thighs, and lower abdomen. The cause of BP is uncertain, but it appears to be related to **radiation exposure, medications,** and **vaccinations** in some cases. Histologically, the blister is formed by separation of the **epidermis** at the subepidermal interface. Immunofluorescence microscopy shows linear deposits of **C3** and/or **IgG** in the basement membrane zone. The IgG autoantibodies show specificity for two **hemidesmosomal proteins** (**BP230** and **BP180**) in the basement membrane zone. Treatment involves systemic steroids, anti-inflammatory drugs, and other immunosuppressive agents.

TABLE 3-2 Features of Epithelium and Their Corresponding Functional and Clinical Correlations

Types of Epithelium	Number of Layers	Type of Cells in the Epithelium	Apical Surface	Main Locations (Lining)	Main Functions	Clinical Correlations
Simple squamous epithelium	1	Flattened, squamous epithelial cells	Smooth	Cornea, blood, and lymphatic vessels—endothelium; surface of body cavities—mesothelium (pleural, pericardial, peritoneal); alveoli in the lung	Fluid transport, lubrication, and exchange	Atherosclerosis (endothelium), mesothelioma (mesothelium)
Simple cuboidal epithelium	1	Cuboidal epithelial cells (height equal to width)	Smooth/short microvilli/ long microvilli depending on location	Kidney tubules, thyroid follicles; small ducts of exocrine glands, and surface of ovary	Absorption, secretion, and transportation	Hyperthyroidism, renal Fanconi syndrome
Simple columnar epithelium	1	Absorptive columnar cells and secretory cells, such as goblet cells	Mostly microvilli; cilia in some locations	Most of digestive tract and gall bladder; oviducts and ductuli efferentes	Secretion, absorption, protection, and transportation	Villous atrophy, malabsorption syndrome, celiac disease (abnormal microvilli), metaplasia, Barrett syndrome

TABLE 3-2 (Continued)

Types of Epithelium	Number of Layers	Type of Cells in the Epithelium	Apical Surface	Main Locations (Lining)	Main Functions	Clinical Correlations
Pseudostratified columnar epithelium	1	Ciliated columnar cells, goblet cells and short basal cells not reaching lumen; all cells rest on the basement membrane	Mostly cilia; stereocilia in some locations	Most of respiratory tract; ductus deferens and epididymis	Secretion, transportation, and absorption	Bronchitis, chronic bronchitis, squamous metaplasia, immotile cilia syndrome
Stratified squamous epithelium	Several	Flattened surface cells, polygonal cells in the middle layers and cuboidal cells in basal layer	Keratinized or nonkeratinized surface layer	Epidermis of the skin; oral cavity, epiglottis and esophagus; vagina	Protection (barrier)	(Keratinized): Squamous cell carcinoma, basal cell carcinoma, psoriasis, bullous pemphigoid, hyperkeratosis. (Nonkeratinized): Barrett esophagus, epithelial dysplasia
Stratified cuboidal epithelium	2–3	Cuboidal cells	Mostly smooth	Large ducts of exocrine glands and ducts of sweat gland (not common type)	Transportation	Salivary gland swelling
Stratified columnar epithelium	2–3	Low columnar surface cells and cuboidal basal cells	Smooth	Large ducts of exocrine glands; conjunctiva of the eye (not common type)	Transportation and protection	Trachoma
Transitional epithelium	4–6 layers (relaxed); 2–3 layers (distended)	Dome-shaped surface cells (relaxed); polygonal in the middle layer; cuboidal cells in the basal layer	Smooth	Urinary tract	Transportation and protection (distensible property)	Transitional cell carcinoma

From Histology to Pathology

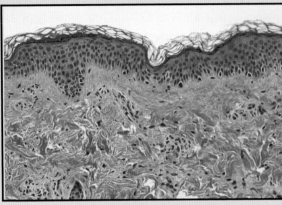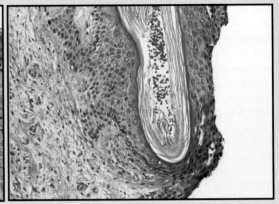

Figure 3-21. Normal stratified squamous epithelium and bullous pemphigoid. (Left) H&E, ×200

Normal stratified squamous epithelium (epidermis of thin skin) on the *left*. **Bullous pemphigoid** (epidermis of thin skin) on the *right*, with a visible blister formed by the separation of the epidermis of the skin. It is a rare, autoimmune skin condition characterized by fluid-filled blisters (bullae).

Clinical Vignette Questions

1. A 65-year-old female complains of epigastric pain, especially after eating for the last year. She awakens from sleep with episodes of regurgitation and a bitter taste in her mouth. She takes antacids for relief and sleeps on several pillows to prevent regurgitation. She sees her primary care physician, who diagnoses the condition as gastroesophageal reflux disease (GERD). She is referred to a gastroenterologist for upper endoscopy, which shows salmon-colored tongues of slightly raised mucosa in the distal esophagus, emanating from the gastroesophageal junction. A biopsy taken from this salmon-colored tissue would most likely show which of the following histologic changes?

A. Change from mucus-secreting columnar epithelium to stratified squamous, nonkeratinized epithelium
B. Change from simple columnar epithelium to keratinized squamous epithelium
C. Change from stratified keratinized epithelium to mucus-secreting columnar epithelium
D. Change from stratified keratinized epithelium to non–mucus-secreting columnar epithelium
E. Change from stratified squamous, nonkeratinized epithelium to mucus-secreting columnar epithelium

2. A 75-year-old man experiences slightly raised, pruritic, scaly (eczematous) lesions on his lower abdomen and arms for several months. He did not seek treatment until the lesions became blistered. A physical examination revealed tense bullae on the flexural surface of his arms and lower abdomen. Punch biopsies are performed on the edge of a blister and submitted for light (H&E) and immunofluorescence microscopy. The pathologist returns a diagnosis of bullous pemphigoid. Which of the following findings would be expected from the immunofluorescence results in this case?

A. IgA deposits in the basement membrane zone
B. "Full house" immunofluorescence with IgG, IgA, IgM, and C3 in the basement membrane zone
C. IgG on the surface of epidermal keratinocytes
D. IgG and/or C3 deposits in the basement membrane zone
E. Negative immunofluorescence result

3. A mother brings her 5-year-old son to your clinic because he has experienced abdominal pain for several months. The symptoms became worse after he visited his grandmother for 2 weeks, where he consumed cakes and homemade bread. The grandmother relates that the boy passed foul-smelling diarrheal stools recently. Evaluation of the boy shows evidence of malnutrition, anemia, and signs of slow growth for his age. Lab tests exclude GI infection but do show serum anti-transglutaminase antibodies. A biopsy of this child's duodenum would most likely show which of the following changes in the mucosal lining?

A. Loss of basal lamina
B. Loss of goblet cells
C. Loss of intercellular junctions
D. Loss of normal villous architecture
E. Loss of mucosa layer of small intestine

Glands

Introduction and Key Concepts for Glands

Glands are composed of epithelial tissue and can be classified as endocrine and exocrine according to how the secretory product leaves the gland. **Endocrine glands** release their products into interstitial fluid or directly into the bloodstream (see Chapter 17, "Endocrine System"). **Exocrine glands** are discussed in this chapter; these glands secrete their products either through ducts into the lumen of an organ or directly onto the body surfaces. Exocrine glands can be classified into several categories according to various criteria.

Exocrine Glands Classified by Product

Exocrine glands can be classified as **serous glands, mucous glands, mixed glands (seromucous),** and **sebaceous glands,** depending on what type of secretion is produced. (1) *Serous glands* secrete a watery proteinaceous fluid. The parotid gland, the gland of von Ebner of the tongue, the pancreas, and sweat glands, are examples of this type of gland. (2) *Mucous glands* secrete mucus, a viscous mixture of glycoprotein and water. Goblet cells in the small and large intestines, respiratory epithelium, some glands in the hard and soft palates, and stomach epithelium are examples of mucous glands. (3) *Mixed glands* have both serous and mucous secretions and include the submandibular gland, sublingual gland, and glands in the trachea and esophagus. (4) *Sebaceous glands* produce lipids. The sebaceous glands in the skin are good examples.

Exocrine Glands Classified by Mechanisms of Secretion

Exocrine glands can be classified into **merocrine secretion, apocrine secretion,** and **holocrine secretion** based on the pathway by which the secretory products are released from the cell. (1) In *merocrine secretion,* the secretory product is released from the cell by exocytosis without the loss of cell material (cytoplasm). The release of secretory zymogen granules by pancreatic acinar cells is an example of merocrine secretion. Merocrine mechanism is the most common mode. (2) In *apocrine secretion,* the secretory product is released together with part of the apical cytoplasm of the secretory cell. The lipid secretion by epithelial cells of the mammary gland belongs to this mode of secretion. (3) In *holocrine secretion,* the secretory product is released by disintegration of the entire cell. The secretory cell dies, and a new secretory cell is formed from a nearby basal cell. The fatty lubricant secretory product, **sebum,** is released by the cells of sebaceous glands by holocrine secretion.

Exocrine Glands Classified by Morphology

The exocrine glands also can be classified into **unicellular** and **multicellular glands** depending upon the number of cells that form the gland.

UNICELLULAR GLANDS are composed of only single cells. The secretory products are released directly onto the surface of an epithelium. Goblet cells are an example of this type of gland.

MULTICELLULAR GLANDS consist of numbers of secretory cells arranged in different organizations. The multicellular glands can be further classified into several subtypes according to their morphology. In general, the terms **simple** and **compound** are tied to their duct shape. *Simple glands* have unbranched ducts or lack ducts. *Compound glands* have branched ducts. The cells of the multicellular glands are arranged into secretory units in the form of **acini** or tubules.

The multicellular glands also can be classified using a combination of duct shape and the shape of secretory units. (1) **Simple tubular glands** have no ducts. The secretory cells are arranged in straight tubules. This type of gland can be found in small and large intestines. (2) **Simple branched tubular glands** do not have ducts, and their secretory cells are split into two or more tubules. This type of gland can be found in the stomach. (3) **Simple coiled tubular glands** have a long duct, and secretory cells are formed by coiled tubules. Sweat glands are examples of this type of gland. (4) **Simple acinar glands** have a short, unbranched duct; the secretory cells are arranged in acini form. The mucus-secreting glands in the submucosa of the penile urethra are examples of this type of gland. (5) **Simple branched acinar glands** have a short, unbranched duct, and their secretory cells are formed into branched acini. The sebaceous glands of the skin belong to this type. (6) **Compound tubular glands** have branched ducts. Their secretory cells are formed into branched tubules as can be found in the Brunner glands of the duodenum. (7) **Compound acinar glands** have branched ducts, and the secretory units are branched acini. The pancreas and mammary glands are examples of this type of gland. (8) **Compound tubuloacinar glands** have branched ducts, and the secretory units are formed by both an acinar component and a tubular component. The submandibular and sublingual glands are good examples of this type of gland.

Duct System

The compound glands often have complex **duct systems.** The secretory **acini** or **tubules** are arranged in **lobules.** The secretory cells empty their products into small ducts called **small intralobular ducts,** which are often referred to as **intercalated ducts.** The small intralobular ducts drain secretory products into **larger intralobular ducts,** which in salivary glands are called **striated ducts.** The striated ducts are so named because the basal cytoplasm of these cells often appears "striped" under the microscope. The striped appearance is a result of the arrangement of the basal cytoplasm into deep folds packed with **mitochondria.** This organization provides the large surface area and generation of energy needed for extensive pumping of ions across the basolateral membrane of the cell. Some glands, such as the pancreas, have intercalated ducts but not striated ducts. In general, the ducts located *inside* of lobules are called **intralobular ducts** and ducts located *between* lobules are called **interlobular ducts.** The large *intralobular ducts* feed into the interlobular ducts; the *interlobular ducts* course through the connective tissue (septa) between the lobules. The secretory products then pass through the major ducts, the **lobar ducts.** Finally, lobar ducts feed into the **main duct** of the gland and the secretory products exit the organ.

Exocrine Glands Classified by Product

The **exocrine glands** can be classified as **serous glands**, **mucous glands**, **mixed glands** (seromucous), and **sebaceous glands**, depending on what **type of secretion** is produced.

Serous Gland

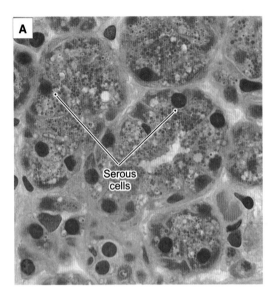

Figure 3-22A. Serous gland, parotid gland. H&E, ×668

An example of a **serous gland** from the parotid gland is shown. Each **serous secretory cell** has a spherical nucleus, the cytoplasm is basophilic, and the secretory vesicles (granules) are located in the apical part of the cytoplasm. These serous cells are organized in acini and produce a watery **proteinaceous** secretion.

Mucous Gland

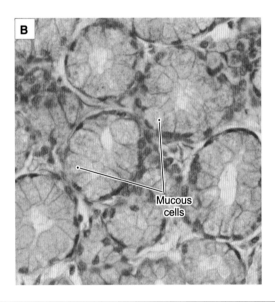

Figure 3-22B. Mucous gland, duodenum. H&E, ×396

An example of a **mucous gland** in the duodenum is shown. The **mucous secretory cell** has a flattened nucleus at the base of the cell and an empty vacuolated appearance of the apical cytoplasm. This reflects the removal of the mucus from the secretory granules during processing of the specimen. These cells are arranged in tubules and produce gel-like **mucin** (**glycoprotein** and water mixture) secretions that usually protect or lubricate epithelial cell surfaces.

Mixed (Seromucous) Gland

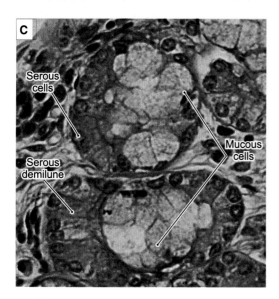

Figure 3-22C. **Mixed (seromucous) gland, sublingual gland.** H&E, ×609

An example of a **mixed gland**, the sublingual gland, containing both **mucous secretory portions** and **serous secretory portions** is shown. The serous cells forming a moon-shaped cap on top of the mucus are called a **serous demilune**.

Sebaceous Gland

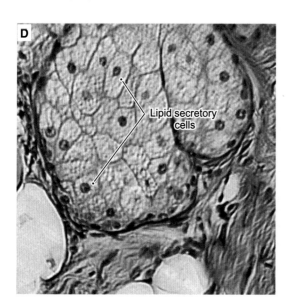

Figure 3-22D. **Sebaceous gland, skin (scalp).** H&E, ×306

An example of a **sebaceous gland** in the scalp is shown. The sebaceous gland cells are tightly packed together in groups. This type of gland produces **sebum**, an oily substance that is a mixture of **lipids** and debris of dead lipid-producing cells.

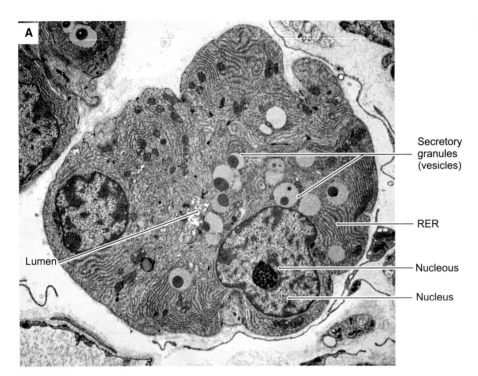

Figure 3-23A. Serous acinus from the parotid gland. EM, ×5,200

Cells that produce **serous** (thin, proteinaceous fluid) secretions have features in common whether they are from one of the salivary glands or from the pancreas. The **nuclei** are relatively large with considerable **euchromatin** and one or more prominent **nucleoli**. The cytoplasm in the basal region is filled with **RER**. The apical cytoplasm contains **secretory vesicles** (**granules**), which vary in their staining characteristics.

Labels for Figure 3-23A:
- Secretory granules (vesicles)
- RER
- Lumen
- Nucleous
- Nucleus

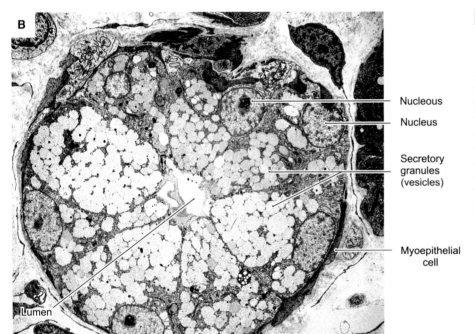

Figure 3-23B. Mucous acinus from the submandibular gland. EM, ×6,300

Although **mucus-secreting cells** have the same general organization as cells that produce serous secretions, there are some distinctions. The **mucous acinus** cell has a **smaller nucleus**, which is located against the basal edge of the cell. In addition, the **secretory granules** are generally more electron lucent than secretory granules of serous secreting cells.

Labels for Figure 3-23B:
- Nucleous
- Nucleus
- Secretory granules (vesicles)
- Myoepithelial cell
- Lumen

SYNOPSIS 3-4 Glands Classified by Product

- ■ Serous glands: Generate serous product, which is a thin, watery fluid containing proteins, glycoproteins, and water.
- ■ Mucous glands: Produce mucin, which is a thick, viscous material containing high concentration of glycosylated glycoproteins and water.
- ■ Mixed glands: Consist of both serous and mucous secretary cells and produce serous and mucous materials.
- ■ Sebaceous glands: Produce lipids (sebum), which contains an oily substance.

Exocrine Glands Classified by Morphology

The **exocrine glands** also can be classified into **unicellular** and **multicellular glands** depending upon the **number** of **cells** that form the gland.

Unicellular Glands

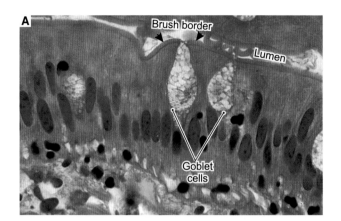

Figure 3-24A. Goblet cell of small intestine. H&E, ×962

Unicellular glands are composed of only a **single cell**. The secretory products are released directly onto the surface of an epithelium. **Goblet cells** are an example of this type of gland. Microvilli with glycocalyx coating form a **brush border** (*arrows*). Note that goblet cells themselves do not have microvilli on their apical surfaces.

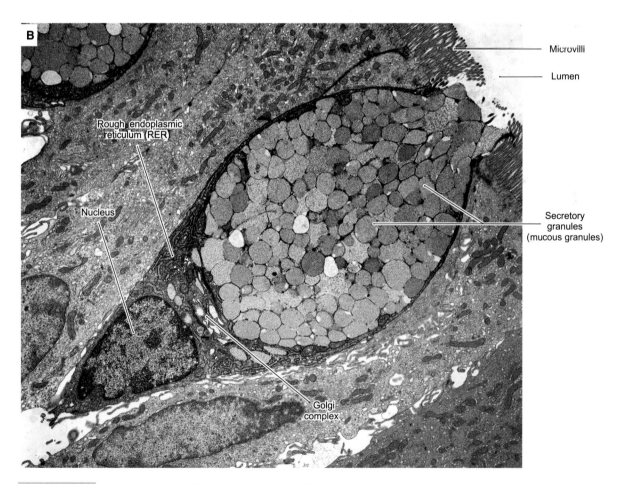

Figure 3-24B. Goblet cell, unicellular glands (single-cell gland). EM, ×5,100

The **goblet cell** can be considered a **single-cell gland** because it is commonly inserted into an epithelium among nonsecretory cells. In this example, the goblet cell is surrounded by **enterocytes**, absorptive cells of the small intestine. Goblet cells are also found among ciliated cells in the respiratory epithelium. Typical features of goblet cells are illustrated here. The relatively small **heterochromatic nucleus** is packed into the narrow base of the cell along with some **RER**. A **Golgi complex** is barely visible adjacent to the apical end of the nucleus. Most of the **cytoplasm** is filled with **secretory vesicles**.

Multicellular Glands

Multicellular glands consist of numbers of secretory cells arranged in different organizations. The multicellular glands can be further classified into several subtypes according to their morphology. In general, the terms **simple** and **compound** are tied to their duct shape. *Simple glands* have unbranched ducts or lack ducts. *Compound glands* have branched ducts. The cells of the multicellular glands are arranged into secretory units in the form of **acini** or tubules.

SIMPLE TUBULAR GLAND

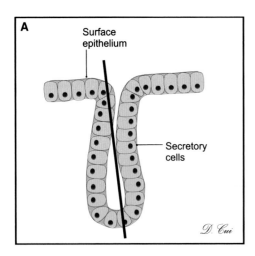

Figure 3-25A. Simple tubular gland.

The **secretory cells** of this **simple tubular gland** are arranged in **straight tubules,** and the gland has **no duct.** The *heavy black line* represents the approximate plane of the section in Figure 3-25B.

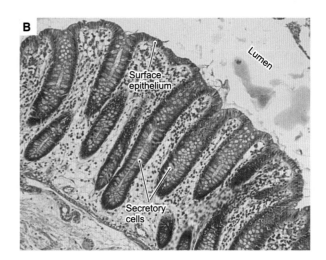

Figure 3-25B. Large intestine. H&E, ×99

An example of the **simple tubular glands** in the large intestine is shown. The **secretory cells (goblet cells)** are arranged in **straight tubules,** and secretory products are released directly into the **lumen** of the intestine. This type of gland also can be found in the small intestine.

SIMPLE BRANCHED TUBULAR GLANDS

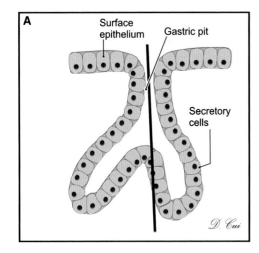

Figure 3-26A. Simple branched tubular gland.

This type of gland has no duct, and the **secretory cells** of the **simple branched tubular gland** are arranged in **two or more branched tubules.** The *heavy black line* represents the approximate plane of the section in Figure 3-26B.

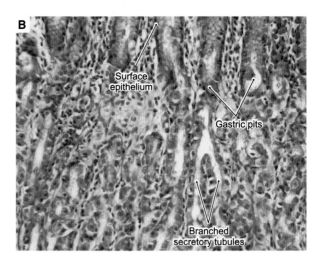

Figure 3-26B. Stomach. H&E, ×198

An example of the **simple branched tubular glands** in the stomach is shown. The **surface epithelium** invaginates to form **gastric pits.** The secretory cells form **branched tubular gastric glands** that empty their secretory products into gastric pits.

SIMPLE COILED TUBULAR GLANDS

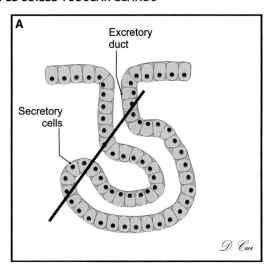

Figure 3-27A. Simple coiled tubular gland.

The **simple coiled tubular gland** has a **long excretory duct** that is **unbranched** (*indicated in blue*). The **secretory portions** are formed by **coiled tubules**. The *heavy black line* represents the approximate plane of the section in Figure 3-27B.

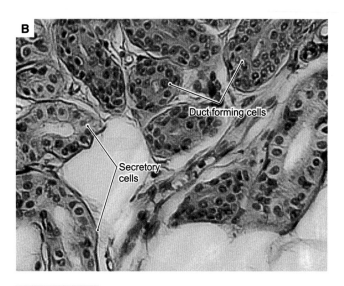

Figure 3-27B. Sweat gland of the skin. H&E, ×377

Sweat glands in the integument (**skin**) are examples of **simple coiled tubular glands**. The **secretory cells** form **coiled tubules** that are lined by simple cuboidal cells. The excretory ducts are lined by stratified cuboidal epithelium. The ducts are long, unbranched, and open at the skin surface.

SIMPLE ACINAR GLANDS

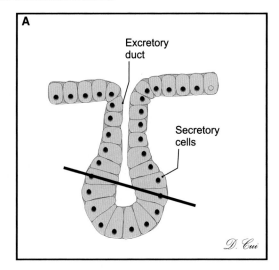

Figure 3-28A. Simple acinar gland.

The **simple acinar gland** has a **short, unbranched duct** (*blue cells*). The secretory portion is formed by **secretory cells** arranged in an **unbranched acinus** or **alveolus** (a small, grape-shaped secretory unit). The *heavy black line* represents the approximate plane of the section in Figure 3-28B.

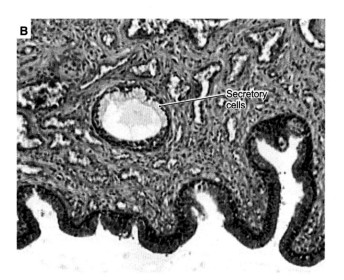

Figure 3-28B. Penis. H&E (perfusion), ×158

Small mucous glands (**Littré glands**) in the submucosa of the male urethra are examples of **simple acinar glands**. They have very short excretory ducts that are directly linked to the surface of the epithelium. The **mucous secretory cells** are arranged in **acinar** form.

SIMPLE BRANCHED ACINAR GLANDS

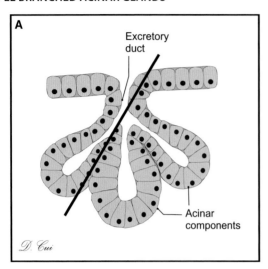

Figure 3-29A. Simple branched acinar gland.

The **simple branched acinar gland** has a short, **unbranched duct** (*blue cells*). The **secretory portions** are **branched acini**. The *heavy black line* represents the approximate plane of the section in Figure 3-29B.

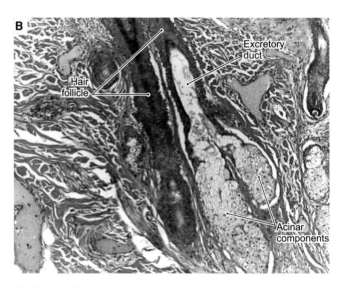

Figure 3-29B. Skin. H&E, ×78

The sebaceous glands in the skin are good examples of a **simple branched acinar gland**. The **secretory cells** are arranged in several **acinar units** and open into a short **excretory duct**. The secretory product, **sebum**, is discharged from the acini through a short duct into the **hair follicle**.

COMPOUND TUBULAR GLANDS

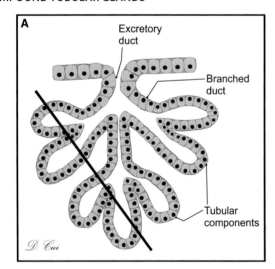

Figure 3-30A. Compound tubular gland.

The **compound tubular gland** has **branched ducts** (*blue cells*). The **secretory portions** are formed by branched **tubules**. The *heavy black line* represents the approximate plane of the section in Figure 3-30B.

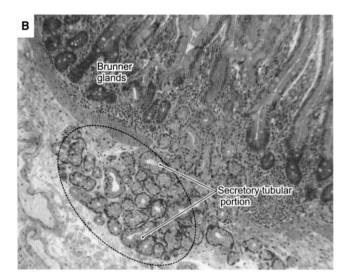

Figure 3-30B. Duodenum. H&E, ×83

The **Brunner glands** in the duodenum are examples of **compound tubular glands**. The **mucous secretory cells** are arranged in **tubular components**. The secretory products exit through branched ducts into the lumen of the duodenum.

COMPOUND ACINAR GLANDS

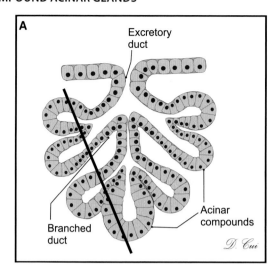

Figure 3-31A. Compound acinar gland.

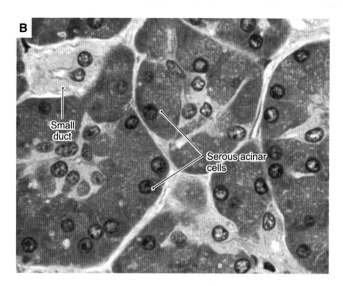

Figure 3-31B. Pancreas. H&E, ×812

The **compound acinar gland** has **branched ducts** (*blue cells*), and the **secretory units** are **branched acini**. The *heavy black line* represents the approximate plane of the section in Figure 3-31B.

Exocrine glands of the pancreas are examples of **compound acinar glands**. The **secretory cells** form numbers of **acinar compounds**, and the secretory products are evacuated into the duodenum through the **duct system** of the glands.

COMPOUND TUBULOACINAR GLANDS

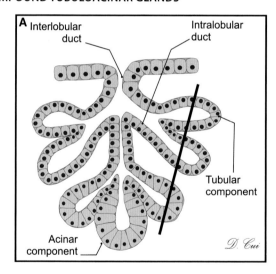

Figure 3-32A. Compound tubuloacinar gland.

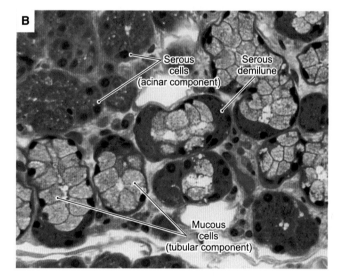

Figure 3-32B. Submandibular gland. H&E, ×436

The **compound tubuloacinar gland** has **branched ducts** (*blue cells*) and **branched secretory portions** of **tubular** and **acinar components**. The *heavy black line* represents the approximate plane of the section in Figure 3-32B.

The submandibular glands and sublingual glands are good examples of this category. The **acinar components** are made up of **serous cells**; the **tubular components** are formed by **mucous cells**. There are several levels of excretory ducts, including **intralobular ducts** and **interlobular ducts**. A serous demilune is also visible.

Duct System of Exocrine Glands

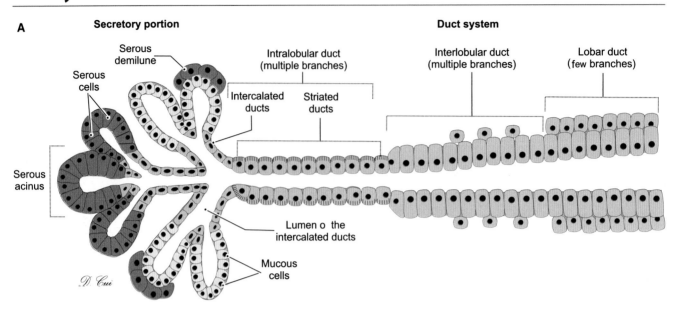

Figure 3-33A. Overview of duct system of exocrine glands.

The compound glands have complex **duct systems**. The secretory **acini** or **tubules** are arranged in **lobules**. The ducts located *inside* of the lobules are called **intralobular ducts,** and ducts located *between* lobules are called **interlobular ducts.** The secretory cells empty their products into small **intralobular ducts (intercalated ducts)** and then drain products into **larger intralobular ducts,** which in salivary glands are called **striated ducts.** Then **large intralobular ducts** drain into interlobular ducts which, in turn, empty in the **lobar ducts and main ducts.**

Epithelial Lining of the Duct System of Exocrine Glands

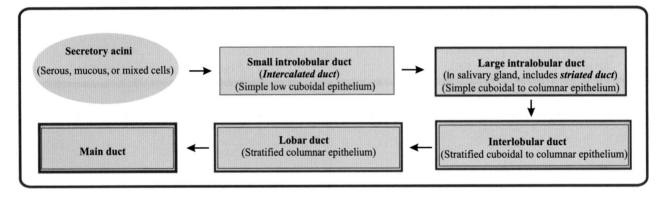

From Histology to Pathology

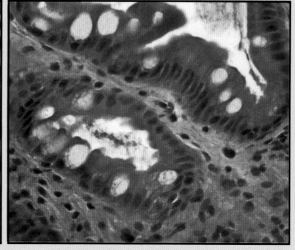

B

Figure 3-33B. Normal gastric glands and metaplasia of gastric glands. H&E, ×400

Normal gastric glands on the *left*. **Metaplasia** of gastric glands (on the *right*), a chronic gastritis with intestinal metaplasia of epithelium in the gastric glands. Goblet cells are usually not present in the normal gastric glands and gastric mucosa. The metaplasia is a reversible change of one type of cells to another due to an environmental stimulus, and in this case, it is the result of **chronic inflammation.**

TABLE 3-3 Exocrine Glands Classified by Morphology

Types of Glands	Shape of the Ducts	Shape of the Secretory Units	Secretory Products	Main Locations
Unicellular glands (Consist of Single Cells)				
Goblet cells	No ducts; products released directly onto surface of an epithelium	Single cell, goblet shaped	Mucus (glycoprotein and water)	Epithelium in respiratory and digestive tracts
Multicellular Glands (Consist of Multiple Secretory Cells)				
Simple tubular glands	No ducts	Single straight tubules	Mucus (glycoprotein and water)	Small and large intestine
Simple branched tubular glands	No ducts	Two or more branched tubules	Mucus (glycoprotein and water)	Stomach (pyloric glands), uterus (uterine glands)
Simple coiled tubular glands	Long, unbranched ducts	Coiled tubules	Watery fluid (sweat)	Sweat glands in the skin

(*Continued*)

TABLE 3-3 (Continued)

Types of Glands	Shape of the Ducts	Shape of the Secretory Units	Secretory Products	Main Locations
Simple acinar glands	Short, unbranched ducts	Unbranched acini/alveoli (grape shaped)	Mucous (glycoprotein and water)	Littré glands in the submucosa of the urethra
Simple branched acinar glands	Short, unbranched ducts	Branched acini/alveoli (grape shaped)	Sebum (mixture of lipids and debris of dead lipid-producing cells)	Sebaceous glands of the skin
Compound tubular glands	Branched ducts	Branched tubules	Mucus (glycoprotein and water)	Brunner glands of duodenum
Compound acinar glands	Branched ducts	Branched acini	Watery proteinaceous fluid	Lacrimal gland in orbit, tarsal gland of eye, pancreas, and mammary glands.
Compound tubuloacinar glands	Branched ducts	Branched tubules and acini	Watery proteinaceous fluid and mucus (glycoprotein and water)	Submandibular and sublingual glands in oral cavity

4 Connective Tissue

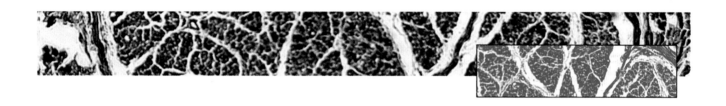

Introduction and Key Concepts for Connective Tissue
Connective Tissue Cells
Connective Tissue Fibers
Ground Substance of Connective Tissue

Types of Connective Tissues

Connective Tissue Cells

Extracellular Matrix

Introduction and Key Concepts for Connective Tissue

Connective tissue provides structural support for the body by binding cells and tissues together to form organs. It also provides metabolic support by creating a hydrophilic environment that mediates the exchange of substances between the blood and tissue. Connective tissue is of mesodermal origin and consists of a mixture of **cells, fibers,** and **ground substance**. The hydrophilic **ground substance** occupies the spaces around cells and fibers. **Fibers (collagen, elastic,** and **reticular)** and the ground substances constitute the extracellular matrix of connective tissue. The classification and function of connective tissue are based on the differences in the composition and amounts of cells, fibers, and ground substance.

Connective Tissue Cells

A variety of cells are found in connective tissue, which differ according to their origin and function. Some cells differentiate from mesenchymal cells, such as adipocytes and fibroblasts; these cells are formed and reside in the connective tissue and are called **fixed cells**. Other cells, which arise from hematopoietic stem cells, differentiate in the bone marrow and migrate from the blood circulation into connective tissue where they perform their functions; these mast cells, macrophages, plasma cells, and leukocytes are called **wandering cells**. Cells found in connective tissue proper include **fibroblasts, macrophages, mast cells, plasma cells,** and **leukocytes**. Some cells, such as *fibroblasts,* are responsible for synthesis and maintenance of the extracellular material. Other cells, such as *macrophages, plasma cells,* and *leukocytes,* have defense and immune functions.

FIBROBLASTS are the most common cells in connective tissue. Their nuclei are ovoid or spindle shaped and can be large or small in size depending on their stage of cellular activity. They have pale-staining cytoplasm and contain well-developed rough endoplasmic reticulum (RER) and rich Golgi complexes. With routine H&E staining, only the very thin, elongated nuclei of the cells are clearly visible. Their thin, pale-staining cytoplasm is usually not obvious. They are responsible for the synthesis of all components of the extracellular matrix (fibers and ground substance) of connective tissue.

MACROPHAGES also called **tissue histiocytes**, are highly phagocytic cells that are derived from blood monocytes. With conventional staining, macrophages are very difficult to identify unless they show visible ingested material inside their cytoplasm. Macrophages may be named differently in certain organs. For example, they are called **Kupffer cells** in the liver, **osteoclasts** in bone, and **microglial cells** in the central nervous system.

MAST CELLS are of bone marrow origin and are distributed chiefly around small blood vessels. They are oval to round in shape, with a centrally placed nucleus. With toluidine blue stain, large basophilic purple staining granules are visible in their cytoplasm. These granules contain and release **heparin, histamines**, and various chemotactic mediators, which are involved in inflammatory responses. Mast cells contain Fc membrane receptors, which bind to immunoglobulin (Ig) E antibodies, an important cellular interaction involved in anaphylactic shock.

PLASMA CELLS are derived from B lymphocytes. They are oval shaped and are able to secrete antibodies that are antigen specific. Their histologic features include an eccentrically placed nucleus, a cartwheel pattern of chromatin in the nucleus, and basophilic-staining cytoplasm due to the presence of abundant RER and a small, clear area near the nucleus. This cytoplasmic clear area (**Golgi zone [GZ]**) marks the position of the Golgi apparatus.

LEUKOCYTES, white blood cells, are considered the transient cells of connective tissue. They migrate from the blood vessels into connective tissue by the process of **diapedesis**. This process increases greatly during various inflammatory conditions. After entering connective tissue, leukocytes, except lymphocytes, do not return to the blood. The following leukocytes are commonly found in connective tissue: (1) **Lymphocytes:** These cells have a round or bean-shaped nucleus and are often located in the subepithelial connective tissue. (2) **Neutrophils (polymorphs):** Each cell has a multilobed nucleus and functions in the defense against infection. (3) **Eosinophils:** Each cell has a bilobed nucleus and reddish granules in the cytoplasm. They have antiparasitic activity and moderate the allergic reaction function. (4) **Basophils:** These cells are not easy to find in normal tissues. Their primary function is like that of mast cells. A detailed account of the structure and the function of leukocytes is given in Chapter 8, "Blood and Hemopoiesis."

ADIPOCYTES (FAT CELLS) arise from undifferentiated mesenchymal cells of connective tissue. They gradually accumulate cytoplasmic fat, which results in a significant flattening of the nucleus in the periphery of the cell. **Adipocytes** are found throughout the body, particularly in loose connective tissue. Their function is to store energy in the form of triglycerides and to synthesize hormones such as **leptin**.

Connective Tissue Fibers

Three types of fibers are found in connective tissue: **collagen, elastic,** and **reticular**. The amount and type of fibers that dominate a connective tissue are a reflection of the structural support needed to serve the function of that particular tissue. These three fibers all consist of proteins that form elongated structures, which, although produced primarily by fibroblasts, may be produced by other cell types in certain locations. For example, collagen and elastic fibers can be produced by smooth muscle cells in large arteries and chondrocytes in cartilages.

COLLAGEN FIBERS are the most common and widespread fibers in connective tissue and are composed primarily of type I collagen. The collagen molecule (**tropocollagen**) is a product of the fibroblast. Each collagen molecule is 300 nm in length and consists of three polypeptide amino acid chains (**alpha chains**) wrapped in a right-handed triple helix. The molecules are arranged head to tail in overlapping parallel, longitudinal rows with a gap between the molecules within each row to form a **collagen fibril**. The parallel array of fibrils forms cross-links to one another to form the collagen fiber. Collagen fibers stain readily with acidic and some basic dyes. When stained with H&E and viewed with the light microscope, they appear as pink, wavy fibers of different sizes. When stained with osmium tetroxide for EM study, the fibers have a transverse banded pattern (light-dark) that repeats every 68 μm along the fiber. The banded pattern is a reflection of the arrangement of collagen molecules within the fibrils of the collagen fiber.

ELASTIC FIBERS stain glassy red with H&E but are best demonstrated with a stain specifically for elastic fibers, such as aldehyde fuchsin. Elastic fibers have a very resilient nature (stretch and recoil), which is important in areas like the lungs, aorta, and skin. They are composed of two proteins, **elastin** and **fibrillin**, and do not have a banding pattern. These fibers are primarily produced by the fibroblasts but can also be produced by smooth muscle cells and chondrocytes.

RETICULAR FIBERS are small-diameter fibers that can only be adequately visualized with silver stains; they are called **argyrophilic fibers** because they appear black after exposure to silver salts. They are produced by modified fibroblasts (**reticular cells**) and are composed of type III collagen. These small, dark-staining fibers form a supportive, meshlike framework for organs that are composed mostly of cells (such as the liver, spleen, pancreas, lymphatic tissue, etc.).

Ground Substance of Connective Tissue

Ground substance is a clear, viscous substance with a high water content, but with very little morphologic structure. When stained with basic dyes (periodic acid-Schiff [PAS]), it appears amorphous, and with H&E, it appears as a clear space. Its major component is **glycosaminoglycans (GAGs)**, which are long, unbranched chains of **polysaccharides** with repeating disaccharide units. Most GAGs are covalently bonded to a large central protein to form larger molecules called **proteoglycans**. Both GAGs and proteoglycans have negative charges and attract water. This semifluid gel allows the diffusion of water-soluble molecules but inhibits movement of large macromolecules and bacteria. This water-attracting ability of ground substance gives us our extracellular body fluids.

Types of Connective Tissues

CONNECTIVE TISSUE PROPER

Dense connective tissue can be divided into **dense irregular connective tissue** and **dense regular connective tissue**. *Dense irregular connective tissue* consists of few connective tissue cells and many connective tissue fibers, the majority being type I collagen fibers, interlaced with a few elastic and reticular fibers. These fibers are arranged in bundles without a definite orientation. The dermis of the skin and capsules of many organs are typical examples of dense irregular connective tissue. *Dense regular connective tissue* also consists of fewer cells and more fibers, with a predominance of type I collagen fibers like the dense irregular connective tissue. Here, the fibers are arranged into a definite linear pattern. Fibroblasts are arranged linearly in the same orientation. Tendons and ligaments are the most common examples of dense regular connective tissue.

Loose connective tissue, also called **areolar connective tissue,** is characterized by abundant ground substance, with numerous connective tissue cells and fewer fibers (more cells and fewer fibers) compared to dense connective tissue. It is richly vascularized, flexible, and not highly resistant to stress. It provides protection, suspension, and support for the tissue. The lamina propria of the digestive tract and the mesentery are good examples of loose connective tissue. This tissue also forms conduits through which blood vessels and nerves course.

SPECIALIZED CONNECTIVE TISSUES

Adipose tissue is a special form of connective tissue, consisting predominantly of **adipocytes** that are the primary site for fat storage and are specialized for heat production. It has a rich neurovascular supply. **Adipose tissue** can be divided into **white adipose tissue** and **brown adipose tissue.** *White adipose tissue* is composed of unilocular adipose cells. The typical appearance of cells in white adipose tissue is lipid stored in the form of a single, large droplet in the cytoplasm of the cell. The flattened nucleus of each adipocyte is displaced to the periphery of the cell. White adipose tissue is found throughout the adult human body. *Brown adipose tissue*, in contrast, is composed of **multilocular adipose cells**. The lipid is stored in multiple droplets in the cytoplasm. Cells have a central nucleus and a relatively large amount of cytoplasm. Brown adipose tissue is more abundant in hibernating animals and is also found in the human embryo, in infants, and in the perirenal region in adults.

Reticular tissue is a specialized loose connective tissue that contains a network of branched reticular fibers, **reticulocytes** (specialized fibroblasts), macrophages, and parenchymal cells, such as pancreatic cells and hepatocytes. Reticular fibers are very fine and much smaller than collagen type 1 and elastic fibers. This tissue provides the architectural framework for parenchymal organs, such as lymphoid nodes, spleen, liver, bone marrow, and endocrine glands.

Elastic tissue is composed of bundles of thick elastic fibers with a sparse network of collagen fibers and fibroblasts filling the interstitial space. In certain locations, such as in elastic arteries, elastic material and collagen fibers can be produced by smooth muscle cells. This tissue provides flexible support for other tissues and can recoil after stretching, which helps to dampen the extremes of pressure associated with some organs, such as elastic arteries. Elastic tissue is usually found in the vertebral ligaments, lungs, large arteries, and the dermis of the skin.

EMBRYONIC CONNECTIVE TISSUE is a type of loose tissue formed in early embryonic development. **Mesenchymal connective tissue** and **mucous connective tissue** also fall under this category.

Mesenchymal connective tissue is found in the embryo and fetus and contains considerable ground substance. It contains scattered reticular fibers and star-shaped mesenchymal cells that have pale-staining cytoplasm with small processes. Mesenchymal connective tissue can differentiate into different types of connective tissues.

Mucous connective tissue exhibits a jellylike matrix with some collagen fibers and stellate-shaped fibroblasts. Mucous tissue is the main constituent of the umbilical cord and is called **Wharton jelly.** This type of tissue does not differentiate beyond this stage. It is mainly found in developing structures, such as the umbilical cord, subdermal connective tissue of the fetus, and dental pulp of the developing teeth. It is also found in the nucleus pulposus of the intervertebral disk in adult tissue.

SUPPORTING CONNECTIVE TISSUE is related to cartilage and bone. Cartilage is composed of chondrocytes and extracellular matrix; bone contains osteoblasts, osteocytes, and osteoclasts and bone matrix. These will be discussed in Chapter 5, "Cartilage and Bone."

HEMATOPOIETIC TISSUE (BLOOD AND BONE MARROW) is a specialized connective tissue in which cells are suspended in the intercellular fluid, and it will be discussed in Chapter 8, "Blood and Hemopoiesis."

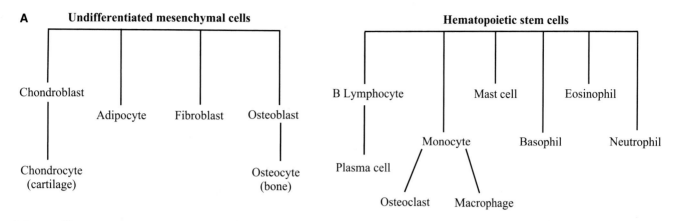

A Undifferentiated mesenchymal cells   Hematopoietic stem cells

Chondroblast   B Lymphocyte   Mast cell   Eosinophil

Adipocyte   Fibroblast   Osteoblast   Monocyte   Basophil   Neutrophil

Chondrocyte   Osteocyte   Plasma cell
(cartilage)   (bone)   Osteoclast   Macrophage

Figure 4-1A. Origin of connective tissue cells.

The *left panel* shows cells arising from **undifferentiated mesenchymal cells**. These cells are formed in, and remain within, the connective tissue and are also called **fixed cells**. The *panel on the right* shows cells arising from **hematopoietic stem cells**. These cells differentiate in the bone marrow and then must migrate by way of circulation to connective tissue where they perform their various functions. They are also called **wandering cells**.

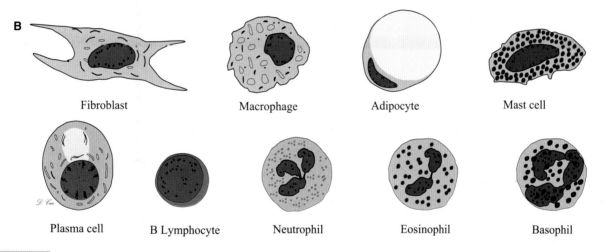

B

Fibroblast   Macrophage   Adipocyte   Mast cell

Plasma cell   B Lymphocyte   Neutrophil   Eosinophil   Basophil

Figure 4-1B. Representation of the main types of connective tissue cells in connective tissue proper.

The nuclei of these connective tissue cells are indicated in *purple*. *Note*: **Mast cells, eosinophils, basophils,** and **neutrophils** all contain granules in their cytoplasm. The *light yellow circle* in the **adipocyte** (fat cell) represents its lipid droplet. These cells are not drawn to scale; the adipocyte is much larger than the others.

SYNOPSIS 4-1 Functions of the Cells in Connective Tissue Proper

- *Fibroblasts* are responsible for synthesis of various fibers and extracellular matrix components, such as collagen, elastic, and reticular fibers.
- *Macrophages* contain many lysosomes and are involved in the removal of cell debris and the ingestion of foreign substances; they also aid in antigen presentation to the immune system.
- *Adipocytes* function to store neutral fats for energy or production of heat and are involved in hormone secretion.
- *Mast cells* contain many granules, indirectly participate in allergic reactions, and act against microbial invasion.
- *Plasma cells* are derived from B lymphocytes and are responsible for the production of antibodies in the immune response.
- *Lymphocytes* participate in the immune response and protect against foreign invasion (see Chapter 10, "Lymphoid System").
- *Neutrophils* are the first line of defense against bacterial invasion.
- *Eosinophils* have antiparasitic activity and moderate allergic reactions.
- *Basophils* have a (primary) function like mast cells; they mediate hypersensitivity reactions (see Chapter 8, "Blood and Hemopoiesis").

Connective Tissue Cells

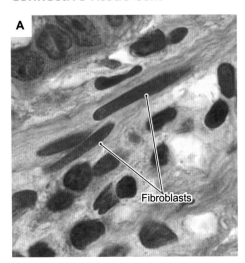

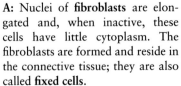

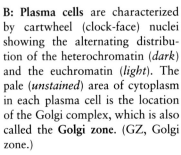

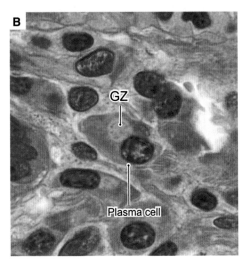

A: Nuclei of **fibroblasts** are elongated and, when inactive, these cells have little cytoplasm. The fibroblasts are formed and reside in the connective tissue; they are also called **fixed cells**.

B: **Plasma cells** are characterized by cartwheel (clock-face) nuclei showing the alternating distribution of the heterochromatin (*dark*) and the euchromatin (*light*). The pale (*unstained*) area of cytoplasm in each plasma cell is the location of the Golgi complex, which is also called the **Golgi zone**. (GZ, Golgi zone.)

C: A **mast cell** has a single, oval-shaped nucleus and granules in its cytoplasm. In paraffin H&E–stained sections, these granules are typically unstained, but they appear red in sections of plastic-embedded tissues stained with a faux H&E set of dyes.

D: An **eosinophil** has a segmented nucleus (two lobes, usually) and numerous eosinophilic (*red*) granules filling the cytoplasm. Eosinophils, mast, and plasma cells are **wandering cells**.

E: Black particles fill the cytoplasm of these active **macrophages**; the nuclei are obscured by the phagocytosed materials.

F: Each **adipocyte** contains a large droplet of lipid, appearing white (*clear*) here because the fat was removed during tissue preparation. The nucleus of each cell is pushed against the periphery of the cell.

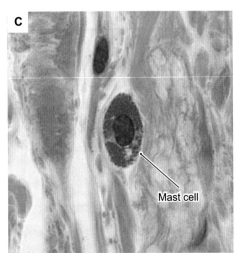

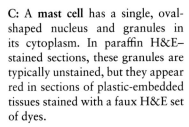

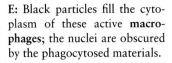

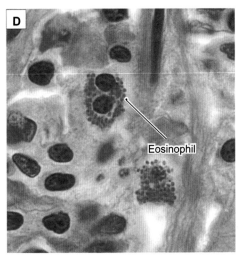

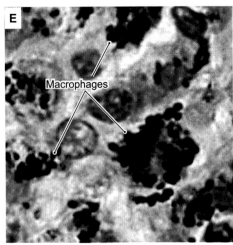

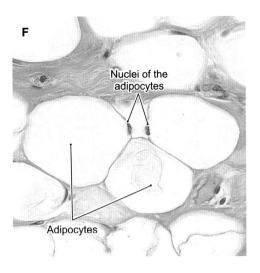

Figure 4-2A–D.   Cells in the connective tissue of the small intestine. Modified H&E, ×1,429

Figure 4-2E.   Macrophages in lung tissue. H&E, ×2,025

Figure 4-2F.   Adipocytes in connective tissue of the mammary gland. H&E, ×373

A

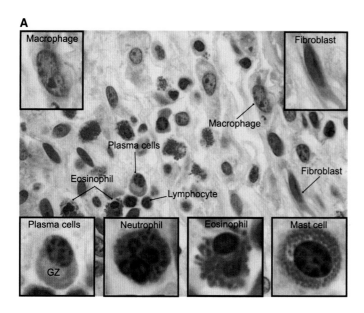

Figure 4-3A. Connective tissue cells in lamina propria. Modified H&E, ×680; inset approximately ×1,200 (GZ, Golgi zone.)

An example of cells in loose connective tissue is shown. **Fibroblasts** are the predominant cells in connective tissue, where they produce procollagen and other components of the extracellular matrix. **Plasma cells** arise from activated B lymphocytes and are responsible for producing antibodies. **Mast cells** have small, ovoid nuclei and contain numerous cytoplasmic granules. When stained with toluidine blue, these granules are metachromatically stained and appear purple. Mast cells are involved in allergic reactions. **Eosinophils** arise from hematopoietic stem cells and are generally characterized by bilobed nuclei and numerous eosinophilic cytoplasmic granules; they are attracted to sites of inflammation by leukocyte chemotactic factors where they may defend against a parasitic infection or moderate an allergic reaction. **Neutrophils** are phagocytes of bacteria; each cell has a multilobed nucleus and some granules in its cytoplasm. For more details on leukocytes, see Chapter 8, "Blood and Hemopoiesis."

B

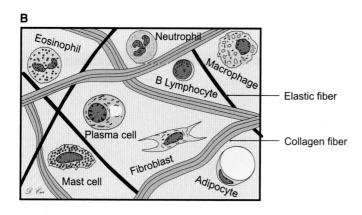

Figure 4-3B. Representation of the cells found in loose connective tissue. (These cells are not drawn to scale.)

(1) **Fibroblasts** are spindle-shaped cells with ovoid or elliptical nuclei and irregular cytoplasmic extensions. (2) **Macrophages** have irregular nuclei. The cytoplasm contains many lysosomes; cell size may vary depending on the level of phagocytic activity. (3) **Adipocytes** contain large lipid droplets, and their nuclei are pushed to the periphery. They are usually present in aggregate. (4) **Mast cells** have centrally located ovoid nuclei and numerous granules in their cytoplasm. (5) **Plasma cells** have eccentric nuclei with peripheral distribution of heterochromatin (clock face) within the nuclei; a clear Golgi area is present within the cytoplasm. (6) **Eosinophils** have bilobed nuclei and coarse cytoplasmic granules. (7) **Neutrophils** and **lymphocytes** are also found in connective tissue, and their numbers may increase in cases of inflammation.

CLINICAL CORRELATION

C

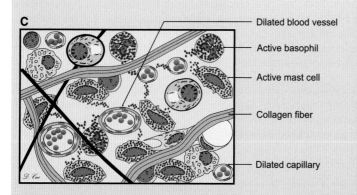

Figure 4-3C. Anaphylaxis.

Anaphylaxis is an allergic reaction that may range from mild to severe and is characterized by increased numbers of **basophils** and **mast cells, dilated capillaries,** and exudates in the loose connective tissue. Symptoms include **urticaria (hives), pruritus (itching),** flushing, shortness of breath, and shock. Anaphylaxis results from the activation and release of **histamine** and **inflammatory mediators** from **mast cells** and **basophils.** Some drugs can cause IgE-mediated anaphylaxis and non–IgE-mediated anaphylactoid reactions. Previous exposure to a suspect antigen is required for the formation of **IgE,** but anaphylactoid reactions can occur even upon first contact in rare cases. Some antibiotics, such as penicillin, can cause severe allergic reactions. Immediate administration of epinephrine, antihistamine, and corticosteroids is the first option of emergency treatment, along with endotracheal intubation to prevent the throat from swelling shut, if necessary.

MAST CELLS

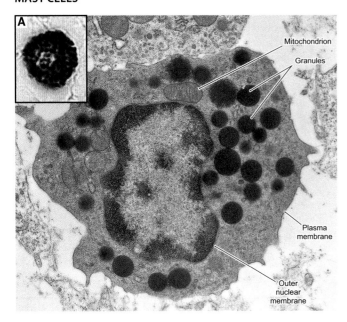

Figure 4-4A. Mast cells. EM, ×42,000; inset toluidine blue ×3,324

The contents of the **granules** that fill the cytoplasm of a **mast cell** are electron dense. **Mitochondria** are the only other prominent constituent of the cytoplasm. These granules are not the only source of signaling molecules released by activated mast cells. The **plasma membrane** and **outer nuclear membrane** are labeled here to highlight their roles in the generation of **eicosanoids**, such as **prostaglandins** and **leukotrienes**. These potent mediators of inflammation are not stored but are synthesized from fatty acids of membranes when the mast cell is stimulated.

The *inset* shows a mast cell in paraffin section stained with toluidine blue. The purple color of the mast cell granules is an example of metachromatic stains.

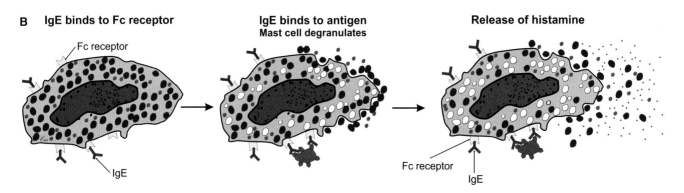

Figure 4-4B. Representation of a mast cell in an allergic reaction (anaphylaxis).

Mast cells derive from bone marrow and migrate into connective tissue where they function as mediators of inflammatory reactions to injury and microbial invasion. The cytoplasm of mast cells contains many granules, which contain **heparin** and **histamine** and other substances. In most cases, when the body encounters a foreign material (**antigen**), the result is clonal selection and expansion of those **lymphocytes** that happen to synthesize an **antibody** that recognizes the antigen. Some of the stimulated lymphocytes will differentiate into **plasma cells** that secrete large amounts of soluble antibody, which enter circulation. Those antibodies that are of the **IgE** class bind to **Fc receptors** on **mast cells** and **basophils**. The **IgE-Fc receptor complexes** can act as triggers that activate the mast cell or basophil if the antigen is encountered again. Binding of the antigen leads to cross-linking of the Fc receptors, which initiates a series of reactions culminating in discharge (**exocytosis**) of the contents of the granules of the mast cell or basophil. The histamine and heparin that are released from the granules contribute to inflammation at the allergic reaction site.

Histamine stimulates many types of cells to produce a variety of responses, depending on where the **allergic reaction** takes place. Effects on blood vessels include dilation due to relaxation of smooth muscle cells (redness and heat) and fluid leakage from venules (**edema**) due to loosening of cell-to-cell junctions between endothelial cells. Histamine can stimulate some smooth muscle cells to contract, as occurs with **asthma** in the respiratory tract, and it can cause excessive secretion in glands. Extremely strong **mast cell–mediated allergic reactions** (also called **allergic** or **type 1 hypersensitivity reactions**) result in **anaphylactic shock**, which can happen very quickly and often requires emergency attention. It can sometimes be fatal.

TABLE 4-1 Connective Tissue Cell Histologic Activities and Clinical Correlations

Type of Cells	Cell Origin	Histologic Activities	Clinical Correlations
Fibroblasts	Mesenchymal cells	Synthesize extracellular matrix (fibers and ground substance)	Wound healing, hypertrophic scarring and keloid formation, healing by fibrosis
Adipocytes	Mesenchymal cells	Synthesize and store fat, synthesize the hormone leptin	Obesity, increased activity in acromegaly, gigantism
Macrophages	Monocytes	Phagocytose particles, present antigens to lymphocytes, release growth factors and cytokines	Phagocytosis of foreign bodies, Langhans giant cells, granuloma formation, mononuclear phagocytic system (MPS)/macrophage system
Mast cells	Hematopoietic stem cells	Contribute to inflammatory responses and allergic reactions and release heparin, histamines, and various chemotactic mediators	Allergic reaction, immediate hypersensitivity reaction, anaphylaxis
Plasma cells	B lymphocytes	Produce antibodies (antigen specific: IgG, IgA, IgM, IgE, and IgD)	Chronic inflammation, multiple myeloma, asthma, autoimmune diseases
Lymphocytes	Hematopoietic stem cells	**B cells:** form plasma cells and produce antibodies (humoral immune response); **T cells:** attack infected cells (cytotoxic T cells, cellular immune response); secrete cytokines that regulate other lymphocytes (regulatory T cells)	Chronic inflammation, human immunodeficiency virus (HIV) infection, lymphoma
Neutrophils	Hematopoietic stem cells	Phagocytosis, defense against bacterial and fungal infections	Bacterial infection, acute suppurative inflammation, neutropenia, agranulocytosis
Eosinophils	Hematopoietic stem cells	Defend against parasitic worms, limit inflammation in various tissues affected by allergic reactions, fight viral infections, and release enzymes, growth factors, and cytokines	Allergic reaction, parasitic infection
Basophils	Hematopoietic stem cells	Contribute to inflammation and allergic reactions	Allergic reaction, immediate hypersensitivity reaction, anaphylaxis

Extracellular Matrix

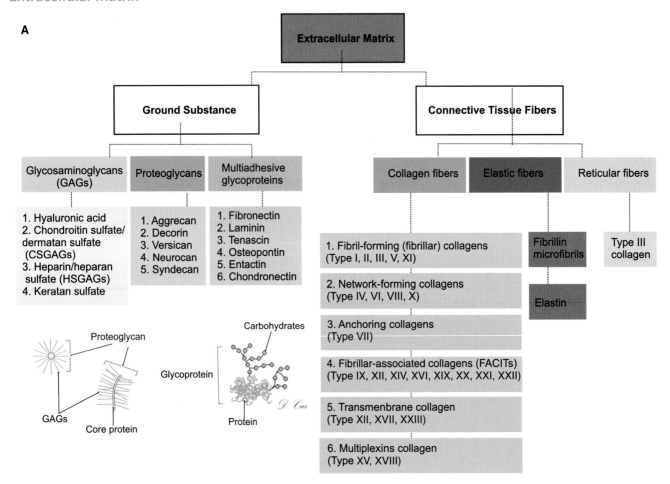

Figure 4-5A. Overview of extracellular matrix.

The extracellular matrix is produced by fibroblasts, and it is composed of **ground substance** and **connective tissue fibers**. It provides mechanical and structural support to the tissue. It also allows for cell movements and transfer of nutrients and waste materials between the tissue and blood circulation. The **ground substance** is composed of **glycosaminoglycans (GAGs)**, **proteoglycans**, and **glycoproteins (multiadhesive glycoproteins)**. **GAGs** can be classified into four groups: (1) hyaluronic acid, (2) chondroitin sulfate/dermatan sulfate (CSGAGs), (3) heparin/heparan sulfate (HSGAGs), and (4) keratan sulfate. **Proteoglycans** are composed of **GAGs** and **central core proteins**. Several of the most common **proteoglycans** associated with the extracellular matrix include (1) aggrecan, (2) decorin, (3) versican, (4) neurocan, and (5) syndecan. **Multiadhesive glycoproteins** include (1) fibronectin, (2) laminin, (3) tenascin, (4) osteopontin, (5) entactin, and (6) chondronectin. **Connective tissue fibers** include **collagen, elastic**, and **reticular fibers**. The collagen fibers can be divided into six main classes and more than twenty types of collagens. (1) **Fibril-forming (fibrillar) collagens** are major components of collagen fibrils. Type I, II, III, V, and XI collagens belong to this category. (2) **Network-forming collagens** form a network in external laminae and basal laminae. Type IV, VI, VIII, and X are examples of these collagens. (3) **Anchoring collagen** links the basal lamina to the connective tissue; this is type VII collagen. (4) **Fibrillar-associated collagens with interrupted triple helices (FACITs)** contain triple helices interspersed with nonhelical domains. This group of collagens is involved in controlling the diameter of collagen fibrils, and they are laterally associated with type I and type II fibrils. They provide stability and maintain the integrity of the extracellular matrix. The collagen types IX, XII, XIV, XVI, XIX, XX, XXI, and XXII belong to this group. (5) **Transmembrane collagens** are associated with basal laminae and hemidesmosomes, as adhesion molecules. Examples include type XIII, XVII, and XXIII collagens. (6) **Multiplexing collagens** form structural links to cells with connective tissue. Type XV and XVIII are examples.

GROUND SUBSTANCE

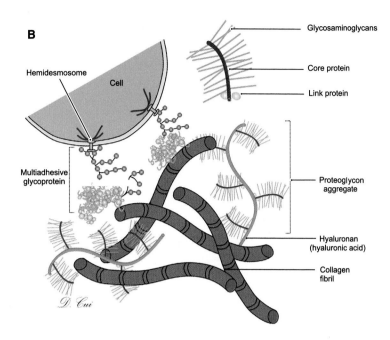

Figure 4-5B. Overview of ground substance.

The ground substance of connective tissue is a clear, gel-like substance with a high water content, but with very little morphological structure. Its main components include **glycosaminoglycans (GAGs)**, **proteoglycans**, and **multiadhesive glycoproteins**. **GAGs** are also known as **mucopolysaccharides**, which are long, unbranched chains of polysaccharides with repeating double sugar (disaccharide) units. **Proteoglycans** are long protein chains with GAGs centrally attached to the core proteins in a bottle-brush-like arrangement. There are small and large **proteoglycans**. **Small proteoglycans** are usually present in equine tendons—examples of which include **decorin, biglycan**, and **fibromodulin**. **Large proteoglycans**, such as **aggrecan** (cartilage), **versican** (blood vessels and skin), **perlecan** (basement membrane), **neurocan** (extracellular matrix), and **brevican** (central nervous system), are present in various locations. The most common **proteoglycans** associated with connective tissue extracellular matrix include **decorin, aggrecan, versican, neurocan**, and **syndecan**. Both **GAGs** and **proteoglycans** are semifluid gel, and they have negative charges that attract water and allow diffusion of water-soluble molecules. **Multiadhesive glycoproteins** are simple proteins with attached carbohydrates. These **multiadhesive glycoproteins** provide adhesion between the cell and the **extracellular matrix**, and they are important for cell migration. (The illustration is not drawn to scale.)

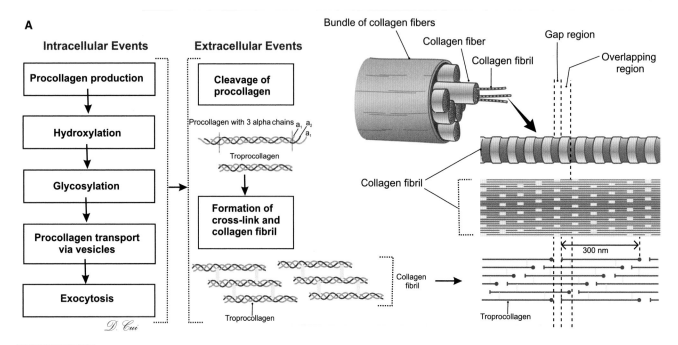

A

Figure 4-6A. Organization of collagen fibers.

Collagen fibers, which are bundles of collagen fibrils, are the most common and abundant fibers in connective tissue. Connective tissue is primarily composed of type 1 collagen. There are more than 20 different types of collagen found in the body. The most basic subunit of all collagen molecules is the α (alpha) **chain**, which is an **amino acid chain**. Amino acid sequences of alpha chains vary among the different collagen types. Each collagen molecule consists of three alpha chains that are coiled into a right-handed triple helix to form a **tropocollagen** molecule. There are series of intracellular events happening during the assembly of tropocollagen. (1) **Procollagen production: Alpha chains** are synthesized in **rough endoplasmic reticulum (RER)**, directed by mRNAs. They include C- and N-terminal propeptides, which will be removed in post-translational processing. Before post-translational processing, the molecule is referred to as **procollagen** (or preprocollagen). (2) **Hydroxylation** of **proline** and **lysine** residues occurs within the RER. **Hydroxyproline** serves as a stabilizer, and **hydroxylysine** provides the interchain cross-link for the triple helix of three alpha chains. This process requires **vitamin C**. Therefore, bleeding gums and joint effusion result when a deficiency of vitamin C exists during this step of collagen synthesis. (3) **Glycosylation**: Addition of the carbohydrates (glycosyl and galactosyl) to hydroxylysine occurs, thus allowing molecules to stick together to form a triple-helix structure of the **procollagen** molecules produced in the RER. (4) **Procollagen transport via vesicles**: The Golgi apparatus transfers and packages procollagen into secretory vesicles that move toward to the cell membrane. (5) **Exocytosis**: Procollagen molecules are transferred from the inside of the cell to the extracellular space via exocytosis. There are two events involved in extracellular collagen formation: (1) **cleavage of procollagen** in which the C- and N-terminal propeptides of alpha chains are removed by peptidases. This completes the transformation of procollagen into the final collagen molecule, which is called **tropocollagen**. (2) **Formation of cross-link and collagen fibril** in which cross-linkage between adjacent tropocollagen molecules occurs, binding them into **collagen fibrils**, stabilized and strengthened by oxidation of the hydroxylysine residues (by the enzyme lysine oxidase).

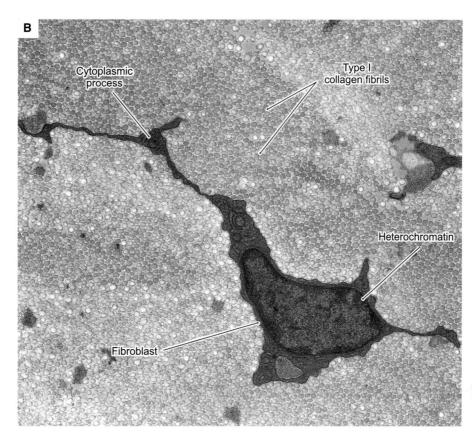

Figure 4-6B. Collagen fibrils and fibroblasts. EM, ×14,000

Sometimes, the term **fibrocyte** is used to designate an **inactive fibroblast** such as the cell seen in this electron micrograph. The quiescent state of the cell can be inferred from the scant cytoplasm and small nucleus in which **heterochromatin** is the predominant form of **chromatin**. The small circles that fill the extracellular space are **type I collagen fibrils**, which are uniformly cut in cross section in this specimen of dura mater, the tough outer layer of the meninges.

There are many types of collagen fibers in humans; types I, II, III, IV, V, and VII are some of the most common types. Collagen fibers are the principal fibers and are most abundant in the connective tissue. Collagen fibers are flexible and have a high tensile strength.

CONNECTIVE TISSUE FIBERS
Collagen fibers

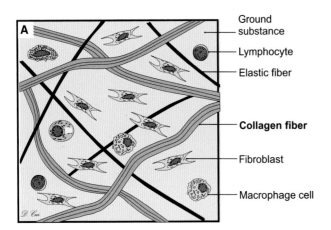

Ground substance
Lymphocyte
Elastic fiber

Collagen fiber

Fibroblast

Macrophage cell

Figure 4-7A. Representation of collagen fibers in loose connective tissue.

Collagen fibers are flexible but impart strength to the tissue. They are arranged loosely, without a definite orientation in loose connective tissue.

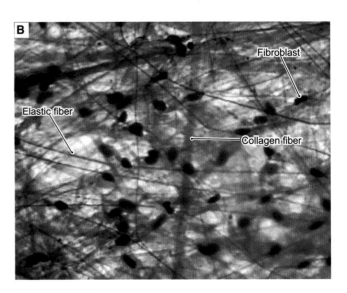

Fibroblast
Elastic fiber
Collagen fiber

Figure 4-7B. Collagen fibers, mesentery spread. Verhoeff stain, ×314

Loose connective tissue, also called **areolar connective tissue**, is shown in a mesentery spread. In this tissue preparation, both collagen fibers and elastic fibers are visible. The **elastic fibers** are thin strands stained deep blue, and **collagen fibers** are thick and stained purple. **Fibroblasts** are seen among the fibers.

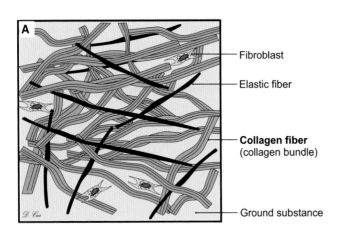

Fibroblast
Elastic fiber
Collagen fiber (collagen bundle)
Ground substance

Figure 4-8A. Representation of collagen fibers in dense connective tissue.

Interwoven bundles of **collagen fibers** interspersed with **elastic fibers** are illustrated here. These fibers are tightly packed together in dense connective tissue.

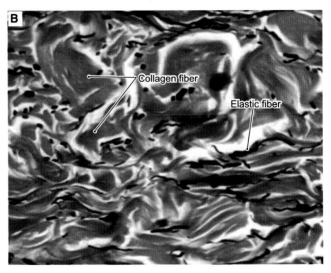

Collagen fiber
Elastic fiber

Figure 4-8B. Collagen fibers, skin. Elastic stain, ×279

An example of **collagen fibers** in the dense irregular connective tissue of the dermis of the skin is shown. Both collagen fibers (*pink*) and **elastic fibers** (*black*) are present. Collagen fibers predominate in dense irregular connective tissue. They are arranged in thick bundles tightly packed together in a nonuniform manner.

TABLE 4-2 Types of Collagen and Associated Collagen Families

Type of Collagen	Synthesizing Cells	Main Locations	Main Function	Examples of Collagen Disorders (Associated Collagen Gene Mutations)
Fibril-Forming Collagens				
I	Fibroblasts, osteoblasts, odontoblasts	Dermis of skin, ligaments, tendons, bone, dentin, interstitial connective tissue, tunics of the digestive tract, muscle fascia, organ capsules, etc.	Resist tension	Osteogenesis imperfecta (*COL1A1, COL1A2*); cardiac valvular type Ehlers-Danlos syndrome (*COL1A2*)
II	Chondroblasts, chondrocytes	Hyaline and elastic cartilage, intervertebral discs, vitreous humor of the eye, notochord	Resist pressure, (coassembled with type XI collagen)	Chondrodysplasias (*COL2A1*), including achondrogenesis, hypochondrogenesis, spondyloepiphyseal dysplasia, spondyloepimetaphyseal dysplasia, Stickler syndrome, Kniest dysplasia; early-onset osteoarthritis
III	Fibroblasts, reticular cells, hepatocytes, smooth muscle cells	Dermis of skin, blood vessel walls, reticular fibers in organs (spleen, lymph node, liver, etc.)	Form structural framework in expansible organs	Vascular deficiency, aortic and arterial aneurysms; vascular type Ehlers-Danlos syndrome (*COL3A1*)
V	Mesenchymal cells, fibroblasts, osteoblasts, cementoblasts	Placenta, dermis, most interstitial tissue, liver, lungs, bone matrix, and cementum	Control the initiation of collagen fibril assembly, associate with type I and III collagen	Skin thickening associated with abnormal collagen deposition in dermis; classical type Ehlers-Danlos syndrome (*COL5A1, COL5A2*)
XI	Fibroblasts, chondrocytes	Tissues containing type II collagen: cartilage, articular cartilage, trachea (interior of type II collagen fibril)	Provide structural support and strength, regulate fibrillogenesis, and maintain space and diameter of type II collagen	Stickler syndrome (*COL11A1, COL11A2*); Marshall syndrome (*COL11A1*); otospondylomega-epiphyseal dysplasia (*COL11A2*)
Network-Forming Collagens				
IV	Endothelial cells, epithelial cells, lens epithelial cells	Basement membrane of epithelium, lens capsule (eye), glomerulus (kidney)	Provide support and filtration, form backbone for basement membrane	Alport syndrome nephropathy (*COL4A3, COL4A4, COL4A5*)
VI	Fibroblasts, chondrocytes, myocytes, cardiomyocytes	Muscles, dermis, cartilage, blood vessel walls (also known as beaded filament collagen)	Form structural link between cells and connective tissue, attach extracellular matrix to chondrocytes, may contribute to fibrogenesis and tissue repair	Ullrich congenital muscular dystrophy (*COL6A1, COL6A2, COL6A3*); Bethlem myopathy (*COL6A1, COL6A2, COL6A3*)
VIII	Endothelial cells	Endothelium, Descemet membrane of cornea	Play roles in structural support and signaling properties during angiogenesis	Fuchs endothelial corneal dystrophy (*COL8A2*)
X	Chondrocytes	Hypertrophic cartilage in epiphyseal plate	Play roles in cartilage calcification during endochondral ossification (long bone growth)	Schmid-type metaphyseal chondrodysplasia (*COL10A1*)

(Continued)

TABLE 4-2 (Continued)

Type of Collagen	Synthesizing Cells	Main Locations	Main Function	Examples of Collagen Disorders (Associated Collagen Gene Mutations)
Anchoring Collagen				
VII	Fibroblasts, keratinocytes	Basement membrane, anchoring fibrils	Anchor epidermal basal lamina to underlying connective tissue, bind type I and III collagen to help stability of extracellular matrix	Dystrophic forms of epidermolysis bullosa (COL7A1, COL17A1); autoimmune diseases systemic lupus erythematosus, systemic sclerosis, Sjögren syndrome
Fibrillar Associated Collagens with Interrupted Triple Helices (FACITs)				
IX	Chondrocytes	Cartilage matrix, vitreous body of the eye	Stabilize matrix and regulate diameter of collagen fibrils, assist in forming a network for cartilage matrix	Osteoarthritis; multiple epiphyseal dysplasia (COL9A1, COL9A2, COL9A3, or other cartilage extracellular matrix gene mutations)
XII	Fibroblasts, chondrocytes	Tissues containing type I collagen: tendons, perichondrium, ligaments, fibrocartilage	Contribute to bone development, interact with type I collagen fibrils and matrix proteins (decorin, tenascin, etc.)	Myopathic Ehlers-Danlos syndrome (COL12A1)
XIV	Fibroblasts, keratinocytes, chondrocytes	Tissues with high mechanical stress: dermis, epidermis, tendons, articular cartilage, endomysium, cornea	Provide tissue with mechanical support, by associating with type I collagen, binding other collagens, and contributing to cell-to-cell adhesion	Palmoplantar keratoderma
XVI	Fibroblasts, chondrocytes, smooth muscle cells, keratinocytes	Papillary dermis of skin, cartilage, heart, intestine, arterial walls, kidney	Anchor microfibrils of epidermis to the basement membrane, stabilize extracellular matrix	Epidermolysis bullosa; scleroderma
XIX	Fibroblasts, rhabdomyosarcoma cells	Colon, kidney, brain, liver, prostate, skin (associated with epithelial, vascular, neural, and mesenchymal tissues)	Play roles as a cross-bridge and maintain the integrity of the extracellular matrix, associated with basement membrane	Antitumor and antiangiogenic activity
XX	Fibroblasts, keratinocytes, mesenchymal cells	Tendons, sternal cartilage, corneal epithelium, embryonic skin	Bind to collagen fibrils (cDNA sequence similarities to types XII and XIV, but smaller)	
XXI	Smooth muscle cells	Blood vessel walls, heart, gingiva, stomach, jejunum	Contribute to blood vessel assembly during vessel formation	
XXII	Fibroblasts,	Skeletal muscle-tendon junctions, cardiac muscle	Bind to integrins and contribute to stability of myotendinous junctions during muscle contraction	Potentially associated with intracranial aneurysms

TABLE 4-2 (Continued)

Type of Collagen	Synthesizing Cells	Main Locations	Main Function	Examples of Collagen Disorders (Associated Collagen Gene Mutations)
Transmembrane Collagens				
XIII	Fibroblasts, chondrocytes	Epidermis, dermal-epidermal junction, intestine, lungs, liver, cartilage, skeletal muscle-tendon junctions, intercalated discs of heart muscle, focal adhesions, and bone	Anchor cells to connective tissue by associating with integrins and actin cytoskeleton in focal contacts. Maintain tissue architecture in development and postnatal growth	Congenital myasthenic syndrome (*COL13A1*)
XVII	Keratinocytes	Epidermis of skin, associated with keratinocyte basal surfaces and hemidesmosomes	Anchor keratinocytes to the basement membrane, play a role in teeth formation	Bullous pemphigoid; junctional epidermolysis bullosa (*COL17A1*)
XXIII		Lungs, heart, cornea, retina, tendons	Maintain cell-to-cell contacts	May play role as a diagnostic tool for prostate and non–small-cell lung cancer patients
Multiplexin Collagens				
XV	Fibroblasts, muscle cells, endothelial cells	Basement membranes, especially of endothelium, skeletal and cardiac muscle, and the nervous system	Associate with microvessels in the cardiac and skeletal muscle tissues	Corneal defects. In animal research: myopathy of heart and skeletal muscle; defects in microvasculature
XVIII	Endothelial cells, epithelial cells, hepatocytes	Vascular and epithelial basement membranes, liver	Associate with basement membrane, inhibit angiogenesis, inhibit tumor growth	Angiogenesis; Knobloch syndrome (*COL18A1*)

Elastic fibers

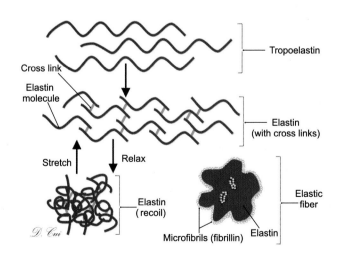

Figure 4-9. Overview of elastic fibers.

Elastic fibers are one of the major connective tissue fibers. They are produced by fibroblasts, smooth muscle cells, and chondrocytes, depending on their locations. Elastic fibers have many branches and connect to one another. They have a very resilient nature and a good capability of stretch and recoil. Unlike collagen fibers, they do not have a banding pattern. Elastic fibers are mainly composed of two proteins: **elastin** and **fibrillin**. **Elastin** forms a central core (elastic core), which occupies about 90% of elastic fiber. The fibrillin components of an elastic fiber include fibrillin-1, fibrillin-2, fibrillin-3, fibrillin-4, and fibrillin-5. **Fibrillin-1** is a glycoprotein, which forms **microfibrils** surrounding the elastic core (peripheral microfibrils) and helps organize elastin into a fiber. **Marfan syndrome** is associated with a fibrillin-1 (FBN1) gene mutation. Elastic molecules consist of hydrophilic and hydrophobic domains that contribute to the stretch and recoil that give them their characteristic elasticity. **Tropoelastin** (without cross-links) is initially secreted by elastin-producing cells, such as fibroblasts. Then it becomes cross-linked via the **lysyl oxidase** process to form elastin.

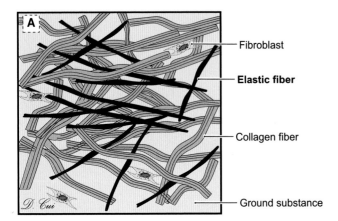

Figure 4-10A. Representation of the elastic fibers in dense connective tissue.

Elastic fibers are thinner than collagen fibers and are interspersed among **collagen fibers**. They are composed of **elastin** and **microfibrillar proteins** and are specialized for stretch and resilience.

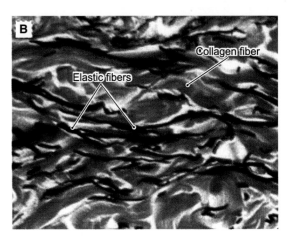

Figure 4-10B. Elastic fibers, skin. Elastic stain, ×408

An example of **elastic fibers** in dense connective tissue of the dermis of the skin is shown. The elastic fibers stain dark with the special stain used in this section. **Collagen fibers** appear as thick, pink bundles.

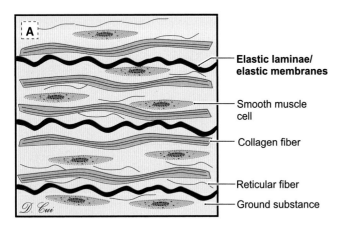

Figure 4-11A. Representation of elastic laminae in a large artery.

Shown is an example of another form of elastic fibers in a large artery, called **elastic laminae (elastic membranes)**. Elastic laminae, as well as **reticular** and **collagen fibers**, are produced by **smooth muscle cells** in the walls of the artery. The collagen fibers, reticular fibers, and **ground substance** lie between the elastic laminae. Smooth muscle cells are interspersed between the fiber layers.

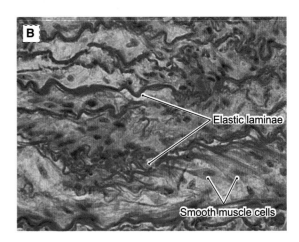

Figure 4-11B. Elastic laminae, elastic artery. H&E, ×426

An example of **elastic laminae** in an elastic artery is shown. The elastic material is arranged in parallel wavy sheets (**lamellar form**) instead of fibers. The **elastin** is eosinophilic and appears red with H&E stain. **Smooth muscle cells** are interspersed between the elastic laminae. Elastic laminae in the large arteries can stretch, allowing these vessels to distend and recoil during the cardiac cycle.

Reticular fibers

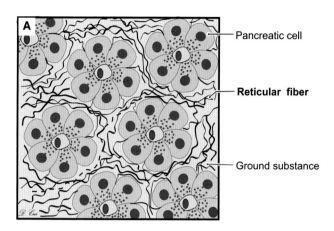

Figure 4-12A. Representation of reticular fibers in the pancreas.

Reticular fibers are composed of **type III collagen**, have small diameters, and do not form large bundles. They form a delicate, architectural framework in the pancreas, liver, and lymph nodes and can be found in many tissues.

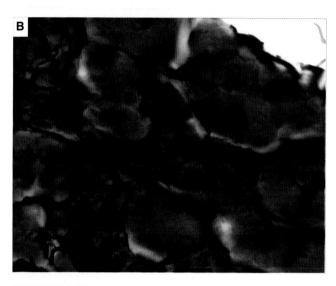

Figure 4-12B. Reticular fibers, pancreas. Silver stain, ×762

An example of **reticular fibers** in the exocrine pancreas is shown. The thin, reticular fibers surrounding pancreatic acinar cells form a netlike supporting framework. In most locations, reticular fibers are produced by reticular cells (fibroblasts); in some places, reticular fibers can be secreted by smooth muscle cells (blood vessels) or by Schwann cells (peripheral nerve tissue).

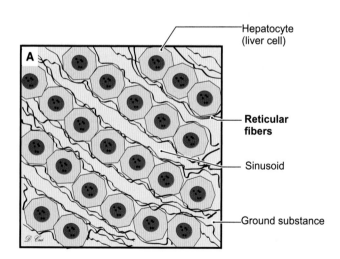

Figure 4-13A. Representation of reticular fibers in the liver.

These **reticular fibers** are arranged in cords (column pattern) to form a fine framework, which holds the **hepatocytes** in place.

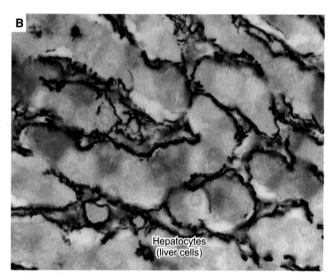

Figure 4-13B. Reticular fibers, liver. PAS/reticular stain, ×544

An example of the **reticular fibers** in the liver is shown. The reticular fibers appear black because of the silver stain. The structure of the **hepatocytes** is difficult to identify because their cytoplasm does not take up silver. The spaces between the reticular fibers are the lumens of **sinusoids** running between the plates of the hepatocytes.

Types of Connective Tissue: Connective Tissue Proper

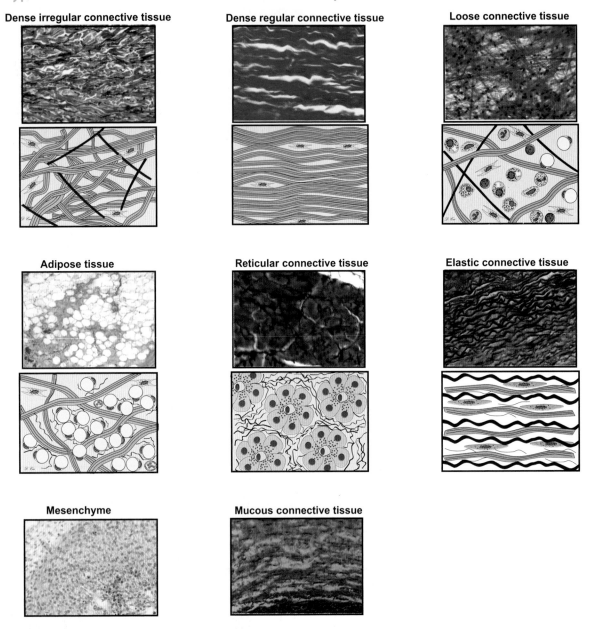

Figure 4-14.   Overview of connective tissue types.

TABLE 4-3   Classification of Connective Tissues

Types of Connective Tissues	Connective Tissue Proper			Specialized Connective Tissue			Embryonic Connective Tissue	
Subtype of connective tissue	Dense irregular	Dense regular	Loose	Adipose	Reticular	Elastic	Mesenchyme	Mucus
Character of the tissue	Fewer cells, more fibers; fibers are arranged without definite orientation	Fewer cells, more fibers; fibers are arranged in uniform orientation	More cells, fewer fibers; fibers are randomly distributed	Adipocytes predominant, supported by reticular fibers	Reticular fibers predominant	Elastic fibers predominant	Mesenchymal cells predominant; hyaluronic acid matrix	Spindle-shaped fibroblasts, jellylike matrix (Wharton jelly) high in heparan sulfate proteoglycan

DENSE IRREGULAR CONNECTIVE TISSUES

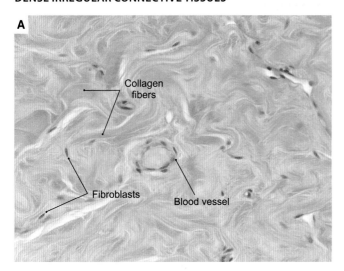

Figure 4-15A. Dense irregular connective tissue, mammary gland. H&E, ×272

Dense irregular connective tissue can be found in the **mammary gland** and also in other places such as capsules of organs. In this example, dense irregular connective tissue in the mammary gland is shown, distributed in between glandular tissues. **Collagen fibers** predominate, appear pink, and are arranged in wavy bundles without a consistent orientation. **Fibroblasts** are visible among these fibers. Occasionally, **blood vessels** and glands can be found in dense irregular connective tissue; however, dense irregular connective tissue is generally not a richly vascularized tissue.

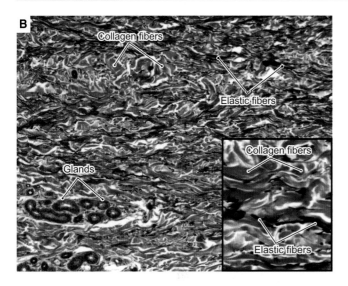

Figure 4-15B. Dense irregular connective tissue, dermis of the skin. Elastic stain, ×68; inset ×151

Collagen fibers are arranged in randomly oriented bundles and appear pink here; they are the principal fibers in **dense connective tissue**. Collagen fibers are flexible and have a high tensile strength. **Elastic fibers** are made visible with a special stain and are seen as thin, dark strands scattered among the collagen fibers. They are able to stretch and return to their original length. Dense irregular connective tissue is a cushion-like tissue, which provides great strength against **pressure-induced stresses** on structures or organs.

CLINICAL CORRELATION

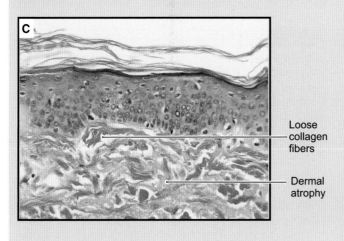

Figure 4-15C. Actinic Keratosis. H&E, ×205

Actinic keratosis, also called **solar elastosis**, is a degenerative skin condition, which mainly affects the **collagen** and **elastic fibers** of the sun-exposed areas of the body. Frequent exposure of the skin to sunlight or ultraviolet light causes and accelerates this degenerative process. Actinic keratosis is a premalignant lesion. Signs and symptoms include loose, wrinkled, dry, and sagging skin. Histologically, the amount of *collagen fibers* present in the affected skin is decreased, whereas the amount of *elastic fibers* increases, but they lose some of their elasticity and flexibility. A bluish discoloration of the papillary dermis is characteristic of ultraviolet damage to the connective tissue of the dermis. **Dermal atrophy** and **loose collagen fibers** are illustrated here. Avoiding unnecessary sun exposure is the most important prevention. Treatment includes liquid nitrogen cryotherapy, surgical curettage, and chemotherapy.

DENSE IRREGULAR CONNECTIVE TISSUES

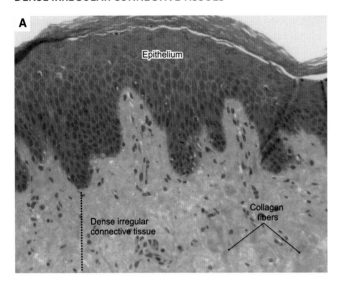

Figure 4-16A. Dense irregular connective tissue, thin skin. H&E, ×193

This is **dense irregular connective tissue** in the dermis of thin skin. The epidermis is composed of **epithelial tissue**; the dermis is composed of dense irregular connective tissue and lies beneath the epidermis. "Dense" refers to the high abundance of collagen fibers (but fewer cells) compared to loose connective tissue. "Irregular" indicates that the orientation of the fiber bundles is in many different directions (or randomly oriented bundles). This type of connective tissue contains mostly **collagen fibers** with a lesser number of other fibers such as elastic fibers. The skin has a thick layer of dense irregular connective tissue, with fibers arranged in various directions to resist stretching forces in any direction. Dense irregular connective tissue is prominent in the dermis of the skin, mammary glands, and capsules of many organs.

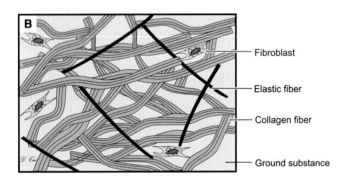

Figure 4-16B. Representation of dense irregular connective tissue.

The background represents **ground substance**. **Collagen fibers** are represented by randomly arranged, thick, pink bundles, and **elastic fibers** are indicated by thinner dark lines. A few **fibroblasts** are scattered sparsely among these fibers. Most collagen and elastic fibers are produced by fibroblasts. Maintaining the normal metabolism of collagen is very important to the body.

Malfunctioning collagen can cause a series of connective tissue diseases such as **Ehlers-Danlos syndrome**. Overproduction of collagen in the dermis of the skin can cause **hypertrophic scars** or **keloids**.

CLINICAL CORRELATION

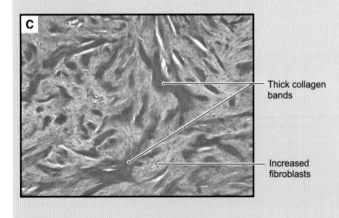

Figure 4-16C. Hypertrophic Scars and Keloids. H&E, ×53

Hypertrophic scars and **keloids** are disorders caused by accumulation of **excessive** amounts of **collagen** deposited in the skin by **hyperproliferation** of fibroblasts. They often occur after burns, radiation injury, or surgical procedures. *Hypertrophic scars* appear raised, are characterized by redness, and usually remain within the margins of the original wound. There is a tendency for spontaneous regression over time. If the scar tissue grows beyond the boundaries of the original wound and does not regress, it is called a *keloid*. A keloid is more severe and more difficult to treat than a hypertrophic scar. Treatments of hypertrophic scars and keloids include cryosurgery (freezing), laser surgery, and steroid injections. This photomicrograph is a keloid on the earlobe; the collagen fibers appear thicker and denser, forming **thick bands**. The number of **fibroblasts** is increased.

DENSE REGULAR CONNECTIVE TISSUES

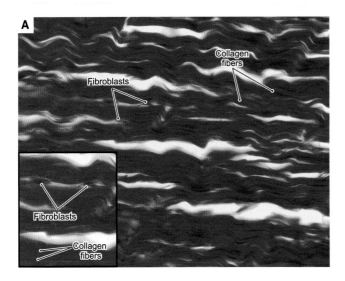

Figure 4-17A. Dense regular connective tissue, tendon. H&E, ×289; inset ×410

This type of tissue is composed of coarse collagen bundles that is densely packed and oriented into parallel cylinders. Long, thin **fibroblasts** are found among the fiber bundles and are oriented in the same direction as the fibers. The nuclei of the fibroblasts are visible, but the cytoplasm is not easily seen. The thick bundles of **collagen fibers** fill the intercellular spaces. **Dense regular connective tissue** provides resistance to traction forces in tendons and ligaments.

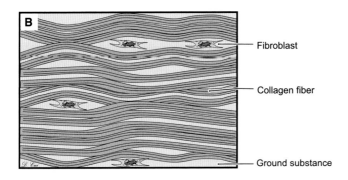

Figure 4-17B. Representation of dense regular connective tissue.

Collagen fibers are represented by uniformly arranged thick, pink bundles that are tightly packed in a parallel fashion. **Fibroblasts** are seen among these fibers. The white background represents the **ground substance**. This tissue architecture can be found in tendons, ligaments, and aponeuroses. The structure formed by this arrangement is particularly strong and resistant to stress such as the intense forces exerted on ligaments and tendons by athletes.

CLINICAL CORRELATION

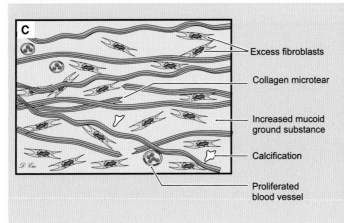

Figure 4-17C. Tendinosis.

Tendinosis is a **degenerative** disease that occurs within the substance of a tendon. This condition is usually associated with age, overexertion, or both. Histologic examination reveals abnormal fibrotic structure including **collagen disorganization, decreased fiber diameter,** and **increased mucoid ground substance.** Additional findings are **collagen microtears, focal hypercellularity, vascular proliferation,** and **focal necrosis** with **calcification.** Tearing of the tendon can occur in severe cases. Treatment includes pain relief, rest, physical therapy, nonsteroidal anti-inflammatory drugs, corticosteroids, and surgical repair, when necessary. The goal is to prevent further degeneration and to preserve function.

LOOSE CONNECTIVE TISSUES

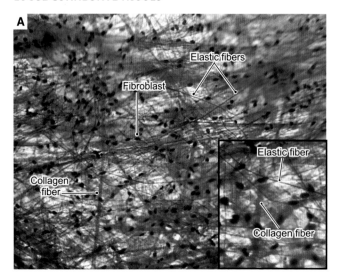

Figure 4-18A. Loose connective tissue, mesentery. Verhoeff stain, ×112; inset ×200

Loose connective tissue, also called **areolar connective tissue**, in a mesentery spread preparation is shown. In this tissue preparation, both **collagen fibers** and **elastic fibers** are visible. The elastic fibers stain deep blue as thin strands and collagen fibers appear as thick, purple bundles. **Fibroblasts** are seen among the fibers. This type of connective tissue has abundant ground substance, with many connective tissue cells and relatively few fibers. It is richly vascularized, flexible, and not highly resistant to stress.

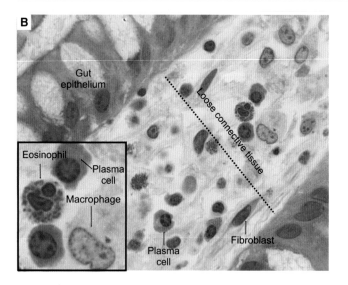

Figure 4-18B. Loose connective tissue, large intestine. H&E, ×680; inset ×1,506

The lamina propria of the digestive tract is an extreme example of **loose connective tissue**. This tissue lies immediately beneath the thin **epithelium of the gut**, which is one place where the body's defense mechanisms initially attack bacteria and pathogens. Therefore, **plasma cells**, mast cells, leukocytes, and **fibroblasts** are common in this area. Loose connective tissue is characterized by loosely arranged, woven connective fibers, abundant ground substance, and tissue fluid, which contains the rich array of connective tissue cells.

SYNOPSIS 4-2 Functions of Connective Tissue

Connective Tissue Proper
■ Dense irregular connective tissue: Provides strong fiber meshwork to resist stress from all directions (e.g., dermis of the skin) and provides protective covering of organs (e.g., capsule of the kidney).
■ Dense regular connective tissue: Provides resistance to traction forces in a single specific direction (e.g., tendons, ligaments).
■ Loose connective tissue: Provides suspension and support for tissues that are not subjected to strong forces and forms conduits in which vessels and nerves course. Cells in loose connective tissue have defense and immune functions (e.g., lamina propria of the digestive tract).

Specialized Connective Tissues
■ Adipose connective tissue: Provides both cushioning for organs and energy storage; some involved in hormone secretion such as leptin (e.g., hypodermis of the skin, mammary glands).
■ Reticular connective tissue: Provides supportive framework for hematopoietic and solid (parenchymal) organs (e.g., liver, pancreas).
■ Elastic connective tissue: Provides distensible support and accommodates pressure changes on the walls of the arteries closest to the heart (e.g., vertebral ligaments, large arteries).

Embryonic Connective Tissues
■ Mesenchymal connective tissue: Gives rise to all types of connective tissues (embryonic mesoderm).
■ Mucous connective tissue: Provides cushioning for the nucleus pulposus of the intervertebral disk and helps prevent kinking in the blood vessels of the umbilical cord.

LOOSE CONNECTIVE TISSUES

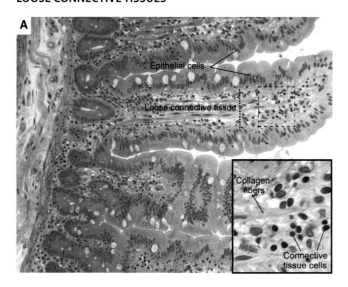

Figure 4-19A. Loose connective tissue, small intestine. H&E, ×136; inset ×384

This is an example of the **loose connective tissue** that lies just below the **epithelium** in the lamina propria of the small intestine. The **collagen fibers** are loosely arranged and inconspicuous. Many cells are tightly packed among the fiber bundles. In comparison, loose connective tissue has more cells and fewer fibers than dense connective tissue. This type of tissue is well vascularized, flexible, and not highly resistant to mechanical stress.

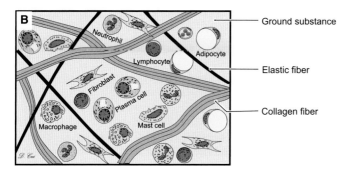

Figure 4-19B. Representation of loose connective tissue.

There are numerous **connective tissue cells** shown among fibers here. They include **fibroblasts, macrophages, adipocytes, mast cells, plasma cells,** and **leukocytes.** If there is a microorganism invasion or mechanical trauma, activation of mast cells and subsequent activation of endothelial cells and vasodilation are among the responses to the tissue injury. Vasodilation promotes delivery of more blood to the local tissue and leads to increased local temperature. Loosening of junctions between endothelial cells enables fluid and serum proteins to leak into the connective tissue. Expression of adhesive molecules (**selectins**) on endothelial cells increases the chance that leukocytes can migrate into the connective tissue from the blood stream. Mast cells and macrophages also increase in number to participate in the repair of tissue damage.

CLINICAL CORRELATION

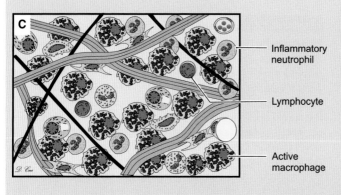

Figure 4-19C. Whipple Disease.

Whipple disease is a multisystemic disease caused by an infection of the bacillus *Tropheryma whipplei*. It primarily affects the small intestine. The clinical symptoms include **abdominal pain, flatulence, malabsorption,** and **diarrhea.** Symptoms are varied and depend upon the organ infected. The lamina propria (loose connective tissue) of the small intestine reveals an increased number of **macrophages.** These macrophages contain large numbers of bacteria within their phagosomes, which are clearly stained by the PAS stain (periodic acid combined with Schiff reagent). Treatment for Whipple disease is antibiotic administration, including intravenous penicillin and streptomycin by mouth.

ADIPOSE TISSUES

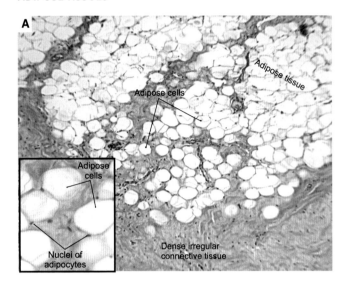

Figure 4-20A. Adipose tissue, mammary gland. H&E, ×68; inset ×178

Adipose tissue is a special form of connective tissue and has a rich neurovascular supply. **Adipocytes** appear white here, and this tissue is referred to as **white adipose tissue**. Each adipocyte contains a single, large lipid droplet in its cytoplasm, so the cells are called **unilocular adipose cells**. Most of the cytoplasm is occupied by the lipid droplet, and the nucleus is displaced to one side. Each adipocyte is surrounded by a basal lamina. This type of adipose tissue is found throughout the adult human body. There is another type of adipose tissue that is highly specialized, called **brown adipose tissue**. It is composed of **multilocular adipocytes**; each adipocyte contains multiple lipid droplets in its cytoplasm. This tissue is mainly found in hibernating mammals and newborn infants but can also be found scattered in some areas in adults, such as the esophagus, trachea, posterior neck, and interscapular areas as vestigial remnant tissue. Tumors sometimes arise from the remnant brown adipose tissue and are called **hibernomas**.

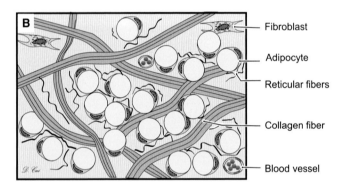

Figure 4-20B. Representation of adipose tissue.

Adipocytes (**fat cells**) are scattered within a loose collagenous supporting tissue in this unilocular adipose tissue. Each adipose cell contains a single large drop of lipid; it has a thin rim of cytoplasm around the lipid, and its flattened nucleus is located in the periphery of the cell. **Adipocytes** are the primary site for **storage of energy**, and lipid deposition and mobilization are regulated by **hormonal factors** (steroids, insulin, thyroid hormone, etc.). Adipocytes also play a role in the synthesis of some hormones such as **leptin**. During childhood, the adipocyte numbers may increase depending on nutrition and other factors, but in adulthood, adipocyte numbers normally remain constant.

CLINICAL CORRELATION

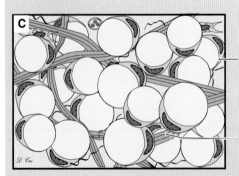

Figure 4-20C. Obesity.

Hypertrophic obesity is a disorder characterized by an increase in total body fat, particularly by expansion (**hypertrophy**) of preexisting fat cells. Obesity increases the risk for several conditions, including diabetes, hypertension, high cholesterol, stroke, and coronary artery disease. Obesity may also increase the risk for some types of cancer, and it is a risk factor for the development of osteoarthritis, pancreatitis, and sleep apnea. Obesity can result from a sedentary lifestyle and the chronic ingestion of excess calories; genetic predisposition may also play a role in the development of obesity. The possible treatments include exercise, diet, medications, and surgery. By contrast, **hyperplastic obesity** is excessive weight gain associated with childhood-onset obesity, characterized by the creation of new fat cells.

RETICULAR CONNECTIVE TISSUES

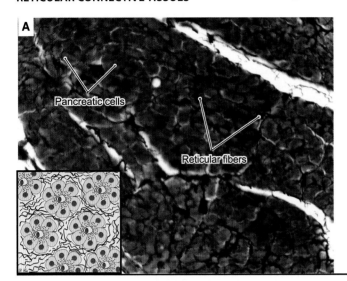

Figure 4-21A. Reticular connective tissue, pancreas. Silver stain, ×136

Reticular tissue is a specialized loose connective tissue that provides a delicate supporting framework for many highly cellular organs, such as endocrine glands, lymphoid organs, the spleen, and the liver. **Reticular fibers** are shown in *black* with a silver stain. These fibers are small in diameter and do not form large bundles. They are arranged in a netlike framework to support **parenchymal cells**, in this example, **pancreatic cells**. The *inset drawing* represents the organization of reticular fibers and pancreatic cells.

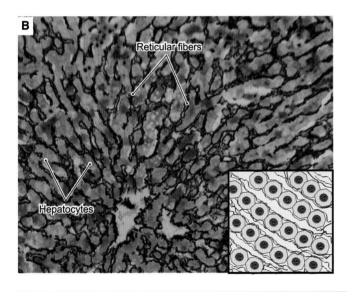

Figure 4-21B. Reticular connective tissue, liver. Silver stain, ×312

The **reticular fibers** can be selectively visualized with a silver stain, that is, they are **argyrophilic**. These fibers consist of **collagen type III**, which forms a meshlike network that supports the liver cells and holds these cells together. The liver cells' cytoplasm is unstained in this preparation, and the structure of the cells is not easy to distinguish here. The *inset drawing* represents the organization of reticular fibers and **hepatocytes**. There is a **sinusoid** running between the reticular fibers, which appears as empty space here.

CLINICAL CORRELATION

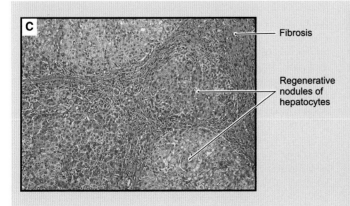

Figure 4-21C. Cirrhosis. H&E, ×100

Cirrhosis is a liver disorder caused by chronic injury to the hepatic parenchyma. The major causes of cirrhosis include alcoholism and chronic infection with hepatitis B or hepatitis C virus. Pathologic changes are characterized by the **collapse** of the delicate supporting **reticular connective tissue** with **increased numbers of collagen** and **elastic fibers**. There is disruption of the liver architecture and vascular bed. **Regenerating hepatocytes form nodules** rather than the characteristic columnar plates. Symptoms include **jaundice, edema,** and **coagulopathy** (a defect of blood coagulation). The resulting damage to the liver tissue impedes drainage of the portal venous system, a condition known as **portal hypertension**, which may eventually lead to **gastroesophageal varices, splenomegaly,** and **ascites**.

ELASTIC CONNECTIVE TISSUE

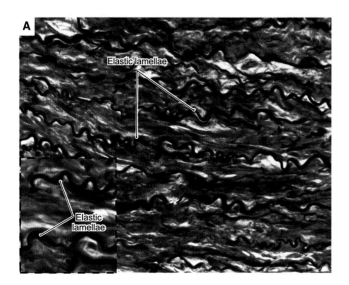

A

Elastic lamellae

Elastic lamellae

Figure 4-22A. **Elastic connective tissue, carotid artery.** Elastic stain (Verhoeff), ×275; inset ×516

This is an example of **elastic connective tissue** in the tunica media of a carotid artery. The wavy **elastic lamellae** are distributed among collagen and smooth muscle cells in the tunica media layer of a large artery. The smooth muscle cells are not visible here because of the type of stain. In general, the **elastic material** (as either **elastic fibers** or **elastic lamellae**) and other connective tissue fibers are produced by **fibroblasts** in the connective tissue, but in blood vessels, **smooth muscle cells** are the principal cells that produce **elastic material** and other connective tissue fibers. Elastic connective tissue consists predominately of elastic material, and this allows distension and recoil of the structure. This tissue can be found in some vertebral ligaments, arterial walls, and in the bronchial tree.

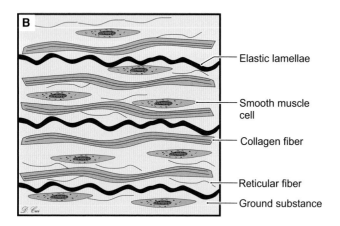

B

— Elastic lamellae

— Smooth muscle cell

— Collagen fiber

— Reticular fiber

— Ground substance

Figure 4-22B. **Representation of elastic connective tissue in the tunica media of a large artery.**

Thick bundles of **elastic lamellae** are arranged in parallel wavy sheets, with the **smooth muscle cells** and **collagen fibers** insinuated between alternating lamellae. The **elastic fibers** are formed by **elastin** and **fibrillin microfibrils**. Elastic connective tissue can recoil after stretching. This property in large arteries helps to moderate the extremes of pressure associated with the cardiac cycle. Abnormal expression of the **fibrillin (FBN1) gene** is associated with abnormal elastic tissue disease.

CLINICAL CORRELATION

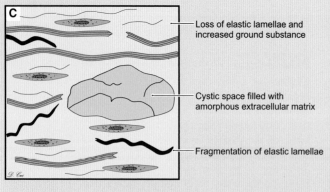

C

— Loss of elastic lamellae and increased ground substance

— Cystic space filled with amorphous extracellular matrix

— Fragmentation of elastic lamellae

Figure 4-22C. Marfan Syndrome—Cystic Medial Degeneration.

Marfan syndrome is an autosomal-dominant disorder caused by an **FBN1 gene mutation**, which affects the formation of elastic fibers, particularly those found in the aorta, heart, eye, and skin. Signs and symptoms include tall stature with long limbs and long, thin fingers and enlargement of the base of the aorta accompanied by aortic regurgitation. There is increased probability of dissecting **aortic aneurysms** and prolapse of the mitral valve. Treatment includes pharmacologic or surgical intervention to prevent potentially fatal or long-term complications, but no permanent cure is yet available. This illustration depicts **cystic medial degeneration (cystic medionecrosis)** of the aorta, including **disruption** and **fragmentation of elastic lamellae** in the tunica media of the aorta, **loss of elastic fibers**, and **increase in ground substance** causing **formation of cystic space**.

EMBRYONIC CONNECTIVE TISSUES

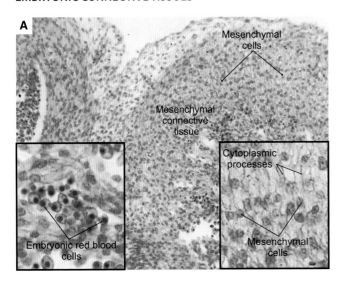

Figure 4-23A. Mesenchyme, embryo. H&E, ×136; inset ×408 (*left*) and ×438 (*right*)

Mesenchyme (**mesenchymal connective tissue**) is found in the developing structures in the **embryo**. It contains scattered **reticular fibers** and **mesenchymal cells**, which have irregular, star or spindle shapes and pale-stained cytoplasm. These cells exhibit **cytoplasmic processes**, which often give the cells a stellate appearance. Mesenchymal cells are relatively unspecialized and can **differentiate** into different cell types in mature tissue cells, such as cartilages, bones, and muscles. **Embryonic red blood cells** can be seen in this specimen. These blood cells contain a nucleus in each cell; this is characteristic of their immature state (anucleated red blood cells are characteristic of the mature state and are found in adult tissues). Interestingly, some vertebrates, such as frogs and chickens, have nucleated red blood cells in the adult state.

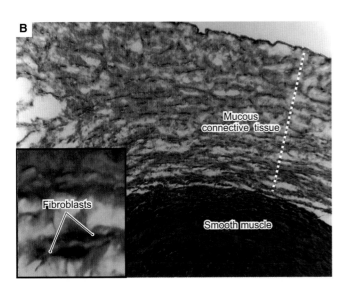

Figure 4-23B. Mucous connective tissue, umbilical cord. Toluidine blue stain, ×68; inset ×178

An example of **mucous connective tissue** that has an abundance of a **jellylike matrix** with some fine aggregates of collagen fibers and stellate-shaped **fibroblasts** is shown. It is found in the umbilical cord and subdermal connective tissue of the embryo. Mucous tissue is a major constituent of the umbilical cord, where it is referred to as **Wharton jelly**. This type of connective tissue does not differentiate beyond this stage. In this example, the viscous ground substance has been stained with a special stain to reveal **jellylike mucin**, which contains **hyaluronic acid** and glycoproteins. Collagen fibers and large stellate-shaped **fibroblasts** (not mesenchymal cells) predominate in the mucous tissue.

SYNOPSIS 4-3 Pathologic Terms for Connective Tissue

■ Urticaria: An itchy skin eruption, also known as **hives**, characterized by wheals with pale interiors and well-defined red margins, often the result of an allergic response to insect bites, foods, or drugs.

■ Pruritus: Itching of the skin due to a variety of causes including hyperbilirubinemia and allergic and irritant contact conditions.

■ Cirrhosis: An abnormal liver condition characterized by diffuse nodularity, due to fibrosis and regenerative nodules of hepatocytes; frequent causes are alcohol abuse and viral hepatitis.

■ Jaundice: Yellow staining of the skin, mucous membranes, or conjunctiva of the eyes caused by elevated blood levels of the bile pigment bilirubin.

■ Coagulopathy: A disorder that prevents the normal clotting process of blood; causes may be acquired, such as hepatic dysfunction, or congenital, such as decreased clotting factors, as seen in inherited conditions like hemophilia.

■ Necrosis: Irreversible cell changes that occur from cell death.

TABLE 4-4 Connective Tissue Types

Type	Connective Tissue Cells	Connective Tissue Fibers	Organization of Fibers and Cells	Main Locations	Main Functions
Connective Tissue Proper					
Dense irregular connective tissue	Predominantly fibroblasts; other connective tissue cells occasionally present	Collagen fibers, elastic fibers, reticular fibers	Fewer cells and more fibers; fibers arranged randomly without a definite orientation in relatively less ground substance	Dermis of the skin, capsules of many organs	Resists stress from all directions; protects organs
Dense regular connective tissue	Predominantly fibroblasts; other connective tissue cells occasionally present	Collagen fibers, elastic fibers, reticular fibers	Fewer cells and more fibers; fibers arranged in uniform parallel bundles	Tendons, ligaments	Provides resistance to traction forces
Loose connective tissue	Fibroblasts, macrophages, adipocytes, mast cells, plasma cells, leukocytes	Collagen fibers predominate; elastic and reticular fibers also present	More cells and fewer fibers; fibers randomly distributed in abundant ground substance	Lamina propria of gastrointestinal tract; around the nerves and vessels (in adventitia layer)	Provides protection, suspension, and support; conduit for vessels and nerves; environment for immune defense function
Specialized Connective Tissues					
Adipose connective tissue	Predominantly adipocytes (fat cells); fibroblasts and other connective tissue cells occasionally present	Collagen fibers and reticular fibers	Fibers form fine meshwork that separates adjacent adipocytes	Hypodermis of the skin, mammary glands, and around many organs	Provides energy storage, insulation; cushioning of organs; hormone secretion
Reticular connective tissue	Fibroblasts, reticular cells, hepatocytes, smooth muscle cells, Schwann cells depending on the location	Reticular fibers	Fibers form delicate meshlike network; cells with process attached to the fibers	Liver, pancreas, lymph nodes, spleen, and bone marrow	Provides supportive framework for hematopoietic and parenchymal organs
Elastic connective tissue	Predominantly fibroblasts or smooth muscle cells; other connective tissue cells occasionally present	Elastic fibers predominate; collagen and reticular fibers also present	Fibers arranged in parallel wavy bundles	Vertebral ligaments, walls of the large arteries	Provides flexible support for the tissue; reduces pressure on the walls of the arteries
Embryonic Connective Tissues					
Mesenchymal connective tissue	Mesenchymal cells	Reticular fibers and collagen fibers	Scattered fibers with spindle-shaped cells having long cytoplasmic processes; mesenchymal cells uniformly distributed	Embryonic mesoderm	Gives rise to all connective tissue types
Mucous connective tissue	Spindle-shaped fibroblasts	Collagen fibers predominate; few elastic and reticular fibers	Fibers and fibroblasts randomly displayed in jellylike matrix (Wharton jelly)	Umbilical cord, subdermal layer of the fetus, dental pulp of the developing teeth, nucleus pulposus of the disk	Provides cushion to protect the blood vessels in the umbilical cord

From Histology to Pathology

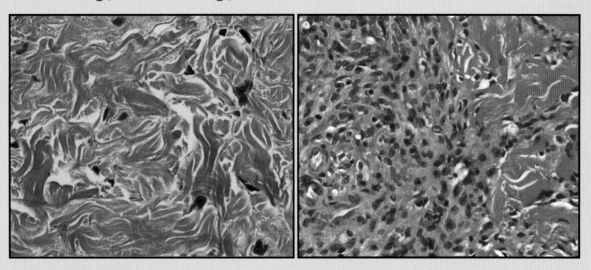

Figure 4-24. Normal dense irregular connective tissue and Kaposi sarcoma. H&E, ×200

Normal dense irregular connective tissue of dermis of the skin is on the *left*. **Kaposi sarcoma** (dermis of the skin) is on the *right*, a vascular neoplasm associated with HIV infection. Neoplastic cells formed a large nodule in the dermis, displacing the normal dense collagen fibers.

Clinical Vignette Questions

1. A 15-year-old female experienced weight loss over a period of 4 months, eventually developing swelling and bleeding of her gums and petechiae (tiny round purple hemorrhages under the skin) around hair follicles, with the eruption of coiled, fragmented hair. After discussing the situation with her parents, the physician determines that the child suffers from an eating disorder and has developed scurvy, caused by deficiency of vitamin C in her diet. Which of the following best describes the role of vitamin C in collagen synthesis?

A. Exocytosis
B. Glycosylation
C. Hydroxylation
D. Production of procollagen
E. Procollagen transport

2. A tall, thin 16-year-old boy comes to your clinic with weakness and shortness of breath. He has disproportionately long arms, legs, fingers, and toes. He also shows severe nearsightedness. Echocardiography indicates dilation of the aortic root. Which of the following gene mutations is most likely the cause of this patient's condition?

A. *Bcl-1* genes
B. *BRCA2* genes
C. *FBN1* genes
D. *p16* genes
E. *p53* genes

3. A 72-year-old farmer had a history of multiple skin lesions removed in the past, including basal cell carcinomas and squamous cell carcinomas. Currently, the patient has a 4-mm, slightly erythematous, scaly lesion on his forehead. Biopsy of the lesion shows hyperkeratosis, loss of the granular layer of the skin, abnormal keratinocytes in the basal layers, and thickened blue-gray fibers within the dermis. Which of the following is the most likely diagnosis?

A. Seborrheic dermatitis
B. Squamous cell carcinoma
C. Verruca vulgaris
D. Seborrheic keratosis
E. Actinic keratosis

5 Cartilage and Bone

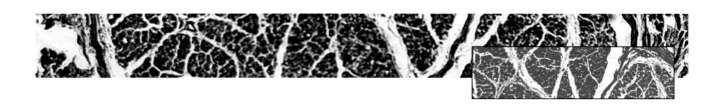

Cartilage
Introduction and Key Concepts for Cartilage
Cartilage Cells
Cartilage Matrix
Types of Cartilage

Cartilage

Introduction and Key Concepts for Cartilage

Cartilage and **bone** are two types of supporting connective tissues. Cartilage is an **avascular** specialized form of connective tissue whose support function is a result of a firm **extracellular matrix** that has variable flexibility depending on its location. This type of tissue is able to bear mechanical stress without permanent deformation. Cartilage has features that are different from other types of connective tissues but, like bone, has the characteristic of isolated cells embedded in extensive matrix. Most cartilage is covered by a layer of dense irregular connective tissue called **perichondrium**, which contains a rich blood supply and is innervated by nerve fibers conveying pain. The exceptions are fibrocartilage and articular cartilage of the joint, which do not have perichondrium. Perichondrium is important for the growth (**appositional growth**) and maintenance of cartilage; it has two layers. The **outer fibrous layer** of the perichondrium contains connective tissue fibers, fibroblasts, and blood vessels. These perichondrial vessels represent an essential blood supply for cartilage. Because cartilage itself is avascular, these vessels are the route through which nutrients access the matrix by diffusion. The **inner cellular layer** of the perichondrium consists of **chondrogenic cells**, which are able to differentiate into **chondroblasts**. The functions of cartilage include the support of soft tissues, the facilitation of smooth movement of bones at joints, and the mediation of growth of the length of bones during bone development.

Cartilage Cells

The main types of cells in cartilage are **chondrogenic cells, chondroblasts**, and **chondrocytes**. (1) *Chondrogenic cells* are located in the **perichondrium** and differentiate into chondroblasts to participate in **appositional growth** of cartilage. These cells are difficult to identify under the light microscope with H&E stain. (2) *Chondroblasts* are young chondrocytes, which derive from **chondrogenic cells**, and are able to actively manufacture the matrix of cartilage. The chondroblasts have ribosome-rich basophilic cytoplasm. They synthesize and deposit cartilage matrix around themselves. As the matrix accumulates and separates the chondroblasts from one another, the cells become entrapped in small individual compartments called **lacunae** and are then referred to as "chondrocytes." (3) *Chondrocytes* are mature chondroblasts that are embedded in the lacunae of the matrix. Chondrocytes retain the ability to divide and often present as an **isogenous group**, two or more chondrocytes arranged in a group that was derived from a single progenitor cell. The isogenous group represents the active division of cells, which contribute to **interstitial growth** (see below, *Cartilage Growth*). In most cartilage, chondrocytes are arranged in an isogenous group. However, in some locations such as in fibrocartilage, chondrocytes are more likely to be arranged in groups of small columns or rows instead of isogenous groups. This is also a sign of interstitial growth.

Cartilage Matrix

The matrix of cartilage is nonmineralized and consists of fibers and ground substance. **Collagen fibers** are mainly **type II** in the matrix, although some cartilage may also contain **type I** or **elastic fibers**. The major components of **ground substance** include glycosaminoglycans (GAGs), proteoglycans, and glycoproteins. The matrix of cartilage surrounding each chondrocyte, or immediately adjacent to chondrocytes of isogenous groups, is called **territorial matrix**. This newly produced matrix has abundant proteoglycans and less collagen and stains more intensely in routine H&E preparations. Another type of matrix, which surrounds the regions of territorial matrix and fills the rest of the space, is called **interterritorial matrix**. This type of matrix stains more lightly than does the territorial matrix.

Types of Cartilage

Cartilage can be classified into three types based on the characteristics of the matrix. All three types of cartilage contain type II collagen; in addition, some types contain type I collagen or elastic fibers in the extracellular matrix. Types of cartilage include **hyaline cartilage, elastic cartilage**, and **fibrocartilage**.

HYALINE CARTILAGE is characterized by the presence of a glassy, homogeneous matrix that contains **type II collagen**, which is evenly dispersed within the ground substance. Most hyaline cartilage is covered by **perichondrium**, except at the articular surfaces of joints. Hyaline cartilage is the most common type of cartilage; is found in the articular ends of long bones, nose, larynx, trachea, bronchi, and the distal ends of ribs; and is the template for endochondral bone formation. Hyaline cartilage covers the smooth surface of joints, providing for free movement, and is also involved in bone formation and long bone growth.

ELASTIC CARTILAGE is similar to hyaline cartilage except for its rich network of **elastic fibers**, arranged in thick bundles in the matrix. This type of cartilage has a **perichondrium**, as does hyaline cartilage, and it also contains **type II collagen** in the matrix. The chondrocytes of elastic cartilage are more abundant and larger than those of hyaline cartilage. Elastic cartilage is located in areas where elasticity and firm support are required, such as the epiglottis and larynx, auditory canal and tube, and the pinna of the ear, which is able to recover its shape after deformation.

FIBROCARTILAGE does not have a perichondrium. It has **type II collagen**, as do the other two types of cartilage. It is characterized by thick, coarse bundles of **type I collagen** fibers that alternate with parallel groups of columns (or rows) of chondrocytes within the matrix. The chondrocytes of fibrocartilage are smaller and much less numerous than in the other two types of cartilage and are often arranged in columns or rows. Because fibrocartilage has no perichondrium, its growth depends on **interstitial growth**. Fibrocartilage is resistant to tearing and compression, can accommodate great pressure, and is often found at connections between bones that do not have an articular surface. It is found in areas where support and tensile strength are required, such as intervertebral disks, the pubic symphysis, and the insertions of tendons and ligaments.

Cartilage Growth

Cartilage grows by either **appositional** or **interstitial growth** or **both**. The growth process is prolonged and involves mitosis and the deposition of additional matrix. (1) *Appositional growth* begins with the **chondrogenic cells** located in the perichondrium. These chondrogenic cells differentiate into **chondroblasts**, also called **young chondrocytes**, and these cells start to elaborate a new layer of matrix at the surface (periphery) region of the cartilage near the perichondrium. Most cartilage growth in the body is appositional growth. (2) *Interstitial growth* occurs during the early stages of cartilage formation in most types of cartilage. It begins with the cell division of **preexisting chondrocytes** (mature chondroblasts surrounded by territorial matrix). Interstitial growth increases the tissue size by expanding the cartilage matrix from within. Fibrocartilage lacks a perichondrium, so it grows only by interstitial growth. In the epiphyseal plates of long bones, interstitial growth serves to lengthen the bone.

SYNOPSIS 5-1 Pathologic and Clinical Terms for Cartilage and Bone

- **Eburnation:** In osteoarthritis, the loss of the articular cartilage results in the exposure of the subchondral bone, which becomes worn and polished.
- **Fibrillation:** Early degenerative change in the process of osteoarthritis by which the articular cartilage becomes worn and produces a papillary appearance; fragments of degenerated cartilage may be released into the joint space.
- **Neoplasm:** Abnormal tissue arising from a single aberrant cell; neoplasms may be benign or malignant. Malignant neoplasms are capable of destructive growth and metastasis.
- **Achondroplasia:** An autosomal-dominant genetic disorder that causes dwarfism. The fibroblast growth factor receptor gene 3 (*FGFR3*) is affected, resulting in abnormal cartilage formation and short stature.
- **Osteoporosis:** A bone disease characterized by reduced bone mineral density, thinned bone cortex, and trabeculae. It causes an increased risk of fracture, especially in postmenopausal women.
- **Osteomalacia:** A bone condition caused by impaired mineralization. It causes rickets in children and bone softening in adults. Vitamin D deficiency and insufficient Ca^{2+} ions are the most common causes of the condition.
- **Paget disease:** A chronic disorder characterized by excessive breakdown and formation of bone tissue that typically results in enlarged and deformed bones. The blood alkaline phosphatase level in patients is usually above normal.
- **Parosteal osteosarcoma:** A malignant bone tumor, usually occurring on the surface of the metaphysis of a long bone.

Overview of Cartilage

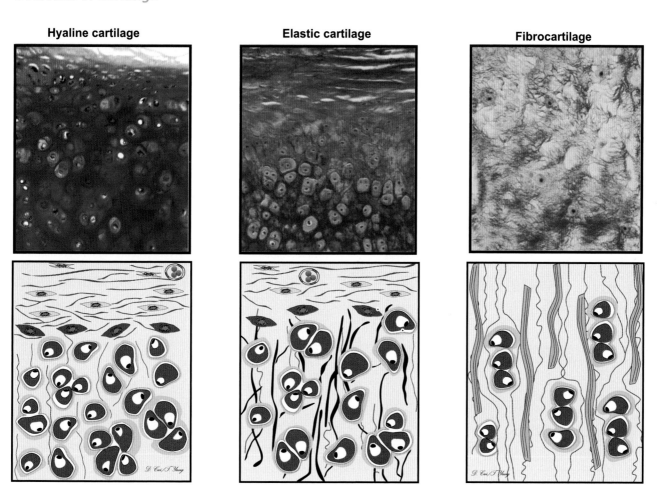

Figure 5-1. Overview of cartilage types. Cartilage can be classified into three types (hyaline, elastic, and fibrocartilage) based on the characteristics of the matrix.

TABLE 5-1   Cartilage

Types of Cartilage	Characteristics of the Extracellular Matrix	Chondrocyte Arrangement	Perichondrium Coverage	Type of Growth	Main Locations	Main Functions
Hyaline cartilage	Type II collagen	Mostly in groups (isogenous groups)	Yes, except articular cartilage surface	Appositional and interstitial growth	Trachea, bronchi, ventral ends of ribs, nose, articular ends and epiphyseal plates of long bones	Confers shape and flexibility (respiratory tract); forms cartilage model for bone growth in the fetus; forms smooth surface to provide free movement in joints
Elastic cartilage	Type II collagen and elastic fibers	Mostly in groups (isogenous groups)	Yes	Appositional and interstitial growth	Epiglottis, larynx, pinna of the ear, and auditory canal and tube	Confers shape and elasticity
Fibrocartilage	Type II and type I collagen	Most are small and sparsely arranged in parallel columns or rows	No	Interstitial growth	Articular disks, intervertebral disks, pubic symphysis, and the insertion of tendons	Provides resistance to compression, cushioning, and tensile strength

Hyaline Cartilage

EXTRACELLULAR MATRIX

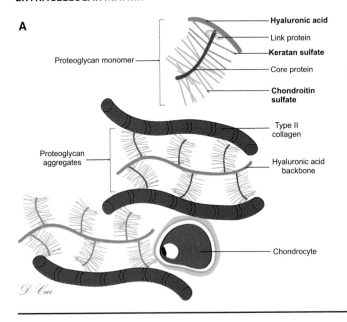

A

- Hyaluronic acid
- Link protein
- **Keratan sulfate**
- Core protein
- **Chondroitin sulfate**
- Type II collagen
- Hyaluronic acid backbone
- Chondrocyte

Proteoglycan monomer

Proteoglycan aggregates

D. Cui

Figure 5-2A.   Overview of extracellular matrix of hyaline cartilage.

The extracellular matrix of hyaline cartilage is composed of ground substance and collagen fibers. The ground substance contains small amounts of **glycoproteins** and large amounts of **glycosaminoglycans (GAGs)** and **proteoglycan**. The **glycosaminoglycans** have three types: **hyaluronic acid, keratan sulfate,** and **chondroitin sulfate.** They are linked to **a core protein** to form a **proteoglycan monomer (proteoglycan aggrecan).** A number of proteoglycan monomers attach to a hyaluronic acid backbone to form a large-sized **proteoglycan aggregate.** In the extracellular matrix, each proteoglycan monomer binds to type II collagen, which provides a scaffolding support for the chondrocytes' attachment and growth. Overall, 75% of hyaline cartilage is composed of water, and 25% is composed of dry weight (organic compounds), 40% of which includes collagen fibers, and 60% of which includes ground substance.

CHONDROCYTES

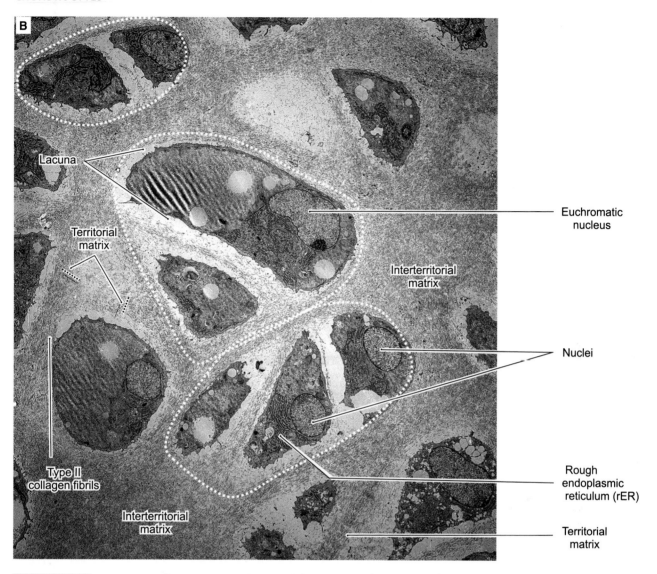

Figure 5-2B. Hyaline cartilage and chondrocytes. EM, ×6,300

When **chondroblasts** of the perichondrium have surrounded themselves with matrix and become embedded in a hyaline cartilage, they are called **chondrocytes**, the cells seen in this electron micrograph. These chondrocytes are still active in synthesizing matrix proteins as indicated by their abundant **rough endoplasmic reticulum** (**RER**) and by the presence of nucleoli and **euchromatin** in their nuclei. Evidence of recent cell divisions is seen in the form of **isogenous groups**, three of which are circumscribed by *dotted lines*. The meshwork of filaments in the matrix is **type II collagen**, which does not aggregate to form fibers.

HYALINE CARTILAGE AND PERICHONDRIUM

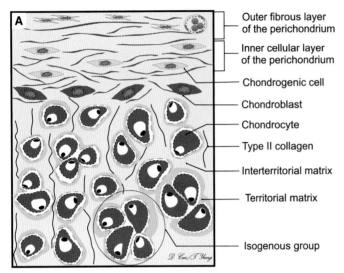

Outer fibrous layer
of the perichondrium

Inner cellular layer
of the perichondrium

Chondrogenic cell

Chondroblast

Chondrocyte

Type II collagen

Interterritorial matrix

Territorial matrix

Isogenous group

Figure 5-3A.   Representation of hyaline cartilage.

Hyaline cartilage is the most common of the three types of cartilage (hyaline cartilage, elastic cartilage, and fibrocartilage). It can be found in the trachea, bronchi, distal ends of ribs, and articular ends and epiphyseal plates of long bones. Most hyaline cartilage is covered by **perichondrium**, a dense irregular connective tissue sheath. However, the hyaline cartilage in the articular joint surfaces of long bones is an exception. Hyaline cartilage is composed of chondroblasts, chondrocytes, delicate **collagen (type II collagen)**, and a homogenous **ground substance (matrix)**, which makes it *glassy* in appearance. The matrices include the **territorial matrix** and the **interterritorial matrix**.

BRONCHUS

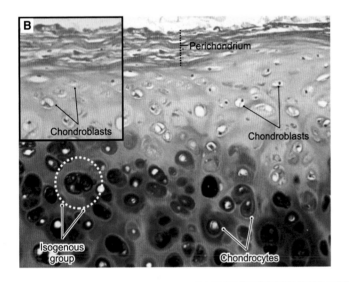

Perichondrium

Chondroblasts

Chondroblasts

Isogenous
group

Chondrocytes

Figure 5-3B.   Hyaline cartilage, bronchus. H&E, ×139; inset ×167

This is an example of **hyaline cartilage** in the bronchus. Cartilage is an **avascular tissue**; nutrients are supplied through matrix diffusion. The **perichondrium**, a dense irregular connective tissue sheath surrounding the surface of the hyaline cartilage, provides the nearest blood supply to the cartilage. The perichondrium consists of (1) an **outer fibrous layer**, which is composed of type I collagen, fibroblasts, and blood vessels, and (2) an **inner cellular layer**, which contains chondrogenic cells that give rise to new **chondroblasts**. These cells are flattened cells, which actively secrete matrix and often are located beneath the perichondrium. Chondrogenic cells are difficult to identify under the light microscope with H&E stain. The chondrocytes are often arranged in small clusters called **isogenous groups**, which contribute to interstitial growth.

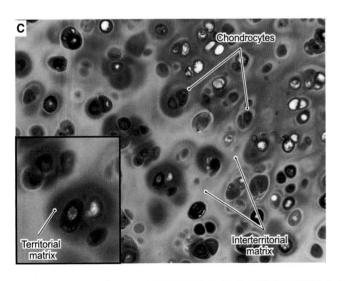

Chondrocytes

Territorial
matrix

Interterritorial
matrix

Figure 5-3C.   Hyaline cartilage, bronchus. H&E, ×136; inset ×251

The **chondrocytes** have small, round nuclei and shrunken, pale-staining cytoplasm, which contains large Golgi apparatuses and lipid droplets. The matrix that surrounds each chondrocyte or isogenous group is called the **territorial matrix**. The matrix that fills in the space between isogenous groups and chondrocytes is called the **interterritorial matrix**. In general, the territorial matrix stains darker than the interterritorial matrix in H&E.

TRACHEA

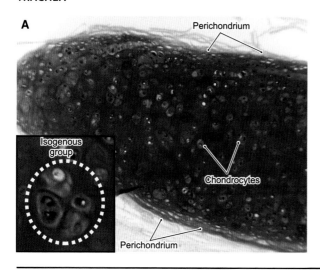

Figure 5-4A. Hyaline cartilage, trachea. H&E, ×68; inset ×276

This is an example of hyaline cartilage in the trachea. The **hyaline cartilage** forms a structural framework to support tissues such as the larynx, trachea, and bronchi in the respiratory tract. The **chondrocytes** are mature chondroblasts that are embedded in the matrix. Each chondrocyte is contained within a small cavity in the matrix called a **lacuna;** sometimes, one lacuna may contain two cells.

ARTICULAR CARTILAGE

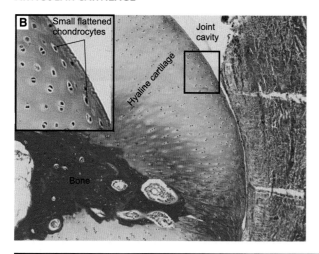

Figure 5-4B. Hyaline cartilage, finger bone. H&E, ×68; inset ×189

This is an example of the **hyaline cartilage** in the articular ends of a long bone (finger bone). The cartilage that covers the articular surface of the bone is called **articular cartilage**. In this particular region, the cartilage is exposed without perichondrium present. The surface area of the articular cartilage is composed of **small, dense, flattened chondrocytes**, which enable it to resist pressure and form a smooth surface to provide free movement in the presence of a lubricating fluid (**synovial fluid**).

CLINICAL CORRELATION

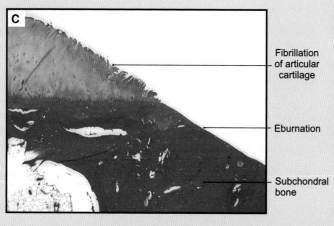

Figure 5-4C. Osteoarthritis. H&E, ×29

Osteoarthritis is a chronic condition that is characterized by a gradual loss of hyaline cartilage from the joints. It commonly affects the hand, knee, hip, spine, and other weight-supporting joints. Risk factors include genetic factors, aging, obesity, female gender, injury, and wear and tear of the joints. Symptoms and signs include joint pain that is worsened by physical activity and relieved by rest, morning stiffness, and changes in the shape of affected joints. There are two types of osteoarthritides: **idiopathic** and **secondary**. *Idiopathic* has no obvious cause, whereas *secondary* has an identifiable cause. Monocyte-derived peptides cause chondrocytes to proliferate. Increased numbers of chondrocytes release degradative enzymes, which cause inadequate repair responses and subsequent inflammation in cartilage, bone, and synovium. Cartilage fragments and soluble proteoglycan and type II collagen can be found in the synovial fluid. This illustration shows the rough surface of the hyaline cartilage with **fibrillations** and **eburnation** as a result of softening, thinning, and loss of the **articular cartilage** and exposure of the **subchondral bone**, which becomes worn and polished.

Elastic Cartilage

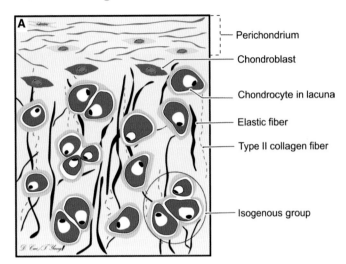

Figure 5-5A. Representation of elastic cartilage.

Elastic cartilage has a rich network of **elastic fibers**, which gives its matrix a rough appearance. It also contains delicate **collagen type II fibers** and ground substance in the matrix, as do other types of cartilage. In general, **chondrocytes** are more abundant in elastic cartilage than in hyaline cartilage and fibrocartilage. Cartilage growth in elastic cartilage includes **appositional growth**, which requires a perichondrium, and **interstitial growth**, indicated by **isogenous groups**. Elastic cartilage provides flexible support for tissue and is located in the areas where flexible stretching is required, such as the epiglottis, larynx, pinna of the ear, and the auditory canal and tube.

EPIGLOTTIS

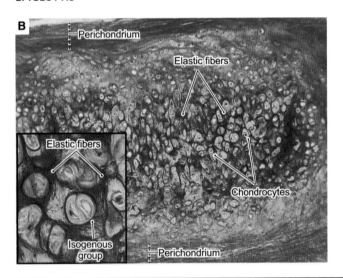

Figure 5-5B. Elastic cartilage, epiglottis. H&E, ×68; inset ×218

An example of **elastic cartilage** in the epiglottis is shown. Elastic cartilage has a **perichondrium** surrounding it as does most hyaline cartilage. The perichondrium protects and provides blood supply for the cartilage tissue. Chondrogenic cells and **chondroblasts** in the perichondrium layer are responsible for appositional growth of the matrix. There are abundant **elastic fibers** and type II collagen fibers in the extracellular matrix. **Isogenous groups** are created by the division of existing cells. The resulting daughter cells that are derived from a single progenitor cell stay in the same lacuna. Elastic cartilage has both **interstitial growth**, which is indicated by the presence of isogenous groups, and **appositional growth**, for which a perichondrium is required.

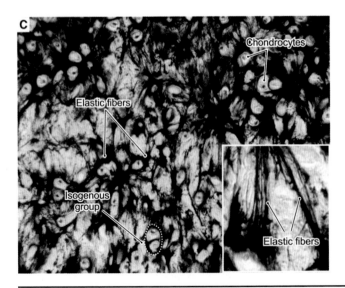

Figure 5-5C. Elastic cartilage, epiglottis. Elastic fiber stain, ×68; inset ×208

An example of **elastic cartilage** in the epiglottis is shown. Elastic cartilage is composed of thick, branching **elastic fibers** with a slight network of **collagen fibers** and **chondrocytes** filling the interstitial space. Elastic cartilage can be found in the epiglottis and pinna of the ear. Elastic fibers presented here with a special stain are seen as thick, dark, elongated profiles. Chondrocytes are arranged in individual and **isogenous groups** among the elastic fibers in the matrix.

Fibrocartilage

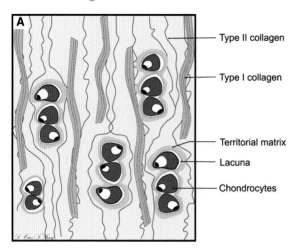

Figure 5-6A. Representation of fibrocartilage.

Fibrocartilage lacks a perichondrium, so no appositional growth takes place. **Chondrocytes** in **lacunae** are often arranged in small groups in parallel columns or rows, which correlate with their method of **interstitial growth**. The chondrocytes are smaller and fewer in number in fibrocartilage than in the other two types of cartilage. Because **type I collagen fibers** are present in its matrix, the matrix has a dense and coarse appearance. Fibrocartilage is less flexible than the other two types of cartilage; it provides firm support, cushioning, and tensile strength.

INTERVERTEBRAL DISK

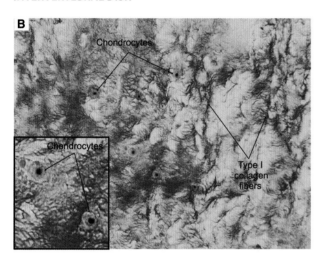

Figure 5-6B. Fibrocartilage, intervertebral disk. H&E, ×136; inset ×292

Fibrocartilage in the intervertebral disk is shown. Fibrocartilage contains **type II** and **type I** collagen fiber bundles in the matrix, which makes the matrix look rough, like an oil painting. Chondrocytes are small and housed in **lacunae**, which are widely scattered in the matrix. There is no perichondrium associated with fibrocartilage; therefore, cartilage growth proceeds by **interstitial growth** only. Fibrocartilage has a firm, dense matrix, and it can be found in the pubic symphysis, intervertebral disks, and insertions of tendons and ligaments.

CLINICAL CORRELATION

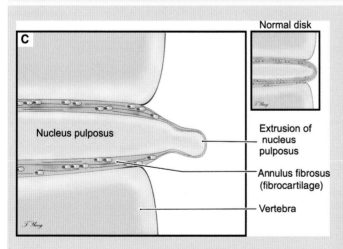

Figure 5-6C. Disk Degeneration and Herniation.

Herniation of an intervertebral disk is a common cause of pain in the lower back and neck. It is most common in people in their 30s and 40s. Risk factors include age, occupation, lifestyle, and genetic propensity. **Degeneration of the intervertebral disk** is because of a combination of factors that may result in changes in hydration of the **nucleus pulposus** (composed of mucous connective tissue) and in the strength of collagen, leading to weakening of the **anulus fibrosus (fibrocartilage)**. The degenerated disk nucleus pulposus loses its cushioning ability and exerts uneven pressure on the surrounding anulus; extrusion of the nucleus pulposus through the weakened anulus is called **herniation**. It happens most often at the L4–L5 (lumbar) and L5–S1 (sacral) vertebral levels, causing back pain and other neurologic symptoms because of compression of the nerve roots. Magnetic resonance imaging is widely used to visualize the herniated disk. Treatment includes bed rest, the McKenzie exercise, steroid injections, open discectomy, and minimally invasive endoscopic discectomy.

Cartilage Growth

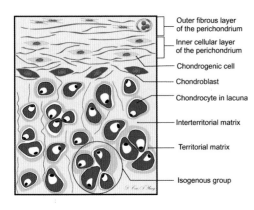
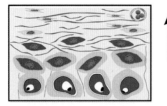
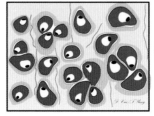

Outer fibrous layer of the perichondrium

Inner cellular layer of the perichondrium

Chondrogenic cell

Chondroblast

Chondrocyte in lacuna

Interterritorial matrix

Territorial matrix

Isogenous group

Figure 5-7. Representation of cartilage growth.

Cartilage grows by either **appositional** or **interstitial growth** or by **both**. The growth process is continuous and involves mitosis and the deposition of additional matrix. *Appositional growth* begins with the **chondrogenic cells** in the **perichondrium**. These chondrogenic cells differentiate into **chondroblasts,** which are also called **young chondrocytes.** Chondroblasts start to elaborate a new layer of matrix at the surface (periphery) region of the cartilage near the perichondrium. Cartilage grows mostly by appositional growth. *Interstitial growth* occurs during the early stages of cartilage formation. The growth begins with the cell division of preexisting chondrocytes (mature chondroblasts, which are surrounded by territorial matrix). Interstitial growth increases the tissue size by expanding the cartilage matrix from within the cartilage mass. This type of growth is indicated by the presence of **isogenous groups** in most cartilage, though sometimes the chondrocytes are arranged in small groups in parallel columns and rows. Articular cartilage lacks a perichondrium, so it enlarges only by interstitial growth. Interstitial growth serves to lengthen the bone such as in the epiphyseal plates of long bones.

SYNOPSIS 5-2 Functions of Cartilage

Hyaline cartilage
- Serves as the **cartilage model** for the formation of bones during bone development.
- Participates in bone-lengthening growth by increasing chondrocyte size and numbers during bone development (**endochondral ossification**).
- Enables free movement by forming smooth surfaces that work with lubricating fluid (**synovial fluid**) in articular cartilage of the joints.
- Provides support and framework for airways in the respiratory tract.

Elastic cartilage
- Provides elastic but stiff framework for pinna and allows it to return to its former shape after stretching.
- Provides elastic support for auditory canals and tube; helps to maintain structural shape.
- Provides a firm and elastic support for the epiglottis and larynx; helps to maintain rigid structure and flexibility.

Fibrocartilage
- Provides tensile strength for connections between the bones such as the pubic symphysis.
- Provides cushioning and resistance between vertebrae, enabling the spinal column to endure great pressure.

SYNOPSIS 5-3 Special Features of Cartilage

- The **function** is to provide firm support with variable flexibility depending on its location.
- The extracellular matrix is **nonmineralized** and consists of fibrillar proteins (collagen) and ground substance (GAGs, proteoglycans, and glycoproteins).
- The extracellular matrix is produced by **chondroblasts** and **chondrocytes.**
- Cartilage grows by both **interstitial** and **appositional** mechanisms.
- It is an **avascular tissue;** the nutrients are supplied through matrix diffusion.
- The **perichondrium** provides the nearest blood supply to the cartilage.
- **Vitamins A, D, and C** are necessary for cartilage growth and matrix formation.

Bone

Introduction and Key Concepts for Bone

Bone is a special type of supporting connective tissue, which has a hard, mineralized, extracellular matrix containing **osteocytes** embedded in the matrix. It is different from cartilage in that bone is calcified and, hence, is harder and stronger than cartilage. In addition, it has many blood vessels penetrating the tissue. Bone protects internal organs, provides support for soft tissues, serves as a calcium reserve for the body, provides an environment for blood cell production, detoxifies certain chemicals in the body, and aids in the movement of the body. In general, the external surface of the bone is covered by **periosteum**, a layer of connective tissue containing small blood vessels, osteogenic cells, and nerve fibers conveying pain information. The inner surface of the bone is covered by **endosteum**, a thin connective tissue layer composed of a single layer of osteoprogenitor cells and osteoblasts that lines all internal cavities within bone; this lining represents the boundary between the bone matrix and the marrow cavities. Bone cells include **osteogenic cells, osteoblasts, osteocytes,** and **osteoclasts**. These cells contribute to bone growth, remodeling, and repair.

Bone Matrix

Bone is primarily characterized by a hard matrix, which contains calcium, phosphate, other organic and inorganic materials, and type I collagen fibers. Compared to cartilage, bone contains only about 25% water in the matrix, whereas cartilage matrix contains about 75% water. This combination makes bone hard, firm, and very strong. **Bone matrix** has **organic** and **inorganic components**. (1) *Organic (noncalcified) matrix* is mainly **type I collagen** with nonmineralized ground substance (chondroitin sulfate and keratan sulfate). It is found in the freshly produced bone matrix, **osteoid** (also called **prebone**), which is produced by **osteoblasts**. This matrix stains light pink in H&E preparations. (2) *Inorganic (calcified) matrix*, mainly in the form of **hydroxyapatite**, contains crystalline mineral salts, mostly of calcium and phosphorus. After osteoid is produced, this fresh matrix undergoes a mineralization process to become the calcified matrix.

Bone Cells

The main types of cells in bone are **osteoprogenitor cells, osteoblasts, osteocytes,** and **osteoclasts**: (1) *Osteoprogenitor cells* are located in the **periosteum** on the surface of the growing bone and can differentiate into osteoblasts. (2) *Osteoblasts* produce the bone matrix. They are cuboidal or low columnar in shape and have a well-developed **Golgi complex** and **RER**, which correlates with their protein-secreting function. The overall process of mineralization relies on the elevation of calcium and phosphate within the matrix and the function of **hydroxyapatite crystals**. This is brought about by complex functions of the osteoblast. (3) *Osteocytes* are small, have cytoplasmic processes, and are unable to divide. These cells originate from osteoblasts and are embedded in the bone matrix. Osteoblasts deposit the matrix around themselves and end up inside the matrix, where they are called "osteocytes." Each osteocyte has many long, thin processes that extend into small narrow spaces called **canaliculi**. The nucleus and surrounding cytoplasm of each osteocyte occupy a space in the bone matrix called a **lacuna**. Thin processes of the osteocyte course through thin channels (canaliculi) that radiate from each lacuna and connect neighboring lacunae. (4) *Osteoclasts* are large, multinucleated cells, which derive from **monocytes**, absorb the bone matrix, and play an essential role in bone remodeling.

Types of Bone

There are several ways to classify bone tissues. Microscopically, bone can be classified as **primary bone** (immature, or "woven" bone) and **secondary bone** (mature, or lamellar bone). Bones can also be classified by their shapes as follows: **long bones, short bones, flat bones,** and **irregular bones**. *Mature bone* can be classified as **compact bone** and **cancellous bone** based on gross appearance and density of the bone. *Compact bone*, also called **cortical bone**, has a much higher density and a well-organized osteon system. It does not have trabeculae and usually forms the external aspect (outside portion) of the bone. *Cancellous bone*, also called **spongy bone**, has a much lower density and contains **bony trabeculae** or **spicules** with intervening bone marrow. It can be found between the inner and the outer tables of the skull, at the ends of long bones, and in the inner core of other bones.

Bone Development

Bone development can be classified as **intramembranous ossification** and **endochondral ossification**, according to the mechanism of its initial formation. (1) *Intramembranous ossification* is the process by which a condensed mesenchyme tissue is transformed into bone. A cartilage precursor is not involved; instead, mesenchymal cells serve as **osteoprogenitor cells**, which then differentiate into **osteoblasts**. Osteoblasts begin to deposit the bone matrix. (2) *Endochondral ossification* is the process by which **hyaline cartilage** serves as a **cartilage model** precursor. This hyaline cartilage proliferates, calcifies, and is gradually replaced by bone. Osteoprogenitor cells migrate along with blood vessels into the region of the calcified cartilage. These cells become osteoblasts, which then begin to deposit the bone matrix on the surface of the calcified cartilage matrix plate. Endochondral ossification involves several events (see Figs. 5-14A and 5-15A for a summary of these processes). The development of long bone is a good example of endochondral formation. In this particular case, the hyaline cartilage undergoes proliferation and calcification in the **epiphyseal plates**. This epiphyseal cartilage can be divided into five recognizable zones: **reserve zone, proliferation zone, hypertrophy zone, calcification zone,** and **ossification zone**.

Overview of Bone

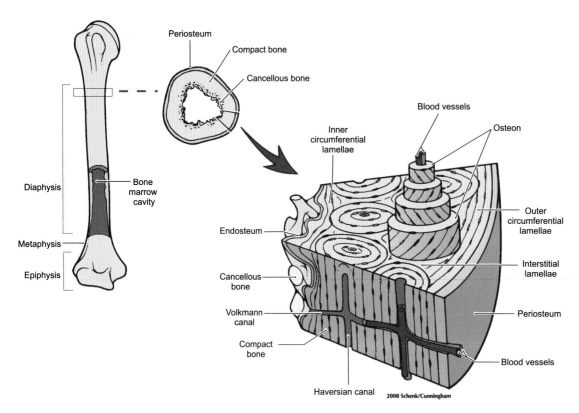

Figure 5-8. Overview of bone structure, long bone.

Bones can be classified as **long bones, short bones, flat bones,** and **irregular bones** according to their shape. *Long bones* are longer than they are wide and consist of a long shaft (**diaphysis**) and two ends (**epiphyses**). *Short bones* are roughly cube shaped, such as wrist and ankle bones. Bone also can be classified as **compact bone** and **cancellous bone** based on gross appearance and bone density. The **diaphysis** of a long bone is composed primarily of *compact bone* and an inner medullary cavity, which is filled with **bone marrow**. The **epiphyses** of long bones are composed mainly of *cancellous (spongy) bone*, and the articular surfaces are covered by articular cartilage, providing a smooth joint surface for articulation with the next bone. The **metaphysis** is a transitional zone between the diaphysis and epiphysis; it represents the level that cancellous bone ends and the bone marrow cavity begins. The external surfaces of compact bone are covered by **periosteum**, a thick layer of dense connective tissue, which contains **blood vessels**. **Endosteum**, a thin layer of connective tissue with a single layer of osteoprogenitor cells and osteoblasts, forms a boundary between the bone and the medullary cavity (this layer may be continuous with the trabeculae of the cancellous bone). The general structure of compact bone includes (1) the **osteon**, a canal surrounded by layers of concentric lamellae; (2) **interstitial lamellae**, lamellae layers in between the osteons; (3) **outer circumferential lamellae**, outer layers of lamellae located beneath the periosteum and surrounding the outside of the entire compact bone; and (4) **inner circumferential lamellae**, layers of lamellae located beneath the endosteum and forming the innermost layer of compact bone. The **haversian canal** is a central space through which blood vessels pass; the **Volkmann canal** is the space that sits perpendicularly to the haversian canals and forms the connection between two haversian canals.

SYNOPSIS 5-4 Functions of Bone

- Provides **protection** for internal organs, such as the brain, heart, lung, bladder, and reproductive organs.
- Provides **supporting framework** for the body (e.g., long bones for limbs and skull for the support of brain and framework for facial features).
- Enables body **movements** in conjunction with the muscles and nervous system.
- Produces blood cells (**hematopoiesis**) within the medullary cavity of long bones and cancellous bone.
- Provides a **calcium** and **phosphorus** reserve for the body.
- Provides **detoxification** for stored heavy metals in the bone tissues. Removes these toxic materials from blood, thereby reducing damage to other organs and tissues.
- Provides **sound transduction** in the middle ear (auditory ossicles: malleus, incus, and stapes).

Types of Bone
COMPACT BONE

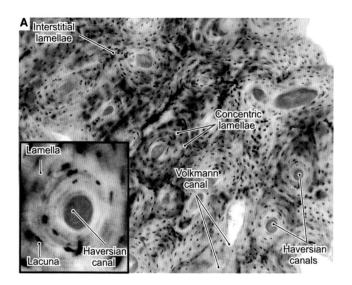

Figure 5-9A. **Compact bone.** Ground specimen (unstained), ×68; inset ×212

A cross section of **compact bone** in a ground specimen (without decalcification of tissue) is shown. **Haversian canals** are round central spaces in the cross-sectional view; a **Volkmann canal** is shown in the longitudinal view. Volkmann canals run perpendicularly to and connect haversian canals with each other. The *inset photomicrograph* shows an **osteon** (**haversian system**), the basic structural unit of compact bone, which includes a **haversian canal**, **lacunae** with housed **osteocytes**, and **concentric lamellae**. Bone matrices located between the osteons are called **interstitial lamellae**.

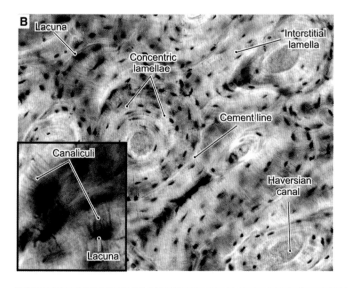

Figure 5-9B. **Compact bone.** Ground specimen (unstained), ×136; inset ×388

A higher power view of compact bone in ground specimen is shown. **Concentric lamellae** and **lacunae** are arranged in rings, which surround the **haversian canal**. Each lacuna has an osteocyte in it. Tiny canals called **canaliculi** contain processes of osteocytes and link the lacunae with each other. The canaliculi permit the osteocytes to communicate via gap junctions where the processes of adjacent osteocytes touch each other inside the canaliculi. A **cement line** forms a boundary between adjacent osteons. Compact bone forms the hard external portion of bone and provides strong support and protection.

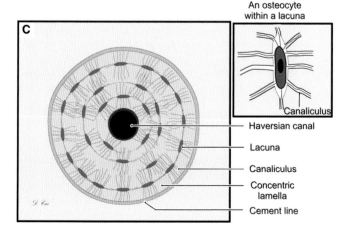

Figure 5-9C. **Representation of an osteon of the compact bone.**

The **osteon**, also called a **haversian system**, is the basic unit of the compact bone structure. It has concentrically arranged laminae (concentric lamellae) surrounding a centrally located haversian canal. The haversian system consists of (1) a **haversian canal** through which blood vessels pass; (2) **concentric lamellae**; (3) **lacunae**, each one of which contains an osteocyte; (4) **canaliculi**, which are small narrow spaces containing osteocyte processes; and (5) a **cement line**, the thin dense, external bony layer that surrounds each osteon.

A schematic drawing illustrates an **osteocyte** occupying a **lacuna** (a space in the bone matrix that houses an osteocyte) and its thin processes within the canaliculi. The hairlike processes of the osteocyte are in contact with the processes of adjacent osteocytes and provide a means of communication between osteocytes.

COMPACT AND CANCELLOUS BONES

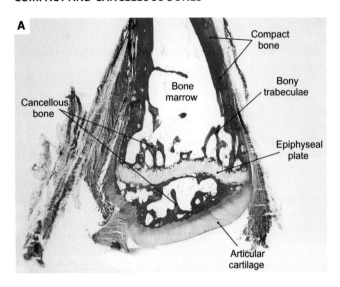

Figure 5-10A.   Compact bone and cancellous bone, finger.
Decalcified bone, H&E, ×11

Bone has a calcified extracellular matrix that is very difficult to cut into thin sections. In order to have thin sections with H&E stain, these bone specimens have to go through a decalcification process that removes calcium compounds from the specimen. Bone can be classified as **compact bone** (**cortical bone**) and **cancellous bone** (**spongy bone**), based on its gross appearance. *Compact bone* has a very high density and a well-organized osteon system. It has no trabeculae and usually forms the external aspect of a bone. *Cancellous bone* (*spongy bone*) has a much lower density and contains **bony trabeculae** or **spicules** with intervening **bone marrow**. It usually forms the inner part of a bone, also called **medullary bone**, and is commonly found between the inner and the outer tables of the skull, at the ends of long bones (limbs and fingers), and in the cores of other bones.

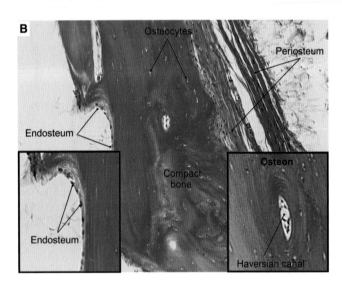

Figure 5-10B.   Compact bone, finger. Decalcified bone, H&E, ×105; inset (*left*) ×154; inset (*right*) ×127

An example of **compact bone** from the diaphysis of the long bone (finger) is shown. The internal surface is covered by a single layer of connective tissue cells forming the **endosteum**. It contains osteoprogenitor cells, which are capable of differentiating into osteoblasts. The external surface is covered by a thicker layer, the **periosteum**, which contains blood vessels, nerves, and osteoprogenitor cells. Osteoprogenitor cells can differentiate into **osteoblasts**, which have the ability to produce bone matrix, **osteoid** (**prebone**). Blood vessels branch to supply bone through a system of interconnected **Volkmann canals** and **haversian canals**. **Osteocytes** are arranged uniformly in compact bone. Each osteocyte occupies one lacuna, which has no isogenous group as it does in cartilage.

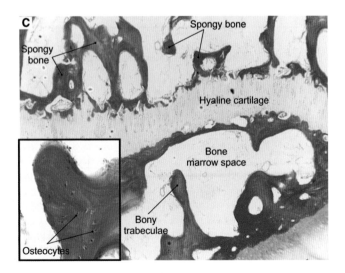

Figure 5-10C.   Cancellous bone (spongy bone), finger.
Decalcified bone, H&E, ×34; inset ×128

Cancellous bone is also called **spongy bone**. It has a lower density than compact bone and consists of **bony trabeculae**, or **spicules**, within a marrow-filled cavity. Osteoblasts line the surface of the bony trabeculae. Cancellous bone displays irregular shapes in the trabecular network. **Bone marrow** fills the space between the bony trabeculae. Most osteocytes in the matrix are arranged in an irregular pattern rather than in circular rings. Cancellous bone mainly forms the inner core of bone and provides (1) a meshwork frame that supports and reduces the overall weight of bone and (2) room for blood vessels to pass through and a place for marrow to function as a hemopoietic compartment, housing and producing blood cells.

Bone Cells

OSTEOBLASTS

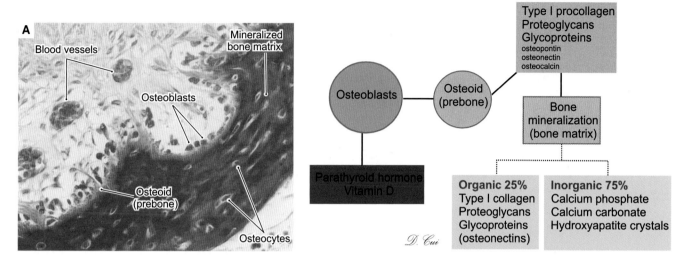

Figure 5-11A. Overview of osteoblasts and bone formation. H&E, ×400 (*left*)

The **bone cells** include **osteogenic cells, osteoblasts, osteocytes,** and **osteoclasts**. The **osteoblasts** are derived from osteogenic cells. Both **parathyroid hormone (PTH)** and **vitamin D** are important factors involved in promoting bone formation. The **osteoid** (also called **prebone**), an uncalcified bone matrix, is produced by **osteoblasts** that contain type I **precollagen, proteoglycans,** and **glyco-proteins. Osteopontin, osteonectin,** and **osteocalcin** are examples of glycoproteins. **Osteocalcin** and **osteonectin** are associated with mineralization of bone matrix. **Osteopontin** is related to the sealing zone of osteoclasts, as it anchors osteoclasts to the mineral bone matrix. The **bone mineralization process** begins a few days after osteoid is formed. It involves the formation of crystalline calcium phosphate mineral in the form of **hydroxyapatite. Extracellular matrix of bone (bone matrix)** is composed of two main substances: (1) **organic matrix** (25% by weight), which includes **collagen** (90% type I, small amounts of type V, and trace amounts of type III, XI, and XIII), **proteoglycans,** and **glycoproteins,** and (2) **inorganic matrix** (75% by weight), which includes (1) **calcium phosphate, calcium carbonate,** and small amounts of magnesium and sodium as well as (2) **hydroxyapatite crystals** (calcium phosphate and calcium hydroxide).

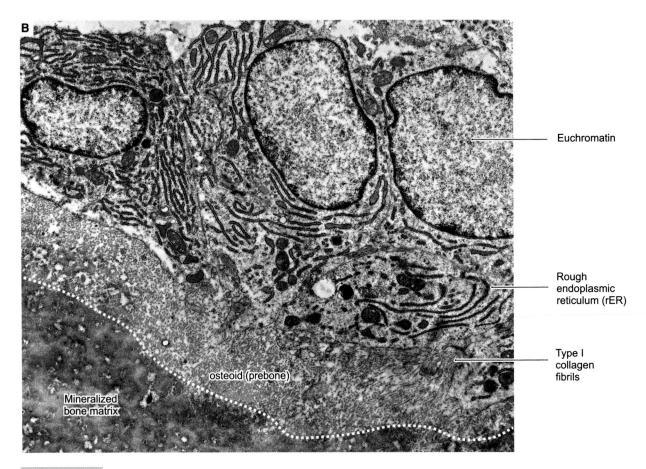

B

Euchromatin

Rough
endoplasmic
reticulum (rER)

Type I
collagen
fibrils

osteoid (prebone)

Mineralized
bone matrix

Figure 5-11B. Osteoblasts. EM, ×19,600

The three **osteoblasts** in this electron micrograph are clearly active in the synthesis and secretion of **type I collagen** and other proteins of bone matrix. Note the high content of **euchromatin** in the nuclei and the predominance of **RER** in the cytoplasm. Minute collagen fibrils (type I collagen) are just discernible in the layer of matrix adjacent to the cells (**prebone** or **osteoid**). The deeper, mineralized bone matrix has a homogeneous appearance that masks the presence of the collagen fibrils. The *dotted white line* indicates the interface between the osteoid above and the **mineralized bone matrix** below.

OSTEOCLASTS

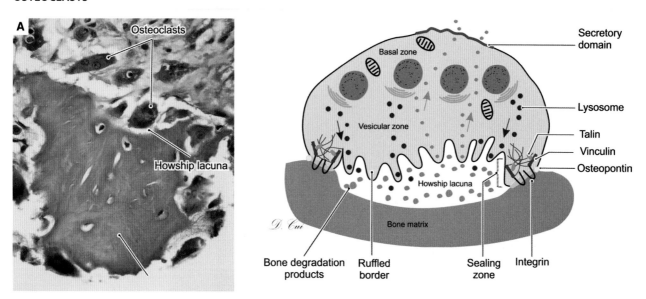

Figure 5-12A. Overview of osteoclasts and their activities. H&E, ×400 (*left*)

Osteoclasts are large multinucleate cells. They derive from monocytes and play an important role in bone resorption and remodeling. The osteoclasts have four regions: basal zone, vesicular zone, ruffled border, and sealing zone. (1) The **basal zone** contains most of the organelles and nuclei. (2) The **vesicular zone** contains vesicles, including lysosomes (lysosomal enzymes) and vesicles for transporting degraded bone products from the Howship lacuna to the inside of the cell via endocytosis. (3) The **ruffled border**, close to the Howship lacuna, is the region that has the folded cell membrane that increases the cell surface area to help increase the efficiency of the resorption of bone matrix. (4) The **sealing zone**, also called the clear zone, is an electron-dense area, free of organelles that surrounds the edge of the ruffled border and provides an attachment between the bone matrix and the cell membrane. Produced by **osteoblasts, osteopontin** is one of the **glycoproteins**, which bind **integrin receptors** and **attachment proteins** (**vinculin** and **talin**) to the **actin filaments** on the edge of the ruffled border. **Osteopontin** plays an important role aiding in the formation of the **sealing zone**, which provides an isolating space for the degrading bone matrix. The Howship lacuna is a space that is formed after bone matrix is reabsorbed by the osteoclast. The vesicles containing degraded bone products are transported from the inside of the osteoclast to the outside environment through a functional secretory domain at the cell membrane close to the basal zone via exocytosis.

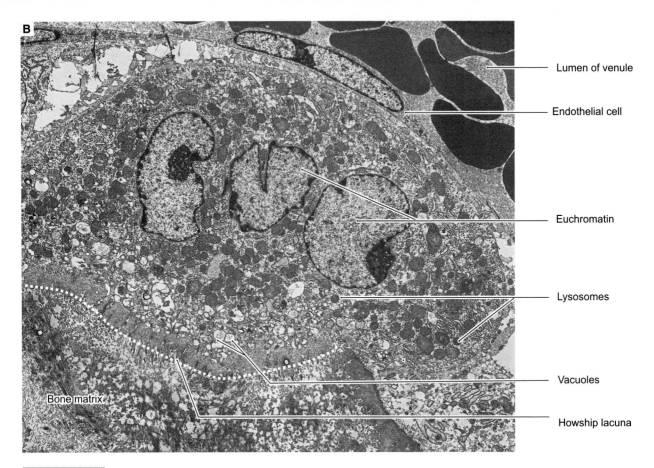

B

— Lumen of venule

— Endothelial cell

— Euchromatin

— Lysosomes

— Vacuoles

— Howship lacuna

Bone matrix

Figure 5-12B. Osteoclast. EM, ×14,000

Osteoclasts are large, multinucleated cells derived from cells seen in circulating blood as monocytes, which are derived, in turn, from progenitor cells in the bone marrow. Key features in identifying an osteoclast are multiple nuclei, abundance of **mitochondria** in the cytoplasm, and intimate attachment to the surface of bone matrix. The mitochondria provide the energy for pumping protons into the space adjacent to the **bone matrix**. The cytoplasm near the matrix contains **lysosomes**, the acid hydrolases of which are secreted into the space adjacent to the bone matrix. This area of the cytoplasm also contains numerous electron lucent **vacuoles** that probably reflect **endocytosis** of degraded matrix components. In an active osteoclast, the **plasmalemma** in the central part of the interface between the cell and the matrix is highly folded into a ruffled border, a structure that is not discernible in this electron micrograph.

BONE REMODELING

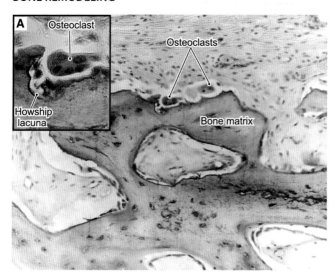

Figure 5-13A. Bone remodeling, nasal. H&E, ×136; inset ×363

Bone remodeling is necessary during bone formation in order to mold the bone into a proper shape to carry out its function. Remodeling usually occurs on the surface of the bone where **osteoblasts** and **osteoclasts** play different roles. In order to achieve a certain shape, bone matrix is continually being deposited by *osteoblasts* in one region, and, at the same time, bone matrix is being absorbed by osteoclasts in another area. *Osteoclasts* are large, multinucleated cells, which originate from monocytes and act as phagocytes. They often sit in the **Howship lacunae** (eroded grooves produced by ongoing reabsorption) on the bone surface. Osteoclasts are under the influence of the hormone **calcitonin**, which is synthesized by the **thyroid gland** and **parathyroid hormone** produced by the **parathyroid gland**. **Calcitonin** directly inhibits osteoclast activity and reduces bone reabsorption. **Parathyroid hormone** indirectly increases osteoclast activity and increases bone reabsorption.

Bone Development and Growth

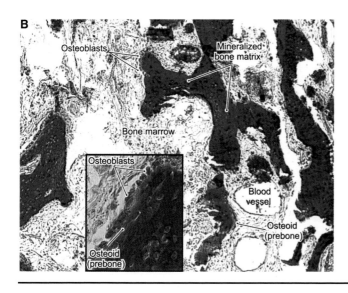

Figure 5-13B. Intramembranous ossification, fetal head. H&E, ×84; inset ×210

Intramembranous ossification is a process of bone formation involving the transformation of condensed **mesenchymal tissue** into bone tissue by differentiation of mesenchymal cells into **osteoblasts** and deposition of **osteoid (prebone)**. *Osteoid* is unmineralized new bone, which contains organic components. Soon after the new bone is deposited, it becomes calcified bone, which is largely composed of **calcium** and **phosphate**. *Osteoblasts* often line up on the surface of the bone matrix. They are cuboidal and low columnar in shape, and each osteoblast contains a large round nucleus and basophilic cytoplasm containing rich **RER** and **Golgi complexes**, indicating their activity in producing protein and organic components. **Mature osteoblasts** are trapped inside the bone matrix to become **osteocytes**. Osteoid appears pink in H&E stain, in contrast to mineralized bone matrix that appears dark red-purple in H&E stain.

INTRAMEMBRANOUS OSSIFICATION

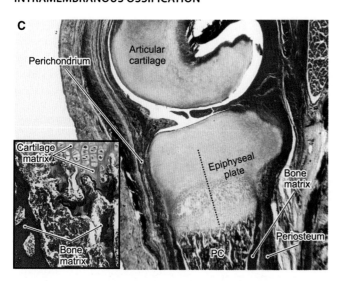

Figure 5-13C. Endochondral ossification, finger. H&E, ×20; inset ×68

Endochondral ossification is a process of bone formation in which hyaline cartilage serves as a cartilage model (precursor). Cartilage proliferation occurs, then calcification, and gradually the cartilage is replaced by bone. This is an example of a long bone (finger), showing the **epiphyseal plate** (cartilage plate) with the **primary ossification center** (primary marrow cavity). There is a thick layer of dense connective tissue covering the peripheral region of the cartilage, called the **perichondrium**. The connective tissue layer that covers the outer surface of the bone is called **periosteum**. The primary ossification center contains blood vessels, newly formed bone tissue, osteoblasts, osteoclasts, calcified cartilage matrix, and dead chondrocytes. (PC, primary ossification center.)

ENDOCHONDRAL OSSIFICATION

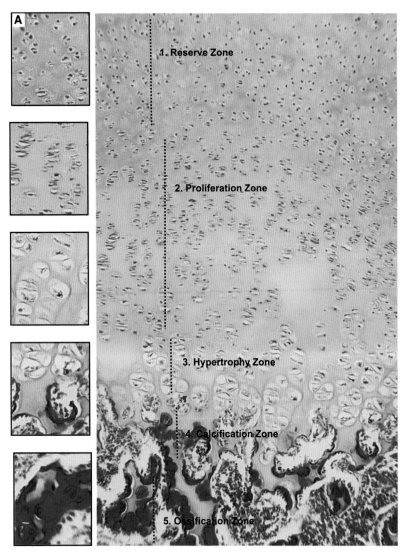

Figure 5-14A. Epiphyseal plate, finger. H&E, ×71; small images ×96

The **epiphyseal plate** is a region of hyaline cartilage at the ends (epiphyses) of the shafts of long bones. Its chondrocytes are undergoing the process of proliferation, hypertrophy, and calcification, during the process of endochondral ossification. The epiphyseal plate can be divided into five functionally distinct zones beginning at the epiphyseal end: (1) In the **reserve zone**, cartilage chondrocytes are inactive and individual cells are not arranged in isogenous groups. These cells are small and randomly scattered in the matrix. (2) In the **proliferation zone**, chondrocytes undergo frequent mitosis and are arranged in groups of columns (indicative of interstitial growth of cartilage) in this region. Chondrocytes are flat, and their size is increased leading to increased length of the cartilage. (3) In the **hypertrophy zone**, chondrocytes become mature, and their size increases markedly (big and fat cells). Isogenous groups are clearly evidenced and cells actively deposit matrix (type X and XI collagen). (4) In the **calcification zone**, cartilage matrix becomes calcified, and chondrocytes die because nutrients and oxygen cannot diffuse through the calcified cartilage matrix. The matrix in this region is filled with hydroxyapatite (a complex phosphate of calcium). (5) In the **ossification zone**, blood vessels invade and create primary marrow; osteoprogenitor cells arrive in this region and differentiate into osteoblasts to start depositing bone matrix (osteoid or new bone) on the surface of the calcified cartilage. Osteoclasts are also present and function as phagocytes to remove unwanted calcified cartilage matrix and dead chondrocytes.

CLINICAL CORRELATION

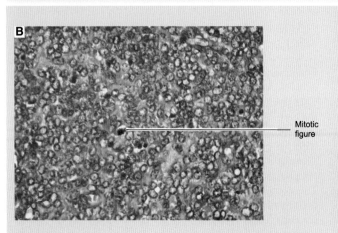

Mitotic figure

Figure 5-14B Ewing Sarcoma of Bone. H&E, ×400

Ewing sarcoma is the second most common bone tumor in children, after osteosarcoma. This sarcoma has a predilection to arise in the diaphysis of long, tubular bones such as the femur. Patients may develop a local mass, pain, and occasional fever. Ewing sarcoma may also arise in soft tissues. If the tumor expresses neural differentiation (expression of antigens typically found in neural-type tissues), the term primitive neuroectodermal tumor (PNET) is preferred, although there is no clinical distinction between the two. Histologically, the tumor shows sheets of small, round, blue cells. If neural differentiation is present, rosettes of cells may be seen. The t(11;22) chromosomal translocation is seen in the majority Ewing sarcoma cases.

EPIPHYSEAL PLATE

ENDOCHONDRAL OSSIFICATION—LONG BONE GROWTH

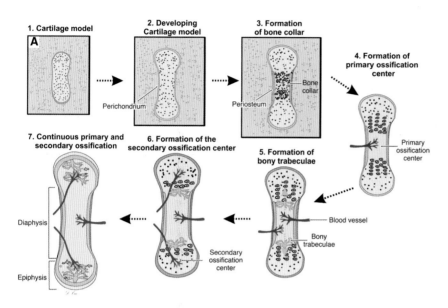

Figure 5-15A. Representation of the development of a long bone.

Most **long bones** are formed by endochondral ossification, a process of bone formation involving hyaline cartilage serving as a cartilage model, cartilage proliferation and calcification, and gradual replacement by bone. Long bone formation includes the following steps: (1) **Cartilage model:** A small piece of hyaline cartilage is formed by mesenchymal tissue, and the outer part of this tissue condenses to form a **perichondrium.** (2) **Developing cartilage model:** Cartilage assumes the shape for the future bone. (3) **Formation of bone collar:** As the cartilage proliferates, the perichondrium in the middle shaft region transforms into **periosteum.** Osteoprogenitor cells in the periosteum differentiate into osteoblasts, which start to form the **bone collar** (periosteal bone) by intramembranous ossification. (4) **Formation of primary ossification centers:** The cartilage plate (epiphyseal plate) continues to proliferate and then calcify. The bone collar (contains bone matrix, osteoblasts, and osteoclasts) triggers blood vessels to invade and create a primary marrow cavity. (5) **Formation of bony trabeculae:** Osteoprogenitor cells in the periosteum migrate with blood vessels into the region of the calcified cartilage. These cells become osteoblasts and begin to deposit **osteoid** (prebone) on the surface of the calcified cartilage matrix. At the same time, osteoclasts remove dead chondrocytes and extra calcified cartilage matrix, thereby producing **bony trabeculae.** (6) **Formation of secondary ossification centers:** A similar bone ossification takes place at the distal ends of long bones (epiphyses) called **secondary ossification centers.** (7) **Continuation of primary and secondary ossification:** Repetition of the endochondral ossification process results in more bone being produced and more cartilage being absorbed in both primary and secondary ossification centers. Finally, the cartilage in the epiphyseal plates disappears, and the primary ossification center meets the secondary ossification center at about age 20 in humans.

CLINICAL CORRELATION

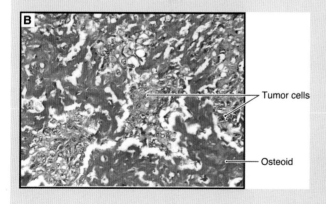

Figure 5-15B Osteosarcoma.

Osteosarcoma, also known as **osteogenic sarcoma**, is the most common primary malignant neoplasm of bone and occurs most commonly in the second decade of life. Conventional osteosarcoma tends to affect the long bones, including the distal femur, proximal tibia, and proximal humerus, and is most often a disease of the **metaphysis.** Clinically, patients may experience pain, decreased range of motion, edema, and localized warmth. Histologically, the **tumor cells** tend to be **pleomorphic** with a variety of sizes and shapes. Central to the diagnosis of osteosarcoma is the presence of **osteoid (prebone)** produced by the malignant cells (tumor cells). Osteoid is a dense, pink, amorphous material. Conventional osteosarcoma is an aggressive tumor and preferentially metastasizes to the lungs. Treatment involves surgery and chemotherapy.

CLINICAL CORRELATION

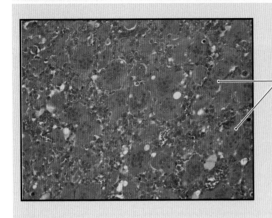

Osteoclast-like
giant cells

Figure 5-16. | Giant Cell Tumor. H&E, ×200

A **giant cell tumor** of bone is a benign, although locally aggressive tumor affecting the metaphyseal and epiphyseal regions of long bones, particularly the distal femur. In young patients, the tumor tends to be limited to the metaphysis. Patients may present symptoms similar to that seen in arthritis, with local pain and swelling. Some patients experience a pathologic fracture due to the local destruction and weakening of the bone. The most common treatment for these lesions is surgery. The histologic appearance shows sheets of osteoclast-like giant cells and mononuclear cells, occasionally associated with necrosis and hemorrhage. The mononuclear cells are thought to be neoplastic primitive stromal cells that express the receptor activator of nuclear factor kappa-B ligand (RANKL), which stimulates the formation of the osteoclast-like giant cells.

TABLE 5-2   Bone

Types of Bone	Gross Appearance (Shape)	Characteristics	Main Locations	Main Functions
Classification Based on Gross Appearance				
Compact bone	Uniform; no trabeculae and spicules	Higher density; lamellae arranged in circular pattern	Outer portion of the bone (cortical bone)	Protection and support
Cancellous (spongy) bone	Irregular shape; trabeculae and spicules present; surrounded by the bone marrow cavities	Lower density; lamellae arranged in parallel pattern	Inner core of the bone (medullary bone)	Support; blood cell production
Classification Based on Shape				
Long bone	Longer than it is wide	Consists of diaphysis (long shaft) and two epiphyses at the ends	Limbs and fingers	Support and movement
Short bone	Short, cube shaped	Thin layer of compact bone outside and thick cancellous bone inside	Wrist and ankle bones	Movement
Flat bone	Flat, thin	Two parallel layers of compact bone separated by a layer of cancellous bone	Many bones of the skull, ribs, scapulae	Support; protection of brain and other soft tissues; blood cell production
Irregular bone	Irregular shape	Consists of thin layer of compact bone outside and cancellous bone inside	Vertebrae and bones of the pelvis	Support; protection of the spinal cord and pelvic viscera; blood cell production
Classification Based on Microscopic Observation				
Primary bone (immature bone)	Irregular arrangement	Lamellae without organized pattern; not heavily mineralized	Developing fetus	Bone development
Secondary bone (mature bone)	Regular arrangement	Well-organized lamellar pattern; heavily mineralized	Adults	Protection and support

From Histology to Pathology

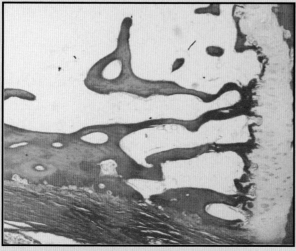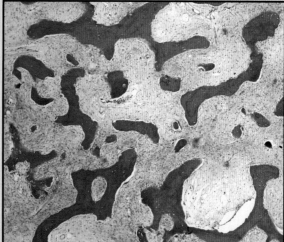

Figure 5-17. Normal bone and fibrous dysplasia. H&E, ×40

Normal long bone on the *left*. **Fibrous dysplasia** on the *right* is a benign bone disease, which affects adolescents during the time of bone growth. It loses the normal trabecular bone pattern and may produce disfiguring deformities with fractures. This image showing curvilinear trabeculae of woven bone among fibrous connective tissue resembles Chinese letters.

Clinical Vignette Questions

1. A 72-year-old man has experienced progressive pain in his right hip for 2 years. He now has difficulty getting out of bed due to pain and stiffness of his right hip joint. The joint remains stiff for about an hour, but the pain seems to get worse during the day, especially when he walks or tries to work in his garden. He gets some relief by resting and taking ibuprofen. At this time, his other joints are mobile and free of pain. Physical exam reveals no tenderness to palpation over the greater trochanter, and a routine x-ray reveals narrowing of the joint space and osteophyte formation. He reports no lower extremity numbness or weakness. Which of the following is the most likely diagnosis?

A. Gout
B. Osteoarthritis
C. Rheumatoid arthritis
D. Spinal stenosis
E. Trochanteric bursitis

2. A 42-year-old youth baseball coach experienced vague right knee pain over the last several months. He took ibuprofen for the pain with minimal results. In practice, while demonstrating a swing, he felt excruciating pain in his right knee area and fell to the ground. In the emergency room, an x-ray revealed a fracture of the distal right femur and a lytic bone lesion in the epiphyseal and metaphyseal areas. A biopsy of the lesion was performed and sent to pathology for an intraoperative consultation. The biopsy revealed sheets of osteoclast-like cells and mononuclear cells with hemorrhage. Based on this information, the most likely diagnosis is which of the following?

A. Aneurysmal bone cyst
B. Giant cell tumor
C. Osteochondroma
D. Osteogenic sarcoma
E. Osteoid osteoma

3. A 14-year-old male complains to his mother of pain around his left knee. His mother notices that the knee area appears swollen and slightly warm to the touch. Fearing he has an infection, she takes him to his pediatrician who obtains an x-ray of the knee region. The x-ray shows an osteolytic lesion involving the diaphyseal area of the distal femur with "onion skinning" of the surrounding periosteum. A bone biopsy is obtained, along with cytogenetic studies revealing a translocation between chromosomes 11 and 22. The bone biopsy of this lesion is most likely to show which of the following?

A. Malignant cells producing osteoid
B. Malignant spindle cells
C. Numerous giant cells
D. Sheets of plasma cells
E. Sheets of small, blue cells

6 Muscle

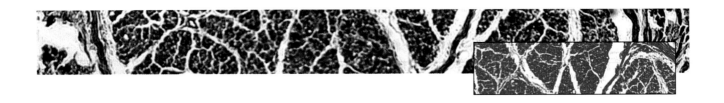

Introduction and Key Concepts for Muscle
Skeletal Muscle
Cardiac Muscle
Smooth Muscle

Introduction and Key Concepts for Muscle

The contraction of **muscle tissue** is the only way in which we can interact with our surroundings and is essential to maintaining life itself. There are three general types of muscles: **skeletal**, **cardiac**, and **smooth**. The voluntary contraction of *skeletal muscle* allows us to move our limbs, fingers, and toes; to turn our head and move our eyes; and to talk. Its name comes from the fact that most skeletal muscle attaches to bones of the skeleton and functions to move the skeleton. However, exceptions include the extraocular muscles, the tongue, and a few others. The continuous, rhythmic contraction of *cardiac muscle* pumps blood through our bodies, without ceasing, for our whole lifetime. Cardiac muscle contraction is involuntary, in contrast to that of skeletal muscle, although its frequency of contraction is modulated by the autonomic nervous system and by hormones and neurotransmitters in the blood. *Smooth muscle* is the most diverse type of muscle. It occurs in different subtypes in different organs and is essential for many involuntary physiological functions, which include regulating blood flow and blood pressure, aiding in the digestion of food, moving food through the digestive system, regulating air flow during respiration, controlling the diameter of the pupil in the eye, expelling the baby during childbirth, and others.

Skeletal Muscle

A single **skeletal muscle**, such as the **biceps**, is composed of numerous bundles of muscle fibers called **fascicles**. The muscle as a whole is surrounded by a sheet of dense connective tissues, called the **epimysium**. Each fascicle is surrounded by a sheet of moderately dense connective tissues, called the **perimysium**, and each individual muscle fiber (muscle cell) in a fascicle is surrounded by a delicate collagen network, called the **endomysium**. A skeletal muscle fiber is a long (as long as 10 cm in some muscles), thin (10–100 μm), tubular structure that contains many nuclei arranged in the cytoplasm (called **sarcoplasm**) just under the cell membrane (called **sarcolemma**). (Many words relating to muscle are derived from the Greek word *sarx*, meaning, "flesh.") A single muscle fiber contains many individual **myofibrils**, tiny bundles of contractile proteins.

CONTRACTION of skeletal muscle is voluntary. Skeletal muscle is characterized by a striped appearance when viewed at higher powers in light microscopy. This pattern of stripes (called **striations**), at right angles to the long axis of the muscle, is more obvious when viewed using polarized light and is striking in electron micrographs. The striations reflect a repeating pattern of contractile elements called **sarcomeres**. Each sarcomere is made up of an orderly array of **actin** and **myosin myofilaments**. Each myofilament consists of a bundle of actin or myosin molecules together with some additional accessory molecules. Sudden, all-or-none contraction occurs in a skeletal muscle fiber when a motor neuron action potential (see Chapter 7, "Nervous Tissue") releases acetylcholine at the neuromuscular junction. This causes a similar action potential to travel along the sarcolemma, triggering the release of **calcium ions** (Ca^{2+}) into the cytosol and initiating a complex interaction between the actin and the myosin myofilaments to produce shortening of the fiber. The necessary Ca^{2+} is stored within the muscle fiber in a modified endoplasmic reticulum called the **sarcoplasmic reticulum**. Calcium channels in the **terminal cisterns** of the sarcoplasmic reticulum open when the electrical action potential that is carried along the sarcolemma travels into the interior of the cell via the **transverse tubule system**. This system consists of many tubular invaginations of the sarcolemma that lie between pairs of terminal cisterns and encircle each myofibril, forming **triads**. In general, skeletal muscle is specialized for rapid contraction under neural control. Although each skeletal muscle fiber contracts at its maximum whenever it contracts, variations of overall force of muscle contraction are achieved by recruiting a greater or lesser number of muscle fibers at any given moment.

Cardiac Muscle

The **muscle of the heart** is similar to skeletal muscle in that it is striated, and the fibers contain sarcomeres made up of arrays of actin and myosin filaments. However, cardiac muscle cells are much shorter than those of skeletal muscle and typically split into two or more branches, which join end to end (or, **anastomose**) with other cells at **intercalated disks**. A transverse tubule system is present in cardiac muscle, but the sarcoplasmic reticulum is not as highly developed as in skeletal muscle. Each cardiac muscle fiber does not receive direct innervation as skeletal muscle fibers do. Excitation spreads from fiber to fiber via **gap junctions**. Contraction is also controlled by a system of **pacemaker nodes** and **Purkinje cells**.

Smooth Muscle

Muscle fibers that do not display striations are termed **smooth muscle**. This type of muscle also contracts by means of a Ca^{2+}-mediated interaction between **actin** and **myosin filaments**, but in contrast to skeletal and cardiac muscles, the filaments are not organized into sarcomeres. Furthermore, the Ca^{2+} enters the cell from the extracellular space rather than the sarcoplasmic reticulum (which is poorly developed in smooth muscle). Small, cup-shaped indentations in the sarcolemma called **caveolae** may play a role in sequestering calcium. Smooth muscle is diverse in its characteristics and is found in many different places in the body, including the gastrointestinal, vascular, respiratory, reproductive, and urinary systems and the ciliary muscle of the eye. For a given volume of muscle tissue, some types of smooth muscles are capable of generating more force and maintaining that force for a longer time than skeletal muscle. In some locations, including the ciliary muscle of the eye, some arteries, and the vas deferens, synapses occur directly between autonomic nerve fibers and individual muscle fibers and contraction is under direct neural control. This type of muscle is termed **multiunit muscle**. In contrast, **unitary** (or **visceral**) smooth muscle has fewer motor nerve endings, the transmitter is released into the intercellular space at multiple **varicosities** along the terminal portion of the axon, and the muscle fibers tend to have spontaneous, rhythmic contractions, modulated but not directed by the autonomic nervous system. Hormones in the bloodstream and stretch of the muscle itself can also influence muscle contractions, and excitation of the muscle fibers can move directly from fiber to fiber via gap junctions that link the membranes of adjacent muscle fibers.

Overview of Muscle Types

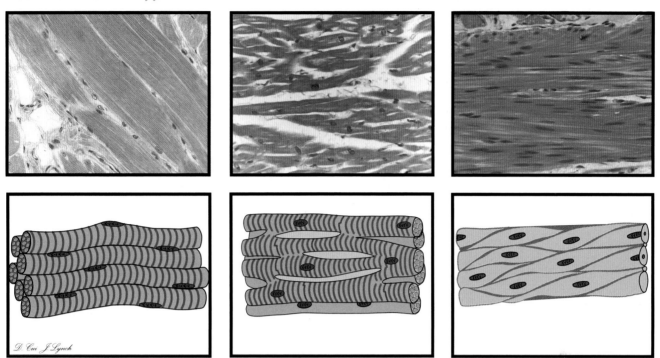

Figure 6-1. Overview of muscle types.

The three major types of contractile tissues in the body, **skeletal muscle, cardiac muscle,** and **smooth muscle,** have many properties in common but differ in many other ways. *Skeletal muscle* is usually, but not always, attached to the bones of the skeleton and is specialized to execute rapid voluntary movements of the limbs, digits, head, etc., in response to signals from the central nervous system (CNS). Skeletal muscle cells are long, thin, tubular structures with multiple nuclei clustered just under the cell membrane. Motor neuron axons form synapses (motor endplates) on each skeletal muscle fiber. Contraction in skeletal muscle is produced by a calcium-mediated interaction between myofilaments that are composed primarily of the proteins actin and myosin. The actin and myosin filaments are arranged into highly organized, repeating units called sarcomeres, which give skeletal muscle a striped ("striated") appearance when viewed at higher magnifications in light microscopy. The calcium necessary to initiate the actin-myosin reaction is stored in modified endoplasmic reticulum structures called the sarcoplasmic reticulum. Calcium is released when electrical charges flow down the transverse tubule system, which is formed by invaginations of the cell membrane, and is located adjacent to parts of the sarcoplasmic reticulum within the muscle cells. *Cardiac muscle*, in contrast, is specialized for repeated, rhythmic, automatic contractions over many years without ceasing. The contractile mechanism is similar to that of skeletal muscle: actin and myosin myofilaments are arranged in sarcomeres and their interaction is mediated by calcium release. However, cardiac muscle cells are short and split into two or three branches; these branching cells are joined end to end by intercalated disks. The overall structure of cardiac muscle is, therefore, one of a meshwork of contractile tissues, instead of being a collection of independent, parallel units such as is found in skeletal muscle. The autonomic axons that innervate cardiac muscle release their neurotransmitters into the intracellular space rather than onto individual cells at motor endplates as in skeletal muscle. The nervous system, therefore, modulates the rhythm of contraction of cardiac muscle but does not command individual contractions. *Smooth muscle* is found in many organ systems including the circulatory, respiratory, gastrointestinal, reproductive, and urinary systems. For the most part, smooth muscle is specialized for automatic, slow, rhythmic contraction, although a few muscles such as the ciliary muscle of the eye are exceptions. Like skeletal and cardiac muscles, smooth muscle uses actin and myosin filaments to produce contraction, but the myofilaments are not organized into sarcomeres. Instead, actin filaments are anchored to dense plaques in the smooth muscle sarcolemma, and a myosin filament contacts several individual actin filaments at both of its ends. These actin-myosin combinations are arranged in a random, crisscross pattern in some muscles and in parallel patterns in other muscles. As in skeletal and cardiac muscles, calcium is a critical factor in initiating a contraction, but in smooth muscle, the calcium is stored in the intercellular space rather than in a sarcoplasmic reticulum. As in cardiac muscle, autonomic motor nerves release neurotransmitters into the intercellular space rather than into motor endplates. The nervous system, therefore, modulates the inherent contractile rhythm of smooth muscle. This rhythm can also be influenced by hormones in the bloodstream and by mechanical stretching of the muscle. Electrical excitation and, hence, muscle contraction can also spread directly from cell to cell via gap junctions between the membranes of adjacent cells.

Skeletal Muscle

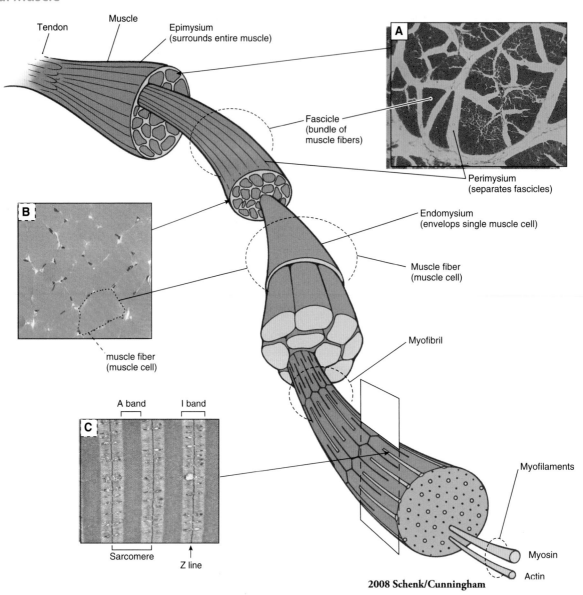

2008 Schenk/Cunningham

Figure 6-2.   Organization of skeletal muscle.

A single skeletal muscle (e.g., the biceps) is composed of numerous **fascicles** ("small bundles"). The muscle as a whole is enveloped in a strong layer of dense connective tissue, the **epimysium.** Each fascicle consists of a large number of **muscle fibers** (cells) and is surrounded by a sheet of less dense connective tissue, the **perimysium** (A). Muscle fibers are unusual among the cells of the body in that each contains a large number of nuclei, and the nuclei are located around the periphery of the cell (B). Each muscle fiber is enveloped by a thin layer of delicate connective tissue, the **endomysium.** An individual muscle fiber contains many **myofibrils,** which, in turn, consist of an array of regularly organized thick and thin **myofilaments,** the contractile elements of the muscle (D). The myofilaments are visible only with the electron microscope (C). Thick myofilaments are composed of clusters of **myosin** molecules, and the thin myofilaments are predominantly **actin** molecules but contain some additional auxiliary molecules that are important for the contraction process. In cross section, the myofilaments are arranged in a repeating pattern so that each threadlike cluster of myosin molecules is surrounded by six actin molecules in a hexagonal array, and the myosin molecule clusters themselves are arranged in a hexagonal array. Longitudinally, the actin and myosin molecules form repeating units called **sarcomeres** (C). Actin filaments are anchored at one end in the **Z line,** a transverse membrane-like structure. Myosin molecules lie parallel to the actin molecules and partially overlap the actin molecules that are attached to two adjacent Z lines. The region in which the myosin and actin overlap is designated the **A band,** and the region in which only actin molecules are present is designated the **I band** (C). Muscle contraction is the result of chemical interactions between the myosin and actin molecules.

DEVELOPMENT OF SKELETAL MUSCLE

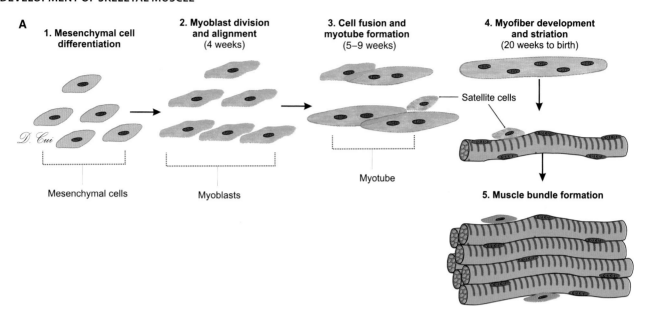

Figure 6-3A. Overview of the development of skeletal muscle (myogenesis).

Skeletal muscle forms from many myoblasts and begins during embryonic development. (1) **Mesenchymal cell differentiation:** Mesenchymal cells elongate, condense, and differentiate into myoblasts in the mesenchymal tissue at about 4 weeks of embryonic development. (2) **Myoblast division and alignment:** Then myoblasts begin to divide and line up in a row (cell alignment). (3) **Cell fusion and myotube formation:** During weeks 5 to 9 of embryonic development, myoblasts fuse together and gradually form an elongated myotube, which undergoes primary and secondary fusion. Some of the myoblasts remain undifferentiated; these cells become satellite cells that serve as stem cells capable of regenerating new muscle fibers in adult tissue. (4) **Myofiber development and striation:** Myotubes continue to lengthen and form myofilaments. Nuclei gradually move from the center to the periphery of the muscle fiber, and striations become more visible. (5) **Muscle bundle formation:** Muscle bundles form as muscle fibers are clustered or grouped together. This process is continuous, beginning at around week 20 of embryonic development and lasting until the birth.

REGENERATION OF SKELETAL MUSCLE

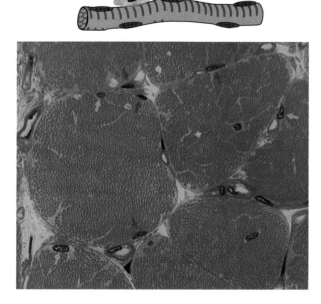

Figure 6-3B. Satellite cells and regeneration of skeletal muscle. H&E, ×272

Satellite cells are undifferentiated cells found within the basal lamina of the muscle fiber. They function similarly to stem cells and play important roles in the regeneration and repair of injured muscle fibers. The number of satellite cells decreases as an individual ages. When adult skeletal muscle tissue incurs damage, satellite cells become activated after a few days and undergo a proliferation process to form myoblasts. Then myoblasts differentiate and undergo alignment and fusion to form myotubes. Next, myotubes are fused together to form a multinucleated skeletal muscle fiber to replace damaged muscle fibers. An intact basal lamina is important for muscle regeneration. This image shows a cross section of a skeletal muscle (*green arrowheads* indicate nuclei of satellite cells; *red arrowheads* indicate nuclei of skeletal muscle fibers, cells).

However, skeletal muscle regeneration is limited. When extensive skeletal muscle damage occurs, connective tissue will replace some of the muscle fibers, and scar tissue will form. Certain diseases can affect skeletal muscle regeneration. For example, the number of satellite cells is greatly decreased in Duchenne muscular dystrophy (DMD), which is associated with the *dystrophin* gene. Dystrophin, a cytoplasmic protein, plays an important role to connect the cytoskeleton of a skeletal muscle fiber to the extracellular matrix.

MYOFIBRILS AND MYOFILAMENTS

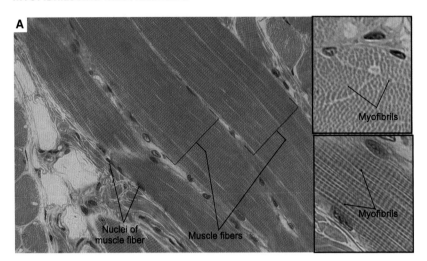

Figure 6-4A. Myofibrils of skeletal muscle. H&E, ×272, insets ×418

This is a longitudinal section of skeletal muscle fibers. Each muscle cell, also known as a muscle fiber or **myofiber**, has multiple nuclei, and it is about 20 cm in length. Each muscle fiber has numbers of **myofilaments** composed of **actin filaments** (**thin filaments**) and **myosin filaments** (**thick filaments**). The uniform organization of these filaments allows for the appearance of striations in skeletal muscle.

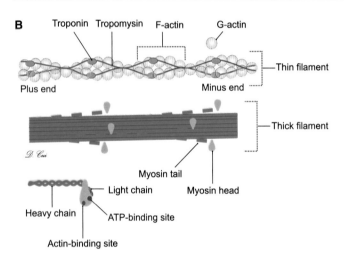

Figure 6-4B. Organization of myofilaments.

The **thin filament** is composed of **F-actin, troponin, tropomyosin**, and associated proteins. (1) **F-actin** is formed by a number of **G-actin** molecules organized into a double helix. F-actin is the core of the thin filament and has a *minus end* and a *plus end*, giving it polarity. The **plus end** binds to the **Z-line** of skeletal muscle, and the **minus end** is located in the **H band** and moves toward the **M line**. F-actin has a myosin-binding site. (2) **Troponin** contains **troponin-T, troponin-C**, and **troponin-I**. It holds **tropomyosin** in place and has a calcium-binding site able to bind **calcium**, which contributes to the initiation of muscle contraction. (3) **Tropomyosin** blocks the myosin-binding site on the thin filament, helping to prevent the muscle from contracting during the resting state. The **thick filament** is mainly composed of **myosin II** and associated proteins (**myomesin, titin**, and **C protein**). Myosin II is a molecule shaped like a golf club, and it includes myosin heavy chains (myosin heads and tails) and light chains. An actin-binding site and an ATP-binding site on the myosin head binds to the actin filament and ATP during muscle contraction.

CLINICAL CORRELATION

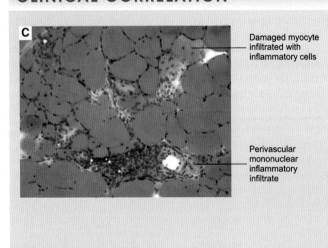

Figure 6-4C. Dermatomyositis, Skeletal Muscle (Deltoid). H&E, ×200

Dermatomyositis is a noninfectious inflammatory myopathy along with polymyositis and inclusion body myositis. **Dermatomyositis**, as the name suggests, is characterized by both skin and muscle findings. Skin changes include **periorbital edema** with a **violaceous to red rash** on the upper eyelids (heliotrope rash). A similar rash may be found on other parts of the body. Muscle weakness typically affects the proximal muscles first, so that patients may have difficulty arising from a chair. Some patients also experience difficulty **swallowing**, or **dysphagia**. Patients appear to be at greater risk for the development of **visceral cancers**. The **antinuclear antibody jo-1** can be detected in some patients with the **inflammatory myopathies**. Biopsy findings include **perifascicular atrophy** of muscle fibers, a predominantly perivascular mononuclear inflammatory cell infiltrate, and **necrosis** of **myocytes**.

STRIATIONS OF THE SKELETAL MUSCLE

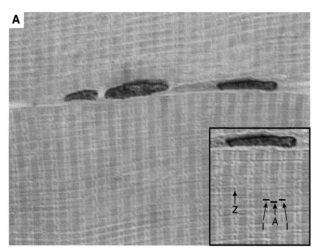

A

Figure 6-5A. Skeletal muscle, striations. H&E, ×1,480; inset ×1,800

A pattern of light and dark stripes is readily apparent in higher magnifications of **skeletal muscle**. This pattern gives skeletal muscle its alternate name, **striated ("striped") muscle**. The names of the striations are based on their behavior under polarized light. The dark bands are named **A bands** because they are **anisotropic** (rotate polarized light strongly), whereas the **I bands** are **isotropic** (rotate polarized light only slightly). The *A bands* correspond to regions in which myosin molecules and actin molecules overlap to a large extent; *I bands* correspond to regions in which actin molecules predominate. In the center of each I band is a thin dark line, the **Z line**, which corresponds to a membrane-like structure to which the ends of actin molecules are attached. This striated pattern was recognized from the early history of light microscopy, but its structural significance was not understood until the advent of practical electron microscope techniques in the 1950s.

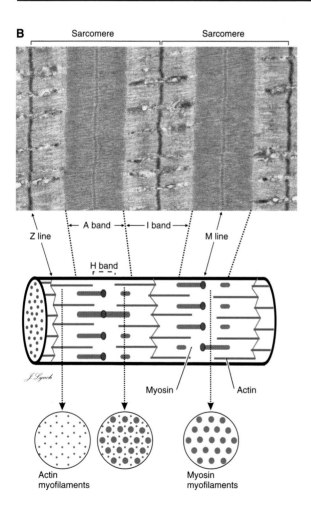

B

Figure 6-5B. Skeletal muscle—sarcomeres, myofilaments. EM, ×17,600

A **sarcomere** is defined as the portion of a myofibril between two adjacent **Z lines**. The electron micrograph at left illustrates two sarcomeres. The basic correspondence between the features on the electron micrograph and the constituent molecules is illustrated in the diagram at left below. **Actin myofilaments** (each consisting of many actin molecules and other accessory molecules) are anchored at the Z lines. **Myosin myofilaments** (each consisting of hundreds of myosin molecules) partially overlap the actin filaments. In cross section, both actin and myosin filaments are arrayed hexagonally.

Figure 6-5C. Muscle contraction.

Myosin and **actin filaments** (1) are not in contact with each other in the resting muscle. (2) When a contraction is initiated, myosin molecules undergo a conformational change and contact adjacent actin filaments. (3) An energy (adenosine triphosphate [ATP]) consuming reaction causes a further conformational change in the "head" of the myosin molecule, which produces a translational movement between the myosin and actin filaments. (4) The myosin molecule is released from the actin filament and the conformational changes are reversed. The process is repeated millions of times in a fraction of a second to produce contraction of the whole muscle.

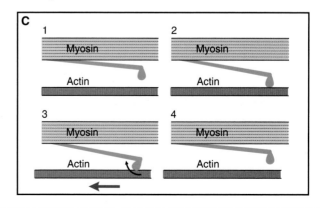

SKELETAL MUSCLE CONTRACTION AND TRANSVERSE TUBULE SYSTEM

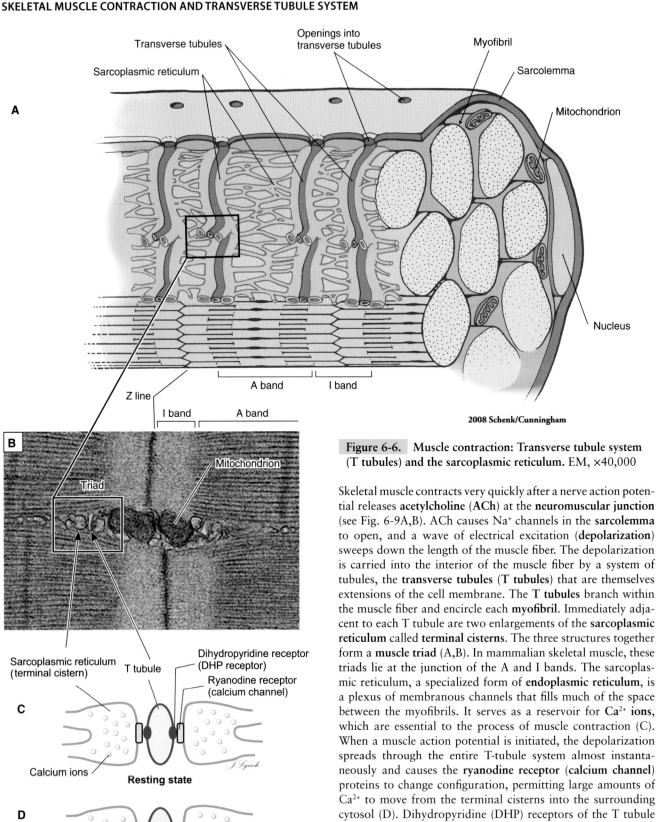

2008 Schenk/Cunningham

Figure 6-6. Muscle contraction: Transverse tubule system (T tubules) and the sarcoplasmic reticulum. EM, ×40,000

Skeletal muscle contracts very quickly after a nerve action potential releases **acetylcholine (ACh)** at the **neuromuscular junction** (see Fig. 6-9A,B). ACh causes Na⁺ channels in the **sarcolemma** to open, and a wave of electrical excitation (**depolarization**) sweeps down the length of the muscle fiber. The depolarization is carried into the interior of the muscle fiber by a system of tubules, the **transverse tubules (T tubules)** that are themselves extensions of the cell membrane. The **T tubules** branch within the muscle fiber and encircle each **myofibril**. Immediately adjacent to each T tubule are two enlargements of the **sarcoplasmic reticulum** called **terminal cisterns**. The three structures together form a **muscle triad** (A,B). In mammalian skeletal muscle, these triads lie at the junction of the A and I bands. The sarcoplasmic reticulum, a specialized form of **endoplasmic reticulum**, is a plexus of membranous channels that fills much of the space between the myofibrils. It serves as a reservoir for Ca^{2+} ions, which are essential to the process of muscle contraction (C). When a muscle action potential is initiated, the depolarization spreads through the entire T-tubule system almost instantaneously and causes the **ryanodine receptor (calcium channel)** proteins to change configuration, permitting large amounts of Ca^{2+} to move from the terminal cisterns into the surrounding cytosol (D). Dihydropyridine (DHP) receptors of the T tubule serve as voltage sensor to control release of calcium. Here, the Ca^{2+} initiates the reaction between the actin and myosin filaments that produces muscle contraction (C). At the end of the contraction, the Ca^{2+} is quickly returned to the sarcoplasmic reticulum by an **ATP-dependent pump** in its membrane.

EVENTS OF SKELETAL MUSCLE CONTRACTION

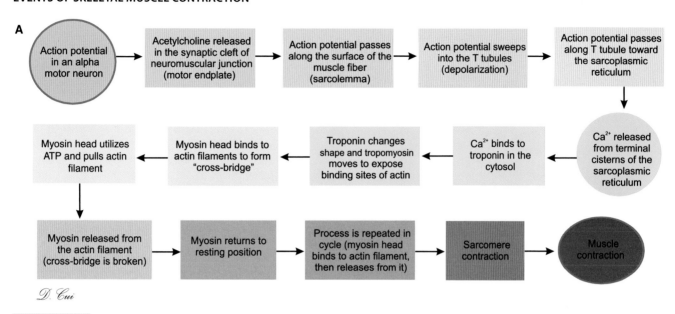

Figure 6-7A. Events of skeletal muscle contraction.

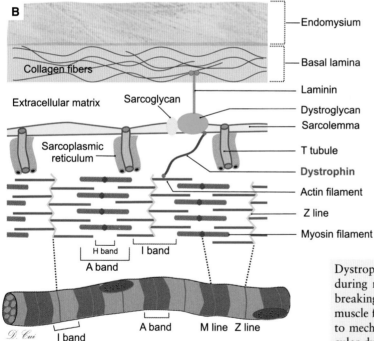

Figure 6-7B. Role of dystrophin in muscle function.

Dystrophin is a critical muscle cytoplasmic protein, which is a core component of the dystrophin-associated protein complex (DAPC). It is found between the inner surface of the cell membrane (sarcolemma), and it links to the cytoskeleton (actin filament) of the muscle fibers. It works with other DAPC proteins (dystroglycan, sarcoglycan, and laminin) to connect the cytoskeleton (actin filaments and myosin filaments) of the muscle cell to the collagen fibers in the basal lamina of the endomysium. This connection helps strengthen the contraction force and protects the sarcolemma from the stresses during muscle contraction.

Dystrophin plays an important role as "shock absorber" during muscle contraction and prevents muscle fibers from breaking down. In the absence of dystrophin, the integrity of muscle fibers is weakened, and they became more susceptible to mechanical injury, leading to necrosis. In Duchenne muscular dystrophy, affected muscle has only 2% of the satellite cells that a normal cell would have, and regenerative muscle capabilities are much lower than in the normal muscle.

CLINICAL CORRELATION

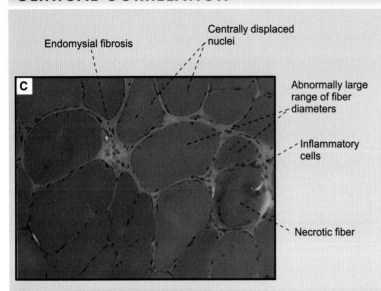

Endomysial fibrosis

Centrally displaced
nuclei

Abnormally large
range of fiber
diameters

Inflammatory
cells

Necrotic fiber

Figure 6-7C. Muscular Dystrophy. H&E, ×136

The **muscular dystrophies** are a group of inherited myogenic disorders characterized by progressive degeneration and weakness of skeletal muscle without associated abnormality of the nervous system. They can be subdivided into various groups based on the distribution and severity of muscle weakness and genetic findings. **Duchenne muscular dystrophy** ([DMD] illustrated here) is the most common and severe form of the disease. It is carried by mutation of an X-linked recessive gene, the **dystrophin** gene. The lack of the dystrophin protein impairs the transfer of force from actin filaments to the cell wall and causes the progressive weakness. Pathologic changes include **large variations in muscle fiber diameter**, extensive **endomysial fibrosis** between the fibers, degeneration and regeneration of fibers with **necrosis** and phagocytosis, **centrally displaced nuclei,** and replacement of muscle by fat and connective tissue. Steroids are the primary drugs used to treat DMD. Gene therapy using a functioning dystrophin protein has not yet been successful.

EXAMPLES OF SKELETAL MUSCLE

A
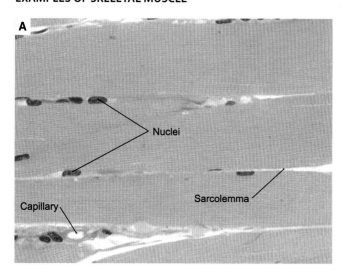

Figure 6-8A. Longitudinal section of striated muscle. H&E, ×400

The cellular units of skeletal muscle are called **muscle fibers**. Each fiber is a long, roughly cylindrical cell bounded by a plasma membrane, the **sarcolemma**. Muscle fibers range from 10 to 100 μm in diameter and may be many centimeters in length in mature muscles. This large size presents a problem for a single cell nucleus serving far distant cytoplasm and cell membrane. In skeletal muscle, this problem is solved by the formation of a **syncytium**, resulting from the fusion of several **myoblasts**, during development. A single muscle fiber will therefore have many nuclei. A distinctive feature of skeletal muscle, visible in this section, is a repeating pattern of dark and light bands oriented at right angles to the length of the fiber. These bands are designated **A bands** and **I bands**. Capillaries and myelinated nerve fibers are often observed in sections of skeletal muscle tissue.

B
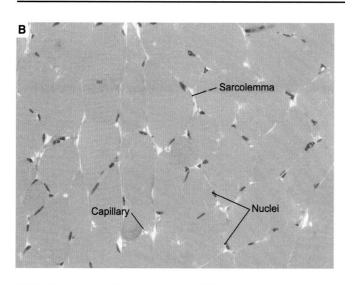

Figure 6-8B. Transverse section of skeletal muscle (tongue). H&E, ×272

Muscle fibers in the tongue run in several different directions, so, although most fibers in this section are cut transversely (in cross section), some are cut diagonally. Skeletal muscle fibers are round or polygonal in cross section, and, in a normal muscle, the fiber diameter is relatively uniform. The nuclei are flattened and lie peripherally in each fiber, just beneath the **sarcolemma**.

SYNOPSIS 6-1 Pathologic and Histologic Terms for Muscle

- **Anastomose:** To join end to end, as in suturing two blood vessels together.
- **Autoimmune disease:** A condition in which an individual's immune system mistakes the individual's own tissue for a foreign invader and attacks the tissue, as in myasthenia gravis or multiple sclerosis.
- **Caveolae:** Small, cup-shaped indentations in the sarcolemma of smooth muscle cells; may be involved in the influx of calcium during contraction.
- **Dystrophin:** A large, rod-shaped protein that plays a critical role in connecting the molecular contractile mechanism of skeletal muscle to the surrounding extracellular matrix so that the force of the actin-myosin contraction can be transferred to other structures to do useful work. The lack of dystrophin is a key feature of some types of muscular dystrophies.
- **Fibrosis:** Abnormal formation of connective tissue, including fibroblasts and connective tissue fibers, to replace normal tissues in response to tissue damage caused by disease or injury.
- **Hyperplasia:** Abnormal proliferation of cells, which may or may not lead to the increase in the size of the affected structure or organ; may be a precancerous condition.
- **Hypertrophy:** An increase in the size of a structure produced by an increase in the size of the cells that make up the structure.
- **Intrafusal:** Structures, particularly muscle fibers, that are found inside the muscle spindle. The word is derived from the Latin "*fusus*," which means "spindle."
- **Necrosis:** Pathologic death of cells or tissues as a result of irreversible damage because of disease or injury.
- **Synaptic cleft:** The small space between a presynaptic axon terminal and the postsynaptic membrane of a muscle cell or a neuron upon which the axon forms a synapse.
- **Varicosity:** A local swelling in a tubelike structure such as an axon.

MOTOR ENDPLATES

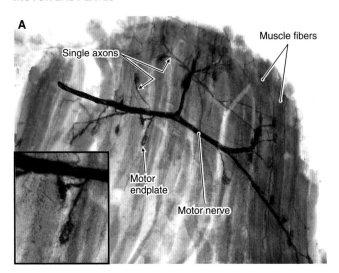

A

Single axons

Muscle fibers

Motor endplate

Motor nerve

Figure 6-9A. **Motor endplates on skeletal muscle.** Silver stain, ×83; inset ×184

A motor nerve (*black*) is shown terminating on skeletal muscle fibers (*violet*). The nerve contains several dozen individual **axons**, which leave the nerve and form multiple **motor endplates**. These endplates are the sites of the **neuromuscular junctions**, where the axon makes synaptic contact with individual muscle fibers. A single axon contacts numerous muscle fibers. The motor neuron, its associated axon, and all of the muscle fibers that it contacts are defined as a **motor unit**. Each time an action potential travels along the axon and causes the release of **Ach** at the neuromuscular junction, a contraction is produced in the muscle fibers innervated by that axon. In small muscles involved in fine movements, a single axon may contact 10 to 100 muscle fibers; in large muscles, which produce great force, the motor units may include 500 to 1,000 muscle fibers.

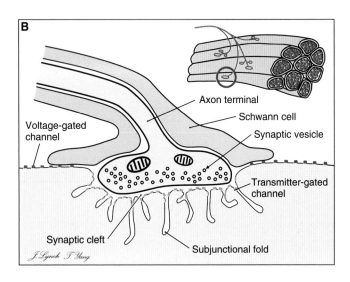

B

Voltage-gated channel

Axon terminal

Schwann cell

Synaptic vesicle

Transmitter-gated channel

Synaptic cleft

Subjunctional fold

J. Lynch T. Yang

Figure 6-9B. **Neuromuscular junction.**

A single motor endplate (*red circle in inset*) is shown in cross section. The nervous system controls muscle contraction using a combination of electrical and chemical signals. When an action potential travels to the end of an axon, the associated electrical charge causes the **synaptic vesicles** clustered in the axon terminal to release a **neurotransmitter, ACh,** into the **synaptic cleft.** The ACh acts upon **receptors** in **transmitter-gated ion channels** (*blue*) in the postsynaptic membrane. When the channels open, a voltage change occurs across the membrane, which, in turn, activates **voltage-gated channels** (*red*) in the sarcolemma. This voltage change sweeps rapidly along the sarcolemma and invades the T-tubule system, in which it causes the release of calcium ions and consequent muscle contraction. The **subjunctional folds** in the postsynaptic membrane serve as a reservoir for the enzyme acetylcholinesterase, which rapidly inactivates the ACh after each transmitter release.

CLINICAL CORRELATION

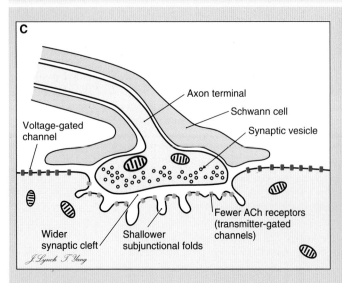

C

Voltage-gated channel

Axon terminal

Schwann cell

Synaptic vesicle

Wider synaptic cleft

Shallower subjunctional folds

Fewer ACh receptors (transmitter-gated channels)

J. Lynch T. Yang

Figure 6-9C. **Myasthenia Gravis.**

Myasthenia gravis is an **autoimmune disease** that affects the neuromuscular junction, causing fluctuating weakness and fatigue of skeletal muscles, including ocular, bulbar, limb, and respiratory muscles. **Acetylcholine receptor antibodies,** which block and attack ACh receptors in the postsynaptic membrane of the neuromuscular junction, are the most common causes, especially for patients who develop the disease in adolescence and adulthood. The mechanism may involve **thymic hyperplasia,** the binding of T lymphocytes to ACh receptors to stimulate B cells to produce autoantibodies, or genetic defects. This illustration shows fewer ACh receptors than normal, reduction in subjunctional fold depth and increased synaptic cleft width. Treatments include using anticholinesterase agents, immunosuppressive agents, and **thymectomy** (surgical excision of the thymus).

A

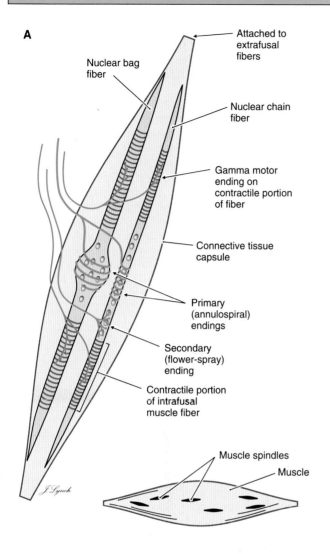

Nuclear bag fiber

Attached to extrafusal fibers

Nuclear chain fiber

Gamma motor ending on contractile portion of fiber

Connective tissue capsule

Primary (annulospiral) endings

Secondary (flower-spray) ending

Contractile portion of intrafusal muscle fiber

Muscle spindles

Muscle

J. Lynch

Figure 6-10A. Simplified schematic diagram of the intrafusal muscle fibers of a muscle spindle receptor.

Muscle spindles (a type of **stretch receptor**) play an important role in the control of voluntary movement, constantly monitoring the length of each muscle and the rate of change of that length. Each spindle contains 10 to 15 specialized muscle fibers (**intrafusal fibers**) innervated by sensory and motor nerve fibers and surrounded by a fluid-filled **connective tissue capsule**. Muscle spindles are generally about 1.5 mm in length and are anchored at each end to connective tissue attached to ordinary muscle fibers (**extrafusal fibers**). The spindle is stretched when the muscle lengthens and is shortened when the muscle itself becomes shorter. A given muscle will contain from a few dozen to a few hundred spindles distributed throughout the bulk of the muscle (*small drawing*). Two general types of muscle fibers are included in spindles: **nuclear bag fibers** (which have a swelling in the middle of the fiber where most of the nuclei are concentrated) and **nuclear chain fibers** (which are smaller in diameter and have a single row of nuclei). A typical human muscle spindle contains three to five nuclear bag fibers and 8 to 10 nuclear chain fibers. There are several highly specialized receptors associated with the sensory nerve endings, which are able to measure (1) muscle length, (2) change in muscle length, and (3) rate of change of muscle length. The sensory axons form two types of endings: (1) **primary** (or **annulospiral**) **endings** (*green*) in which the axon wraps around the equator of nuclear bag or nuclear chain fibers and (2) **secondary** (**flower-spray**) **endings** (*green*), which are more common on nuclear chain fibers. The two ends of each intrafusal fiber consist of contractile muscle very similar to that of the extrafusal fibers (*striated region in drawing*). These contractile portions of the intrafusal fibers are innervated by small-diameter myelinated motor axons (**gamma motor neurons** or **fusimotor neurons** [*blue*]). This innervation causes the intrafusal fibers to shorten when the muscle as a whole shortens and to relax when the muscle as a whole lengthens, therefore maintaining the sensitivity of the length-sensitive stretch receptors in their optimum range and providing accurate information about the state of the muscle to the motor centers of the CNS.

B

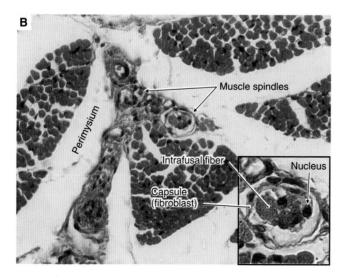

Perimysium

Muscle spindles

Intrafusal fiber

Nucleus

Capsule (fibroblast)

Figure 6-10B. Skeletal muscle—muscle spindle, cross section. H&E, ×272; inset ×680

Fascicles of skeletal muscle separated by **perimysium** are illustrated. Several **muscle spindles** can be seen in tangential section in the central fascicle. The flattened **fibroblasts** making up the capsule can be seen in the *inset*, as well as five or six **intrafusal fibers**. In general, muscles that are used in delicate, highly controlled movements contain the largest numbers of muscle spindles. The intrinsic muscles of the hand, for example, contain a relatively larger number of spindles than do larger muscles, such as the quadriceps and gluteus maximus, which are specialized for producing large amounts of force.

Cardiac Muscle

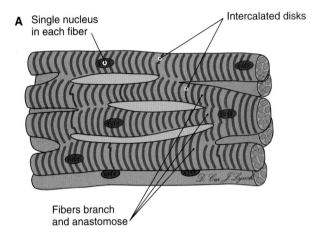

A Single nucleus in each fiber

Intercalated disks

Fibers branch and anastomose

D. Cui J. Lynch

Figure 6-11A. Organization of cardiac muscle—a branching network of interconnected muscle cells.

Cardiac muscle fibers split and branch repeatedly and join other muscle fibers end to end to form an **anastomosing** network of contractile tissues. In contrast to skeletal muscle, cardiac muscle fibers contract and relax spontaneously. The **intercalated disks** at the boundaries between fibers contain gap junctions, which permit electrical depolarization to move directly and rapidly from one myocyte to the next. The **sympathetic** and **parasympathetic innervation** of the heart serves to *increase* or *decrease* the rhythm of contraction rather than to command individual contractions as the peripheral nervous system does for skeletal muscle. This modulation of heart rate occurs via a system that includes the **sinoatrial** and **atrioventricular (AV) nodes** and specialized, highly conductive muscle fibers (**AV bundle** and **Purkinje fibers**) that connect the AV node with the contractile myocytes.

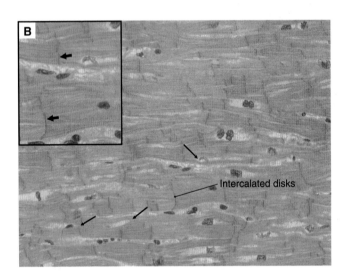

B

Intercalated disks

Figure 6-11B. Cardiac muscle, longitudinal section. H&E, ×272; inset ×418

Cardiac muscle is like skeletal muscle in that it is **striated**. Actin and myosin filaments are arranged into sarcomeres, with A bands, I bands, H bands, and Z lines. However, cardiac muscle is different in several respects. Actin and myosin filaments are not arranged in discrete myofibrils. **Cardiac muscle fibers** are much shorter than skeletal muscle fibers and typically split into two or more branches (*thin arrows*). The branches are joined, end to end, by **intercalated disks** (*thick arrows in inset*) and form a meshwork of muscle fibers. Each fiber has a single, centrally located nucleus, occasionally, two nuclei. Cardiac muscle tissue is highly vascularized and contains many more mitochondria than other muscle types, owing to its constant activity and resulting high metabolic requirements.

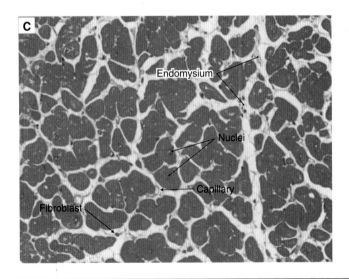

C

Endomysium

Nuclei

Capillary

Fibroblast

Figure 6-11C. Cardiac muscle, transverse section. H&E, ×272

Cardiac muscle fibers (**myocytes**) are elliptical or lobulated in transverse section. Each fiber (cell) has a single nucleus, which is irregular in shape and centrally located in the fiber, occasionally, two nuclei. Many **capillaries** traverse the tissue, and the **endomysium** is typically more prominent than in skeletal muscle.

CHARACTERISTIC OF CARDIAC MUSCLE

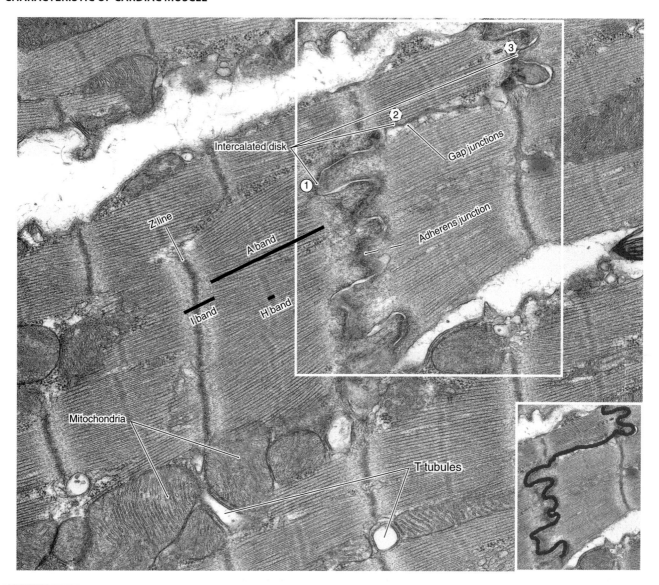

Figure 6-12. Cardiac muscle. EM, ×24,800

Cardiac muscle is similar to skeletal muscle in many respects. Both have similar arrangements of **actin** and **myosin filaments** that interact to produce contraction. The actin filaments are anchored at Z lines, and myosin filaments occupy a central position between two successive Z lines. The structures between two Z lines form a **sarcomere**. The resulting **A band, I band, H band,** and **Z line** are analogous in the two muscle types. However, there are several notable structural differences. The most obvious is that cardiac myocytes are much shorter than are skeletal muscle fibers and are joined to each other by complex structures called **intercalated disks.** The intercalated disks are specialized regions of the sarcolemma that contain regions of **fascia adherens,** which bind the adjacent cells together against the stress of contraction, and **gap junctions** which provide a path for the muscle action potential to travel directly from one cell to the next. The fascia adherens anchor actin filaments of one cardiocyte to another, while desmosomes anchoring intermediate filaments (desmin, in muscle) of the two adjacent cells. In the human heart, components of the fascia adherens and desmosomes are often mixed in one place, called **area composita.** A single intercalated disk typically includes portions that are oriented transversely with respect to the muscle fiber (1 and 3) and a portion that is oriented longitudinally (2). The path of this intercalated disk is indicated by the *red line in the inset.* **Gap junctions** are found predominantly in the longitudinal sections. A second major difference is in the T-tubule system. **T tubules** (invaginations of the cell membrane) are prominent in cardiac muscle, although there is only one tubule per sarcomere (located at the Z line) instead of two tubules per sarcomere (located at the A–I junctions) as in skeletal muscle. In addition, the **sarcoplasmic reticulum** is not as prominent in cardiac muscle and its function in contraction is not as well understood. Nevertheless, the release of Ca^{2+} is critical to contraction, just as in skeletal muscle. The muscle action potential travels along the cell membrane and T tubules and triggers the flow of Ca^{2+} into the cell from the extracellular space and from the sarcoplasmic reticulum. There is also a slow leakage of Ca^{2+} into the muscle fibers that is responsible for the spontaneous contraction and relaxation rhythm of isolated cardiac muscle. This natural rhythm is modified by **neuronal** (**autonomic**) and **hormonal influences.** Heart rate increases during physical exercise or stress and decreases during periods of rest and sleep.

Smooth Muscle

A

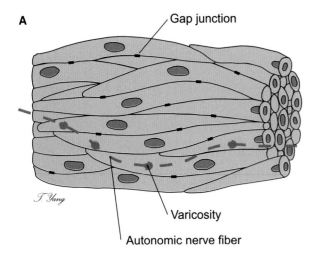

Gap junction

Varicosity

Autonomic nerve fiber

T. Yang

Figure 6-13A. **A representation of smooth muscle.**

Smooth muscle is similar to skeletal and cardiac muscle in that contraction is produced by the interaction of **actin** and **myosin filaments** in the presence of Ca²⁺. However, there are many differences. Smooth muscle fibers are short (15 to 500 μm) and **spindle shaped** and have single, centrally placed nuclei. Smooth muscle lacks the striations observed in skeletal and cardiac muscle because the arrangement of the actin and myosin filaments is not as orderly. Smooth muscle is innervated by sympathetic and parasympathetic axons, but transmitter molecules are released into the intercellular space at swellings in the axon (**varicosities**), rather than at specific neuromuscular junctions ("endplates") as in skeletal muscle. The sarcolemmas of some smooth muscles contain **gap junctions** that permit electrical excitation to move directly from one fiber to adjacent fibers, therefore producing a moving wave of contraction.

B

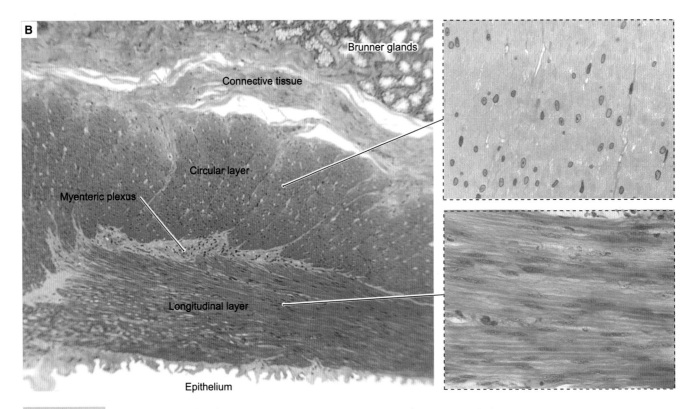

Brunner glands

Connective tissue

Circular layer

Myenteric plexus

Longitudinal layer

Epithelium

Figure 6-13B. **Smooth muscle, duodenum.** H&E, ×117; upper inset ×485; lower inset ×259

In the gastrointestinal tract, **smooth muscle** is important for keeping food moving at the proper rate to enhance digestion, to permit the absorption of nutrients, and to prepare waste to be expelled from the body. A low-power section through the duodenum of the small intestine is shown (*left*). Brunner glands are seen at the top of the image; beneath them is a layer of connective tissue. Bands of smooth muscles encircle the duodenum. A transverse section through this **circular layer** is shown at higher power in the *upper inset*. The nuclei are scattered randomly through the section. Many muscle fibers are cut through a portion of the fiber that does not contain a nucleus. A second layer of smooth muscle is oriented along the length of the duodenum and here, it is cut longitudinally. The *lower inset* shows a longitudinal section at higher power. Note the long, spindle-shaped nuclei. The smooth muscle of the gut is classified as **visceral** or **unitary smooth muscle** and has many gap junctions. Spontaneous waves of contraction move along the length of the gut, modulated by signals from pacemaker ganglia or **plexuses** in the autonomic nervous system. One such plexus, a **myenteric plexus**, is visible in the low-power photomicrograph.

UTERUS

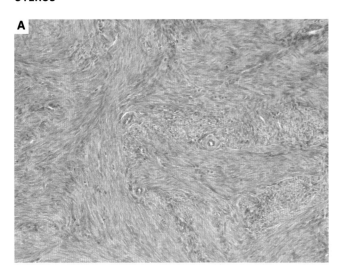

Figure 6-14A. Smooth muscle in the wall of the uterus. H&E, ×136

In most locations, fascicles of smooth muscle are oriented in the same direction. However, in hollow organs in which the overall size of the organ is reduced by smooth muscle contraction, such as the **uterus**, the fascicles are intertwined and run in all different directions. In this section, some fascicles are cut in a longitudinal plane, some in a tangential plane, and others are cut diagonally.

The large forces generated by uterine smooth muscle are important in **expelling the fetus during childbirth** and are also critical for **clamping down on blood vessels** to stop bleeding after the placenta is pulled away from its attachment to the wall of the uterus. Contraction of this smooth muscle can be enhanced by the administration of **oxytocic agents** (e.g., **oxytocin, ergonovine**) after delivery to stimulate myometrial contractions and prevent or treat **postpartum hemorrhage.**

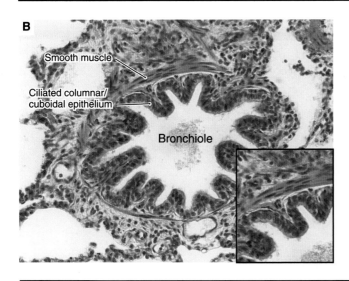

Smooth muscle

Ciliated columnar/ cuboidal epithelium

Bronchiole

Figure 6-14B. Smooth muscle in a bronchiole. H&E, ×136; inset ×160

Smooth muscle lines the walls of the bronchioles in the respiratory system. It relaxes to increase the size of the airway passages under the influence of the sympathetic nervous system and hormones controlled by the sympathetic nervous system, and it contracts to reduce the size of the airway passages under the influence of the parasympathetic nervous system. This smooth muscle aids in expelling air from the lungs during breathing. It is also important in the cough reflex, which helps to expel foreign matter such as dust, smoke, and excess mucus from the lungs. With age, and in response to irritants such as tobacco smoke, the contractility of smooth muscle may be reduced, causing respiratory insufficiency. Note the long, thin, spindle-shaped nuclei of the smooth muscle cells in the *inset*.

CLINICAL CORRELATION

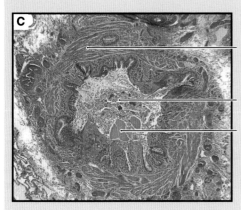

Thickening (hypertrophy and hyperplasia) of smooth muscle layer

Airway plugged by cell debris and mucus

Figure 6-14C. Chronic Asthma. H&E, ×27

Asthma is a chronic condition characterized by wheezing, shortness of breath, chest tightness, and coughing. Respiratory airways are hypersensitive and hyperresponsive to a variety of stimuli. Clinical findings include airflow obstruction caused by smooth muscle constriction around airways, airway mucosal edema, intraluminal mucus accumulation, inflammatory cell infiltration in the submucosa, and basement membrane thickening. During acute asthma attacks, spasms of smooth muscle together with excessive mucous secretion may close off airways and may be fatal. Pathologic findings include **smooth muscle thickening (hypertrophy** and **hyperplasia)** and remodeling of nearby small and mid-sized pulmonary blood vessels. Treatment includes using combinations of drugs and environmental and lifestyle changes.

CHARACTERISTIC OF SMOOTH MUSCLE

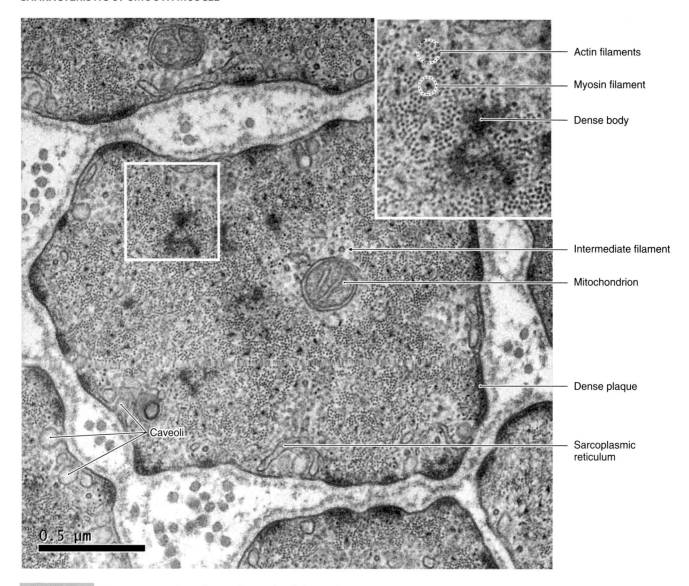

— Actin filaments

— Myosin filament

— Dense body

— Intermediate filament

— Mitochondrion

— Dense plaque

— Sarcoplasmic reticulum

Caveoli

0.5 µm

Figure 6-15. Transverse section of smooth muscle of the trachea. EM, ×14,750

Although contraction of smooth muscle is produced by a calcium-mediated interaction between **actin** and **myosin filaments** similar to that described in Figure 6-5C, there are significant differences in the structure of smooth muscle cells and striated (skeletal and cardiac) muscle cells. Actin and myosin filaments are clearly visible (*see inset*), but their arrangement is not as orderly as in skeletal muscle. Actin filaments are anchored to the cell walls at **dense plaques** or at **dense bodies** in the interior of the cell. The actin filaments contact myosin filaments to produce contraction, but the organization is more random and more changeable than in skeletal or cardiac muscle. Smooth muscle has the property of being able to produce relatively constant contractile force over a greater range of cell lengths than striated muscle. Skeletal muscle, for example, cannot produce maximum contraction force when it is fully extended because there is not sufficient overlap between the actin and myosin filaments. This property of smooth muscle is important in organs such as the stomach and uterus where strong contraction may be needed when the organ is distended and the muscle cells already considerably stretched. Some smooth muscles have the ability to remodel their contractile architecture in response to different conditions of muscle extension. **Intermediate filaments** provide mechanical and structural integrity for many types of cells, including smooth muscle. They are composed primarily of the proteins vimentin and desmin. Lack of these proteins impairs the contractility of smooth muscle. Contraction of smooth muscle can be initiated by **neural signals** (e.g., iris, respiratory system), **mechanical stretch** (e.g., gut, urinary tract), **electrical signals** traveling from one smooth muscle fiber to another via gap junctions (e.g., gut, respiratory system), or **hormones** in the blood stream (e.g., respiratory system, uterus). The calcium necessary to initiate contraction enters the cell from the **extracellular space** rather than from the **sarcoplasmic reticulum** as in striated muscle. Smooth muscle fibers have a poorly developed **sarcoplasmic reticulum** and no T-tubule system at all. Cup-shaped indentations in the sarcolemma (**caveolae**) may play a role in sequestering calcium.

SMOOTH MUSCLE FIBERS AND MUSCLE CONTRACTION

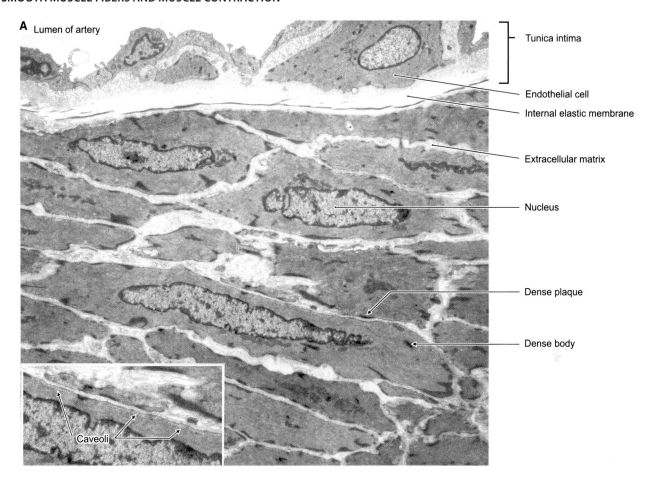

A Lumen of artery

Tunica intima

Endothelial cell

Internal elastic membrane

Extracellular matrix

Nucleus

Dense plaque

Dense body

Caveoli

Figure 6-16A. Smooth muscle fibers in the tunica media of a medium artery. EM, ×4,260; inset ×6,530

The smooth muscle fibers in this illustration are cut obliquely to their long axis. The thickenings of the cell membrane, which are termed **dense plaques**, can be clearly seen. Actin myofilaments are attached to these structures and the force of the actin-myosin contraction is transmitted to the cell wall at these points. Actin myofilaments are also sometimes anchored to **dense bodies** within the cytoplasm. In some types of smooth muscles (e.g., in the intestine), the myofilaments seem to be arranged randomly, in a criss-cross fashion. In other types (e.g., in the airway), myofilaments seem to be arranged in parallel. Smooth muscle cells transmit force from one to another via the **extracellular matrix** and, in some cases, via gap junctions between the cell membranes of adjacent cells. The extracellular matrix in smooth muscle is composed of elastin, collagen, and other elements, but in contrast to other tissues, it is secreted by the myocytes themselves rather than by fibroblasts. In some tissues, such as in elastic arteries and in the airway, smooth muscle fibers may, with age or disease, gradually lose their ability to contract and become more and more like fibroblasts.

B

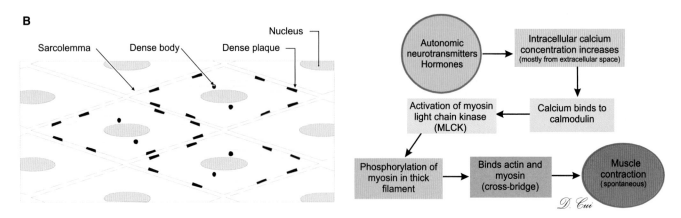

Figure 6-16B.   Contractile mechanism of smooth muscle.

Actin filaments (*red*) in smooth muscle are anchored in **dense plaques** in the cell walls, and the corresponding myosin filaments (*green*) are suspended between two or more actin filaments. This arrangement is much less orderly than the arrangement of actin and myosin in skeletal and cardiac muscles, thus preventing the appearance of striations. Furthermore, the organization is, to some extent, dynamic and can be rearranged in response to changing demands on the muscle. The cells are attached to each other via junctions with the collagen and elastin fibers in the extracellular matrix. The diagram on the *right* shows the events of smooth muscle contraction.

Nonmuscle Contractile Cells

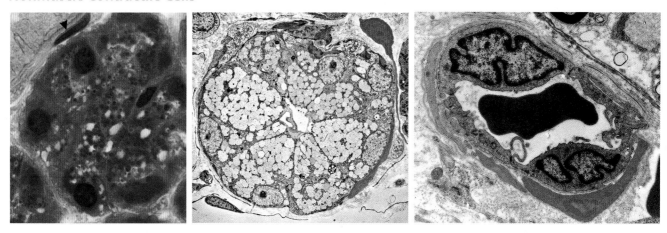

Figure 6-17. **Contractile nonmuscle cells.** H&E, ×1,079 (A); EM (B), ×6,818; EM (C), ×5,100

Here are some examples of contractile cells that do not belong to muscle cells but have contractile function. They can be found in glandular tissue, microvessels, and many other locations. (1) **Myoepithelial cells** contain actin and myosin, which is similar to the smooth muscle cell. Each cell has a flat nucleus located beneath a glandular, secretory cell within the basal lamina. The mechanism of contraction of myoepithelial cell is similar to that of smooth muscle. These cells can be found in the salivary glands (e.g., A & B: submandibular gland), mammary glands, and lacrimal glands. (2) **Pericytes** are elongated perivascular cells found in the microvessels (capillaries and small blood vessels). They are mesenchymal-like cells, having contractile function, and they play important roles in angiogenesis and blood flow regulation (C: capillary). (3) **Myofibroblasts** have features of both fibroblasts and smooth muscle cells. They contain actin and myosin in their cytoplasm and have contractile abilities. These cells differentiate from fibroblasts after tissue injury and contribute to tissue repair during wound healing.

TABLE 6-1   Muscle Characteristics

Features	Skeletal Muscle	Cardiac Muscle	Smooth Muscle
Striations	Yes	Yes	No
Fibers	Long, cylindrical, unbranched	Short, branched, anastomosing	Short, spindle shaped
Nuclei	Multiple, peripheral in cell	Single, central in cell	Single, central in cell
Cell junctions	No	Intercalated disks (fasciae adherents, desmosome/macula adherens, gap junctions)	Gap (nexus) junctions, adherens junctions
T tubules	Well developed	Well developed	No
Sarcoplasmic reticulum	Highly developed; has terminal cisterns	Less well developed; small cisterns	Present, but poorly developed
Regeneration	Yes, satellite cells	No	Yes, mitosis
Contraction	Initiated by nerve action potential	Spontaneous; pacemaker system; modulated by the nervous system and hormones	Spontaneous; modulated by the nervous system and hormones
Main function	Voluntary movement of limbs, digits, face, tongue, and other muscles	Involuntary rhythmic contractions; pumps blood to muscles and organs; modulated by physiologic and emotional factors	Involuntary control of blood vessel diameter, gut peristalsis, uterine contractions during childbirth, airway diameter, and others
Clinical correlations	Muscular dystrophy, Duchenne muscular dystrophy, myasthenia gravis, sarcopenia, muscular hypertrophies, desmin-related myofibrillar myopathy, amyotrophic lateral sclerosis (ALS)	Myocardial infarction, desmin-related cardiomyopathy, myocardial necrosis, cardiac troponins (troponin I and T) as markers for diagnosis of myocardial damage	Chronic asthma, leiomyoma, abnormal contractions of smooth muscle in blood vessels can cause hypertension, ischemia, and infarction

From Histology to Pathology

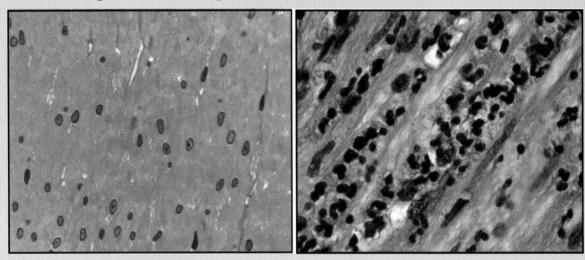

Figure 6-18. Normal smooth muscle and acute inflammation of smooth muscle. H&E, ×1,000

Normal smooth muscle is on the *left*. **Acute inflammation of smooth muscle** on the *right* shows an infiltration of neutrophils within the smooth muscle in acute appendicitis. During the acute inflammation, blood flow increases, and inflammatory cells migrate from the blood circulation into the tissue due to the immune response.

Clinical Vignette Questions

1. A 46-year-old female began to notice swelling and the appearance of a bluish rash on her upper eyelids. Weeks later, she experienced listlessness and muscle weakness that made it difficult for her to get out of a chair. In addition, after several more weeks, she began to have difficulty swallowing. At this point, she presented to her primary care physician who noted the continued periorbital swelling and rash. Physical exam also revealed swelling, erythema, and scaling over her knuckles and elbows. Laboratory tests were unremarkable except for a positive antinuclear antibody screen with subsequent tests revealing specificity for anti-Jo-1. A muscle biopsy shows perifascicular atrophy, a perivascular inflammatory infiltrate, and occasional damaged myocytes containing inflammatory cells. Based on this information, what is the most likely diagnosis?

A. Dermatomyositis
B. Myotonic dystrophy
C. Polymyositis
D. Sjögren syndrome
E. Systemic lupus erythematosus

2. A 3-year-old boy having difficulty running, jumping, and walking up steps was brought to the clinic by his mother. Physical examination reveals pseudohypertrophy of the calf and quadriceps muscles, lumbar lordosis, a waddling gait, shortening of the Achilles tendons, hypotonia, and hyporeflexia. When rising from the floor, the boy uses his hands to push himself to an upright position (positive Gower sign). The boy is shorter than average. Laboratory examination of peripheral blood reveals elevated creatine kinase (CK), and a muscle biopsy shows pathologic changes including large variations in muscle fiber diameter, muscle fiber necrosis, and centrally displaced nuclei. Which of the following is most likely the cause of this patient's condition?

A. Mutations in the alpha-tropomyosin gene
B. Mutations in the dystrophin gene
C. Mutations in the fibrillin 1 gene (*FBN1*)
D. Type I collagen (*Col1A*) defects
E. Type II collagen (*Col2A*) defects

7 Nervous Tissue

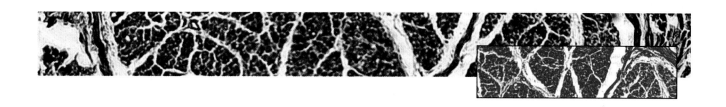

Introduction and Key Concepts for the Nervous System
Neurons and Synapses

Overview of the Peripheral and Central Nervous Systems
Peripheral Nervous System
Central Nervous System
Autonomic Nervous System

Introduction and Key Concepts for the Nervous System

It is difficult to consider the tissue of the nervous system separately from the nervous system itself. In most organ systems, the purpose of the tissue is to filter, secrete, or transfer gases or digest and absorb nutrients. The histologic structure of one small region of the liver or kidney or small intestine is very much like the structure of any other region of that organ, and the function of one portion of the organ is very much like the function of any other portion. By contrast, the purpose of the nervous system is to carry sensory information from the sensory organs to the brain; to process that sensory information in the brain to produce perceptions, memories, decisions, and plans; and to carry motor information from the brain to the skeletal muscles in order to exert an influence on the individual's surroundings. In truth, all we know of the world that surrounds us is carried as electrical impulses over our sensory nerves; the only way we have of interacting with that world is via electrical impulses carried by motor nerves from our brains to our muscles.

Neurons and Synapses

The building blocks of the nervous system are cells called **neurons**. These cells have a long, thin process, the **axon**, in which the cell membrane incorporates specialized protein **ion channels** that enable the axon to conduct an electrochemical signal (**action potential**) from the cell body to the **axon terminals**. Axon terminals of one neuron make synaptic contacts with other neurons, generally on processes called **dendrites** or on the cell body itself. When the action potential reaches the axon terminals, a **neurotransmitter** is released from **synaptic vesicles** into the terminals. The neurotransmitter molecules act on **receptor molecules** that are part of ion channels in the dendrites and soma of the next neuron in a chain. The constant interplay of excitatory and inhibitory influences at the many billions of synapses in the nervous system forms the basis of our ability to be aware of our surroundings and to initiate actions to influence our surroundings.

Overview of the Peripheral and Central Nervous Systems

By definition, the brain and spinal cord are classified as the **central nervous system (CNS)**, and the nerves and ganglia outside these structures are classified as the **peripheral nervous system (PNS)**. Collections of axons that carry action potentials from one place to another are called **nerves** in the PNS and **tracts** within the CNS. Clusters of neuron cell bodies are called **ganglia** in the PNS and **nuclei** or **cortices** in the CNS.

Peripheral Nervous System

Nerves in the **PNS** carry sensory information from receptors located in the skin, muscles, and other organs and carry motor commands from the CNS to muscles and glands. Nerves consist of clusters of axons surrounded by protective connective tissues. Nerve axons range in diameter from about 0.5 to 22 μm, with the conduction velocity being higher for larger axons. In addition, larger axons generally have a dense, lipid-rich coating, **myelin**, which further increases conduction velocity. The cell bodies associated with the sensory neurons are clustered in a swelling of the posterior spinal root, the **posterior (dorsal) root ganglion**.

Central Nervous System

The spinal cord consists of large bundles of myelinated and unmyelinated axons arranged into **ascending (sensory)** and **descending (motor) tracts**. The *ascending tracts* carry information from peripheral receptors to nuclei in the brainstem and thalamus and from there to the cerebral cortex. The *descending tracts* carry motor information from the cerebral cortex and motor centers in the brainstem to interneurons (relay neurons) in the motor pathways and directly to spinal motor neurons.

These motor neurons innervate muscles directly to produce movement. The tracts are clustered around a central region, the **spinal gray matter**, which contains large numbers of **sensory** and **motor interneurons, spinal motor neurons,** and **preganglionic autonomic visceromotor neurons**.

The higher levels of the CNS include large groups of **nuclei** including the **thalamus** and the **basal nuclei** as well as sensory and motor nuclei in the brainstem associated with cranial nerves. The **cerebellum** is a large, specialized structure composed of nuclei and cortex, and the **cerebral cortex** envelops the surface of the cerebral hemispheres.

MENINGES are brain hemisphere and spinal cord coverings with three layers of connective tissue membranes that protect the nervous system, provide mechanical stability, provide a support framework for arteries and veins, and enclose a space that is filled with cerebrospinal fluid (CSF), a fluid that is essential to the survival and normal function of the CNS. The meninges include the **dura mater**, the **arachnoid**, and the **pia mater**.

GLIAL CELLS are nonneural cells that provide a variety of support functions for the neurons that relate to nutrition, regulation of the extracellular environment including the blood-brain barrier, immune system, myelin insulation for many axons, and a host of other support functions.

Autonomic Nervous System

The **autonomic nervous system (ANS)** is composed of three divisions: **sympathetic, parasympathetic,** and **enteric**. The *sympathetic* and *parasympathetic divisions* function under direct CNS control; the *enteric division* functions somewhat more independently. The ANS, together with the **endocrine system** and under the general control of certain systems within the CNS, maintains the **homeostasis** of the internal environment of the body. That is, the autonomic and endocrine systems ensure that the levels of nutrients, electrolytes, oxygen, carbon dioxide, temperature, pH, osmolarity, and many other related variables are maintained within optimal physiological limits.

Neurons and Synapses

STRUCTURE OF A NEURON

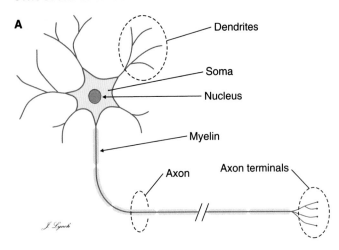

Figure 7-1A. Neurons: Building blocks of the nervous system.

Neurons contain the organelles that are common to all cells: a cell membrane, nucleus, endoplasmic reticulum, and cytoplasm. In addition, neurons possess two types of specialized processes, **dendrites** and **axons**. The plasma membranes of dendrites and of the cell body itself contain specialized receptors that react to the release of **neurotransmitters**. These molecules produce a change in polarization of the membrane. The membrane of axons, by contrast, is specialized to transmit electrochemical signals called **action potentials**. An action potential is a wave of membrane depolarization that maintains its size as it travels along the axon. When the action potential reaches the end of the axon, neurotransmitters are released from the **axon terminals** that influence the next neuron in line. Some axons are surrounded by a lipid-rich sheath called **myelin**, which facilitates the rapid conduction of action potentials.

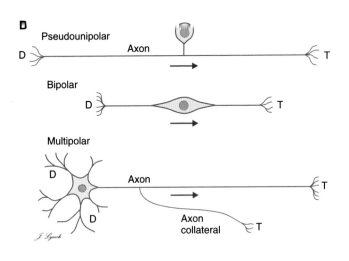

Figure 7-1B. Types of neurons.

Neurons can be classified on the basis of the shapes of their cell bodies and the general arrangement of their axons and dendrites. **Unipolar** or **pseudounipolar neurons** have a single process attached to a round cell body. This process typically divides and forms a long axon extending from sensory receptors in the various tissues of the body to synaptic terminals in the CNS. **Bipolar neurons** have a process extending from each end of the cell body. This type of neuron is found primarily in the eye, ear, vestibular end organs, and olfactory system. **Multipolar neurons** have many dendrites extending from the cell body and a single axon (although the axon may split into two or more **collateral axons** after it leaves the cell body). Multipolar neurons are the most numerous in the nervous system and have many different shapes and sizes. (D, dendrites; T, axon terminals ["terminal boutons" or "boutons terminaux"] with synaptic endings. *Red arrows* indicate the direction of information transmission.)

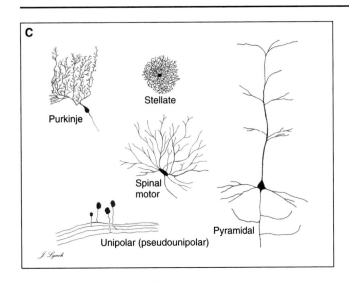

Figure 7-1C. Some representative neurons. Drawings from Golgi-stained tissue.

Neurons come in a wide variety of shapes and sizes, depending on their function and location. **Purkinje cells** are found in the cerebellar cortex. **Pyramidal cells** are the most numerous cells in the cerebral cortex. **Stellate cells** are also located in the cerebral cortex. Multipolar motor neurons are found in the anterior horn of the spinal cord (**spinal motor neurons**) and in the motor nuclei of cranial nerves. Other types of multipolar neurons are found in many central and autonomic nervous system sites. **Unipolar neurons** have cell bodies in the posterior root ganglia of the spinal cord. Their peripheral processes contact sensory receptors in the skin, muscles, and internal organs; their central processes form synapses on neurons in nuclei of the CNS. There are many additional types of neurons in the nervous system, but these represent some of the most common types and demonstrate the wide variety that exists.

TYPES OF STAINS FOR NEURONS

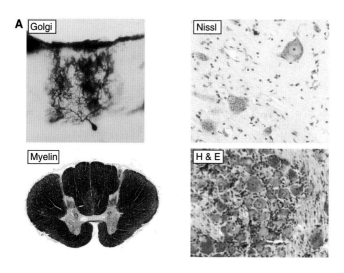

Figure 7-2A. Types of stains for neurons.

The various features of nervous tissue are more difficult to visualize than are the features of most other histological tissues. Consequently, several **special stains** are commonly used with nervous tissue. **Golgi preparations** stain all of the processes of an individual neuron (dendrites, cell body, and axon) but react with only a very small percentage of the total number of neurons (Purkinje cell, *upper left*). **Nissl stains** react with rough endoplasmic reticulum and, therefore, allow the shape and size of cell bodies to be visualized but do not stain dendrites and axons (spinal motor neurons, *upper right*). **Myelin stains** allow the visualization of myelinated fibers but do not react with cell bodies or dendrites (spinal cord, *lower left*). Myelinated fiber tracts are, therefore, dark, and areas with high concentrations of neuron cell bodies are light. **H&E stains** are often used in the diagnosis of pathological conditions and sometimes used to stain normal nervous tissue (posterior root ganglion, *lower right*).

SYNAPSE AND INFORMATION TRANSMISSION

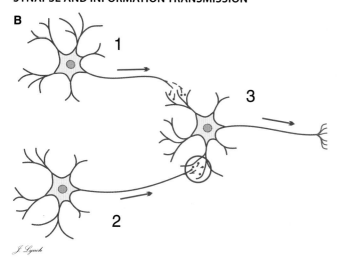

Figure 7-2B. Information transmission in the nervous system.

The primary functions of the **nervous system** are to **transfer information** (in the form of **action potentials**) from one place to another and to **process that information** to generate sensory experience, perceptions, ideas, and motor activity. Information is carried in the form of action potentials along **axons** (*red arrows 1 and 2*). At the ends of axons, there are **axon terminals**, where the electrochemical action potential causes the release of molecules called **neurotransmitters**. These molecules act upon **receptor complexes** in the dendrites and somas of the next neuron in a series (e.g., *3*) at regions of **synapses** (*red dashed circle*). The action of the neurotransmitters may be either excitatory or inhibitory on the **postsynaptic membrane**. When the excitatory influences on a neuron exceed the inhibitory influence by a certain threshold amount, that neuron generates an action potential that is then transmitted onto yet another neuron.

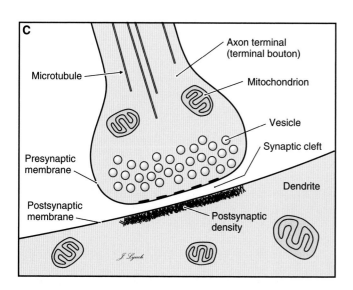

Figure 7-2C. Elements of the synapse.

A typical **chemical synapse** consists of a **terminal bouton** (a swelling at the end of an axon terminal) that includes a **presynaptic membrane**, a specialized **postsynaptic membrane**, and a space between the two (the **synaptic cleft**). The terminal bouton contains many **synaptic vesicles** that contain neurotransmitter molecules. When an action potential arrives at the axon terminal, a complex chemical process is initiated that culminates in the fusion of some vesicles with the presynaptic membrane and the discharge of their neurotransmitter molecules via **exocytosis** into the synaptic cleft where they can act on **receptors** in the postsynaptic membrane. The postsynaptic membrane is thickened in the immediate vicinity of the synapse as a result of the dense concentration of receptor protein complexes in that region. Both the presynaptic and postsynaptic regions contain numerous mitochondria, which supply the energy needed by the synaptic transmission process.

STRUCTURE OF THE SYNAPSE

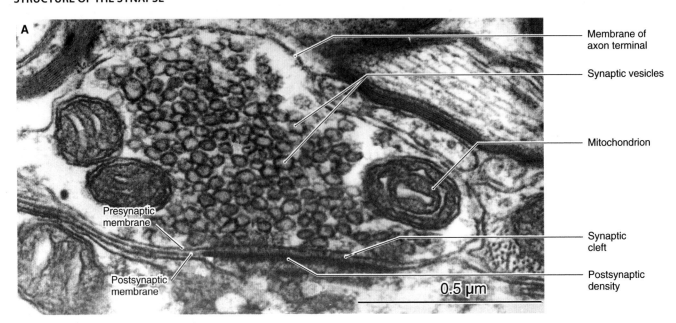

A

Membrane of
axon terminal

Synaptic vesicles

Mitochondrion

Presynaptic
membrane

Synaptic
cleft

Postsynaptic
membrane

Postsynaptic
density

0.5 μm

Figure 7-3A. Structure of the synapse. EM, scale line = 0.5 μm; ×104,000

A high magnification electron micrograph of an **axon terminal** and adjacent **postsynaptic membrane** is shown. Many **synaptic vesicles** and three **mitochondria** are visible within the axon terminal. When an action potential reaches the axon terminal, some synaptic vesicles fuse with the **presynaptic membrane** and empty their neurotransmitter molecules into the **synaptic cleft**. The transmitter molecules bind with receptor complexes in the postsynaptic membrane leading to either **depolarization** (excitatory influence) or **hyperpolarization** (inhibitory influence) of the postsynaptic membrane. The sum of the excitatory and inhibitory influences upon the postsynaptic neuron determines whether it will fire an action potential or not. The large difference in the thickness of the presynaptic and postsynaptic membranes makes this contact an **asymmetric synapse**. Differences in regions of **postsynaptic density** in different synapses are probably a reflection of different types of receptors in different postsynaptic membranes.

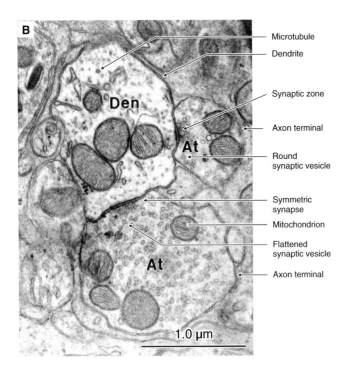

B

Den

At

At

Microtubule

Dendrite

Synaptic zone

Axon terminal

Round
synaptic vesicle

Symmetric
synapse

Mitochondrion

Flattened
synaptic vesicle

Axon terminal

1.0 μm

Figure 7-3B. Structure of the synapse. EM, scale line = 1.0 μm; ×35,000

Two **axon terminals** (*At*) form synaptic contacts with a **dendrite** (*Den*). The dendrite contains many **microtubules**, which are more concentrated in dendrites than in axon terminals. The smaller terminal contains predominantly **round vesicles**, which are generally associated with excitatory neurotransmitters, whereas the larger terminal contains many **flattened vesicles**. Such vesicles are usually associated with inhibitory neurotransmitters. A mixture of round and flattened vesicles is termed a **pleomorphic** distribution. The larger axon terminal forms a synapse in which the postsynaptic membrane is about the same thickness as the presynaptic membrane (**symmetric synapse**). This type of synapse is thought to indicate an **inhibitory synapse**, whereas a synapse in which the postsynaptic membrane is significantly thicker than the presynaptic membrane is an **asymmetric synapse** and is thought to be **excitatory** in its action. Numerous **mitochondria** are present in both the dendrite and the axon terminals. Other types of synapses not illustrated here include axon terminals that contact neuron cell bodies or the initial segment of axons, axon terminals that contact other axon terminals, and reciprocal synapses at which two adjacent dendrites form synaptic contacts with each other. In addition, terminal bundles of axons sometimes make multiple contacts through **boutons en passage** rather than terminal boutons.

TYPES OF SYNAPSES

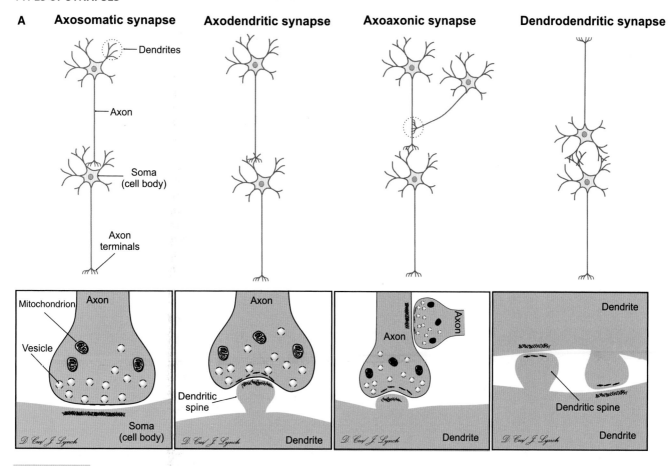

Figure 7-4A. Overview of types of synapses.

The synapse is a special region where an **electrochemical signal** in a **presynaptic neuron** causes the release of an **ionic current** and/or a **chemical substance (neurotransmitter)** that produces an electrochemical signal (postsynaptic potential) in the postsynaptic neuron. Synapses can be divided into several types based on their synaptic arrangement. (1) With **axosomatic synapses**, the signal transmits between an axon and the soma (cell body of the neuron). (2) With **axodendritic synapses**, the signal transmits between an axon and a dendrite. (3) With **axoaxonic synapses**, the signal transmits between axons. (4) With **dendrodendritic synapses**, the signal transmits between dendrites. (5) With **axosecretory synapses**, an axon terminal secretes directly into the bloodstream. (6) With **axoextracellular synapses**, an axon terminal with no connection secretes into the ECF. (7) With **axosynaptic synapses**, an axon terminal ends on another axon terminal. Others include somatodendritic, dendrosomatic, and somatosomatic synapses. The most common types of synapses are shown here.

NEUROMUSCULAR JUNCTION

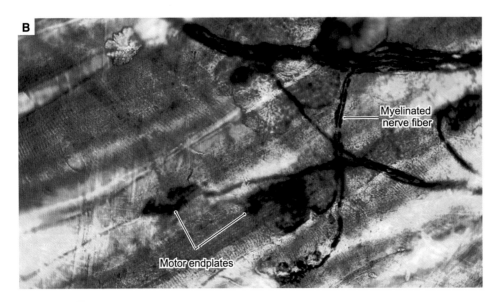

Figure 7-4B. **Chemical synapse: neuromuscular junction.** Silver stain, ×400

There are two main types of synapses based on their methods of transmitting signals: **electrical** and **chemical**. Electrical synapses transmit signals using electrical impulses, such as an ionic current. Chemical synapses use chemical molecules (neurotransmitters) to transmit signals. A neuromuscular junction (motor endplate) is the site of the chemical synapse between a motor nerve axon terminal and a skeletal muscle fiber. The neurotransmitter **acetylcholinesterase (ACH)** is released from the motor nerve axon terminal into the synaptic cleft, the space between the axon terminal of the motor nerve and the skeletal muscle fiber.

Overview of the Nervous System

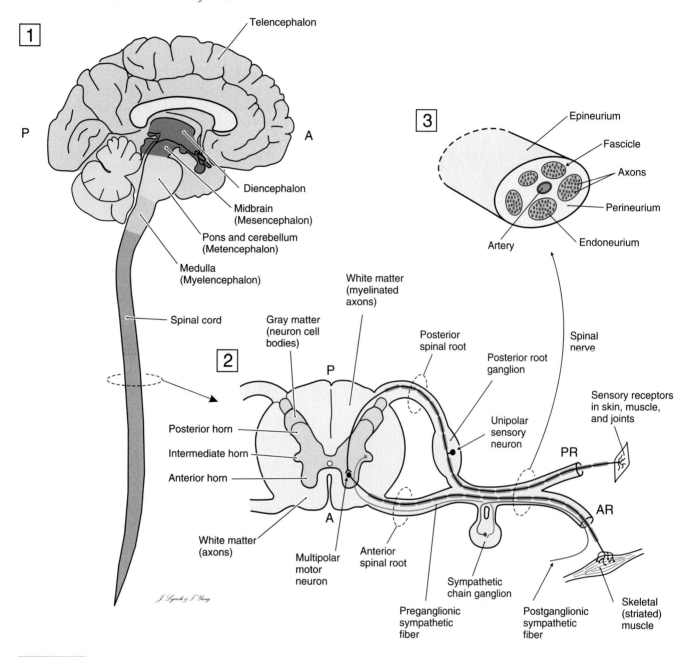

Figure 7-5. Overview of the central and peripheral nervous systems.

The nervous system is divided into three general divisions: the **CNS**, the **PNS**, and the **ANS**. The *CNS* consists of the brain and spinal cord (*1*). The brain is divided into five regions, labeled above, based on developmental considerations. A typical cross section through the spinal cord is illustrated in (*2*). The *PNS* includes all of the peripheral nerves, which join or exit the spinal cord as 31 sets of **spinal roots** and 12 sets of **cranial nerves**. In general, the **posterior spinal roots** carry sensory information from the body back to the CNS; the **anterior roots** carry motor signals from the CNS to the muscles and internal organs. The spinal cord includes large bundles of axons (**white matter** in *2*) that carry sensory signals to the brain or motor signals to motor neurons located in the gray matter of the spinal cord. The **gray matter** is composed of concentrations of neuron cell bodies. These neurons include interneurons in sensory and motor pathways, as well as motor neurons, which directly innervate muscle fibers. The color of the white matter derives from the shiny white lipid, **myelin**, that coats many of the axons. This coating is sparse in regions of concentrated neuron cell bodies, resulting in the gray color of those regions. **Peripheral nerves** (*3*) are composed of several bundles (**fascicles**) of axons surrounded by connective tissue. The *ANS* is devoted to the control of internal organs, glands, blood vessels, and associated structures and is diagrammed in Figure 7-14. It includes **sympathetic**, **parasympathetic**, and **enteric** subdivisions. (In *2*, A, anterior; P, posterior; AR, anterior ramus; PR, posterior ramus. Both the anterior and the posterior rami contain sensory, motor, and autonomic nerve fibers.)

Peripheral Nervous System
PERIPHERAL NERVE

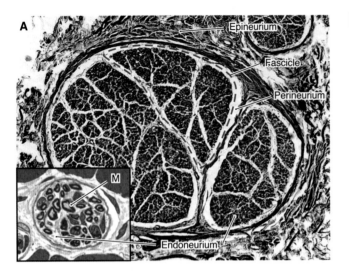

Figure 7-6A. **Cross section of a peripheral nerve.** Trichrome, ×68; inset toluidine blue, ×336

Peripheral nerve fibers carry motor, sensory, and autonomic nerve fibers. Peripheral nerves are surrounded by a sheath of dense, irregular connective tissue, the **epineurium**. Blood vessels that run with peripheral nerve trunks typically lie in the epineurium. The axons in a nerve are arranged into clusters called **fascicles** (*red dashed line*). Each fascicle is surrounded by a layer of connective tissue, the **perineurium**, containing many flattened fibroblasts. These cells are connected with each other, forming a **blood-nerve barrier** similar to the blood-brain barrier. Within fascicles, a loose, delicate connective tissue, the **endoneurium**, surrounds each axon. The *inset* shows a small branch of a motor nerve within a skeletal muscle. Many of the axons in this branch are surrounded by a dense layer of myelin (*M*). There are no separate fascicles within this small nerve branch but only myelinated axons each surrounded by endoneurium.

POSTERIOR ROOT GANGLION

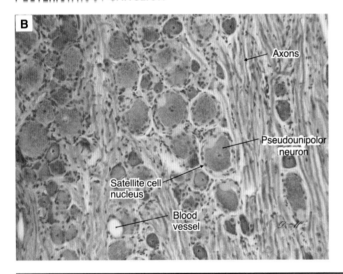

Figure 7-6B. **Posterior root ganglion.** H&E, ×146

Posterior root ganglia (**sensory ganglia**) are enlargements in the posterior peripheral nerve roots of the spinal cord and contain the cell bodies of **Pseudounipolar sensory neurons** and their axons. The cell bodies are generally round in shape with centrally located nuclei. There is a wide range of sizes of neuron cell bodies, with the largest having axons that are heavily myelinated and carry touch or muscle stretch information and the smallest having axons that are lightly myelinated or unmyelinated and that carry pain and temperature information. Small glialike cells, **satellite cells**, surround the neuron cell bodies and regulate the extracellular ionic environment. Schwann cells provide myelin for the myelinated axons. The posterior root contains only sensory neurons, whereas the anterior root contains axons of motor neurons. In contrast to autonomic ganglia (see below), there are no synapses in posterior root ganglia.

CLINICAL CORRELATION

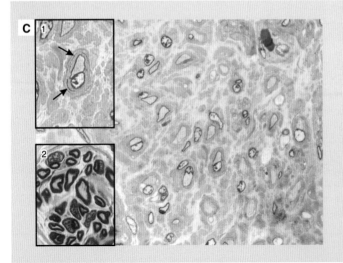

Figure 7-6C. **Hereditary Sensory Motor Neuropathy, Type III (HSMN III).** Paragon stain of epon section, ×680; *inset 1*, paragon, ×1,150; *inset 2*, toluidine blue, ×907

The profound loss of large myelinated axons, shown here in a **hereditary demyelinating neuropathy**, is best appreciated when compared with the density of large myelinated axons in a normal peripheral nerve (*inset 2*). Surviving large axons are remyelinated, encircled by thin sheaths of compact myelin, which are in turn surrounded by layers of Schwann cell processes such as the layers of an onion (*onion bulb*, *inset 1*, *arrows*). Note the Schwann cell nuclei, marked by sparse central chromatin (open chromatin) and large nucleoli. **HSMN III** is both autosomal dominant and recessive. Affected children are **ataxic** and have difficulty walking. They may have **scoliosis**, a curvature of the spine. Sometimes peripheral nerves become so hypertrophic that they can be palpated beneath the skin.

MYELINATED AND UNMYELINATED AXONS

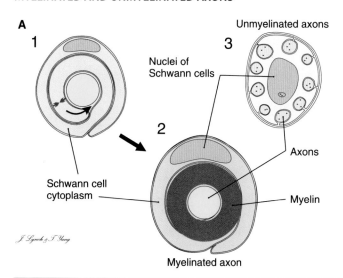

Figure 7-7A. Myelinated and unmyelinated axons.

The **myelin sheath** consists of a tight spiral wrapping of the lipid-rich cell membrane of a **Schwann cell** in the PNS or an **oligodendrocyte** in the CNS. As the Schwann cell envelops the axon, the wrapping process proceeds from outside to inside (*black arrow, 1*) and the cytoplasm is excluded, bringing the inner surfaces of the cell membrane together (*red arrows, 1*). The closely apposed inner surfaces of the membrane form the **major dense line** in the spiraling myelin. When the myelination is complete, the axon is surrounded by many layers of membrane, which function as "insulation," increasing the speed and efficiency of nerve conduction (*2*). The smallest axons in the PNS and CNS lack the thick coating of myelin that is present in medium and large axons. These axons lie in grooves in the cell bodies of supporting Schwann cells and have much slower conduction velocities than myelinated axons.

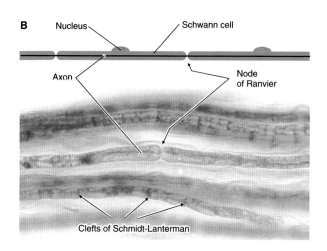

Figure 7-7B. Myelinated peripheral nerve axons (**nodes of Ranvier**). Trichrome stain, ×272

A preparation of teased **myelinated axons** is shown here. The myelin coating is not continuous. Each axon is enveloped by numerous Schwann cells, each covering a distance of between a few millimeters and a few tens of millimeters. Between each pair of Schwann cells is a gap, the **node of Ranvier**, where the bare axon membrane is exposed to the extracellular environment. Voltage-gated channels are concentrated at these nodes, and the membrane becomes active during nerve conduction. Action potentials jump from one node to the next, a process that increases both the speed and the metabolic efficiency of nerve conduction in large myelinated nerves. The **clefts of Schmidt-Lanterman** contain cytoplasm that provides metabolic support for the membrane of the myelin coating.

CLINICAL CORRELATION

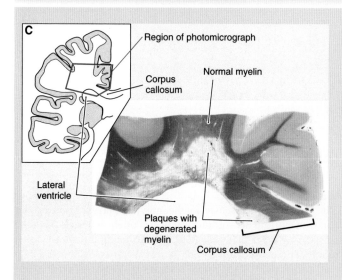

Figure 7-7C. Multiple Sclerosis. Luxol fast blue stain.

Multiple sclerosis (MS) is an **autoimmune inflammatory demyelinating disease** of the CNS, in which the body's immune system destroys the myelin sheath that covers and protects the nerves. It most often affects young women between 20 and 40 years of age. Signs and symptoms depend on the location of affected nerves and severity of the damage and may include numbness or weakness of limbs, visual impairments (double or blurring vision), unusual sensations in certain body parts, tremor, and fatigue. A typical case would have multiple episodes with some resolution between episodes. Genetics and childhood infections may play a role in causing the disease. Pathologically, MS produces **multiple plaques of demyelination** (illustrated) with the loss of oligodendrocytes and astroglial scarring and possible axonal injury and loss. Glucocorticoids and immunomodulatory agents are treatments of first choice.

NODE OF RANVIER

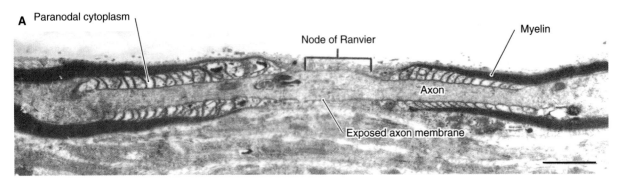

Figure 7-8A. Node of Ranvier between two adjacent Schwann cells. EM, scale bar = 1.0 μm; ×14,000

The **node of Ranvier** is a region **between two Schwann cells** where the axon membrane lacks a thick coating of insulating myelin. This region is therefore able to carry out the complicated exchange of sodium and potassium ions across the membrane that is the basis of the conduction of the action potential. Zones of **paranodal cytoplasm** are visible in this section. Each layer of the spiral wrapping of myelin is associated with one of these zones, which provides metabolic support for the attached thin membranous layer of myelin. Cytoplasm enclosed in the **incisures (clefts) of Schmidt-Lanterman** plays a similar metabolic support role to the myelin at various points along the length of the myelin coating.

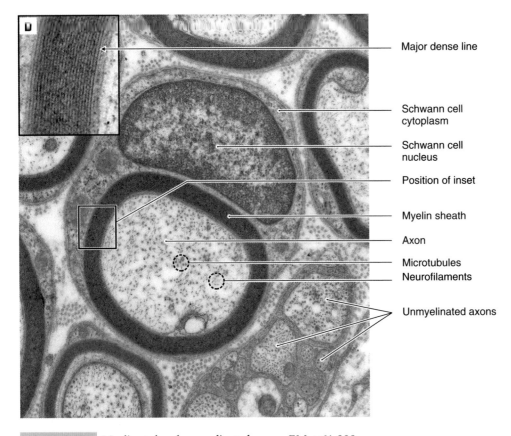

Figure 7-8B. Myelinated and unmyelinated axons. EM, ×61,000

A medium-sized **myelinated axon** together with its associated **Schwann cell** and **myelin sheath** is illustrated in the center of this photomicrograph. The *small rectangle* shows the position of the *inset*. The *higher power inset* shows the individual layers of the myelin sheath, indicated by **major dense lines. Microtubules** are important in transporting neurotransmitters and other materials from the cell body to the axon terminals (**anterograde transport**) and for transporting other materials (e.g., growth factors) from the axon terminals back to the cell body (**retrograde transport**). Both microtubules and **neurofilaments** are part of the cytoskeleton and help maintain the structural integrity of the neuron. In the lower right-hand corner of the illustration, several small, **unmyelinated axons** are lying in grooves in the body of a single Schwann cell.

PERIPHERAL NERVE

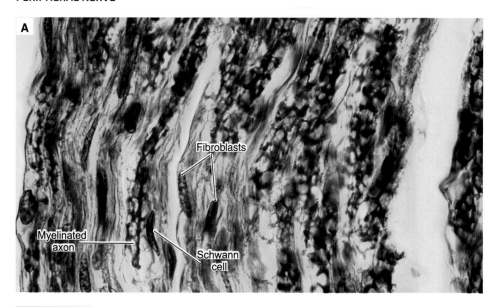

Figure 7-9A. Peripheral nerve. Trichome, ×1,000

This figure depicts a longitudinal section of **peripheral nerve fibers. Collagen fibrils** of **the endoneurium** are stained blue in this photomicrograph. The endoneurium is a loose connective tissue layer that surrounds each individual dark **myelinated axon**. A few **fibroblasts** are visible; these cells produce collagen fibrils. A **Schwann cell** with a small and flat nucleus is also visible close to the labeled axon. The myelin sheath surrounding each axon is produced by Schwann cells. Schwann cells are capable of proliferating and contributing to nerve repair and regeneration.

PERIPHERAL NERVE REPAIR AND REGENERATION

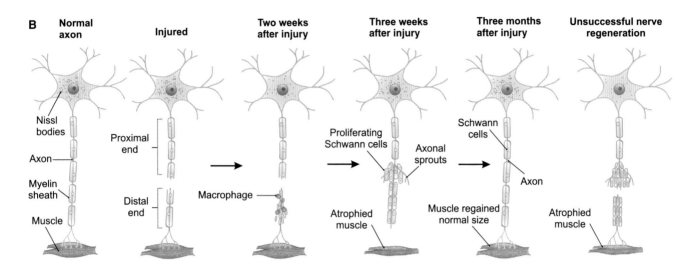

Figure 7-9B. Overview of peripheral nerve repair and regeneration.

Although **nerve fibers** (tracts) in the central nervous system (i.e., nerve fibers within the **brain** and **spinal cord**) are not able to regenerate, peripheral nerves have an ability to repair and regenerate. Each **axon** has a thin layer of surrounding connective tissue called **endoneurium**, which contains numerous Schwann cells. Schwann cells are supporting cells (glia cells) found in peripheral nerves, and they play an essential role in nerve repair and regeneration. A **spinal nerve** is an example of a peripheral nerve that contains sensory and motor fibers. The **cell bodies** of somatic motor **neurons** are located inside the **spinal cord** (**anterior horn**), and their **axons** are very long, extending to **skeletal muscles**, where they synapse on skeletal muscle fibers. (1) A **normal neuron** has many **rough endoplasmic reticula** (**RER**) in its cytoplasm. These RER appear under the microscope as a series of highly organized, parallel folds called Nissl bodies (Nissl substances), which are aptly named because they are viewed with the application of a special stain called a Nissl stain during slide preparation. Each axon is also covered by a myelin sheath. (2) After a nerve is damaged, in about **2 weeks**, the distal portion of the axon undergoes degeneration and loses its surrounding myelin sheath. The proximal axon (attached to the cell body) undergoes **chromatolysis**, which is an induced response that greatly reduces and redistributes Nissl bodies. The distal axon undergoes apoptosis, and the remaining debris is cleaned by macrophages. (3) **Three weeks** after injury, **Schwann cells proliferate** and form cord-like structures called **bands of Büngner**, and the connective tissue basement membranes remaining after the nerve degeneration form **endoneurial tubes** that provide a column-like framework that guides the growth of regenerating axons. The new budding axonal tissue called **axonal sprouts** penetrate the **bands of Büngner** and grow along the endoneurial tubes. The growth of axons is a continuous process, and the growth rate in the human body is 2 to 5 mm/day. During this time, when skeletal muscle tissue has lost nerve innervation, it undergoes atrophy. (4) About 3 months after injury, the axons have been completely repaired and regenerated, the myelin sheaths are formed, and each renewed axon is covered with a connective tissue layer, **endoneurium**. Once the axons reach and innervate skeletal muscle tissue, the skeletal muscle function is restored. With the neuromuscular junctions restored, the skeletal muscles regain their size and capability of contraction.

In the clinic, **peripheral nerve reconstruction surgery** can greatly increase the success rate of nerve repair and regeneration.

PERIPHERAL SENSORY RECEPTORS

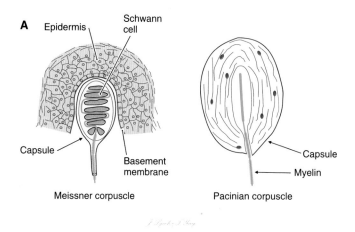

Figure 7-10A. Peripheral sensory receptors.

Axons of the neuron cell bodies in the posterior root ganglia carry information from **sensory receptors** in the skin, muscles, joints, viscera, blood vessels, mesenteries, and other connective tissues. Sensory receptors associated with these axons may consist of **encapsulated axon endings**, specialized endings around **hair follicles**, endings in conjunction with specialized cells (e.g., **Merkel cells**), **muscle spindles**, and specialized regions of axonal membranes termed **free nerve endings**. **Meissner corpuscles** and **Pacinian corpuscles** are two types of encapsulated endings and are easier to see using light microscopy than other receptors in the skin. In these receptors, the axonal membrane is specialized to change its permeability in response to mechanical pressure (the regions of specialization are indicated by the *thicker blue lines*). The connective tissue capsules help to focus mechanical force on the axonal membrane.

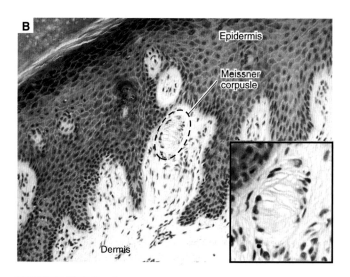

Figure 7-10B. Meissner corpuscle, thick skin of palm.
H&E, ×136; inset ×360

Meissner corpuscles are encapsulated, quickly adapting mechanoreceptors that are sensitive to light touch and low-frequency vibration. They are important for the sensation of discriminative touch. Meissner corpuscles are located in the **dermal ridges**, at the interface of the **dermis** and **epidermis**. Only the nuclei of the capsular connective tissue cells are visible after H&E stains. Using special stains, the corpuscle looks like a stack of pancakes (Schwann cells) with one or more axons intertwining among them. The main axons associated with Meissner corpuscles are large (6–12 μm) and heavily myelinated, hence their rapid conduction velocities. Meissner corpuscles are found in all parts of the skin of the hand and foot, in the lips, and in a number of other locations but are most concentrated in thick, hairless (**glabrous**) skin.

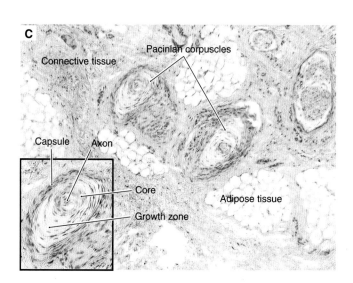

Figure 7-10C. Pacinian corpuscle, thick skin of palm.
H&E, ×68; inset ×105

Pacinian corpuscles are large, encapsulated structures that detect very light touch and vibration. They are located primarily in the **hypodermis** of the palms of the hands and fingers and the soles of the feet but are also found in other areas of skin as well as in the periostea and mesentery. They are much larger than Meissner corpuscles, sometimes reaching 2 mm in length (note different magnification). Pacinian corpuscles consist of a specialized zone of axonal membrane that is exquisitely sensitive to pressure, surrounded by a layered cellular structure that consists of a **central core** immediately surrounding the axon, an **intermediate growth zone**, and an **outer capsule**. Around 60 to 100 layers are formed by very thin cells that overlap at their edges, giving the Pacinian corpuscle the appearance of an onion when sectioned. This sample is from the hypodermis of the skin.

Central Nervous System

SPINAL CORD

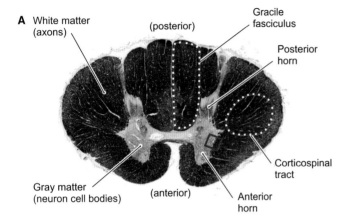

A White matter (axons)
(posterior)
Gracile fasciculus
Posterior horn
Corticospinal tract
Gray matter (neuron cell bodies)
(anterior)
Anterior horn

Figure 7-11A. Spinal cord. Myelin stain, ×7

In this section through an upper thoracic level of the **spinal cord**, the **white matter** (fiber pathways) has been stained dark brown with a myelin stain. The **gray matter** is a region of densely packed neuron cell bodies, and this stain has consequently left the gray matter in the center of the cord relatively unaffected. The **anterior horn** of the gray matter contains motor neurons that innervate muscle fibers; the **posterior horn** contains interneurons in both sensory and motor pathways. The white matter consists of nerve fibers carrying sensory information from receptors in skin and muscles up to the brain (e.g., the **gracile fasciculus**) or nerve fibers carrying motor information down from the brain to interneurons and motor neurons in the gray matter of the spinal cord (e.g., the **corticospinal tract**). The *red rectangle* indicates the position of the tissue in Figure 7-11B that has been stained with a Nissl stain for neuron cell bodies.

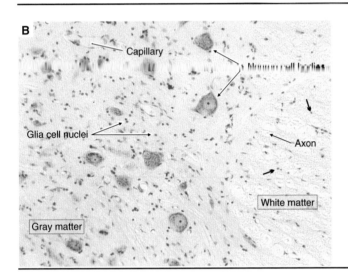

B Capillary
Neuron cell bodies
Glia cell nuclei
Axon
White matter
Gray matter

Figure 7-11B. Spinal cord. Nissl stain, ×136

Nissl stains, such as **thionin** or **cresyl violet**, react with **nucleic acids (RNA, DNA)** and, therefore, stain the **rough endoplasmic reticulum**, **nuclei**, and **nucleoli** of neurons. This renders the neuron cell bodies visible, along with the **nuclei of glial cells** and nuclei of epithelial cells in blood vessels. The large cell bodies in this section belong to motor neurons in the anterior horn of the **spinal cord** (*red rectangle* in Fig. 7-11A). Also visible are the nuclei of glial cells (**astrocytes** and **oligodendrocytes**) in the **gray matter** on the left side of the picture and in the **white matter** on the right side of the picture (*small arrows*). It is important to keep in mind when looking at myelin-stained sections such as in Figure 7-11A that the light-colored areas, where nothing seems to be stained, are in fact filled with neuron cell bodies similar to the ones illustrated here.

BRAINSTEM

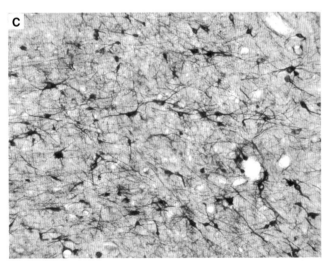

C

Figure 7-11C. Neurons in the reticular formation of the brainstem. NADPH histochemical stain, ×68

Neurons use a wide variety of **neurotransmitters**. In addition to stains that react with structural components of a nerve cell, it is possible to use **histochemical reactions** to visualize the presence of particular neurotransmitters. This photomicrograph illustrates an example of such a reaction, in which only those neurons that generate the neurotransmitter **nitric oxide (NO)** are visualized. In this case, an enzyme necessary for the synthesis of NO, **NADPH diaphorase**, was labeled using a blue chromogen (colored substance). The neurons are colored in their entirety because NO is a novel neurotransmitter that is not bound in vesicles as are most neurotransmitters, but rather is synthesized everywhere in the cell and leaks through the cell membrane when it is released. It often functions to modulate the action of other neurotransmitters.

CEREBRAL CORTEX

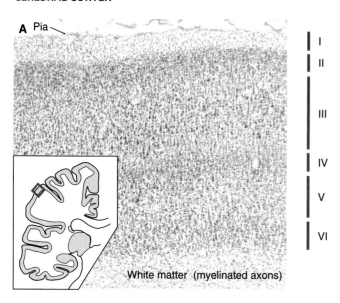

Figure 7-12A. Cerebral cortex. Nissl stain, ×24

The **cerebral cortex** is a layer of densely packed neurons about 2 mm thick that forms the surface of the hemispheres of the brain. The cortex is organized into **layers** (indicated by *red lines* and *Roman numerals*) on the basis of the **size, shape**, and **packing density** of the neurons in different regions of the cortex. For example, **layers II** and **IV** in this photomicrograph consist of small, tightly packed neurons (mainly granule cells), whereas **layers III** and **V** consist of larger neurons (mostly pyramidal cells). This example is taken from the association cortex of the parietal lobe (*red box in inset*). **Layer I** consists predominantly of horizontally running dendrites and axons; the nuclei in this region belong to glial cells. The white matter consists of axons entering and leaving this small region of cortex and connecting it with other cortical regions, with subcortical structures such as the thalamus and with the spinal cord.

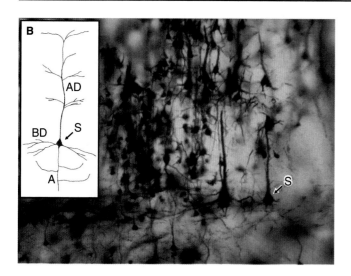

Figure 7-12B. Cerebral cortex, pyramidal cells. Golgi preparation, ×136

The most numerous neurons in the **cerebral cortex** are **pyramidal cells**, named for their triangular cell bodies (singular, **soma**; plural **somata**; *S* in the *inset* and photomicrograph). Pyramidal cells are also characterized by a long **apical dendrite** (*AD*) that extends into layer I and has many lateral branches; several **basal dendrites** (*BD*) that extend laterally from the base of the soma; and a long **axon** (*A*) that leaves the cortex and extends, in the white matter, either to some other region of the cortex or to subcortical structures, such as the basal nuclei, brainstem, or spinal cord. Pyramidal cells are found in layers II through VI of the cortex but are most obvious in layers III and V. Somata range in size from 10 to over 50 μm, with the largest located in layer V of primary motor cortex. The sample shown here is taken from layer III. It includes several medium pyramidal cells and many small pyramidal cells.

CLINICAL CORRELATION

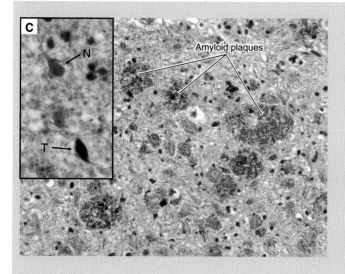

Figure 7-12C. Alzheimer Disease. Bielschowsky stain, ×272; inset ×550

Alzheimer disease is the most common form of **dementia** in the elderly (60%–80% of cases). Patients show **progressive memory loss, personality changes**, and **cognitive impairments**. Pathologically, Alzheimer disease is characterized by extracellular deposition of **Aβ protein (plaques)**, **intracellular neurofibrillary tangles** (*inset*: N, normal neuron; T, neuron cell body filled with dark-staining tangles), and **loss of neurons** and synapses in the cerebral cortex and some subcortical regions. Gross anatomy shows **atrophy** of the affected regions. The most prominent theory is that mutation of genes such as those located on chromosome 21 lead to overproduction of Aβ precursor. There is no cure for Alzheimer disease. Treatments include pharmaceutical and psychosocial therapies and supportive caregiving.

CEREBELLUM

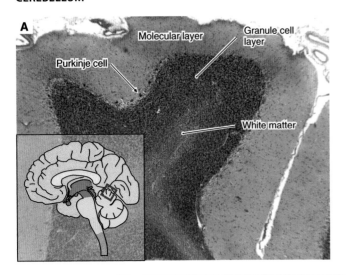

Figure 7-13A.   Cerebellar folium. Nissl stain, ×34

The **cerebellum** (*green structure* in *inset*) is a large, complex structure that lies beneath the posterior portion of the cerebral hemispheres. Its name means "little brain." It is critical for smooth, coordinated movements and participates, to a lesser extent, in many other functions. The structural organization of the cerebellum is similar to that of the cerebrum in which it consists of **white matter**, a **cortex**, and **subcortical nuclei**. However, the organization of the cortex is very different from that of the cerebral cortex. There are only three layers, the **granule cell layer**, the **Purkinje cell layer**, and the **molecular layer**. The granule cell layer contains an enormous number of very small, tightly packed cells and their dendrites. The Purkinje cell layer, at the interface of the granule cell and molecular layers, is only one cell deep. The molecular layer contains primarily axons and dendrites, with only very few neuron cell bodies. The *red rectangle* indicates the position of the tissue in this figure.

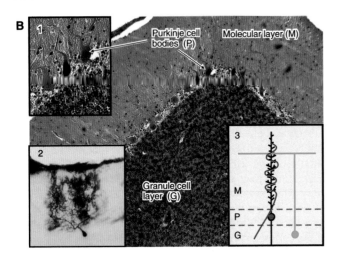

Figure 7-13B.   Cerebellar cortex. Nissl stain, ×68, *inset 1*, ×124; *inset 2*, Golgi, ×74

Purkinje cells and **granule cells** are the most obvious neurons in the cerebellar cortex. Purkinje cells, among the largest neurons in the CNS, lie between the granule cell layer and the molecular layer (*inset 1*). Purkinje cells have widely branching dendritic trees that extend through the entire depth of the molecular layer (*inset 2*). The dendritic tree of a Purkinje cell is shaped like a paper fan. The wide part of the "fan" is seen when cutting across the long axis of a folium (*inset 2*). The edge of the fan is seen when cutting parallel to the long axis of the folium (*inset 3*). *Granule cells* (*blue, inset 3*) send their axons into the molecular layer in which they divide and run parallel to the long axis of the folium, making synaptic contact with hundreds or thousands of Purkinje cell dendrites. Another major element in the basic cerebellar cortex circuitry is the **climbing fiber** (*red, inset 3*). These axons originate in the inferior olivary nucleus. Each climbing fiber encircles the dendrites of a single Purkinje cell. Purkinje cell axons provide the sole output pathway of the cerebellar cortex.

CLINICAL CORRELATION

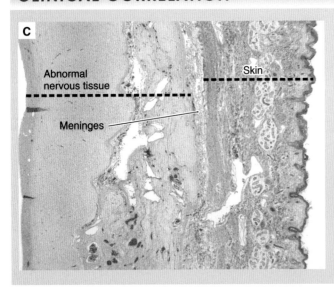

Figure 7-13C.   Encephalocele. H&E, ×17

In some embryos, the **neuroectoderm** does not separate from the **surface ectoderm** during early stages of development. A defect in the **calvarium** may occur as the bone of the skull is formed, through which CSF, meninges, and brain tissue may protrude. This case illustrates immature brain tissue and its meningeal covering, which have herniated through a bony defect in the occipital bone. These neuroectodermal tissues are found directly beneath the dense subcutaneous connective tissue of overlying skin. **Encephaloceles** are most frequently found in the occipital region. In their several variations, they may contain (1) only CSF and meninges, (2) CSF, meninges, and brain substance (occipital lobe or cerebellum), or (3) CSF, meninges, brain, and part of the ventricular system. The more elaborate the encephalocele, the more debilitating and difficult it is to treat.

MENINGES

A

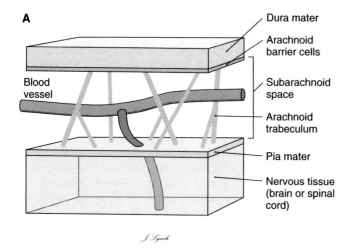

Dura mater

Arachnoid barrier cells

Blood vessel

Subarachnoid space

Arachnoid trabeculum

Pia mater

Nervous tissue (brain or spinal cord)

J. Lynch

Figure 7-14A. Dura mater, arachnoid, and pia mater.

The leathery outer meningeal layer, the **dura mater** (or **dura**), consists of elongated fibroblasts and large amounts of extracellular collagen. It is tenuously attached to the **arachnoid barrier layer**; there is no "subdural space" in the normal state. The dura is tenaciously attached to the skull at the base of the brain and at the sutures and is less tightly adherent to the skull in other regions. The arachnoid barrier layer consists of two to three layers of cells that are attached to each other by many continuous tight junctions, hence its "barrier" nature to CSF. The subarachnoid space (SAS) is located between the arachnoid and the pia, contains blood vessels and CSF, and is traversed by **arachnoid trabeculae**. The **pia mater** generally consists of one to two layers of flattened fibroblasts that are adherent to the surface of the brain and spinal cord. Blood vessels located in the SAS are frequently covered by thin layers of pia. The interface between the pia and the nervous tissue is characterized by a **glial limiting membrane (glia limitans)**, as shown in Figure 7-15A.

B

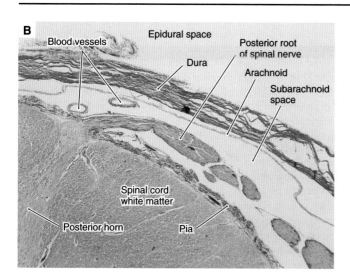

Blood vessels

Epidural space

Posterior root of spinal nerve

Dura

Arachnoid

Subarachnoid space

Spinal cord white matter

Posterior horn

Pia

Figure 7-14B. Spinal meninges in the region of the posterior roots. H&E, ×34

At spinal levels, the **dura mater** forms a tubular sac enclosing the spinal cord. However, in contrast to the cranial dura, which adheres to the skull, the spinal dura is separated from the vertebral bodies by an **epidural space**. Both the spinal and the cranial dura consist of many elongated fibroblasts and abundant extracellular collagen. The **arachnoid barrier cell layer** is basically the same at cranial and spinal levels. In the normal state, the barrier cell layer is attached to the dura, although only weakly. There is no naturally occurring subdural space; what appears to be a space here is a tissue preparation artifact. The **pia mater** on the cord is continuous with the **epineurium** on the posterior root, the latter representing a part of a peripheral nerve. The SAS is located between the pia and the arachnoid and at this point contains the posterior roots.

CLINICAL CORRELATION

C

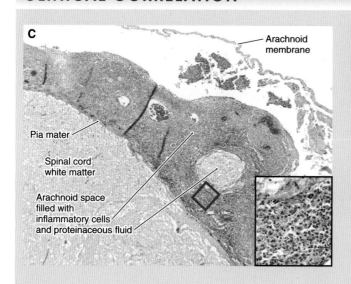

Arachnoid membrane

Pia mater

Spinal cord white matter

Arachnoid space filled with inflammatory cells and proteinaceous fluid

Figure 7-14C. Meningitis. H&E, ×34; inset ×147

Meningitis is an inflammatory disease of the meninges that is largely sequestered in the **SAS**. The inflammation is usually caused by infection by **viruses, bacteria, or fungal agents**. Signs and symptoms include fever, headache, irritability, photophobia, neck stiffness (**meningismus**), vomiting, altered mental status, and cutaneous hemorrhages (**purpura**). Complications may lead to deafness, epilepsy, and hydrocephalus. Pathologically, the meningitis affects the pia-arachnoid and the CSF in the SAS and may extend into the cerebral ventricles. Characteristic findings include perivascular cuffs of acute and chronic inflammatory cells (*inset, from red box*), which distend the arachnoid space. **Lumbar puncture** (spinal tap) for CSF is an important diagnostic tool. Treatment is usually supportive for viral meningitis and includes antibiotics or other agents that can cross the blood-brain barrier for bacterial or fungal meningitis.

GLIAL CELLS

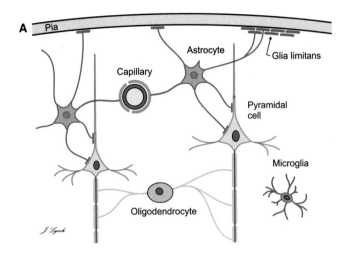

Figure 7-15A. Types of glial cells.

Glial cells (also called **neuroglia** or **glia**) are nonneuronal cells that aid in transferring nutrients from capillaries to neurons, maintain the blood-brain barrier, regulate the intercellular environment, provide myelin insulation for axons, provide mechanical support to neurons, act as phagocytes to remove pathogens and dead neurons, play a role in presenting antigens in the immune system, and perform numerous other functions. Recent evidence suggests that glial cells even participate in some aspects of synaptic transmission. It is thought that there are as many as 10 times the number of glial cells as neurons in the nervous system. The major types of CNS glial cells are **astrocytes** (described below), **oligodendrocytes** (which produce myelin), and **microglia** (which act as phagocytes and elements of the immune system). Other glialike cells include **radial glia cells** and **ependymal cells** in the CNS and **Schwann cells** and **satellite cells** in the PNS.

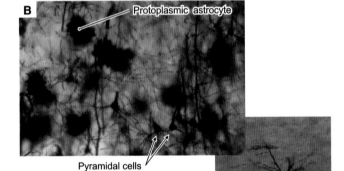

Figure 7-15B. **Astrocytes.** Golgi preparations, upper left, ×136; lower right, ×204

Astrocytes are found throughout the CNS. Astrocyte processes called **end-feet** form contacts with capillaries that help produce the blood-brain barrier and form contacts on neurons that play a role in supplying nutrients to these cells. Astrocytes regulate the ionic composition and pH of the extracellular environment and secrete various neuroactive substances. Astrocyte end-feet form the **glia limitans**, a coating of the inner surface of the pia mater that surrounds the brain and spinal cord (Fig. 7-13A). Finally, astrocytes play an important role in neurotransmitter metabolism and in the modulation of synaptic transmission. There are two types of astrocytes. **Protoplasmic astrocytes**, in gray matter, have short, thick processes that are densely clustered and highly branched, giving them a cloudlike appearance. **Fibrous astrocytes**, in white matter, have long, thin processes with relatively few branchings. The two types of astrocytes have similar functions but differ in some special properties.

CLINICAL CORRELATION

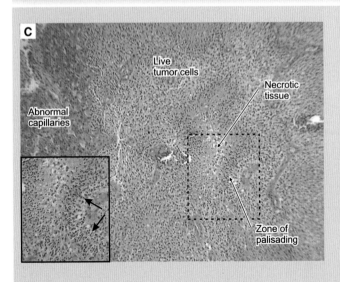

Figure 7-15C. **Glioblastoma.** H&E, ×68; inset ×84

Glioblastoma (a form of **astrocytoma**) is a highly malignant tumor that arises in the brain from **neoplastic astrocytes**. Several features of this tumor help the pathologist arrive at the diagnosis. In the center of this micrograph, the tumor cells are necrotic. At the edges of the zone of necrosis, nonnecrotic tumor cells align themselves in a striking parallel array, like the pickets of a fence. This configuration is called **palisading** (*arrows, inset*). Beyond the area of palisading, living tumor cells commonly surround complex abnormal vascular structures (**glomeruloid vascular structures**) that resemble the glomeruli of the kidney in their tortuous arrangement of capillaries. **Increased mitosis** among the viable tumor cells also aids in the diagnostic process. Increasing the life span of patients with glioblastoma is currently an area of intensive research.

Autonomic Nervous System

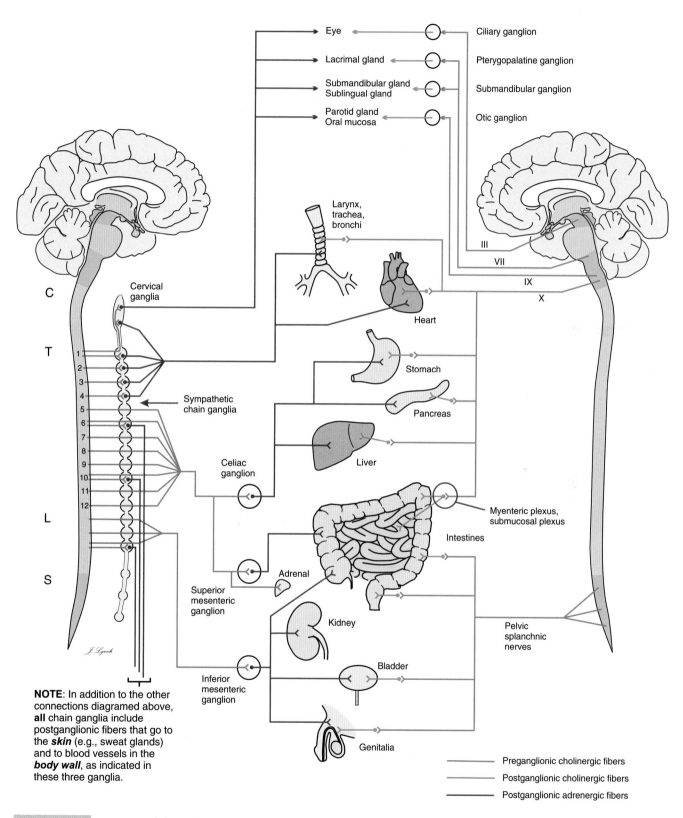

Eye

Ciliary ganglion

Lacrimal gland

Pterygopalatine ganglion

Submandibular gland
Sublingual gland

Submandibular ganglion

Parotid gland
Oral mucosa

Otic ganglion

Larynx,
trachea,
bronchi

III

VII

IX

X

Cervical
ganglia

Heart

C

T

Stomach

Pancreas

Sympathetic
chain ganglia

Liver

Celiac
ganglion

Myenteric plexus,
submucosal plexus

Intestines

L

Adrenal

S

Superior
mesenteric
ganglion

Kidney

Pelvic
splanchnic
nerves

Bladder

Inferior
mesenteric
ganglion

Genitalia

NOTE: In addition to the other
connections diagramed above,
all chain ganglia include
postganglionic fibers that go to
the **skin** (e.g., sweat glands)
and to blood vessels in the
body wall, as indicated in
these three ganglia.

——— Preganglionic cholinergic fibers

——— Postganglionic cholinergic fibers

——— Postganglionic adrenergic fibers

J. Lynch

Figure 7-16. Overview of the autonomic nervous system. (continues on next page)

Autonomic Ganglia

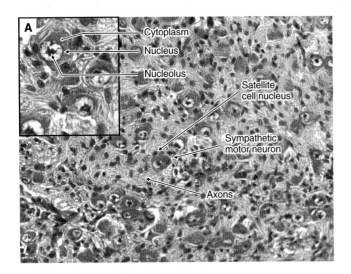

Figure 7-17A.   Sympathetic ganglion. H&E, ×272; inset ×520

This section from a **sympathetic chain ganglion** shows small- to medium-sized visceromotor neuron cell bodies that give rise to **postganglionic axons**. These neurons receive synapses from **preganglionic sympathetic axons** that originate in the lateral horn of the thoracic and upper lumbar spinal cord. The *preganglionic axons* are myelinated; the *postganglionic axons* are unmyelinated. These **motor neurons** are **multipolar** (in contrast to the unipolar sensory neurons in the posterior root ganglia), although the dendrites are not visible in this H&E stain. The sizes of the cell bodies are more uniform than in the sensory ganglia, and the cell bodies and axons are distributed more evenly across the ganglia rather than being grouped into clumps as in the sensory ganglia. The **satellite cells** are not distributed so evenly around the neuron cell bodies as they are in the sensory ganglia.

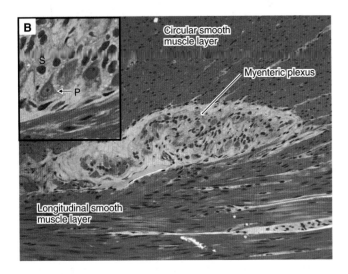

Figure 7-17B.   Myenteric plexus (Auerbach plexus). H&E, ×136; inset ×300

The enteric division lacks the discrete, encapsulated ganglia that characterize the sympathetic division. Its visceromotor neurons are distributed in a network of plexuses that are distributed within the walls of the gastrointestinal tract. Most neurons in the enteric division are found in the **myenteric and submucosal plexuses**. The myenteric plexuses lie between the **circular smooth muscle layer** and the **longitudinal smooth muscle layer** of the intestine (see Chapter 15 "Digestive Tract"; see also Chapter 6, "Muscle"). These plexuses are clusters of parasympathetic postganglionic motor neurons; sensory neurons, which receive input from chemoreceptors and mechanoreceptors in the intestinal wall; and **local circuit neurons (interneurons)**. Interneurons can process neural signals within a plexus and can also mediate the coordination of multiple plexuses. (*Inset*: P, multipolar postganglionic motor neuron; S, satellite cell.)

Figure 7-16.   Overview of the autonomic nervous system. (*continued*).

The autonomic nervous system is composed of three divisions: **sympathetic, parasympathetic,** and **enteric.** The sympathetic and parasympathetic divisions function under direct CNS control; the enteric division functions somewhat more independently. The *sympathetic division* includes **preganglionic neurons** with cell bodies in the **lateral horn** of the thoracic and upper lumbar spinal cord. Some of these neurons synapse on **postganglionic neurons** in the **sympathetic chain ganglia**; others continue past these ganglia and synapse in **prevertebral sympathetic ganglia** (e.g., celiac ganglion, mesenteric ganglia) near the organs to be innervated. Postganglionic neurons send axons to internal organs, glands, and blood vessels. Effects of sympathetic activity include increasing cardiac output, blood pressure, and bronchial diameter; decreasing gut peristalsis; and, in general, preparing the individual for strenuous activity, sometimes called the "fight-or-flight" reaction. The *parasympathetic division* has a markedly different organization. Preganglionic fibers originate in brainstem nuclei associated with cranial nerves III, VII, IX, and X and in the **sacral parasympathetic nucleus** (which occupies a position in the sacral spinal cord similar to that of the lateral horn in the thoracic cord). The **parasympathetic preganglionic fibers** that supply the head region synapse in discrete ganglia and the postganglionic fibers end in glands and smooth muscle. By contrast, parasympathetic preganglionic fibers that travel in cranial nerve X (vagus nerve) and the pelvic splanchnic nerves send signals to the viscera and blood vessels within the body cavity. These fibers do not synapse in discrete ganglia but rather in small **plexuses** of postganglionic cell bodies that lie in or adjacent to the walls of their target organs. The general effect of parasympathetic activity is the opposite of sympathetic activity and tends to return the internal organs and cardiovascular system to a baseline level of function. The *enteric division* consists of a vast number of neurons arranged in a network of plexuses in the walls of the gut. Some of these plexuses are shared with the parasympathetic division. The activity of the enteric division is modulated in a general way by the sympathetic and parasympathetic divisions, but it is able to act independently and reflexively to move boluses of food substances through the gastrointestinal tract by peristaltic action and to control absorption, local blood flow, and secretion in response to the chemical composition of the bolus.

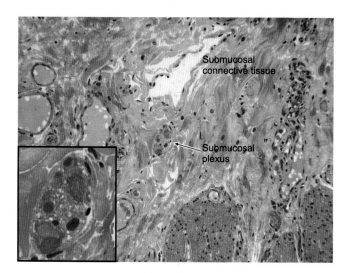

Submucosal connective tissue

Submucosal plexus

Figure 7-18. Submucosal plexus (of Meissner). H&E, ×136; inset ×453

The **submucosal plexuses (of Meissner)** are located in the submucosal layer of the intestine (see Chapter 15, "Digestive Tract"). These plexuses are similar to the myenteric plexuses in that they are unencapsulated clusters of **parasympathetic postganglionic motor neurons; sensory neurons,** which receive input from chemoreceptors and mechanoreceptors in the intestinal wall; and **local circuit neurons (interneurons).** The postganglionic motor neurons may innervate smooth muscle to either increase or decrease muscle activity and may also innervate secretory cells in the walls of the intestine.

TABLE 7-1 Comparison of Posterior Root and Autonomic Ganglia

Type of Ganglion	Cell Body Arrangement	Cell Body Characteristics	Satellite Cells	Synapses in Ganglion
Posterior root (sensory)	Arranged into groups within ganglion, cell bodies variable in size	Round cell body, central nucleus	Complete capsule of satellite cells	No synapses
Autonomic (visceromotor)	Evenly distributed within ganglion, uniform in size	Multipolar cell body, eccentric nucleus	Incomplete capsule of satellite cells	Numerous synaptic contacts

SYNOPSIS 7-1 Pathologic and Clinical Terms for the Nervous System

■ *Ataxia:* Inability to coordinate the muscles properly in the execution of a voluntary movement.

■ *Gliosis:* The multiplication of astrocytes as a response to injury in the brain, as exemplified by the feltwork of astrocytic cell bodies and processes in a demyelinated plaque of MS.

■ *Glomeruloid vascular structures:* Complex arrays of capillaries that resemble the glomeruli of a kidney are another hallmark of the glioblastoma.

■ *Neurofibrillary tangle:* The helical arrangement of abnormally phosphorylated neurofilaments found in many hippocampal and cortical neurons of an Alzheimer patient.

■ *Neuropathy:* A disease involving the cranial or spinal nerves.

■ *Onion bulb:* After repeated cycles of demyelination and remyelination, thin layers of Schwann cell cytoplasm form concentric circles around a central axon. The appearance of the structure resembles a cross section of an onion bulb and its nested leaves.

■ *Palisading:* The alignment of viable tumor cells at the edge of a necrotic focus in glioblastoma, a diagnostic hallmark of this grade 4 (most malignant) astrocytoma, a family of glial tumors derived from the astrocyte.

■ *Plaque:* This word indicates a lesion, in several pathological contexts. (1) An atherosclerotic plaque is the hard, calcified buildup of fatty material in large arteries, such as the coronary arteries or aorta. (2) A neuritic plaque is the extracellular knot of phosphorylated axons and dendrites, often with a central deposit of amyloid protein, found in great numbers in brains of patients with Alzheimer disease. (3) In MS, a demyelinated plaque is an irregular zone of axons, often in a periventricular location, that have lost their sheaths of myelin.

From Histology to Pathology

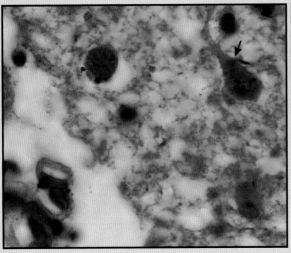 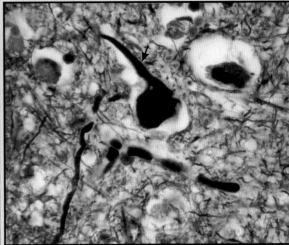

Figure 7-19.   Normal neuron and neurofibrillary tangles. Bielschowsky stain (left) ×400; Silver stain, (right) ×400

Black arrows indicate a **normal neuron** on the *left* and a **neuron with neurofibrillary tangles** on the *right*. These neurofibrillary tangles resemble a twisted, black helix in the cytoplasm of a neuron from a patient with

Alzheimer disease. Neurofibrillary tangles are formed by microtubule-associated tau proteins and abnormally phosphorylated neurofilaments.

Clinical Vignette Questions

1. A 28-year-old female with progressive vision impairment for 3 months comes to your office for a check-up. She also complains of weakness and tingling in her lower extremities, which she describes as sometimes worse and sometimes better (waxing and waning). She is alert without showing any cognitive disorder. Physical examinations show nystagmus, tremor, and muscle weakness in both lower extremities. MRI reveals numerous cerebral plaques in the periventricular region and corpus callosum. Lumbar puncture shows oligoclonal bands on the electrophoresis. Assuming a histologic examination on the plaques was conducted, which of the following is the most significant finding?

A. Demyelination and perivascular infiltration of lymphocytes and macrophages
B. Elevated myelin protein and well-preserved axons
C. Increased astrocytes and glial cells
D. Increased oligodendrocytes with elevated myelin protein
E. Neovascularization with increased Schwann cells

2. An 84-year-old Caucasian female walked away about a mile from her home one early morning and could not find her way back. Her husband died 5 years ago, and she has lived alone ever since. One of her daughters reported that, in the last 6 months, her mother seemed to have difficulty communicating with

her. She could not correctly remember her children's names. Examination reveals obvious memory loss and changes in personality. Assuming microphotographs were taken from her cerebral cortex, which of the following would be the most prominent finding?

A. Decrease in amyloid protein and intracellular neurofibrillary tangles
B. Decrease in oligodendrocytes
C. Increase in amyloid plaques and intracellular neurofibrillary tangles
D. Increase in astrocytes in the cerebral cortex
E. Increase in neurons in the cerebral cortex

3. A 19-year-old male college student suddenly became ill about 38 hours ago. He was brought into the emergency department after suffering a seizure. He complains of a severe headache, and he is running a fever of 103°F. Before arriving to the hospital, the patient had a single episode of vomiting. A physical examination shows neck stiffness, photophobia, and irritability. You order a CT scan and lumbar puncture. CSF findings reveal a white blood cell count of 4,800/μL (88% are neutrophils), and protein of 420 mg/dL. The Gram stain is positive. Which of the following is the most likely diagnosis?

A. Bacterial meningitis
B. Cryptococcal meningitis
C. Tuberculous meningitis
D. Viral encephalitis
E. Viral meningitis

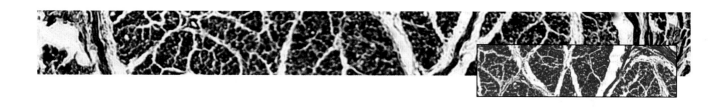

8 Blood and Hemopoiesis

Peripheral Blood Cells

Clinical Vignette Questions

Peripheral Blood Cells

Introduction and Key Concepts for Peripheral Blood Cells

Blood smears are prepared so that the morphology of the formed elements can be assessed, and the relative numbers of the leukocytes can be calculated (**differential leukocyte count**). If a person is anemic, examination of erythrocyte morphology can help classify the type of anemia. If a person has an elevated leukocyte count, a **differential white cell count** can provide valuable information toward determining what kind of infection or leukemia the person has. All formed elements serve critically important functions. **Erythrocytes** function in transport of respiratory gases, **platelets** function mainly in hemostasis, and **leukocytes** function in various ways to protect from infection by a wide variety of potential pathogenic organisms.

ERYTHROCYTES deliver oxygen from the lungs to all the tissues of the body, although they are also involved in carbon dioxide transport and pH regulation. Because erythrocytes are anucleate and lack membrane-bounded organelles, their internal structure is homogeneous. An erythrocyte is essentially a plasmalemma bag containing a highly concentrated (30%) hemoglobin solution. In addition, erythrocytes have a membrane-associated complex of cytoskeletal proteins that renders the biconcave disk shape.

PLATELETS (thrombocytes) are small fragments of cytoplasm with a complex and highly organized structure. They normally range in number from 200,000 to 400,000/μL. If the platelet number falls below 60,000/μL ("thrombocytopenia"), the integrity of the smallest blood vessels is compromised. Platelets function to minimize loss of blood when there is a breach in the circulatory system.

LEUKOCYTES are much less abundant than erythrocytes, 4,500 to 11,000/μL in contrast to about 5 million/μL. However, white cell numbers can increase markedly in some circumstances, such as infection or leukemia. Leukocytes have a wide range of life spans—from a few days (neutrophils) to years (some lymphocytes). All leukocytes are involved in defense against microorganisms and other foreign agents and in tissue responses to injury. Usually, they perform their functions only after leaving the blood stream and entering the conventional connective tissue through processes of attachment to endothelial cells and active movement through gaps in the endothelium (**diapedesis**). Leukocytes are constantly released from the bone marrow to be delivered by the cardiovascular system to the vascular beds of all peripheral tissues. Leukocytes are classified as either **nongranular** (**agranular**) or **granular** depending on whether specific cytoplasmic granules are evident when the cells are stained with Romanowsky-type stains like Wright stain. The three types of *granulocytes*—basophils, eosinophils, and **neutrophils**—are named and identified by the staining reaction of their specific granules. The two types of *nongranular leukocytes*, **lymphocytes** and **monocytes**, also have granules, but the granules are only nonspecific granules (**lysosomes**). All granulocytes are **terminal cells**; that is, they will never again divide because they have lost that capacity during differentiation. Monocytes and lymphocytes have the potential for further division.

Lymphocytes are the second most abundant leukocyte, amounting to about 25% to 33% of leukocytes. These are the cells that mediate specific immunity against foreign molecules and organisms. **B lymphocytes** produce immunoglobulins, and their derivatives, **plasma cells**, are specialized to secrete soluble antibodies. **T lymphocytes** are the agents of cell-mediated specific immune responses, and they comprise several types. Among these, **cytotoxic T cells** function to kill virus-infected host cells, and **helper T cells** and **suppressor T cells** regulate immune responses. For null cells, see Chapter 10, "Lymphoid System."

Monocytes the largest of the leukocytes, constitute about 3% to 7% of circulating white blood cells. Monocytes are not functionally or structurally mature when they are circulating in blood. Rather, they are an intermediate form of a cell lineage that starts differentiation in the bone marrow (like all blood cells) but does not fully complete differentiation until arrival in a peripheral tissue. There are several functional cell types that are derived from monocytes, including **tissue macrophages**, **Kupffer cells, microglial cells, osteoclasts**, and **antigen-presenting cells**.

Neutrophils are by far the most abundant leukocytes. Typically, 54% to 62% of leukocytes are mature neutrophils, and an additional 3% to 5% of leukocytes are immature (band) forms. Neutrophils are the main cellular weapon for destroying bacteria, and the total number of circulating neutrophils can rise sharply in response to bacterial infections. Once a neutrophil makes contact with a bacterium, the neutrophil attaches to the bacterium and engulfs it (**phagocytosis**) within a phagosome. The primary and secondary granules of the neutrophil fuse with the phagosome, thereby exposing the bacterium to an array of bactericidal compounds and enzymes. Another bacteria-killing mechanism employed by neutrophils is the generation of reactive oxygen compounds in a process termed the **respiratory burst**.

Eosinophils amount to about 1% to 3% of circulating leukocytes, and, like basophils, their numbers tend to rise in response to parasitic infections and allergic reactions. The functions of eosinophils are not fully understood, but they clearly function in defense against infection by parasitic worms such as schistosomes. Eosinophils are recruited to sites of parasitic infection, and some of their granule contents (e.g., major basic proteins) are highly toxic to parasites. They also appear to function in dampening and limiting inflammation at sites of allergic reactions.

Basophils are the least numerous (<1%) of the leukocytes. Basophils are functionally similar to the mast cells found in connective tissue. Neither cell type functions by phagocytosis, so they are quite unlike neutrophils. Instead, their functions in defense against microbial invasion are indirect. When activated, they secrete (or **exocytose**) a variety of inflammatory mediators from their granules and synthesize and release a number of arachidonic acid derivatives, such as **leukotrienes** and **prostaglandins**. These signaling molecules intensify inflammation by (1) increasing local blood flow, (2) enhancing leakage of plasma proteins from blood, (3) promoting recruitment of other leukocytes to a site of infection, and (4) enhancing the activity of the other leukocytes.

SYNOPSIS 8-1 Life Spans, Counts, and Sizes of Blood Cells

- **Leukocytes:** Total number count is 4,500 to 11,000/mm³.
- **Erythrocytes:** Life span is about 120 days; count is 4,200,000 to 5,900,000/mm³ (male 4,500,000–5,900,000/mm³; female 4,200,000–5,400,000/mm³); size is 7 to 8 µm (in diameter).
- **Platelets (thrombocytes):** Life span is 8 to 12 days, count is 150,000 to 400,000/mm³; size is 1 to 4 µm.
- **Monocytes:** Duration in circulation is a few hours to a few days before differentiating (a macrophage's life span is up to several months); count is 200 to 900/mm³; size is 12 to 15 µm.
- **Lymphocytes:** Life span is a few days to years; count is 1,000 to 4,000/mm³; size is 6 to 12 µm.
- **Neutrophils:** Duration in circulation is a few hours, life span is about 8 days; count is 3,500 to 7,000/mm³; size is 9 to 12 µm.
- **Eosinophils:** Life span is uncertain, likely a few days; count is 50 to 450/mm³; size is 9 to 14 µm.
- **Basophils:** Life span is uncertain, likely a few days; count is 0 to 200/mm³; size is 8 to 10 µm.
- Clinical lab blood counts measure *total number* count of white blood cells ([WBCs] leukocytes/mm³) and *differential counts* (percent of each type of leukocyte). *Absolute numbers* of WBCs can be calculated by multiplying total number/mm³ times percent of each type of leukocyte.
- **Shift to left:** Increase in number of immature leukocytes (especially neutrophils in band forms), which suggests high demand because of infection or acute inflammation (normal range of band leukocyte is 2%–6%).
- **Shift to right:** Absence of immature leukocytes in differential count of leukocytes.

Blood Composition

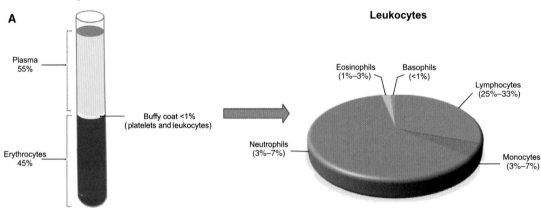

Figure 8-1A.   Overview of composition of peripheral blood.

Blood fractionation is usually done by centrifuging whole anticoagulated blood in a small tube. In this process, blood is separated into three layers: (1) **Erythrocytes** (about 45%) at the bottom of the tube, (2) a **Buffy coat** (<1%) in the middle, and (3) **plasma** (about 55%) on the top (including water, proteins, and solutes) (*left side of figure*). The **Buffy coat** contains **platelets** and **leukocytes** that include neutrophils (54%–62%), lymphocytes (25%–33%), monocytes (3%–7%), eosinophils (1%–3%), and basophils (<1%) (*right side of figure*).

B

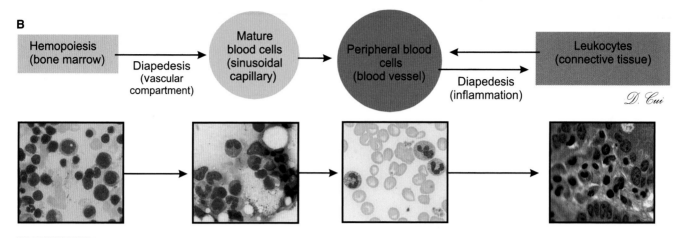

Figure 8-1B. Blood cell maturation and migration diagram.

Blood cells develop in the **hematopoietic compartment** of **bone marrow** and then move into the **vascular compartment** of **bone marrow,** which contains many **sinusoidal blood vessels** that allow mature blood cells to migrate into the blood circulation by **diapedesis. Leukocytes** move into connective tissue when **inflammation** happens due to infection and tissue damage, or antigens are present in the tissue. **Diapedesis** is also known as **leukocyte extravasation.** Some leukocytes (lymphocytes) may move back into circulation after they encounter the antigen.

CLINICAL CORRELATION

C

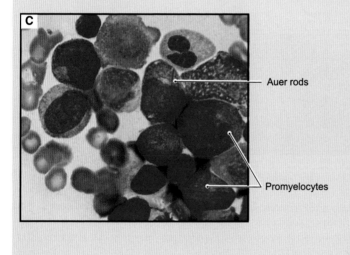

Auer rods

Promyelocytes

Figure 8-1C. Acute Myeloid Leukemia. H&E, ×1,000

Acute myeloid leukemia (AML) is a heterogeneous group of **malignant myeloid neoplasms** that occur due to genetic mutations leading to alterations in the normal maturation process. Many of the genetic defects are **translocations,** such as **t (15;17)** seen in acute **promyelocytic leukemia (APL),** one form of AML. As immature precursors accumulate in the marrow, normal hematopoietic cells are reduced, leading to **anemia, thrombocytopenia,** and a reduction in normal white blood cells. Patients often present with **petechiae,** round red or purple spots on the skin from bleeding, due to a decrease in platelets (**thrombocytopenia**). The peripheral white blood count is often markedly elevated due to the presence of the abnormal, immature cells. The cells of AML have the qualities of blasts with nucleoli and show different degrees of differentiation. One histologic hallmark of AML is the presence of rod-shaped cytoplasmic inclusions called **Auer rods.**

Peripheral Blood Cell Types

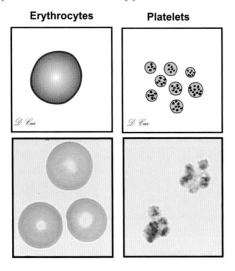

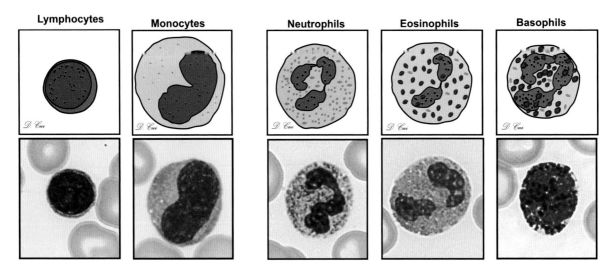

Figure 8-2. Overview of peripheral blood cell types (mature blood cells), blood smear. Wright stain, ×1,569

Blood is a specialized connective tissue composed of **blood cells** suspended in intercellular fluid (or **plasma**). Blood cells include **erythrocytes (red blood cells)**, **platelets (thrombocytes)**, and leukocytes **(white blood cells)**. *Erythrocytes* are the most numerous. They are biconcave disk–shaped cells without nuclei and are important in transportation of gases. *Platelets* are very tiny cell fragments that have no nuclei, cannot reproduce, and come from huge cells called **megakaryocytes**. Platelets play an important role in hemostasis. *Leukocytes* can be classified as either **agranulocytes** or **granulocytes** based on the absence or presence of specific granules in their cytoplasm. Granulocytes are also called **polymorphonuclear leukocytes** because of the multiple lobes of their nuclei, but the term is often used specifically for neutrophils. (1) *Agranulocytes* lack specific cytoplasmic granules but have the ability to divide. **Lymphocytes** and **monocytes** fall into this category. *Lymphocytes* are the smallest cells in the leukocyte series. Each has a round nucleus and a small amount of cytoplasm. They can be found outside of the blood stream in lymphoid organs and connective tissues. Lymphocytes can be classified as **T lymphocytes**, **B lymphocytes**, and **null cells**. They are associated with immunological defense functions. B lymphocytes can further differentiate into **plasma cells**. *Monocytes* are the largest cells in the leukocyte series. They have large, elongated, and often kidney-shaped nuclei. They can differentiate into **phagocytes**, including **macrophages**, **Kupffer cells**, **microglia**, and **osteoclasts**. (2) *Granulocytes* contain specific granules in their cytoplasm, and their nuclei are segmented. They are terminal cells without the capability to divide further. Granulocytes include **neutrophils**, **eosinophils**, and **basophils**. *Neutrophils* are the most abundant leukocytes in circulating blood. Each cell has a multilobed nucleus and a pale pink cytoplasm that contains primary and secondary (specific) granules. Neutrophils play an important role in defense against bacterial infection. *Eosinophils* contain large, specific granules that stain red with eosin dye. They usually have a bilobed, or occasionally a trilobed, nucleus. Eosinophils function in controlling allergic reactions and in combating parasitic infections. *Basophils* are the rarest of the leukocytes (<1%). They contain large, specific granules that are deep violet with a Wright stain. Each basophil has a nucleus with two to three lobes that are not completely separated. Basophils, along with mast cells, are instigators of allergic reactions (see the introduction to this chapter).

Erythrocytes and Platelets

A

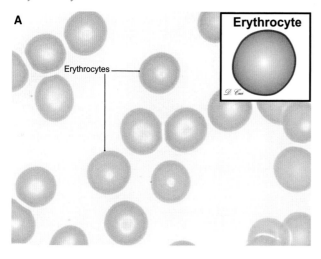

Erythrocytes

Erythrocyte

D. Cui

Figure 8-3A. Erythrocytes (red blood cells), blood smear. Wright stain, ×1,576

Erythrocytes are the most abundant cells in blood. They have a unique **biconcave** disk appearance, are **anucleate** (without nuclei), and have no organelles after they mature. Here, red blood cells are seen as *pink circles with pale centers* in a Wright stain. Erythrocytes are produced in the red bone marrow and are transported into the blood circulation through the walls of sinusoidal capillaries in the marrow. Their life span is about 120 days. Aged erythrocytes are destroyed by macrophages in the spleen, liver, and bone marrow. Erythrocytes contain highly concentrated hemoglobin (Hb). They appear bright red in color when oxygen content is high and are more purple when they are depleted of oxygen. Their function is to transport oxygen to peripheral tissues and carry carbon dioxide out of tissues. Hemoglobin binds with oxygen to form oxyhemoglobin when the O_2 level is high (lung) and binds with CO_2 to form carbaminohemoglobin when the CO_2 level is high (tissue).

B

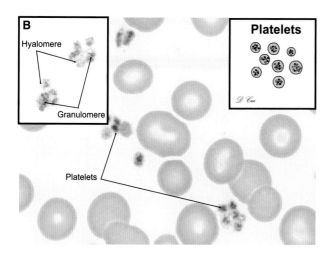

Hyalomere

Granulomere

Platelets

Platelets

D. Cui

Figure 8-3B. Platelets (thrombocytes), blood smear. Wright stain, ×1,576; inset ×1,570

Platelets, also called **thrombocytes**, are very small, lens-shaped fragments of cells. They have some functional characteristics of whole cells, even though they do not have nuclei. Each platelet has a surface membrane covering cytoplasm that contains microtubules, microfilaments, mitochondria, and several types of granules. The central region where granules stain purple is termed the **granulomere**; the peripheral region, which stains light blue, is called the **hyalomere**. The two main types of granules in platelets are **alpha granules** and **delta granules** (**dense bodies**). These play a role in the adhesion and aggregation of platelets in blood coagulation. If damage occurs to the vascular endothelium, platelets adhere to the vessel wall, releasing granules and aggregating to stop bleeding.

The absence of alpha granules can cause **gray platelet syndrome**, whereas reduced numbers or absence of delta granules will lead to **storage pool deficiency**.

CLINICAL CORRELATION

C

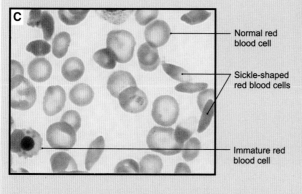

Normal red blood cell

Sickle-shaped red blood cells

Immature red blood cell

Figure 8-3C. Sickle Cell Anemia, Blood Smear. Wright stain, ×1,035

Sickle cell anemia is an autosomal recessive disorder characterized by the production of defective hemoglobins, which aggregate and polymerize when deoxygenated. The red blood cells become longer and curved, similar to a "sickle." Sickle cells block blood vessels, causing **ischemia** of the tissues and severe pain. Symptoms and signs, which start in early childhood, include anemia, vasoocclusive complications, and chronic **hyperbilirubinemia**. This disease is more common in people of African, Turkish, Arabian, and Mediterranean ancestry. Dehydration, infection, hypertonicity, and decreased pH can trigger an onset. In a sickle cell patient, the average life span of red blood cells is 17 days, as compared to 120 days in normal persons. Bone marrow transplants can cure a small number of people. **Normal** and **sickle cell** forms are shown here.

ERYTHROCYTES AND PLATELETS IN THE BLOOD VESSELS

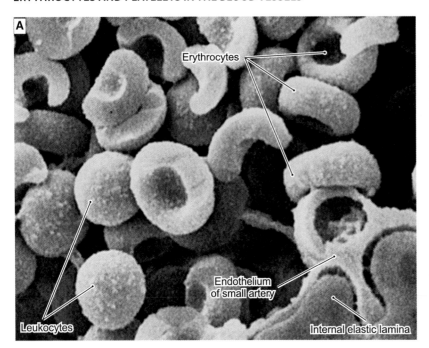

Figure 8-4A. Erythrocytes, small artery. SEM, ×1,140

This scanning electron micrograph demonstrates the various shapes of the blood cells contained in the lumen of a **small artery**. The **erythrocytes** appear as biconcave disks; that is, "doughnuts" with thin diaphragms across the holes. By contrast, the **leukocytes** are spherical, and the different types cannot be distinguished. No platelets are visible in this view. The inner layer of the artery wall is tunica intima, composed mainly of **endothelium** and a thin **internal elastic lamina**.

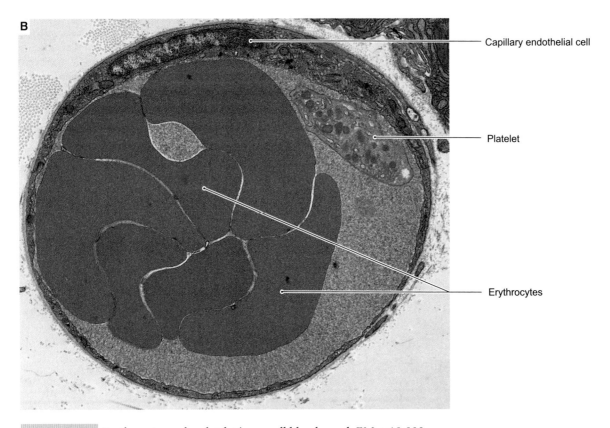

Figure 8-4B. Erythrocytes and a platelet in a small blood vessel. EM, ×10,000

The lumen of this **capillary** (or **venule**) contains profiles of several **erythrocytes** and a **platelet**. The erythrocytes in this thin section present a variety of profile shapes owing to two effects: the random orientation of the plane of section and the flexibility that allows the cells to bend in compliance with surrounding pressures. The platelet here is cut transversely through its biconvex shape, which is maintained by microtubules arranged as a hoop at the edge of the disk. The magnification of this view is not quite sufficient to reveal the microtubules. It can be seen here that the platelet contains a variety of granules and tubules.

Leukocytes: Agranulocytes

LYMPHOCYTES AND MONOCYTES

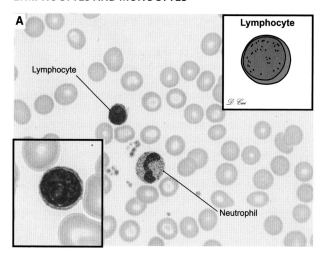

Figure 8-5A. Lymphocytes, blood smear. Wright stain, ×754; inset ×1,569

Most **lymphocytes** in the blood are small- to medium-sized cells. Each has a relatively large, round nucleus with a thin rim of cytoplasm (which is often crescent shaped). Lymphocytes originate in the bone marrow and thymus and circulate throughout the body in the blood and lymph circulation systems. Lymphocytes are motile and play an important role in immunological defense. They can be classified into **B lymphocytes**, **T lymphocytes**, and **null cells** based on their immunologic functions. *B lymphocytes* are responsible for the **humoral immune response**, in which immunoglobulins are secreted after they differentiate into plasma cells. *T lymphocytes* are responsible for the **cellular immune response**. T and B lymphocytes are morphologically indistinguishable in blood smears. *Null cells* are large cells that are morphologically similar to other lymphocytes but lack the characteristic surface markers of the B and T cells (see Chapter 10, "Lymphoid System").

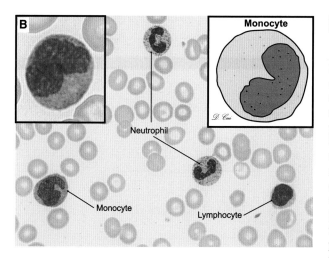

Figure 8-5B. Monocytes, blood smear. Wright stain, ×754; inset ×1,569

Monocytes are the largest agranular cells in the peripheral blood. Each cell has a large, elongated nucleus, often assuming kidney or horseshoe shapes. The cytoplasm of monocytes is blue-gray and contains a variable number of dark blue-purple granules that are called **azurophilic granules**, so named because they attract azure (blue-purple) dyes in stains used for blood smears. Azurophilic granules are lysosomes, so they are nonspecific granules present in the cytoplasm of both agranular and granular leukocytes. They are distinct from the specific granules found in granular leukocytes. Monocytes originate from the bone marrow and remain in the blood circulation in an immature (precursor) state for 1 to 2 days. They then enter peripheral tissues to complete their differentiation. They become **macrophages** (**tissue phagocytes**) in connective tissue, **Kupffer cells** in the liver, **microglia** in the nervous system, and **osteoclasts** in bones.

CLINICAL CORRELATION

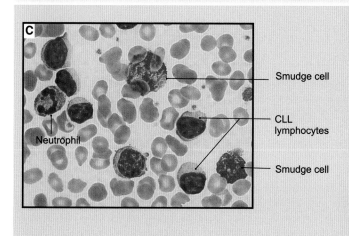

Figure 8-5C. Chronic Lymphocytic Leukemia, Smear. Wright stain, ×736

Chronic lymphocytic leukemia (CLL) is a type of blood cancer characterized by abnormally high numbers of mature lymphocytes in certain tissues and peripheral blood. **Lymphocytes** infiltrate the liver, spleen, lymph nodes, and the bone marrow. Signs and symptoms include **petechiae** ("pinpoint" hemorrhages) in the skin and soft palate; enlargement of the liver, spleen, and lymph nodes; anemia; fever; infections; bone pain; and weight loss. In some patients, CLL will transform into an aggressive lymphoma. The cause of CLL is not clear, but it may be associated with chromosomal disorders, radiation, benzene exposure, and chemotherapy. CLL progresses slowly but is not considered curable. Treatment includes chemotherapy and bone marrow transplant. In the peripheral blood, CLL cells are small lymphocytes with clumped chromatin and little cytoplasm. **Smudge cells**, although not specific for CLL, are commonly seen on peripheral blood smears.

Leukocytes: Granulocytes
NEUTROPHILS

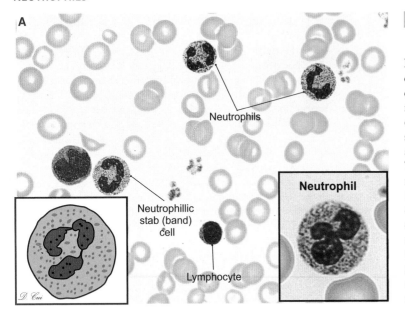

A

Neutrophils

Neutrophillic
stab (band)
cell

Lymphocyte

Neutrophil

Figure 8-6A. **Neutrophils, blood smear.** Wright stain, ×754; inset ×1,569

Neutrophils are the most abundant cells in the leukocyte series. They have a multilobed (two to five interconnected lobes) nucleus and pale pink cytoplasm with many granules (or **vesicles**). There are two main types of granules in neutrophils: **primary** (**nonspecific**) and **secondary** (**specific**) **granules.** *Primary granules* are azurophilic granules, which are modified **lysosomes**. The neutrophils' primary granules are larger and less numerous than specific granules. *Secondary granules* (**specific** or **neutrophilic granules**) are more numerous than primary granules, and they contain a variety of antibacterial compounds. They stain lavender or salmon-pink with Wright stain, but they are difficult to distinguish because of their small size. Like other granular leukocytes, neutrophils are terminally differentiated cells unable to divide. They play a primary role in defense against bacterial and fungal infections.

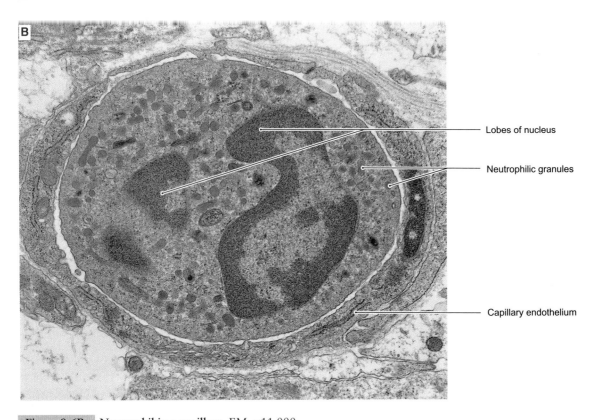

B

Lobes of nucleus

Neutrophilic granules

Capillary endothelium

Figure 8-6B. **Neutrophil in a capillary.** EM, ×11,000

This **leukocyte** fills the lumen of the **capillary** in which it resides. Although the thickness of the section is only about one two-hundredth of the diameter of the cell, the features of the neutrophil are readily apparent. Profiles of three **lobes of the nucleus** can be seen, and the cytoplasm has an abundance of small granules that vary in electron density. The shapes of the granules also vary from spherical to rice shaped. It is difficult to unequivocally distinguish the two main types of granules strictly on the basis of morphology. However, the smallest and most numerous granules are **specific** (**neutrophilic, secondary**) **granules,** and the largest granules are **nonspecific** (**azurophilic, primary**) **granules.** The neutrophilic granules are difficult to discern in the light microscope because their size is close to the limit of resolution of light microscopy.

NEUTROPHIL PHAGOCYTOSIS

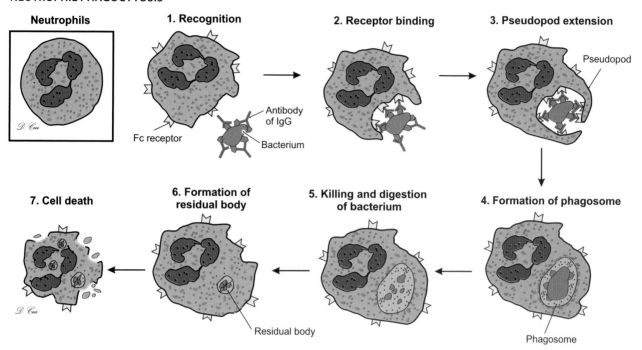

Figure 8-7. Representation of neutrophil phagocytosis of bacteria.

Neutrophils play a central role in cellular defense against bacterial and fungal infections. They are highly motile cells and respond quickly to inflammation in cases of microbial invasion. Acute inflammation, one of the body's defense mechanisms, occurs in the very early stage of tissue response to injuring agents, such as bacteria and fungi. During acute inflammation, microvessels dilate, and their permeability increases as a result of histamine and other inflammatory chemicals, which are released into the connective tissue by mast cells (see Chapter 4, "Connective Tissue"). Neutrophils quickly enter tissues from the blood circulation by adhering to activated endothelial cells of capillaries and venules at the site of the inflammation. Bacteria are neutralized by several mechanisms, which include the complement system and antibodies. Neutrophil phagocytosis of bacteria occurs in several steps: (1) **Recognition:** The process begins with recognition of the bacterium by **opsonins** (IgG and complement C3b fragments) that coat the bacterium and render it more susceptible to phagocytes. (2) **Receptor binding:** Fc receptors of neutrophils recognize and bind IgG that has bound to the bacterium, or complement C3b receptors bind C3b fragments on the surface of the bacterium. (3) **Pseudopod extension:** Pseudopods are slender cytoplasmic processes of neutrophils, which engulf (or "phagocytose") the bacterium that has been recognized and bound by receptors. (4) **Formation of phagosome:** The engulfment of the bacterium sequesters it in a membrane-bound vesicle, the **phagosome** (food vacuole). (5) **Killing and digestion of bacterium:** Immediately after or even during formation of the phagosome, the **proton pumps** in the membrane of the phagosome generate an acidic pH; both primary and secondary neutrophil granules fuse with the phagosome and release their components into the phagosome to kill the bacterium and break down the constituents (proteins, carbohydrates, nucleic acids) of the bacterium. Lysosomal enzymes and other products may leak into the extracellular space, causing damage to endothelial cells and nearby tissues. (6) **Formation of the residual body:** Most of the remaining digested materials form **residual bodies** (vesicles containing leftover products of indigestible materials after fusion with the contents of a lysosome) inside the cells. (7) **Cell death:** Soon after neutrophils have finished their job of killing and digesting bacteria, they die. The dead neutrophils may be phagocytosed by macrophages, or they may accumulate locally with tissue debris and fluid to form pus.

Neutrophils use **oxidative** and **nonoxidative mechanisms** in killing bacteria and destroying other microbes. The *oxidative mechanism*, also known as **respiratory burst** or **oxygen-dependent mechanism**, involves generation of hydrogen peroxide by the NADPH (nicotinamide adenine dinucleotide phosphate) oxidase system and generation of hypochlorous acid by myeloperoxidase (components of primary granules). The *nonoxidative mechanism* is involved in **phagocytosis** in the following manner: Primary and secondary granules fuse with the phagosome, and their granule components are released directly onto the microbe (see above steps 4 and 5). These components include **defensins, neutral serine protease,** and **lysozyme** from the primary granules as well as **lactoferrin** and **lysozyme** from the secondary granules. They perform their antimicrobial function by disrupting the phagosomal membrane, degrading bacterial membranes, breaking down the protein and carbohydrate of the bacterium, and binding iron (which is needed for bacterial growth) to prevent bacterial growth. Both oxidative and nonoxidative mechanisms work in concert to facilitate killing of the microbes.

A pathologic condition known as **myeloperoxidase deficiency** is caused by a defect in the NADPH oxidase complex. This condition results in the inability to produce "superoxides" in neutrophils and other phagocytic cells. Affected individuals are unable to kill invading microbes that are normally engulfed by these phagocytic cells. People with this defect can have frequent and prolonged bacterial and fungal infections.

EOSINOPHILS AND BASOPHILs

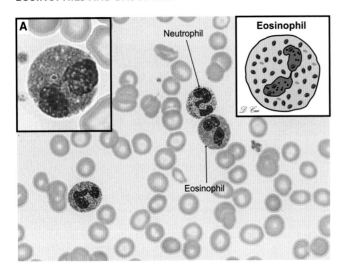

Figure 8-8A. **Eosinophil, blood smear.** Wright stain, ×754; inset ×1,569

Eosinophils have a two- to three-lobed (segmented) nucleus, numerous **specific (eosinophilic) granules**, and a few **azurophilic granules** in the cytoplasm. *Specific granules* contain **acid hydrolases, peroxidase, histaminase, basic protein, and eosinophil cationic proteins,** which have antihelminthic properties. *Azurophilic granules* contain mainly **lysosomal enzymes.** Normally, the bone marrow contains a large reserve pool of eosinophils (and other granulocytes) ready for deployment on demand. Eosinophils have a life span of a few days in circulating blood, although they can survive longer in the tissues. They are commonly found in the connective tissue of the digestive tract. Some of the granules in eosinophils are highly toxic to parasitic worms such as schistosomes. Eosinophils also play a role in moderating inflammation resulting from an allergic reaction. They selectively ingest and degrade antigen-antibody complexes and also degrade histamine, therefore limiting inflammation.

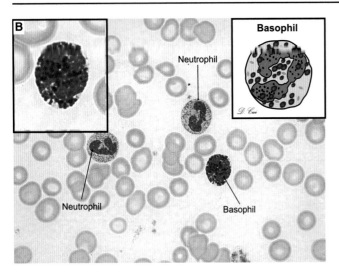

Figure 8-8B. **Basophil, blood smear.** Wright stain, ×754; inset ×1,569

Basophils are the least numerous in the blood circulation, comprising less than 1% of the leukocytes. It is therefore difficult to find them in normal blood smears. They have a two- to three-lobed nucleus and large granules in the cytoplasm. These granules stain deep violet with Wright stain and are distributed unevenly in the cytoplasm. **Specific granules** in basophils contain **heparin, histamine, peroxidase, and eosinophil and neutrophil chemotactic factors** (attracts eosinophils and neutrophils to the site). **Azurophilic granules** are also present in basophils. Basophils have a similar function to mast cells in connective tissue. They contribute to allergic reactions by releasing histamine and heparin to produce inflammation at the allergic reaction site. (For details, see Fig. 4-4B).

CLINICAL CORRELATION

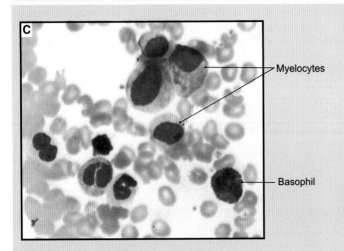

Figure 8-8C. **Chronic Myelogenous Leukemia.** Wright-Giemsa, ×50

Chronic myelogenous leukemia (CML) is a myeloproliferative disorder characterized by a **chimeric BCR-ABL gene** composed of the BCR gene on **chromosome 22** and the ABL gene on chromosome 9. In more than 90% of cases, this chimeric gene arises due to a reciprocal translocation, **t(9;22)(q34;q11)**, also known as the Philadelphia chromosome (part of chromosome 9 and part of chromosome 22 break off and trade places). Clinically, patients may present with slowly progressive weakness, fatigability, weight loss, and splenomegaly. Laboratory studies reveal an elevated **white blood count** and **anemia.** A differential count of the white blood cells typically reveals **neutrophils, band** forms, **metamyelocytes, myelocytes, eosinophils,** and **basophils.** Within months, a patient may enter an accelerated phase with increasing **anemia** and **thrombocytopenia** (decrease in platelets), and ultimately enter the blast phase with acute leukemia. The blasts may be of myeloid or lymphoid origin. Treatment includes **BCR-ABL inhibitors,** which can result in sustained remissions in the majority of patients.

EOSINOPHILS

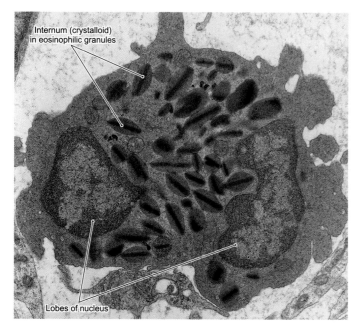

Internum (crystalloid) in eosinophilic granules

Lobes of nucleus

Figure 8-9. Eosinophil in connective tissue. EM, ×12,000

The irregular surface contours of this cell suggest that it was in motion at the time the specimen was obtained. The **two lobes** typical of the nucleus of an **eosinophil** are present in the section, and the relatively large specific granules have the features that are characteristic of eosinophilic granules. The profiles of the granules have two-dimensional shapes that are consistent with a biconvex three-dimensional shape. Each granule has a crystalline core (**internum**) composed of a major basic protein, one of the cationic proteins sequestered within eosinophilic granules.

TABLE 8-1 Leukocytes with Functional and Clinical Correlations

Types of Leukocytes	Approximate % of WBCs	Nucleus	Granules in Cytoplasm	Main Functions	Clinical Correlations
Lymphocyte	25%–33%	Round, relatively large compared to cell size	If present, only a few azurophilic granules	Play an important role in immune defense	Chronic inflammation, human immunodeficiency virus (HIV) infection, lymphoma
Monocyte	3%–7%	Large, kidney shaped or horseshoe shaped; nonsegmented	Azurophilic granules only (lysozyme, endogenous pyrogens/IL-1)	Phagocytosis of any recognizable nonself agents after becoming mature tissue phagocytes (macrophages, kupffer cells, microglial cells, dust cells, osteoclasts)	Whipple disease, malakoplakia, tuberculosis, Langerhans cell histiocytosis, heart failure
Neutrophil	54%–62%	Multilobed (five or more); segmented	Azurophilic (primary) granules contain lysosome, myeloperoxidase, and superoxide; small, salmon-pink, specific (secondary) granules contain major basic proteins, lactoferrin, lysozyme, collagenase, and proteases	Defend against bacterial and fungal infection	Bacterial infection, acute suppurative inflammation, neutropenia, agranulocytosis
Eosinophil	1%–3%	Two to three lobes; segmented	Azurophilic granules; large red, specific granules contain major basic proteins, acid phosphatase, peroxidase, arylsulfatase, and β-glucuronidase	Defend against infection by parasitic worms; moderate inflammation in allergic reaction; fight viral infection	Allergic reaction, parasitic infection
Basophil	<1%	Two to three lobes; segmented	Azurophilic granules; large violet (or purple-blue), specific granules contain histamine, heparin, peroxidase, eosinophil/neutrophil chemotactic factor	Involved with inflammation and allergic reactions (similar to mast cells)	Allergic reaction, immediate hypersensitivity reaction, anaphylaxis

Hemopoiesis

Introduction and Key Concepts for Hemopoiesis

All formed elements, with the exception of some lymphocytes, have a finite life span in circulation, so there must be an ongoing replacement throughout the life of an individual. The magnitude of the task for a given cell type can be appreciated if the approximate required daily production rate is calculated from estimates of the total number in circulation and the rate of turnover for the cell type. For **erythrocytes**, with a life span of about 120 days, the daily production rate is roughly 250 billion, for **neutrophils**, with a time in circulation of less than a day, the daily production rate is normally roughly 60 billion, and for **platelets**, with a life span of about 10 days, the daily production rate is ~150 billion. The development of each type of blood cell involves numerous cell divisions and a series of differentiation steps so that a small number of completely undifferentiated stem cells produce enormous numbers of cells that have the specific equipment necessary for the particular mature cell to perform its functions. Although all blood cells originate from a common **pluripotential hemopoietic stem cell**, each blood cell type has its own lineage of cell generations committed to proliferate and, at the same time, differentiate only into that cell type. Cells that can be recognized morphologically as undertaking differentiation into a particular blood cell are called **precursor cells**. Precursor cells are produced by cells that are committed to a specific lineage (i.e., they are determined to give rise to, e.g., only erythrocytes) but show no morphological signs of differentiation. These are called **progenitor cells**. Some progenitor cells are not restricted in potential to just one blood cell lineage but rather to two lineages. Progenitor cells are also termed **colony-forming cells (CFCs)**. A commonly used abbreviation system for designating specific progenitor cells uses the first letter of the blood cell name after the letters CFC, for example, CFC-E for **erythrocyte colony–forming cell** and CFC-B for **basophil colony–forming cell**. Development of blood cells occurs mostly in the specialized environment of the bone marrow. Because extensive cell proliferation is required, the process is very vulnerable to irradiation, so protection within the cores of bones is clearly advantageous. The development of each type of blood cell involves a series of precursor cells that can be recognized in smears of the red bone marrow that have been stained with the same procedures used for peripheral blood smears. **Lymphocytes** and **monocytes** are little differentiated, so the morphological appearance of their precursors (**lymphoblasts** and **promonocytes**, respectively) is not easily distinguished. By contrast, the precursors of **erythrocytes**, **granulocytes**, and **platelets** exhibit relatively distinct features as they differentiate in a series of steps that involve predictable changes and identifiable stages. The red bone marrow is a hemopoietic compartment where blood cells (except lymphocytes) develop and mature.

ERYTHROCYTE DEVELOPMENT is called **erythropoiesis**. The appearances of the **precursors** of **erythrocytes** reflect the processes that must take place to generate, from an undifferentiated cell, a cell that is essentially a plasmalemma bag of hemoglobin. In the initial stage, the **proerythroblast**, the main event is generation of free ribosomes that will be needed to synthesize the globin that will combine with heme to form hemoglobin. Therefore, the intense basophilic staining of the cytoplasm in the next stage, the **basophilic erythroblast**, results from a peak concentration of free ribosomes that begin translation of globin mRNAs. In the **polychromatophilic erythroblast**, enough hemoglobin has accumulated to confer some **eosinophilia** to the cytoplasm, whereas the concentration of **ribosomes** has decreased from dilution that accompanies cell division. Continuation of cell division, dilution of ribosomes, and accumulation of more hemoglobin account for the strong eosinophilic staining of the cytoplasm in the **orthochromatophilic erythroblast (normoblast)**. Concurrent with the successive changes in staining of the cytoplasm during erythrocyte development in the cytoplasm are changes in the appearance of the nucleus. Production of ribosomes and transcription of mRNA for globin and other proteins are manifested by a large **euchromatic nucleus** with prominent nucleoli in the **proerythroblast**; subsequent stages have progressively smaller, less active nuclei, and the nucleus is ultimately extruded at the end of the **orthochromatophilic erythroblast** stage. The mitochondrion, another key organelle, is required to synthesize **protoporphyrin** and combine it with iron to form the heme of **hemoglobin**.

PLATELET DEVELOPMENT is called **thrombopoiesis**. Although **platelets** are small (2–4 μm in greatest diameter) fragments of highly organized cytoplasm, they are produced by very large cells called **megakaryocytes**. These cells measure up to 100 μm or more in diameter. Megakaryocytes develop from precursor cells (called **megakaryoblasts**) through a series of incomplete cell cycles (**endomitosis**) that do not include division of the nucleus or cytoplasm. The result is that the nucleus of a mature megakaryocyte has up to 64N chromosomes, instead of the usual 2N chromosomes. The nucleus is large and lobular, but it remains one nucleus. The cytoplasm develops numerous mitochondria, a variety of granules, and microfilaments and microtubules. As the megakaryocyte reaches maturity, its cytoplasm becomes cordoned off by an elaborate system of membranes, called **demarcation membranes** or **channels**, which subdivide the cytoplasm into platelet zones—like perforations in a sheet of stamps.

GRANULOCYTE DEVELOPMENT (GRANULOCYTOPOIESIS) proceeds through an orderly sequence of events that result in cytoplasm that is packed with granules containing a wide variety of substances related to inflammation and destruction of pathogenic organisms. As is the case with erythrocyte development, the initial discernible event is generation of components (ribosomes and **RNA**) needed for protein synthesis, but in granulocyte development, the proteins will be packaged in **vesicles (granules)**. Accordingly, packaging of the proteins requires development of an extensive **endoplasmic reticulum** and **Golgi complex**. These events are prominent in the **myeloblast** and **promyelocyte** stages, both of which have relatively large, active nuclei with nucleoli and cytoplasm that is basophilic owing to its content of ribosomes. Granule generation occurs sequentially, the **nonspecific (lysosomal) granules** first, in the promyelocyte stage, and the **specific granules** second, in the myelocyte stage. Because specific granules first appear in the myelocyte stage, this is the earliest stage at which the precursors of the three granulocytes can be distinguished from each other. Other notable changes during granulocyte maturation are progressive condensation, elongation, and segmentation of the nucleus.

Erythropoiesis

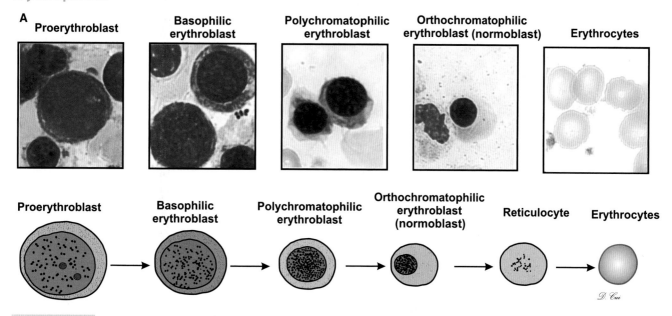

Figure 8-10A. Representation of erythropoiesis (red blood cell formation), bone marrow. Wright stain, ×1,569

Erythrocyte formation includes several stages of cell changes during differentiation. Erythrocytes derive from **progenitor cells (CFC-Es)** that give rise to the first recognizable erythrocyte precursor, the **proerythroblast**. The proerythroblast is a large cell, which has a large active nucleus with nucleoli. Each proerythroblast divides into two **basophilic erythroblasts**. Each basophilic erythroblast divides into two **polychromatophilic erythroblasts**, each of which then divides to form **orthochromatophilic erythroblasts**, which do not divide. These, in turn, differentiate into **reticulocytes**, which finally become **erythrocytes**. There are some general tendencies accompanying differentiation of erythrocytes: (1) the overall size of the cells decreases, (2) the nucleus size decreases and the condensation of the chromatin increases, (3) nucleoli disappear, and (4) the color of the cytoplasm changes from blue to gray to pink because of a reduction of ribosomes and an increase of hemoglobin. When the ribosomes are diluted by cell division and the hemoglobin concentration rises to a near mature level, the cell becomes an orthochromatophilic erythroblast (or **normoblast**). When the nucleus is extruded and only a few organelles (polyribosomes and mitochondria) remain in the cytoplasm, the cell is called a **reticulocyte**. The reticulocyte completes maturation and enters the blood circulation to become a **mature erythrocyte (red blood corpuscle)**.

Thrombopoiesis

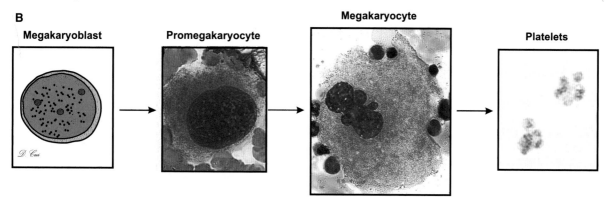

Figure 8-10B. Thrombopoiesis (platelet formation process), bone marrow. Wright stain, ×843, ×586, and ×1,570 (*from left to right*)

Platelets are very small fragments of cells that have no nuclei. They are also called **thrombocytes**. Their differentiation from a large cell, the **megakaryocyte**, takes place in the bone marrow. **Megakaryoblasts** are the precursor cells. They have a large, round nucleus, undergo mitosis, and become **promegakaryocytes**. These cells have a large, round nucleus and develop through growth and a series of endomitoses into **megakaryocytes**. A megakaryocyte has a large, multilobed nucleus with a huge amount of cytoplasm containing numerous granules. The maturation process includes the development of a demarcation membrane system and the subdivision of the cytoplasm to form platelets.

Erythropoiesis

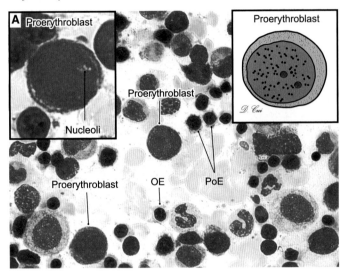

Figure 8-11A. Proerythroblasts, bone marrow smear. Wright stain, ×710; inset ×1,569

The **proerythroblast** is a relatively large cell with a large, round nucleus containing two to three nucleoli. The cytoplasm appears **basophilic** (blue) because of the presence of a large number of ribosomes. At this stage, the cell is beginning to accumulate the necessary components for the production of **hemoglobin**. Proerythroblasts are precursor cells, which develop from two functionally identifiable progenitor cells: **burst-forming unit–erythroid (BFU-E) cells**, which take about a week to mature to become **colony-forming unit–erythroid (CFU-E) cells** and another week to become proerythroblasts. Proerythroblasts undergo mitosis to produce two daughter cells that will develop the features of **basophilic erythroblasts**.

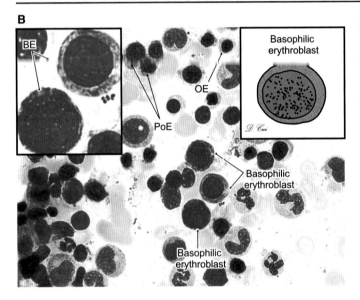

Figure 8-11B. Basophilic erythroblasts, bone marrow smear. Wright stain, ×710; inset ×1,569

The **basophilic erythroblast** is smaller than the proerythroblast, and its cytoplasm is deep blue because of a high content of tightly packed **ribosomes**. Compared to proerythroblasts, basophilic erythroblasts have smaller nuclei with a coarser texture because most of the chromatin is in the heterochromatin form. At this stage, nuclei are less active than in proerythroblasts, and their nucleoli disappear. These cells undergo mitosis and divide into daughter cells, which mature to become **polychromatophilic erythroblasts**. (OE, orthochromatophilic erythroblast; PoE, polychromatophilic erythroblast; BE, basophilic erythroblast.)

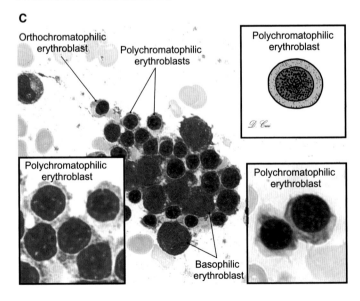

Figure 8-11C. Polychromatophilic erythroblasts, bone marrow smear. Wright stain, ×710; inset ×1,569

The **polychromatophilic erythroblast** is smaller than its parent cell (**basophilic erythroblast**). The nucleus is smaller, and it has no nucleoli. The condensed nucleus is densely stained, and it displays a patchy pattern because of condensation of chromatin. The cytoplasm of the cell is usually grayish in overall color because, at this stage, significant amounts of **hemoglobin** have been produced and accumulated in the cytoplasm, so that the staining of the cytoplasm reflects the presence of both ribosomes (basophilic) and hemoglobin (eosinophilic). Therefore, the cytoplasm is mottled with mixed patches of blue and pink (**polychromatophilic** means "attracting multiple colors"). Polychromatophilic erythroblasts undergo mitosis and divide into daughter cells that develop into **orthochromatophilic erythroblasts**.

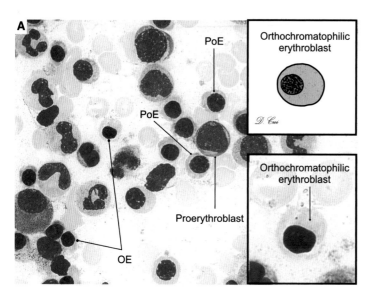

Figure 8-12A. Orthochromatophilic erythroblasts, bone marrow smear. Wright stain, ×710; inset ×1,569

The **orthochromatophilic erythroblast**, also called a **normoblast**, is a very small cell, close to the size of an erythrocyte. The nucleus is small and so condensed that it looks like a dark dot because of the extreme condensation of the chromatin. The cytoplasm appears pinker than that of the **polychromatophilic erythroblast**. Hemoglobin production and accumulation are almost complete, with few ribosomes left in the cytoplasm. At this stage, the cell is unable to divide. Orthochromatophilic erythroblasts become reticulocytes after losing their nuclei.

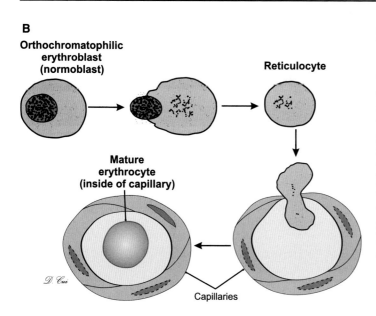

Figure 8-12B. Reticulocytes: final step of erythrocyte formation.

Orthochromatophilic erythroblasts have small and highly condensed nuclei. In the next stage, the nucleus is extruded and phagocytosed by **macrophages**. Although the cells lose their nuclei, they retain some **polyribosomes** in their cytoplasm. When stained supravitally with cresyl blue or new methylene blue, the ribosomes aggregate into a blue reticular network; therefore, the cells are called **reticulocytes**. Reticular cells appear the same as mature erythrocytes with Wright stain. Reticulocytes enter the blood circulation through the bone marrow sinusoidal capillaries and become mature erythrocytes in 1 or 2 days. Mature erythrocytes have neither nuclei nor organelles and appear as a biconcave disk.

CLINICAL CORRELATION

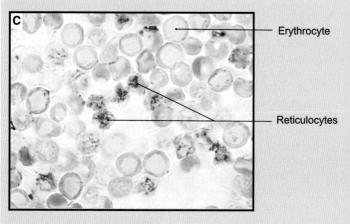

Figure 8-12C. Reticulocytosis, peripheral blood smear. New methylene blue stain, ×1,020

Reticulocytosis is a condition characterized by an increased number of reticulocytes. **Reticulocytes** are premature red blood cells. The normal percentage of reticulocytes is 0.5% to 1.5%. **Hemolytic anemia** usually increases erythropoietin production, which in turn causes the bone marrow to produce more red blood cells, resulting in a reticulocyte percentage of above 4% to 5%. An increased number of reticulocytes in peripheral blood is an important indication of **hemolysis (red blood cell rupture)** or **bleeding**. It can also be the consequence of treating the anemia of chronic kidney disease with erythropoietin. This illustration shows the increased number of reticulocytes with new methylene blue stain after hemolytic anemia.

Thrombopoiesis

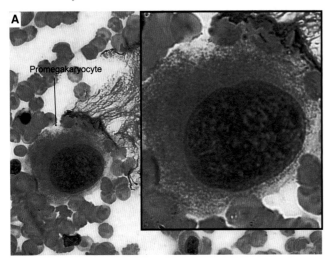

Figure 8-13A.　Promegakaryocytes (immature megakaryo-cytes), bone marrow smear. Wright stain, ×754; inset ×1,605

Promegakaryocytes develop from megakaryoblasts in the bone marrow. **Megakaryoblasts** lose their ability to undergo cytokinesis but undergo a series of incomplete cell cycles called "endomitosis" that results in replication of DNA up to 64N without division of nuclei or cytoplasm. Each megakaryoblast has a large nucleus, multiple nucleoli, and basophilic cytoplasm. **Promegakaryocytes** can be recognized by their large size, round (or oval) nuclei, and large amount of cytoplasm. Development of a **demarcation membrane system** is an important feature of thrombopoiesis and begins at a very early stage. The demarcation membrane system is produced by the invagination of plasma membranes to form branched interconnected channels through the cytoplasm. This system may play an important role in later subdivision of the cytoplasm into platelet zones.

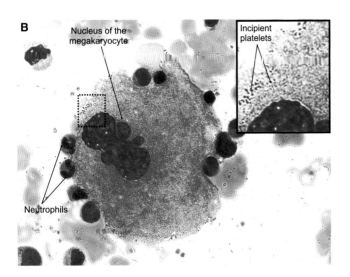

Figure 8-13B.　Megakaryocytes, bone marrow smear. Wright stain, ×754; inset ×2,827

Because of their very large size, **megakaryocytes** are sometimes called **giant cells**. They have a large indented (partially lobulated) nucleus and an extremely voluminous cytoplasm containing a variety of granules. In this stage, the **demarcation membrane system** is complete, and the megakaryocytes are ready to release platelets. Megakaryocytes tend to move toward and attach to the **marrow sinusoids** (capillaries in the bone marrow) after they become mature. The platelets are released into the blood circulation through the wall of the marrow sinusoids. Note the neutrophils on the surface of the megakaryocyte for size comparison. The *inset* shows **incipient platelets** (fragments of cytoplasm beginning to become platelets) in the surface region of the megakaryocyte that are ready to be released. **Thrombopoietin,** a humoral factor produced in the liver, is believed to regulate megakaryocytes and the production of platelets.

CLINICAL CORRELATION

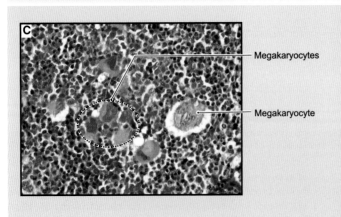

Figure 8-13C.　Essential Thrombocytosis, Bone Marrow Smear. Wright stain, ×304

Essential thrombocytosis, also called **essential thrombocythemia,** is one of the myeloproliferative disorders, characterized by overproduction of platelets by megakaryocytes in the bone marrow without an identifiable cause. The platelet counts exceed 600,000/μL, but the platelets do not function properly. Symptoms and signs include headache; bleeding from gums, nose, and gastrointestinal tract; throbbing and burning pain of the hands and feet caused by thrombosis of small arterioles; and **splenomegaly** (enlarged spleen). Treatment includes using low-dose aspirin to control headache and other vasomotor symptoms and anticancer agents such as **hydroxyurea** to maintain proper platelet count. Bone marrow smears show increased numbers of megakaryocytes. Large platelets, similar in size to red blood cells, may be found in the peripheral blood.

Blood Cell Migration

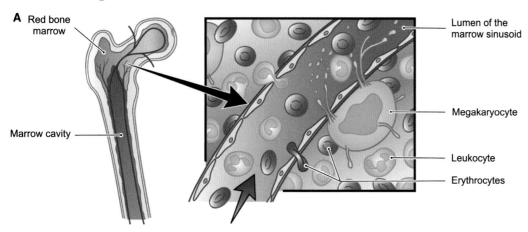

Figure 8-14A. Blood cell migration from bone marrow into blood circulation.

After developing blood cells complete a series of differentiation steps, most of **erythrocytes** and **leukocytes** are mature and ready to be released from bone marrow to the blood circulation. Mature **erythrocytes** have no organelles and mainly contain **hemoglobin**. They are not able to actively move by themselves, but the pressure gradient pushes them through the wall of marrow **sinusoids**. Marrow **sinusoids** are **discontinuous capillaries**, which have incomplete basal laminae and gaps between the endothelial cells comprising their endothelial lining. **Platelets** are released into sinusoids from **megakaryocytes** after the **demarcation membrane system** is completed. Mcgakaryocytes move and attach to the marrow sinusoids and release numbers of platelets from their surface regions of cytoplasm into the lumen of the capillary. **Leukocytes** are capable of actively moving from the bone marrow into sinusoids. Mature blood cells as well as platelets migrated or released into the blood circulation system are called **formed elements** and blood cells called **peripheral blood cells**. Normal peripheral blood cells circulate within the blood vessels for the duration of their **life spans**. If inflammation occurs, **leukocytes** can migrate to the local infected or damaged tissue via **diapedesis**, a process in which leukocytes pass through the endothelial cells and migrate from the postcapillary venules into the interstitium of connective tissue. Some **leukocytes**, such as **lymphocytes**, may move from the tissue back to the circulation after encountering **antigens**.

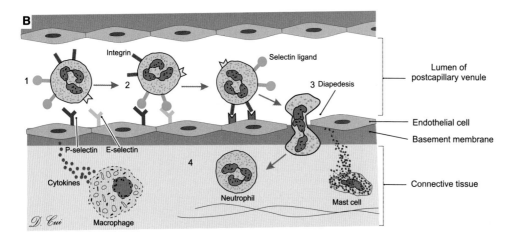

Figure 8-14B. Events of leukocyte diapedesis (extravasation).

In a situation of inflammatory response involving bacterial infection, activating substances released by bacteria cause tissue damage. Histamine and heparin released from tissue mast cells cause microvessel dilation and loosening of junctions between endothelial cells, which allows leukocyte extravasation. Neutrophils are a type of leukocyte and the first cell type to migrate from the circulation into the tissue. Neutrophils circulating in postcapillary venules migrate through the vessel walls, the most common sites of diapedesis. Neutrophil extravasation involves the following events: (1) **chemoattraction:** released by activated macrophages, cytokines (IL-1 and TNF-a) activate selectins (P- and E-selectin) that are found on endothelial cells. (2) **Rolling** and **adhesion:** ligands on the surface of neutrophils bind to selectins, which allow neutrophils to slowly roll on the endothelial cell inner surface and adhere transiently. Integrins, which are involved in cellular adhesion, are expressed on the neutrophils. (3) **Diapedesis:** neutrophils cross the endothelium in order to infiltrate the connective tissue through loosening junctions between the endothelial cells. (4) **Infiltration:** Neutrophils cross the basement membrane and enter the connective tissue.

Granulocytopoiesis

A

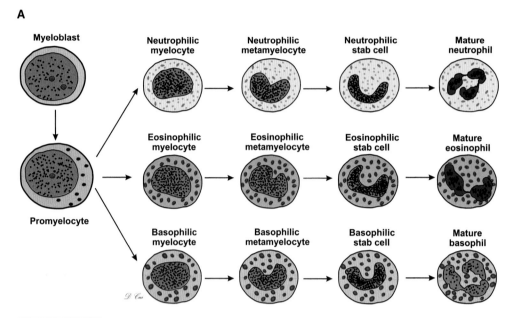

Figure 8-15A. **Figure 8-15A.**   Representation of granulocytopoiesis.

In addition to **erythropoiesis**, **leukopoiesis** also occurs in the bone marrow. Here are examples of the development of **granular leukocytes** (**granulocytopoiesis**). The **myeloblast** is the earliest morphologically recognizable precursor cell. Cell division occurs in myeloblasts, promyelocytes, and myelocytes. The myelocyte is the last stage that is capable of dividing. The generation of nonspecific granules occurs in the promyelocyte stage and specific granules in the myelocyte stage. Maturation of granulocytes follows this sequence: **myeloblasts, promyelocytes, myelocytes, metamyelocytes,** and **stab (band) cells.** The following morphologic changes occur during granulocyte maturation: (1) **nucleoli** are present only before and during the promyelocyte stage; (2) the nucleus takes the following shapes in different developmental stages: oval, elongated, indented, arched, and then segmented (lobed); and (3) **specific granules** are first present at the myelocyte stage.

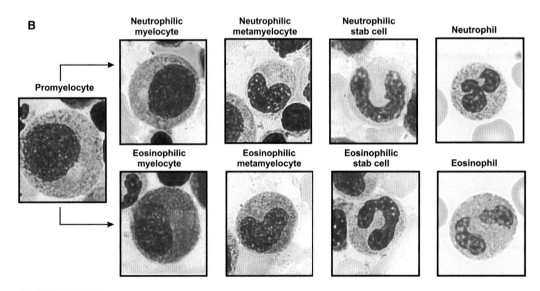

Figure 8-15B.   Overview of stages of granulocytes in development, bone marrow smear. Wright stain, ×1,569

These are examples of microphotographs that show various stages of **granulocyte maturation** in the **neutrophilic** and **eosinophilic** series.

Granulocytopoiesis

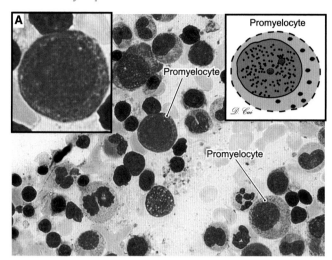

Figure 8-16A. **Promyelocytes, bone marrow smear.** Wright stain, ×710; inset ×1,569

Promyelocytes (also called **progranulocytes**) have a round or oval-shaped nucleus with one to three nucleoli. The cytoplasm is light blue, containing some dark purple granules (**azurophilic granules**). At this stage, specific granules have not been produced. Promyelocytes vary in size and are produced by the division of **myeloblasts**. Their nuclei have a smooth, fine texture because of the fact that most of the chromatin is **euchromatin**, which is delicately dispersed. **Promyelocytes** divide to form **myelocytes**.

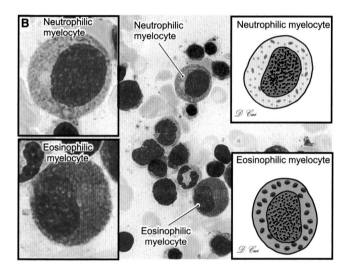

Figure 8-16B. **Myelocytes, bone marrow smear.** Wright stain, ×710; inset ×1,569

The **myelocyte** has an oval or kidney-shaped nucleus that has no nuclei and a coarse texture because of increasing heterochromatin content. The cytoplasm contains **azurophilic granules** and **specific granules**. In this stage, the cell has stopped producing azurophilic granules. In addition, these granules have also been diluted during cell division, so they are not as prominent as in the promyelocyte stage. At the same time, the cell has begun to make and accumulate specific granules so that the cytoplasm starts to take the characteristic appearance of a mature granulocyte. The specific granules in neutrophilic myelocytes are small and appear pinkish, granules in eosinophilic myelocytes are large and stain red, and granules in basophilic myelocytes are blue-purple. Basophilic myelocytes are least numerous and, therefore, difficult to find. In general, myelocytes are smaller than promyelocytes, and their nuclear shape and size may vary. This stage is the longest in **granulocytopoiesis**.

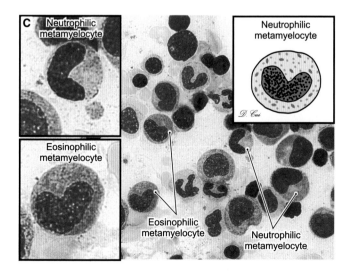

Figure 8-16C. **Metamyelocytes, bone marrow smear.** Wright stain, ×710; inset ×1,569

Metamyelocytes are small cells. They have condensed nuclei, which are elongated with various degrees of indentation and contain clumped chromatin. Metamyelocytes are unable to divide (myelocytes are the last stage in cell division). The cytoplasm of metamyelocytes contains both types of granules. Their cytoplasm and granules are similar to those of mature granulocytes. At this stage, cells have their distinguishing features, but their nuclei have not yet become segmented.

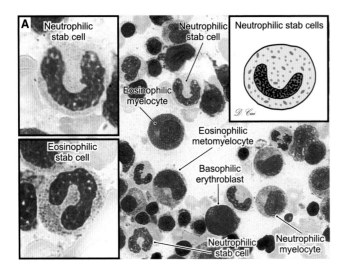

Figure 8-17A. Stab (band) cells, bone marrow smear. Wright stain, ×710; insets ×1,569

Granular **metamyelocytes** mature to become **stab cells**, which are also called **band cells**. The stab cells (mainly neutrophilic stab cells) can be found in both the bone marrow and the peripheral blood. Their nuclei are elongated and become band and arch (or "C") shaped, and the cytoplasm is the same as that of mature neutrophils. These cells are the last stage of granulocyte maturation without division, and in function and structure, they are very close to mature neutrophils. The nuclei of mature neutrophils become multilobulated (segmented), contain dense **heterochromatin**, and often are described as **polymorphonuclear (or segmented) neutrophils**.

Bone Marrow and Blood Cells

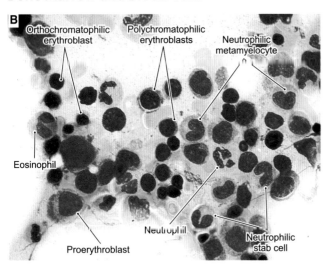

Figure 8-17B. Bone marrow cells, bone marrow smear. Wright stain, ×710

This is an example of blood cells at various stages of development in the **bone marrow**, which includes both the **erythrocyte** and the **granulocyte series**. These cells, at various stages of development, are densely packed together and can be found randomly distributed in the bone marrow. During the maturation process, the cell size becomes smaller and nuclei denser. In the *erythropoiesis series*, the cytoplasm of cells becomes light blue and then pinker, and nuclei become much denser and smaller and finally disappear. In the *granulocytopoiesis series*, the cytoplasm becomes less blue, primary (nonspecific) granules are produced, and then specific granules are produced and are present in myelocytes, which give these cells the appearance characteristic of their identity as a neutrophil, eosinophil, or basophil. In other changes, nuclei become progressively denser, and the shape changes from round to oval, elongated, indented, and then lobed (segmented).

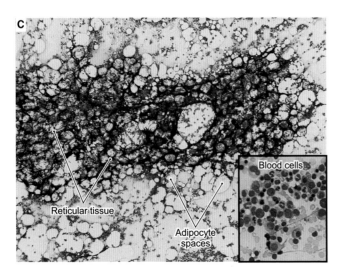

Figure 8-17C. Bone marrow, bone marrow smear. Wright stain, ×35; inset ×184

Bone marrow is a specialized example of a **reticular connective tissue**, a loose connective tissue in which numerous cells are supported by a delicate network of reticular fibers. It resides in cavities within bones. Bone marrow can be categorized into **red bone marrow** and **yellow bone marrow**. The term *red bone marrow* denotes active **hematopoiesis**; *yellow bone marrow* refers to a marrow composed chiefly of **adipocytes (fat cells)**. Pictured is a smear of red bone marrow, which contains many developing blood cells, a few **adipocytes**, and some thin-walled blood vessels (sinusoidal capillaries). The red bone marrow is organized into a **hemopoietic compartment** and a **vascular compartment**. The hemopoietic compartment is a network of reticular fibers in which immature and mature blood cells are suspended. The vascular compartment is composed of mainly sinusoidal capillaries, which allow mature blood cells to enter the blood circulation.

DEVELOPING BLOOD CELLS IN THE HEMATOPOIETIC COMPARTMENT

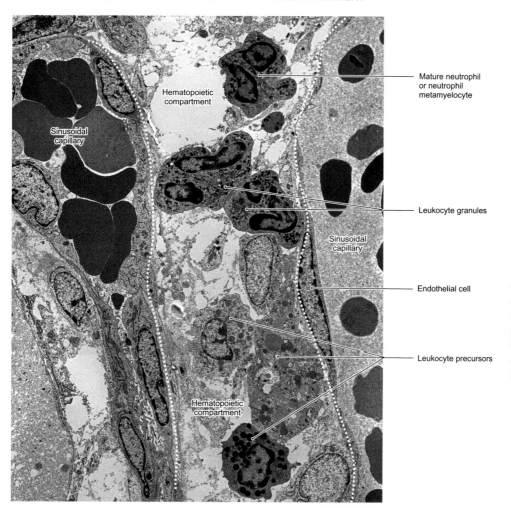

Hematopoietic compartment

Sinusoidal capillary

Sinusoidal capillary

Hematopoietic compartment

Mature neutrophil or neutrophil metamyelocyte

Leukocyte granules

Endothelial cell

Leukocyte precursors

Figure 8-18. Developing blood cells in the bone marrow. EM, ×5,000

The two compartments of the red (hematopoietically active) **bone marrow** can be distinguished here. The **vascular compartment** is composed of **sinusoidal capillaries**, which in this view contain numerous mature erythrocytes. The **hematopoietic compartment** is composed of blood cells and the precursors and progenitors of blood cells suspended in a loose network of support cells and reticular fibers. The cells seen in the hematopoietic compartment here appear to be mostly developing or mature granulocytes. The exact stage of differentiation of individual cells is not as clear here as it is in a bone marrow smear.

CLINICAL CORRELATION

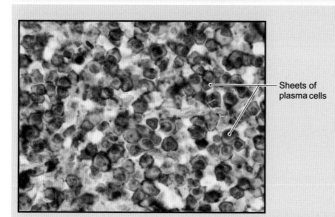

Sheets of plasma cells

Figure 8-19. **Plasma Cell Myeloma.** Immunohistochemical preparation for kappa light chains, ×400

Plasma cell, or **multiple myeloma**, is a malignant tumor of plasma cells that typically affects older individuals and is usually associated with the production of monoclonal proteins composed of intact immunoglobulin or immunoglobulin light chains. These monoclonal proteins, or "m proteins" may be detected electrophoretically in serum and urine. In light chain disease, the clonal expansion of plasma cells produces only immunoglobulin light chains of the kappa or lambda type. These light chains are rapidly filtered into the urine, where they are called "Bence-Jones" proteins. Patients often present with bone pain and fatigue due to the infiltration of the bone marrow by malignant plasma cells, causing dissolution of the bone partly by the stimulation of osteoclasts. Bone marrow biopsy typically reveals sheets of plasma cells, which may vary from histologically normal to bizarre.

SYNOPSIS 8-2 Hematopoiesis

Stem, Progenitor, and Precursor cells
■ *Stem cells* are capable of differentiating into multiple cell lineages and can undergo proliferation indefinitely.
■ *Progenitor cells* are only capable of differentiating into a single cell lineage (restricted to one or two blood cell types) and are morphologically undifferentiated.
■ *Precursor cells* can be recognized morphologically as undergoing differentiation along a particular blood cell lineage.

Erythropoiesis
■ *Cytoplasm* becomes progressively less basophilic because of dilution of ribosomes during the erythropoiesis process.
■ *Nucleus size* progressively decreases because of increased condensation of chromatin.
■ *Cell size* progressively decreases during the erythroid differentiation.
■ *Cytoplasm* becomes progressively more eosinophilic because of increased accumulation of hemoglobin.
■ *The nucleus* retains a round shape and no indentation occurs before it disappears.

Granulocytopoiesis
■ *Cell size* decreases and nucleus becomes more condensed as in erythropoiesis.
■ *Nucleus shape* changes from round or oval (promyeloblasts) to kidney shaped/slightly indented (myelocytes) and then changes from deeply indented (metamyelocytes) to band shaped (band cells) and finally to lobed (mature granulocytes).
■ *Promyelocytes* do not have specific granules (only azurophilic granules); at this stage, it is too early to tell which granular leukocytes they will become.
■ *Myelocytes* are the last developmental stage capable of dividing; specific granules accumulate in this stage.

SYNOPSIS 8-3 Pathologic and Clinical Terms for Mature and Developing Blood Cells

■ *Gray platelet syndrome:* This condition is characterized by a deficiency or absence of the alpha granules and contents in blood platelets, giving platelets a gray appearance in a Wright stain smear.
■ *Platelet storage pool deficiency:* Disorder caused by a decrease or absence of platelet delta granules (dense bodies), which normally store and release adenine nucleotides and 5HT. "Platelet-type" bleeding is common with this deficiency.
■ *Petechiae:* Minute red or purple spots on the skin or mucous membranes caused by capillary hemorrhage; common causes include physical trauma and decreased platelets (thrombocytopenia).
■ *Smudge cell:* Damaged lymphocytes seen on a peripheral blood smear caused by mechanical stress in the process of producing the smear; although nonspecific, smudge cells are encountered more frequently on blood smears of patients with chronic lymphocytic leukemia.
■ *Reticulocytosis:* Increased reticulocytes in the blood, often in response to blood loss, stimulation by erythropoietin treatment, or treatment of iron deficiency anemia with iron supplementation.
■ *Thrombocytosis:* Increased platelet count in the blood, which may be reactive or neoplastic, as in the disease essential thrombocytosis.

From Histology to Pathology

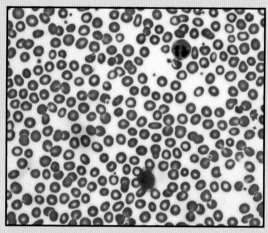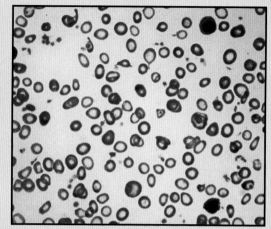

Figure 8-20. Normal erythrocytes and iron deficiency anemia. Wright stain, ×600.

Normal erythrocytes on the *left*. Iron deficiency anemia (IDA) on the *right*, with small (microcytic) erythrocytes (red blood cells) with an enlarged area of central pallor (hypochromic). A large bluish polychromatophilic erythroblast (immature erythrocyte) is present due to the fact that bone marrow is attempting to replenish the lost or dysfunctional red blood cells.

Clinical Vignette Questions

1. A 62-year-old man presents to a physician with complaints of easy fatigability and a 15-lb unintentional weight loss. A physical examination shows pale conjunctivae, but it is otherwise unremarkable. A complete blood count reveals an elevated white blood cell count and low hemoglobin and hematocrit. A peripheral blood smear shows not only mature neutrophils and band forms but also metamyelocytes, myelocytes, eosinophils, and basophils. No blasts are identified. Cytogenetic analysis of the peripheral blood reveals a characteristic translocation, and the patient is diagnosed with chronic myelogenous leukemia (CML). Which of the following is the characteristic translocation seen in more than 90% of CML patients?

A. t(4;11)
B. t(9;22)
C. t(11;14)
D. t(12;21)
E. t(14;18)

2. A 66-year-old man presented to his primary care physician with complaints of worsening fatigue and low back pain over the last several months. Physical examination was unremarkable except for pallor of the conjunctivae. Laboratory examination revealed anemia, hyperproteinemia, and hypercalcemia. Due to these laboratory findings, the physician ordered radiographic studies as well as electrophoresis of the serum and urine. An x-ray study of the spine revealed discrete radiolucent lesions of the vertebral bodies. The serum protein electrophoresis showed a prominent abnormal discrete band in the gamma region, and the urine protein electrophoresis revealed mild, nonselective proteinuria with a similar band paralleling that was seen in the serum. Based on this information, the most appropriate diagnosis is which of the following?

A. Chronic lymphocytic leukemia (CLL)
B. Metastatic adenocarcinoma of the prostate gland
C. Monoclonal gammopathy of undetermined significance (MGUS)
D. Plasma cell myeloma
E. Waldenstrom macroglobulinemia

3. A 42-year-old female with a 3-month history of progressive fatigue and malaise presented to the emergency room after she noticed small red spots, mainly over her upper extremities and trunk. Physical examination revealed a markedly pale woman with petechial hemorrhages in the aforementioned distribution. No lymphadenopathy was identified, and the remainder of the physical examination was unremarkable. A complete blood count (CBC) revealed anemia and thrombocytopenia with a markedly elevated white blood cell count. The white cell differential count showed an abnormal population of large cells with fine chromatin, prominent nucleoli, cytoplasmic granules, and occasion rod-shaped cytoplasmic inclusions. Based on this information, the diagnosis is most likely which of the following?

A. Acute myeloid leukemia (AML)
B. Chronic lymphocytic leukemia (CLL)
C. Chronic myeloid leukemia (CML)
D. Follicular lymphoma
E. Hodgkin lymphoma

9 Circulatory System

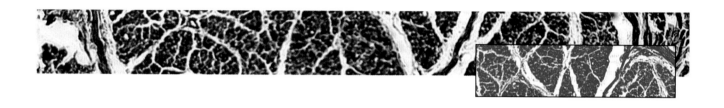

Introduction and Key Concepts for the Circulatory System

Cardiovascular System
Heart
Types of Blood Vessels

Lymphatic Vascular System
Lymphatic Vessels

Cardiovascular System

Systemic and Pulmonary Circulation Systems
Anatomy of the Heart

Layers of the Heart Wall

General Structure of the Blood Vessel Layers

Types of Blood Vessels

Arterial System

Capillary System

Venous System

Lymphatic Vascular System

From Histology to Pathology

Clinical Vignette Questions

Introduction and Key Concepts for the Circulatory System

The **circulatory system** (postnatal circulation) includes the **cardiovascular system** and the **lymphatic vascular system**. The *cardiovascular system* includes the **heart** and the **arterial, capillary,** and **venous systems**. Blood is transported from the heart through the arterial system to the capillaries, where exchange of gases, nutrients, and other substances takes place. Blood is carried back to the heart by the venous system. Blood flows through two routes: (1) The **systemic circulation system** transports oxygenated blood from the heart to the capillaries in the tissues and organs of the body and then collects and carries the blood back to the heart. (2) The **pulmonary circulation system** transports deoxygenated blood from the heart to the capillaries of the lungs. After gas exchange, blood is carried back to the heart. The *lymphatic vascular system* consists of **lymphatic capillaries, lymphatic vessels,** and **lymphatic ducts**. This system collects **lymph** (excess tissue fluid) from the tissues of all organs (except the nervous system, bone marrow, and hard tissues) by lymphatic capillaries and then transports it through lymphatic vessels to the lymphatic ducts, which eventually empty the lymph into the venous system. The collected lymph passes through lymph organs, where it is filtered, and lymphocytes are exposed to antigens. Lymphopoiesis and the immune response occur here.

Cardiovascular System

Heart

The **heart** contains four chambers: the left and right atria and the left and right ventricles. The **atria** receive blood flow discharged from the venous system, whereas the **ventricles** pump blood into the arterial system. The wall of the heart is composed of three layers: **endocardium** (innermost layer), **myocardium** (middle layer), and **epicardium** (outermost layer). (1) *Endocardium* consists of **endothelium, subendothelial connective tissue,** and **subendocardium** (Purkinje fibers, small coronary blood vessels, and nerve fibers). (2) *Myocardium*, the thickest layer of the heart, contains an abundance of **cardiac muscle cells**. Cardiac muscle contracts producing heart beats, which are generated and regulated by the heart conductive system including the **sinoatrial (SA) node**, the **atrioventricular (AV) node**, the **AV bundle**, and **Purkinje fibers**. (3) *Epicardium* is covered by **mesothelium** and contains fibrous connective tissue, nerves, coronary vessels, and adipose tissue.

Types of Blood Vessels

ARTERIAL SYSTEM is composed of **large (conducting)** arteries, **medium (distributing)** arteries, **small arteries,** and **arterioles**. The arterial system conducts blood (under higher pressure than veins) from the ventricles to the capillary networks. The walls of arteries can be generally divided into three layers: **tunica intima, tunica media,** and **tunica adventitia**.

Large arteries are also called **elastic arteries** because of the large quantity of elastic material in their walls. They have a thick tunica media with numerous elastic membranes. The **internal** and **external elastic laminae** are hard to distinguish from the nearby elastic membranes. Large arteries conduct blood from the ventricles into the medium arteries. Rich elastic materials in large arteries enable the vessels to recoil to accommodate pressure changes and maintain a continuous flow of blood during ventricular diastole (relaxation). Examples of large arteries include the aorta, pulmonary arteries, common carotid artery, the subclavian artery, and common iliac arteries.

Medium arteries are also called **muscular arteries** because of their thick tunica media, which contains circularly arranged multiple layers of **smooth muscle cells** in a distinct sheath. Internal and external elastic laminae are easy to distinguish from nearby tissues. Examples of medium arteries include the radial, ulnar, femoral, and splenic artery as well as branches of the external carotid and popliteal arteries.

Small arteries and *arterioles* are smaller-diameter vessels. The walls of small arteries contain two to six layers of smooth muscle cells. *Arterioles* are the smallest components of the arterial system, with only one or two layers of smooth muscle cells. They control the blood flow into the capillaries. Examples of small arteries include vessels found in the tongue, digestive tract, and Fallopian tubes.

CAPILLARY SYSTEM contains continuous capillaries, fenestrated capillaries, and discontinuous (sinusoidal) capillaries. They provide sites for gases, nutrients, metabolic wasters, hormones, and signaling molecules exchange between the blood and tissue. Capillaries are the smallest vessels in the circulation system. They connect arterioles and venules to form a microvessel network, which allows blood movement in the microcirculation and material exchange between the blood and tissue.

Continuous capillaries have a continuous basal lamina and complete endothelial cells. These structures only allow a very limited amount of material to pass through the capillary walls. Examples include capillaries in the muscle tissue, connective tissue, lung, exocrine glands, and thymus.

Fenestrated capillaries have a continuous basal lamina and fenestrated endothelial cells (perforated by small pores), which allow a great range of substances to pass through the capillary walls. Their endothelial cells often bridged by a diaphragm except capillaries in the glomerulus of the kidney. Examples of fenestrated capillaries include capillaries in the endocrine organs, kidney, pancreas, and digestive tract.

Discontinuous (sinusoidal) capillaries have a discontinuous (or missing) basal lamina and incomplete (perforated by large pores), which allow proteins and other materials, even cells, to pass through freely the capillary walls. Examples include capillaries in the bone marrow, liver, and spleen.

VENOUS SYSTEM is composed of **venules** and **small, medium,** and **large veins**. Veins collect blood (under lower pressure than arteries) from capillaries and transport it to the heart. Veins have larger, flat lumens and thinner walls than their companion arteries.

Venules and *small veins* have very thin walls and few valves. Venules drain exchanged blood from the capillaries to the small veins. Venules are the primary sites of many inflammatory reactions.

Medium veins have various diameters, and their structure varies based on their size and location. Segments of medium veins in some locations have a thick **tunica adventitia** with a few **longitudinal smooth muscle bundles**. Valves are prominent in medium veins, with an abundance in the extremities to prevent blood from flowing backward.

Large veins have a thick **tunica adventitia** with numerous **longitudinal smooth muscle bundles,** which help to force blood to flow toward the heart. There are some large valves in the large veins.

Lymphatic Vascular System

Lymphatic Vessels

The **lymphatic vascular system** is composed of lymphatic capillaries, lymphatic vessels, and lymphatic ducts, which collect and drain interstitial fluid from body tissues into larger veins. Functions include the transfer of proteins, hormones, antibodies, fluid, and lymphocytes. Lymphatic vessels are found in most types of connective tissue and lymphatic organs, but they are not found in the central nervous system and nonvascular tissues. The route of lymph drainage is from lymphatic capillaries to lymphatic vessels, and it enters the lymph nodes via the afferent lymphatic vessels while exiting via efferent lymphatic vessels. Most of the lymphoid organs do not have both afferent and efferent lymphatic vessels, except lymph nodes. Collected lymph from lymphoid organs drains into the thoracic duct and the right lymphatic duct and then empties into the subclavian veins.

Lymphatic capillaries have very thin walls and have larger lumens than the blood capillaries. Between the endothelial cells lining lymphatic capillaries, there are small spaces that allow interstitial fluid and lymphocytes to be transferred into the lymphatic capillaries.

Lymphatic vessels have a structure like that of small veins. They have a large lumen and numerous valves. These valves are present in all sizes of lymphatic vessels. Lymphocytes and lymph materials may be present in the lumen of lymphatic vessels.

Lymphatic ducts are large lymphatic vessels that have a few layers of smooth muscle cells in their walls. They have lumens that are structurally similar to those of small veins, except their lumens are larger, and prominent valves are present. Lymphocytes and lymph materials are often present in the lumens of lymphatic vessels.

SYNOPSIS 9-1 Pathologic and Clinical Terms for the Circulatory System

- *Vasculitis:* Inflammation and damage to blood vessels often resulting in ischemia of the tissue served by the affected vessels; may be related to infection, medications, and various autoimmune disorders.
- *Angina:* Chest pain associated with ischemia of the myocardium, most often due to severe atherosclerosis of the coronary arteries; the pain of angina, often described as pressure, is typically substernal but may radiate to the arms or neck.
- *Myocardial infarction:* Necrosis of cardiac muscle due to interruption of its blood supply, most often due to coronary artery atherosclerosis.
- *Atherosclerosis:* The most clinically significant form of arteriosclerosis ("hardening of the arteries"), characterized by the accumulation of lipid within the intima of arteries producing plaques that cause narrowing, or "stenosis," of the artery.
- *Arteriosclerosis:* A general term referring to any hardening (loss of elasticity) of arteries, especially small arteries. High blood pressure is the most common cause. Atherosclerosis is one form of arteriosclerosis.
- *Thrombus:* A blood clot formed within an artery or vein as a result of endothelial injury, abnormal blood flow, or an increased tendency to form clots (hypercoagulability); rupture of an atherosclerotic plaque in a coronary artery promotes the formation of a thrombus.

Cardiovascular System

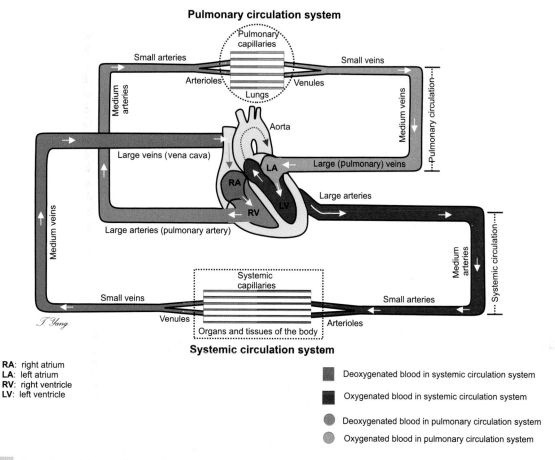

RA: right atrium
LA: left atrium
RV: right ventricle
LV: left ventricle

■ Deoxygenated blood in systemic circulation system
■ Oxygenated blood in systemic circulation system
● Deoxygenated blood in pulmonary circulation system
● Oxygenated blood in pulmonary circulation system

Figure 9-1. Overview of the cardiovascular system.

The **cardiovascular system** consists of the **heart, arterial system, venous system**, and **capillary system**. The *heart* is composed of two **atria** and two **ventricles**. The **right atrium** receives blood from the body, and the **left atrium** receives blood from the lungs; the **left ventricle** pumps blood to the body, and the **right ventricle** pumps blood to the lungs. The *arterial system* conducts blood from the heart to capillaries in the body and the lungs. This system includes large arteries (elastic arteries), medium arteries (muscular arteries), small arteries, and arterioles. The *venous system* carries blood from the capillary system in the body and lungs to the heart. It includes venules, small veins, medium veins, and large veins. The *capillary system* is located between arterioles and venules and often forms capillary beds where exchange of gases and various substances and movement of blood cells (**diapedesis**) take place. It includes **continuous, fenestrated**, and **sinusoidal (discontinuous) capillaries**. Blood flows through two routes: (1) the **systemic circulation system**, which supplies oxygenated blood from the heart to the organs and tissues of the body and then carries deoxygenated blood back to the heart and (2) the **pulmonary circulation system**, which sends deoxygenated blood from the heart to the lungs for gas exchange and then returns oxygenated blood to the heart.

Systemic and Pulmonary Circulation Systems

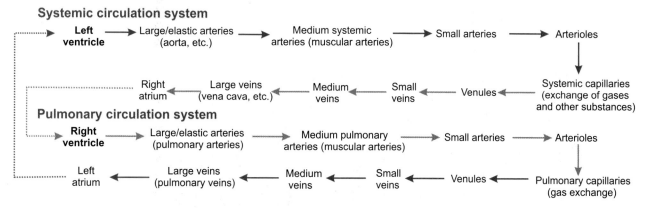

Anatomy of the Heart

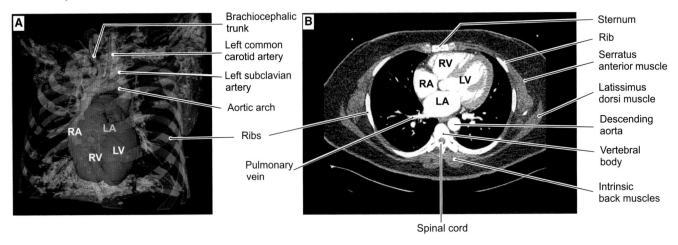

Figure 9-2A,B. **Anatomy of the heart.** 3D stereoscopic model image (A); computed tomography angiography (B)

The heart is a four-chambered muscular organ that lies within the pericardium in the mediastinum. It's a pyramid-shaped structure, resting on the top of the diaphragm. The heart has three surfaces and an apex. The anterior surface, or the **sternocostal surface**, of the heart mainly consists of the **right atrium** (**RA**) and the **right ventricle** (**RV**). The diaphragmatic surface is formed mainly by the **right atrium** (**RA**) and **left ventricle** (**LV**). The posterior surface or the base of the heart is formed mainly by the **LA**. The apex of the heart consists of the **LV**, pointing to the left and downward. The heart is connected to several major blood vessels. The **pulmonary arteries** branch out from the **pulmonary trunk** to deliver deoxygenated blood from the **RV** to the **lungs**. In turn, the **pulmonary veins** bring oxygenated blood back to the **LA** from which the oxygenated blood flows into the **LV**. Oxygenated blood is then pumped from the **LV** to the **aorta** by which it is then distributed to the other parts of the body. The **coronary arteries** supply blood to the heart muscle. There are two coronary arteries, the left and the right coronary arteries. They are branches of the ascending aorta immediately above the right and left cusps of the **aortic semilunar valve**, respectively.

CLINICAL CORRELATION

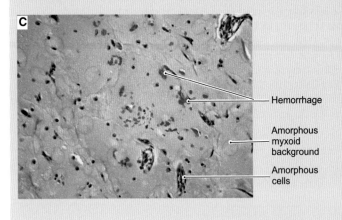

Figure 9-2C. **Cardiac Myxomas.** H&E, ×200

Cardiac myxomas are benign neoplasms that typically arise in the atria of the heart, particularly the **left atrium** in the region near the **fossa ovalis**. These **neoplasms** are often pedunculated (on a stalk) and may cause obstruction to blood flow through a valve and may cause valve damage in the long term. These lesions may become clinically apparent if a portion of the **myxoma** breaks apart from the main lesion causing systemic embolization (clot formation). Grossly, **myxomas** appear soft and gelatinous. Histologically, **myxomas** are characterized by myxoma cells arranged singly and in groups, often with an appearance of a blood vessel. The background is an amorphous and **eosinophilic mucopolysaccharide ground substance**, often showing **hemorrhage** and occasional **mononuclear inflammatory cells**. Treatment involves surgical removal, which is usually curative.

CLINICAL CORRELATION

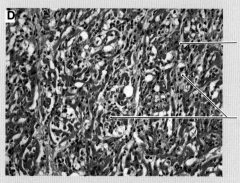

Remaining normal cardiac muscle cells

Myocardium with diffuse lymphocytes

Figure 9-2D. **Myocarditis.** H&E, ×200

Myocarditis represents inflammation of heart muscle due to a variety of causes including infectious agents, hypersensitivity reactions due to drugs, autoimmune diseases, transplant rejection, and sarcoidosis (growth of tiny collections of inflammatory cells). Among infectious etiologies, viruses are the most common cause in the United States, particularly **enteroviruses** like **coxsackieviruses A and B.** Viral infection of the heart typically elicits an immune reaction with infiltration of myocardial tissue by lymphocytes (lymphocytic myocarditis). Myocytes are damaged, either directly by the virus or indirectly by the immunological response. Other forms of **myocarditis**, such as hypersensitivity myocarditis, feature eosinophils as a part of the inflammatory response. Myocarditis has a wide range of clinical presentation, from clinically silent to severe with sudden death.

IMPULSE CONDUCTIVE FUNCTION OF THE HEART

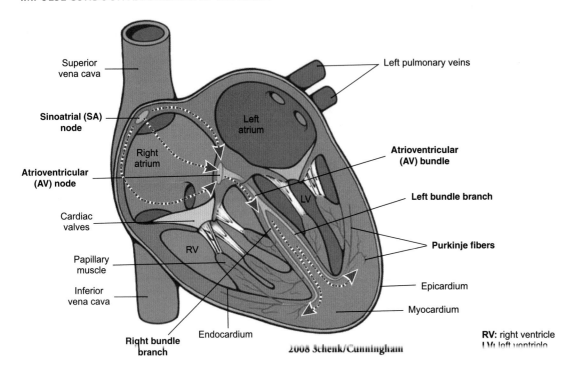

Left pulmonary veins

Superior
vena cava

Sinoatrial (SA)
node

Atrioventricular
(AV) node

Atrioventricular
(AV) bundle

Left
atrium

Right
atrium

Left bundle branch

LV

Cardiac
valves

RV

Purkinje fibers

Papillary
muscle

Inferior
vena cava

Epicardium

Myocardium

Endocardium

RV: right ventricle

Right bundle
branch

2008 Schenk/Cunningham

LV: left ventricle

Figure 9-3.   Impulse conductive function of the heart.

The contractions of the right and left **atria** and **ventricles** must be coordinated precisely in order for blood to be pumped efficiently to the lungs for oxygenation and then to the rest of the body. A network of specially modified cardiac muscle fibers generates and conducts electrical impulses that provide the necessary coordination. This network includes the **SA node**, the **AV node**, the **AV bundle**, and **Purkinje fibers**. (1) The *SA node* is located in the right atrial wall near the opening of the **superior vena cava**. The SA node is important for initiating the heartbeat impulse and controlling its frequency; it is also called the "pacemaker" of the heart. (2) The *AV node* is also located in the right atrial wall, medial to the right AV valve, and along the lower part of the interatrial septum. (3) The *AV bundle* arises from the AV node and divides into two branches (right and left) to run along the sides of the interventricular septum. (4) *Purkinje fibers* are the terminal branches of the right and left branches of the AV bundle. Purkinje fibers run along the inferior and lateral wall of the ventricle and extend to the **papillary muscles**. These fibers are modified large cardiac muscle cells, which contain numerous **gap junctions** and well-developed **intercalated disks**. The SA node generates the heartbeat signal, which quickly spreads to adjacent cardiac muscle cells in the **myocardium** of both atria to cause the atria to contract. Impulses are also picked up by the AV node and travel along the AV bundle. These impulses pass through the **right** and **left bundle branches** to Purkinje fibers in the ventricles, where they induce contraction of the cardiac muscles of the ventricles. There is a time delay, which allows the atria to contract first to empty blood into the ventricles, before the ventricles contract. This time delay ensures that blood flows smoothly from the atria to the ventricles and then to the conductive arteries.

SYNOPSIS 9-2 Structure and Functions of the Heart

■ The heart is composed of two **atria** (singular: *atrium*) and two **ventricles**.
■ The wall of the heart consists of **endocardium** (inner layer), **myocardium** (cardiac muscle layer), and **epicardium** (outer layer).
■ **Endocardium** is composed of endothelium, subendothelium (a thin layer of connective tissue), and subendocardium. Purkinje fibers are located in the subendocardium.
■ **Myocardium** is composed of cardiac muscles, the thickest layer of the heart; cardiac muscles are branched and connected to each other end to end by intercalated disks (junction complexes). Cardiac muscle fibers require high oxygen supply.
■ **Epicardium** is composed of mesothelium and a thicker layer of connective tissue, which contains coronary vessels, nerves, and adipose tissue.
■ The **conductive system** of the heart consists of groups of specially modified cardiac muscle fibers, the **SA node**, **AV node**, **AV bundle**, and **Purkinje fibers**.

Layers of the Heart Wall

ENDOCARDIUM

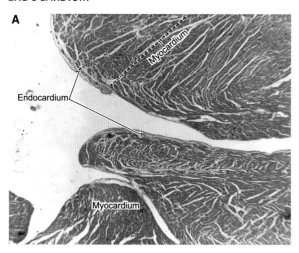

A

Figure 9-4A. Layers of the heart wall: endocardium, ventricle. H&E, ×68

The wall of the heart is much thicker than the wall of the large vessels and is composed of three basic layers, as are the blood vessels: **endocardium** (equivalent to the **tunica intima**), **myocardium** (equivalent to the **tunica media**), and **epicardium** (equivalent to **the tunica adventitia**). The *endocardium* is the innermost layer of the heart wall, which lines the lumen of the heart. This layer consists of **endothelium** (simple squamous epithelium), **subendothelial connective tissue**, and **subendocardium**. The subendocardium is in contact with the cardiac muscle and contains small coronary blood vessels, nerves, and **Purkinje fibers** in certain areas. Some adipose cells are also present within the connective tissue. The endocardium provides a smooth lining for the four chambers of the heart and provides a covering for the **AV valves**.

MYOCARDIUM

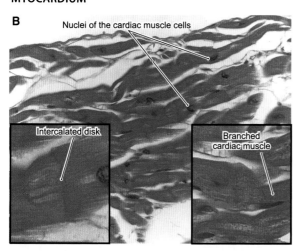

B

Figure 9-4B. Layers of the heart wall: myocardium, ventricle. H&E, ×272; insets ×786

Myocardium is the thickest layer of the heart wall and makes up the bulk of the heart. It consists of **cardiac muscle cells** that are arranged in branching columns. The ends of the cardiac muscle cells are connected to each other by **intercalated disks**. The *inset* shows cardiac muscles with their characteristic striations and an intercalated disk. These muscles contract to pump blood out of the ventricles of the heart and distribute blood to the tissues and organs of the body. Myocardium of the LV wall is the thickest because it must pump the blood a great distance and overcome the high pressure and resistance of the systemic circulation. In general, the atria have thinner walls than the ventricles. Myocardium of the right atrium is the thinnest because of the relatively low pressure and resistance of the blood circulation.

EPICARDIUM

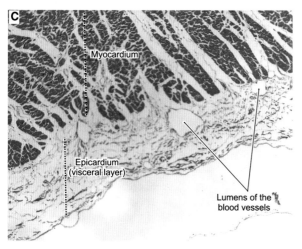

C

Figure 9-4C. Layers of the heart wall: epicardium, ventricle. H&E, ×68

Epicardium surrounds the heart. It is a layer of connective tissue that contains nerves, blood vessels, and adipocytes. The inner surface of the epicardium is connected with cardiac muscle, and the outer surface is covered by **mesothelium** that faces the **pericardial cavity**. Mesothelium secretes a fluid known as **pericardial fluid**, which provides lubrication and reduces friction between the **epicardium** (visceral pericardium) and the **parietal pericardium** during the movements caused by heart contraction. Epicardium covers and protects the heart and allows small blood vessels and nerves to pass through to provide nutrients and nerve innervation.

Pericardial effusion refers to excess fluid in the pericardial cavity due to inflammation of the pericardium (**pericarditis**); **hemopericardium** is a condition in which blood is trapped in the pericardial cavity. In either case, compression of the thin-walled atria and vena cava can result in cardiac tamponade and failure of circulation.

PURKINJE FIBERS AND INTERCALATED DISK

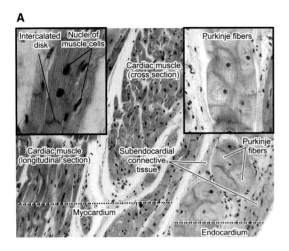

A

Intercalated disk
Nuclei of muscle cells
Purkinje fibers
Cardiac muscle (cross section)
Cardiac muscle (longitudinal section)
Subendocardial connective tissue
Purkinje fibers
Myocardium
Endocardium

Figure 9-5A. Purkinje fibers and intercalated disks, ventricle. H&E, ×136; inset (*right*) ×198, inset (*left*) ×229

Purkinje fibers (impulse-conducting fibers) are large, modified cardiac muscle cells, which are part of the heart conducting system. They are terminal branches of the AV bundle branches, located in **subendocardial connective tissue**. Purkinje fibers often appear large in size and cluster as groups. Each cell has only one or two nuclei and pale-staining cytoplasm because it has fewer **myofibrils** than regular cardiac muscle cells. Purkinje fibers work together with other impulse-conducting structures to regulate the heartbeats by conveying impulses to neighboring **cardiac muscle cells**. **Intercalated disks** are specialized **junctional complexes** that contain **fascia adherens, desmosomes (macula adherens)**, and **gap junctions**, which provide connection and communication between the cardiac muscle cells. Intercalated disks bind cardiac muscle cells together in an entire unit to prevent muscle cells being pulled apart during contraction. They also provide **ion exchange** through gap junctions, allowing electrical impulses to pass from one cell to another.

CARDIAC VALVES

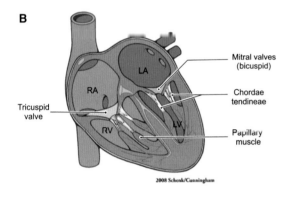

B

LA
RA
Tricuspid valve
RV
LV
Mitral valves (bicuspid)
Chordae tendineae
Papillary muscle
2008 Schenk/Cunningham

Figure 9-5B. Cardiac valves.

There are four valves in the heart: two AV valves (bicuspid, or mitral, and tricuspid valves) between the atria and ventricles of the heart and two semilunar valves (aortic and pulmonary valves) in the arteries leaving the heart. AV valves control blood flow from the atria into the ventricles and prevent the flow of blood back into the atria during ventricular contraction. The aortic valve controls blood flow from the LV into the aorta and prevents the flow of blood back into the LV. The pulmonary valve controls blood flow from the RV into the pulmonary artery and prevents the flow of blood back into the RV. In general, the heart valves open and close to allow the blood to flow through the openings and to prevent the backflow of blood. The tricuspid and bicuspid, or mitral, valves are anchored to the ventricular walls by fibrous stringlike structures called chordae tendineae, which are attached to papillary muscles.

Common heart valve diseases include **calcific aortic valve disease, valvitis**, and **rheumatic heart disease**. These diseases can lead to aortic stenosis, aortic regurgitation, embolism, and mitral valve stenosis.

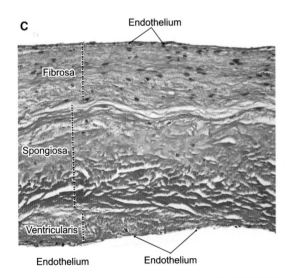

C

Endothelium
Fibrosa
Spongiosa
Ventricularis
Endothelium
Endothelium

Figure 9-5C. Cardiac valves, aortic valve. H&E, ×134

Heart valves consist of connective tissues, and both surfaces are covered by endothelium. They are composed of three layers: (1) **Fibrosa**, covered by endothelium, contains dense irregular connective tissue. This layer is continuous with the ventricular surface of AV valves and the arterial surface of the semilunar valves. AV valves are continuous with the chordae tendineae, which provide tensile support to the leaflets of the valves. (2) **Spongiosa**, the core of the heart valve, consists of loosely arranged collagen and elastic fibers. This layer serves as a shock absorber and provides flexible support to the valve. (3) **Ventricularis**, or **atrialis**, is a dense connective tissue layer with many elastic and collagen fibers. The surface of the ventricularis (atrialis) is covered by **endothelium**. The atrialis is continuous with the atrial surface of the AV valves, and the ventricularis is continuous with the ventricular surface of the semilunar valves. Shown here is an example of the **aortic valve**. The *aortic valve* has three cusps and lies between the LV and the aorta.

General Structure of the Blood Vessel Layers

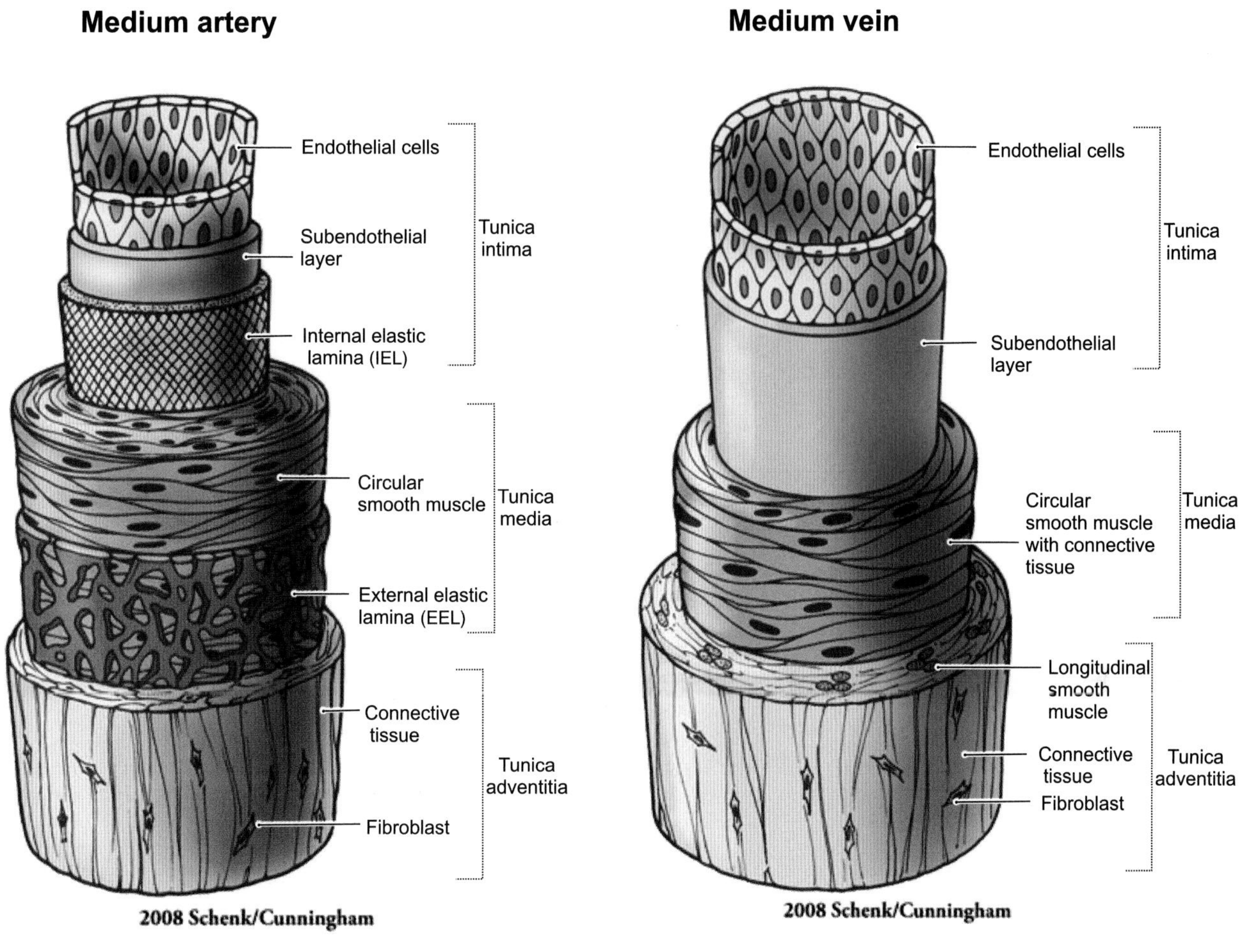

Figure 9-6. Representation of the general structure of blood vessel layers (tunicae) and a comparison of a medium artery and a medium vein.

The walls of the **blood vessels** can be divided into three **layers** (**tunicae**). The innermost layer in contact with the blood is called the **tunica intima**. This layer contains endothelium and subendothelial connective tissue and may contain an **internal elastic lamina** (IEL) in some vessels, particularly arteries. The **endothelium** is a layer of simple squamous cells, which forms the smooth surface of the lumen. **Subendothelial connective tissue** is a thin layer of connective tissue beneath the endothelium. The IEL, if present, is a sheet of elastic material that divides the tunica intima from the tunica media. The middle layer is called the **tunica media**. It primarily contains circularly arranged smooth muscle cells (except in elastic arteries). Contraction and relaxation of these smooth muscle cells will change the vessel diameter and affect blood pressure. The outermost layer, the **tunica adventitia**, is a layer of connective tissue dominated by collagenous and elastic fibers. In large and some medium veins, the tunica adventitia may also contain **longitudinal smooth muscle bundles**. Tunica adventitia surrounds and covers the vessels for protection. Occasionally, small blood vessels called **vasa vasorum** are found in the tunica adventitia of large vessels. The vasa vasorum provides oxygen and nutrients for the large vessel walls when the distance from the lumen is great and it is difficult to get nutrients from diffusion. Some differences between a medium artery and a medium vein are listed here: (1) the artery has a smaller and more rounded lumen, whereas the vein has a larger and oval or irregular-shaped lumen; (2) the artery has a thicker wall than does the vein; (3) in the artery, the tunica media is much thicker than the tunica adventitia, but in the vein, the tunica adventitia is much thicker than the tunica media; (4) circularly oriented smooth muscle cells form uniform sheets in the tunica media of the artery; however, smooth muscle cells are fewer and do not form a distinct sheet in the vein; (5) there are a few longitudinal smooth muscle bundles in the tunica adventitia of medium veins in some locations, whereas these smooth muscle bundles are more abundant in large veins. This pattern does not occur in arteries. Longitudinal smooth muscle bundles in the tunica adventitia of the vein contract to help push blood back to the heart; and (6) valves are present in many veins, especially in the medium veins of the extremities. Their function is to prevent gravitational backflow of the blood and to help blood return to the heart. Arteries do not have valves (except the aortic and pulmonary valves).

Types of Blood Vessels

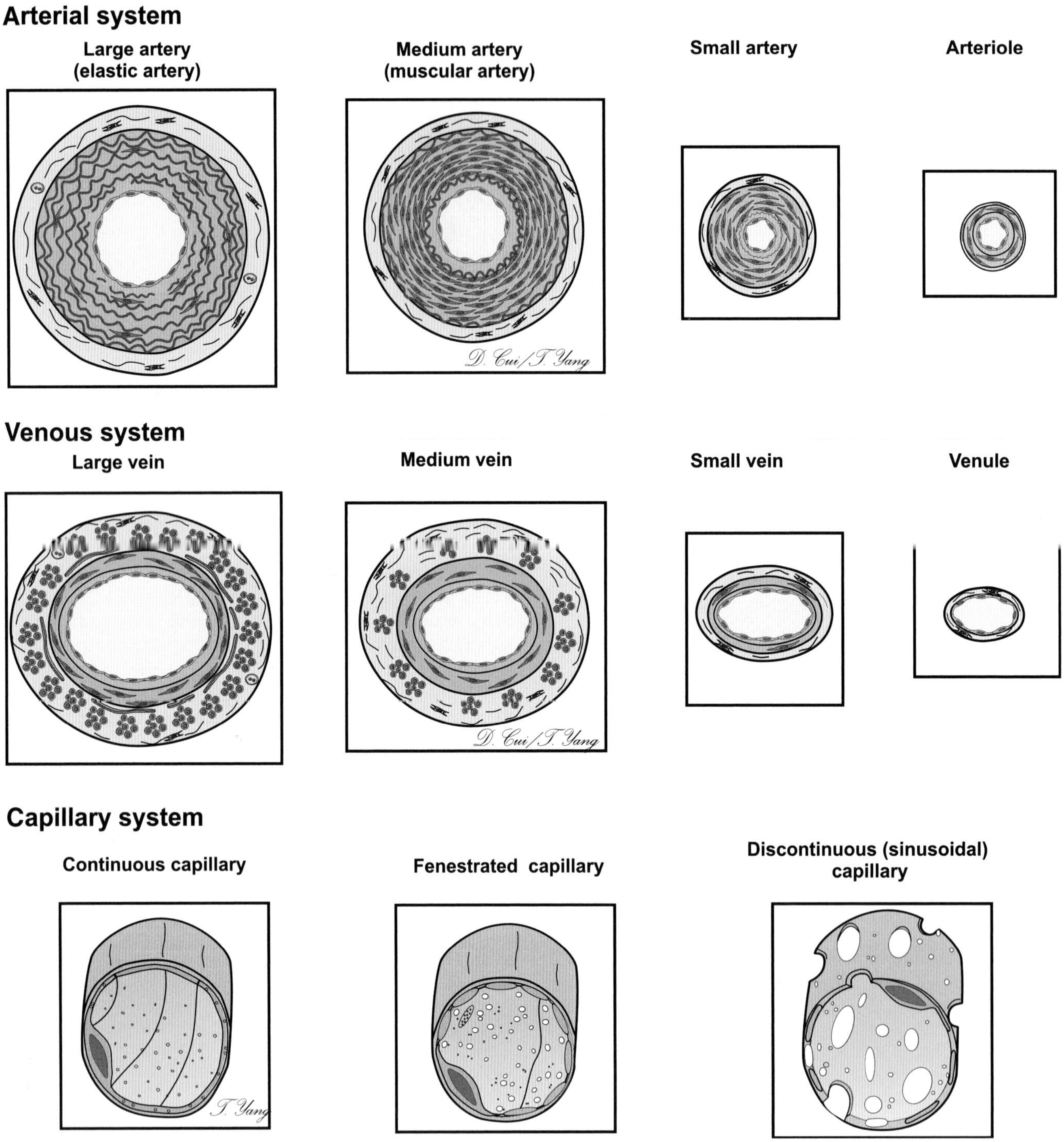

Arterial system

**Large artery
(elastic artery)**

**Medium artery
(muscular artery)**

Small artery

Arteriole

D. Cui / T. Yang

Venous system

Large vein

Medium vein

Small vein

Venule

D. Cui / T. Yang

Capillary system

Continuous capillary

Fenestrated capillary

**Discontinuous (sinusoidal)
capillary**

T. Yang

Figure 9-7. Representation of types of blood vessels: arteries, veins, and capillaries.

Blood vessels make up the **arterial**, the **venous**, and the **capillary systems**. In general, arteries have smaller, rounder lumens than veins; their tunica media are thicker than the tunica adventitia, and the IEL are prominent. Veins have larger, flatter lumens than arteries; longitudinal smooth muscle bundles may be present in the tunica adventitia, which is the most dominant layer in large and some medium veins. The tunica adventitia is much thicker in the veins than the tunica media. For details, also see Table 9-1. Exchange of gases, nutrients, and materials occurs in the capillaries. Three types of capillaries are illustrated here. **Continuous capillaries** have complete endothelial cells and continuous basal laminae. **Fenestrated capillaries** have continuous basal laminae with fenestrated endothelial cells (perforated by small pores); **discontinuous (sinusoidal) capillaries** have incomplete endothelial cells perforated by large pores, and part of the cytoplasm may be missing. The basal lamina is discontinuous. Discontinuous capillaries have gaps between endothelial cells, and their lumen sizes are much larger than the other two types. Blood vessel sizes are not drawn to scale.

Arterial System

LARGE ARTERIES

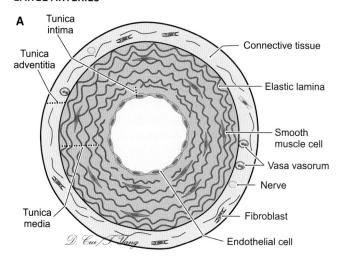

A

Tunica intima

Tunica adventitia

Tunica media

Connective tissue

Elastic lamina

Smooth muscle cell

Vasa vasorum

Nerve

Fibroblast

Endothelial cell

D. Cui/T. Yang

Figure 9-8A. Representation of a large/elastic (conducting) artery.

Large arteries (**elastic arteries**) are also referred to as **conducting arteries**, because of their function in conducting blood flow out of the heart. There are abundant **elastic laminae** (thick bundles of elastic fibers) in the **tunica media** of large arteries, which enable the walls to recoil to resist pressure as well as to maintain arterial pressure during diastole when the ventricles are relaxed, and pressure is not generated by the heart. Small vessels located in the **tunica adventitia** are called **vasa vasorum**; they supply the tissue of the artery wall with oxygen and nutrients when they are far from the lumen and diffusion of nutrients is difficult. The aorta, pulmonary arteries, and their main branches are good examples of elastic arteries.

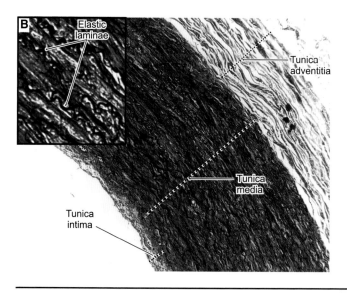

B

Elastic laminae

Tunica adventitia

Tunica media

Tunica intima

Figure 9-8B. Large/elastic (conducting) artery, carotid artery. Elastic stain, ×68; inset ×242

This is an example of a **large artery** (elastic artery) from a portion of the **carotid artery**. The carotid artery generally has the characteristics of elastic arteries. The **tunica media** of the vessel wall has multiple layers of **elastic lamina** that are well organized in concentric fashion. These elastic laminae are sheets of fenestrated elastic material produced by smooth muscle cells in the tunica media. These cells are interspersed between the elastic laminae. The elastic laminae in this specimen are revealed as parallel wavy black sheets by a special elastic stain; smooth muscle cells are not visible here with this type of stain. The **tunica adventitia** of an elastic artery consists of loosely arranged connective tissue fibers. These fibers are mainly **collagen fibers**, with a small number of **elastic fibers** that are produced by **fibroblasts**.

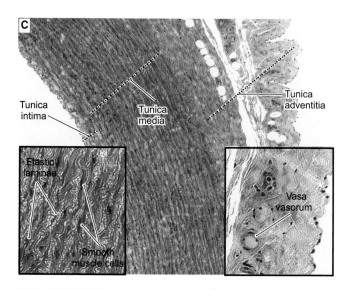

C

Tunica intima

Tunica media

Tunica adventitia

Elastic laminae

Smooth muscle cells

Vasa vasorum

Figure 9-8C. Large/elastic (conducting) artery, aorta. H&E, ×68; insets ×198

An example of a **large artery** (aorta) is shown. The **elastic laminae** are pink and are more difficult to distinguish with routine H&E stain than they are with elastic stains. The dark nuclei in the **tunica media** belong to **smooth muscle cells** (*left inset*), which produce the elastic membrane. There are some **vasa vasorum** deep in the tunica adventitia (*right inset*), which provide oxygen and nutrients for the tunica media and tunica adventitia of the large artery wall. Nerves belonging to the autonomic nervous system may occasionally be found in the **tunica adventitia**.

MEDIUM ARTERIES

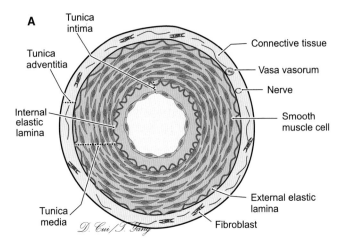

A

Tunica intima

Tunica adventitia

Internal elastic lamina

Tunica media

Connective tissue

Vasa vasorum

Nerve

Smooth muscle cell

External elastic lamina

Fibroblast

D. Cui/S. Fang

Figure 9-9A. Representation of a medium artery (muscular or distributing artery).

The **medium arteries** are also called **muscular arteries**, referring to the fact that the arterial wall is dominated by smooth muscle. There are about 6 to 40 layers of smooth muscle cells that form a distinct sheath in the **tunica media**. In general, the tunica media is much thicker than the **tunica adventitia**. **Vasoconstriction** can be caused by smooth muscle contraction that is controlled by the sympathetic nervous system. Internal and external elastic laminae are obvious in medium arteries. The IEL separates the tunica intima from the tunica media; the **external elastic lamina** (EEL) separates the tunica media from the tunica adventitia. The **tunica adventitia** is composed of connective tissues (fibroblasts and connective tissue fibers). **Vasa vasorum** may also be present. Medium arteries, also sometimes called **distributing arteries**, distribute blood to the small arteries in various organs of the body.

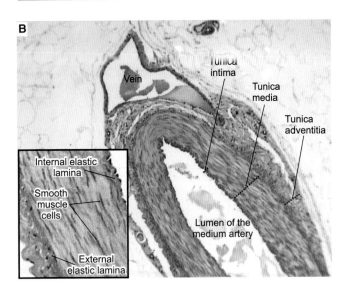

B

Vein

Tunica intima

Tunica media

Tunica adventitia

Internal elastic lamina

Smooth muscle cells

External elastic lamina

Lumen of the medium artery

Figure 9-9B. Medium artery (small muscular artery). H&E, ×68; inset ×207

The size of medium arteries (muscular arteries) varies depending upon the location. This is an example of a small segment, which has 10 to 12 layers of smooth muscle cells in the **tunica media**. Smooth muscle cells are arranged in a **circular orientation** around the lumen, are connected to each other by **gap junctions**, and are surrounded by a network of **extracellular matrix**. This arrangement allows the smooth muscle cells to function as one unit. When smooth muscle contracts, the lumen size decreases and blood pressure increases, thereby keeping blood moving forward from medium arteries to small arteries. Smooth muscle cells in the tunica media are the targets of various **neural** and **endocrine substances**. Both the IEL and EEL are prominent, appearing red-pink with H&E stain.

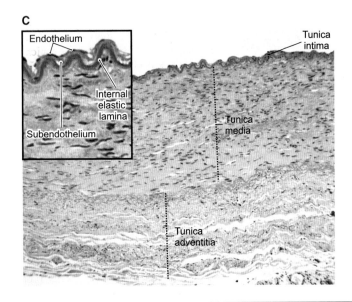

C

Endothelium

Internal elastic lamina

Subendothelium

Tunica intima

Tunica media

Tunica adventitia

Figure 9-9C. Medium artery (large muscular artery). H&E, ×68; inset ×218

This is an example of a large segment of a **medium artery**, which has about 20 to 40 layers of smooth muscle cells. The **tunica intima** is composed of **endothelium, subendothelial connective tissue**, and an IEL. The thin subendothelial connective tissue layer may become thicker with age and in **atherosclerosis**. The IEL is a wavy pink sheet forming the boundary between the tunica intima and tunica media. In general, the **tunica media** is the thickest layer, composed of smooth muscle cells. The **tunica adventitia** is composed of a layer of dense irregular connective tissue. **Vasa vasorum** and **nerve fibers** can be found in this layer but are not as prominent as in elastic arteries.

Damage to **endothelial cells** can lead to various types of cardiovascular diseases, such as **atherosclerosis** and **arteriosclerosis**.

MEDIUM AND SMALL ARTERIES

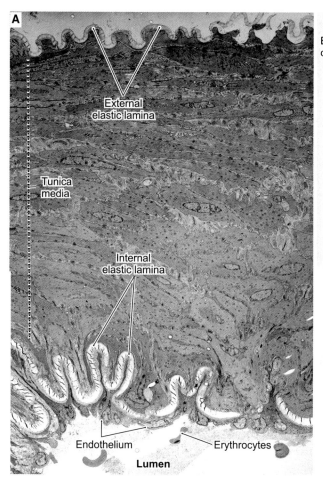

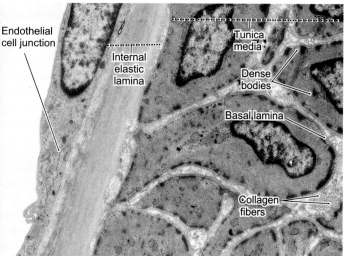

Figure 9-10A. Medium artery. TEM, ×1,000 left; ×8,700 above

In the wall of the healthy **medium artery** on the left, the layer of squamous **endothelial cells** adheres closely to the prominent, highly corrugated, **internal elastic membrane**. The **external elastic membrane** is also corrugated but thinner. The thick **tunica media** is composed of many layers of closely apposed smooth muscle cells. In the higher magnification view on the right, the **dense bodies** and **basal laminae** that are characteristic of smooth muscle cells are readily apparent. The amorphous appearance of the **internal elastic membrane** is typical of elastic membranes in transmission electron micrographs.

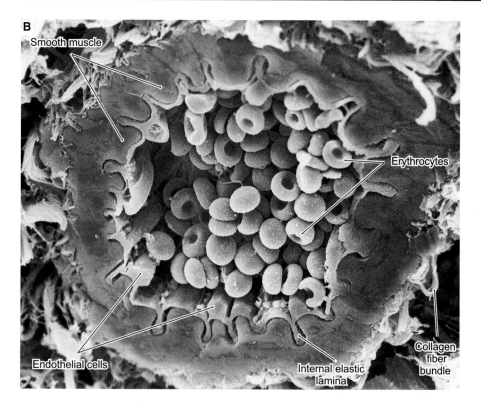

Figure 9-10B. Small artery. SEM, ×1,300

In this scanning electron micrograph of a **small artery**, the **endothelial cells** are extremely squamous, and they are so closely apposed to the **internal elastic membrane** that the interface between the two layers is indistinguishable. The **smooth muscle cells** of the tunica media are also closely apposed to each other so that boundaries between cells are difficult to discern. The ground substance of the tunica adventitia and the surrounding connective tissue has been removed during specimen processing so that only some **bundles of collagen fibers** remain.

SMALL ARTERIES AND ARTERIOLES

A   Small artery

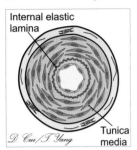

Arteriole

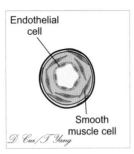

Figure 9-11A.   Representation of a small artery and an arteriole.

Small arteries (*left*) have the general structure of muscular arteries but with a smaller diameter and no EEL. The **tunica media** usually contains about three to six layers of smooth muscle cells. An **IEL** is usually present but not prominent. Small arteries help control and modulate blood pressure. **Arterioles** (*right*) are the smallest arteries, leading blood flow into capillary beds. They play an important role in regulating blood pressure and controlling the blood flow entering capillaries. Arterioles have a very small diameter and narrow lumen. There are only one to two layers of **smooth muscle cells** in the arteriolar walls, and the tunica adventitia is barely visible. Both an IEL and a subendothelial layer are often absent.

Small arteries and arterioles are sometimes referred to as **resistance vessels** because of their function in reducing and stabilizing blood pressure before blood flows into the capillary network.

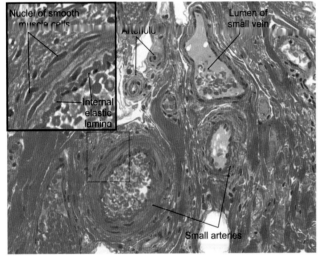

Figure 9-11B.   Small arteries, small intestine (ileum). H&E, ×136; inset ×408

An example of a small artery in the tissue of the small intestine is shown. Small arteries can be found in various types of tissues and organs where oxygen, nutrients, and other materials must be exchanged. Small arteries have a thin tunica intima and tunica adventitia. The **tunica media**, the most obvious layer in small arteries, contains three to six layers of circularly arranged **smooth muscle cells**. An IEL is often present. Smooth muscle is innervated by the autonomic nervous system and regulates blood pressure by causing vasoconstriction (sympathetic nervous system) and vasodilation (parasympathetic nervous system).

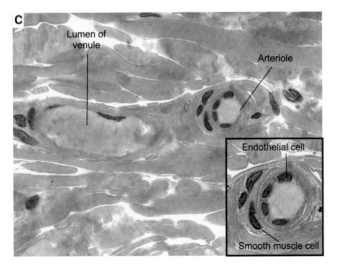

Figure 9-11C.   Arterioles, tongue. H&E, ×680; inset ×1,020

Arterioles have a very small, round **lumen** (<0.5 mm in diameter) and one or two layers of **smooth muscle cells** in the arteriolar wall. Arterioles are the last segment of the arterial system. They connect small arteries to the capillary network. The **endothelium** of these small vessels is able to sense changes in blood pressure, blood flow, and oxygen tension and to respond to these changes by releasing signals, such as **endothelin (vasoconstrictor)** and **nitric oxide (vasodilator)**. These signals regulate the tone of adjacent smooth muscle cells. Changes in muscle tone control blood flow into the capillaries. Arterioles can be structurally distinct depending on their location. For example, arterioles in the lung are not structured identically to those in the kidney. A venule accompanying an arteriole is shown here. Venules have very thin walls consisting mainly of endothelium. Smooth muscle cells are not prominent in venules.

ARTERIOLES

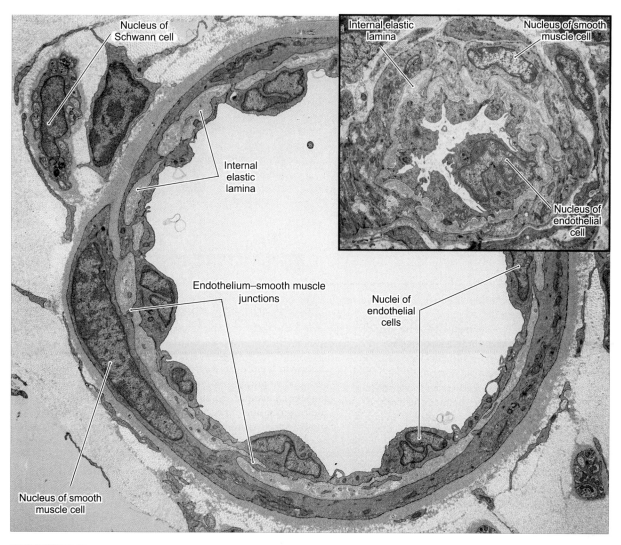

Figure 9-12. Arteriole. TEM, ×5, 800; inset ×3,800

The **arteriole** in the larger image was fixed in a dilated state, whereas the *inset* shows a slightly smaller arteriole that was fixed in a contracted state. In both vessels, a thin elastic lamina separates the endothelium from the smooth muscle cells of the tunica media. The state of contraction of the smooth muscle cells is regulated largely by signals from the endothelial cells. In addition to chemical messengers, such as nitric oxide and endothelin, signaling may also involve direct contacts between endothelial and smooth muscle cells. The cell in the upper left corner of the larger micrograph is a **Schwann cell** with several unmyelinated axons embedded in its cytoplasm.

SYNOPSIS 9-3 Functions of Endothelium in Blood Vessels

■ Endothelium provides a permeability barrier and controls the composition of interstitial tissue fluid.
■ Endothelium allows the movement of leukocytes, fluid, and immunoglobulins into tissues.
■ Endothelium provides for angiogenesis in the formation and differentiation of new blood vessels.
■ Endothelium provides signals that regulate the tone of adjacent vascular smooth muscle cells that control blood pressure by vasoconstriction (endothelin) and vasodilation (nitric oxide, prostacyclin).
■ Endothelium provides anticoagulant signals (thrombomodulin, nitrous oxide, and prostacyclin) that inhibit platelet attachment and aggregation to prevent blood clotting and allow unobstructed flow of blood in normal conditions.

When endothelial cells are injured, they reduce the production of platelet inhibitors and increase the release of stimulators of platelet activation (e.g., von Willebrand factor, tissue thromboplastin). Exposure of the underlying basal lamina and connective tissue further stimulates platelets to adhere and aggregate. Damage to the endothelium will slow down oxidation and clearance of low-density lipoprotein, leading to many cardiovascular diseases such as **atherosclerosis**.

MICROCIRCULATION

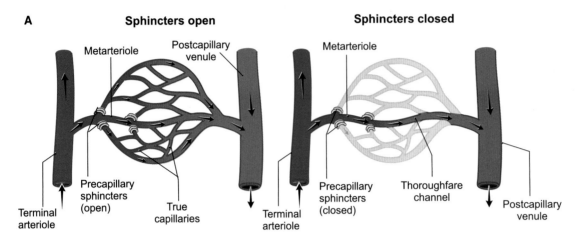

A

Sphincters open   Sphincters closed

Metarteriole   Postcapillary venule   Metarteriole

Precapillary sphincters (open)   True capillaries

Terminal arteriole   Terminal arteriole   Precapillary sphincters (closed)   Thoroughfare channel   Postcapillary venule

Figure 9-13A. Overview of microcirculation

The process of **microcirculation** involves the transfer of oxygen and nutrient-rich blood from the **arterioles** to **venule** through the **capillary bed**. A **capillary bed** is a vascular network of tiny vessels that includes the terminal parts of **arterioles, metarteriole, capillaries,** and the initial parts of venules. **Metarterioles** are branches from a terminal arteriole, which connect the arteriole to the capillary bed. They contain **precapillary sphincters** that are formed by **pericytes,** and their function is to control blood flow. (1) **Sphincters open:** Open precapillary sphincters allow blood to flow into the capillary bed, promote oxygen and nutrient exchange from the blood to the tissues, and allow carbon dioxide and metabolic waste products to cross from tissues into the blood. (2) **Sphincters closed:** Closed precapillary sphincters only permit blood to flow through the metarterioles into the thoroughfare channel and bypass the capillary bed. The blood flows directly from the terminal arterioles into the venules. This system of shunting blood from arterioles to venules directly is important for maintaining a stable body temperature by conserving heat during environmental changes to cooler temperatures. For instance, the direct shunting of blood between arterioles and venules within the dermis of the skin reduces the loss of heat to the surroundings.

CLINICAL CORRELATIONS

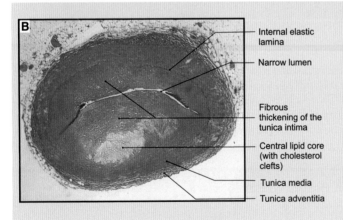

B

Internal elastic lamina

Narrow lumen

Fibrous thickening of the tunica intima

Central lipid core (with cholesterol clefts)

Tunica media

Tunica adventitia

Figure 9-13B. Coronary Artery Atherosclerosis. H&E, ×21

Coronary artery atherosclerosis (CAD) is characterized by the presence of atherosclerotic changes within the walls of the coronary arteries. These changes include accumulation of lipid, formation of atherosclerotic plaques, and thickening of arterial tunica intima. Eventually, normal blood flow to the heart muscle is impaired or obstructed. Rupture of an atherosclerotic plaque promotes the formation of a blood clot, or **thrombus,** which may occlude the lumen of the coronary artery. Angina (cardiac chest pain), even myocardial infarction (heart muscle death), can develop when blood flow is reduced below a certain level. CAD is a progressive disease process that generally begins in childhood and manifests clinically in mid-to-late adulthood. Lifestyle changes to lower blood cholesterol and control hypertension and diabetes are important in preventing the disease and reducing the severe consequences.

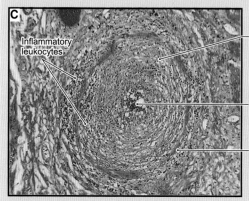

C
Inflammatory leukocytes

Fibrous thickening of the tunica intima

Diminished lumen of the small artery

Disrupted internal elastic lamina

Figure 9-13C. Polyarteritis Nodosa (Vasculitis), Small Artery in Intestine. H&E, ×71

Polyarteritis nodosa is a multisystem **necrotizing vasculitis** of small- and medium-sized muscular arteries in which involvement of renal and visceral arteries is characteristic. Classic polyarteritis nodosa spares the pulmonary arteries. The cause of the disease is not clear, but it is associated with hepatitis B virus infection in 20% to 30% of cases. Symptoms may be nonspecific, making it difficult to diagnose. Fever, weight loss, and **malaise** are present in more than 50% of cases. Patients may present with fever, headache, weakness, abdominal pain, and **myalgias**. Histologically, affected arteries are characterized by segmental transmural inflammation. Internal and external elastic laminae are disrupted, which may lead to aneurysms and bleeding. Polymorphonuclear leukocytes and mononuclear leukocytes are visible in the cellular infiltrate. Steroids are the major drugs used to control disease progression.

Capillary System

CONTINUOUS CAPILLARIES

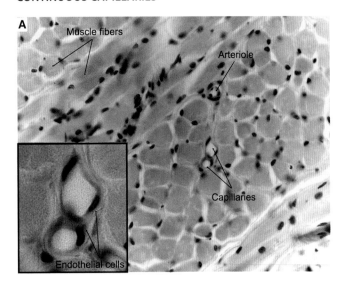

Figure 9-14A. Continuous capillaries, skeletal muscle. H&E, ×272; inset ×870

Capillaries, the smallest vessels (5–10 μm in diameter) in the blood circulatory system, connect arterioles to venules. Capillaries contain one layer of endothelial cells with a basal lamina sometimes wrapped by pericytes. According to the structure of the endothelial cells and the continuity of the basal lamina, capillaries can be classified into three types: (1) **continuous capillaries,** (2) **fenestrated capillaries,** and (3) **discontinuous (sinusoidal) capillaries.** *Continuous capillaries* have **complete endothelial cells** (no pores), interrupted only by **intercellular clefts** between the cells, and a **continuous basal lamina** with no breaks in the endothelial barrier between the vascular compartment and the surrounding tissues. Such structures in the continuous capillaries allow very limited amounts of materials to pass through their walls. Continuous capillaries can be found in muscles, connective tissues, nervous tissues, lungs, exocrine glands, and the thymus.

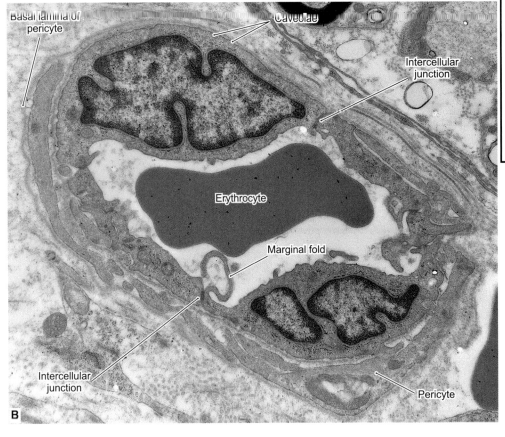

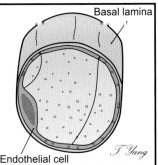

Figure 9-14B. Continuous capillary, loose connective tissue. TEM ×5,100

The caliber of this **continuous capillary** can be inferred from the **erythrocyte** that occupies the lumen. Nuclei of two endothelial cells are prominent, and portions of **pericytes** can be seen external to the endothelial cells. A continuous layer of endothelial cell cytoplasm forms a barrier between the capillary lumen and the surrounding tissue compartment. **Junctions** between adjacent endothelial cells can be of both the **occludens** and the **adherens** types. **Marginal folds,** such as the one beneath the erythrocyte, are typical features at the junctions between capillary endothelial cells. Each endothelial cell has numerous **caveolae** beneath its plasmalemma, although these structures are difficult to discern at this magnification. The caveolae are a manifestation of active transcytosis of materials between the plasma and the tissue space.

FENESTRATED CAPILLARIES

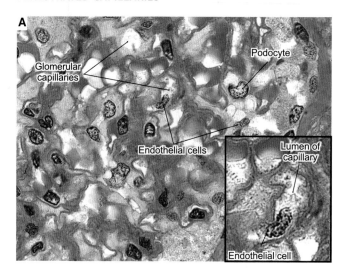

Figure 9-15A. Fenestrated capillaries, kidney. H&E, ×680; inset ×1,405

Fenestrated capillaries have endothelial cells that are perforated by **small pores**, often bridged by **diaphragms**, a very thin membrane across the small pores. The glomerulus of the kidney is an exception, which does not have a diaphragm. The **basal laminae** beneath the endothelial cells are **continuous**. This type of capillary allows a greater range of substances to pass freely through the capillary wall. Examples of fenestrated capillaries are the capillary beds in the intestine (where nutrients are absorbed), the glomerulus of the kidney (where blood is filtered and urine is formed), and the capillaries in the endocrine organs, such as in the pituitary gland and endocrine pancreas (where hormones are secreted and released into the capillaries). The glomerular capillaries in the kidney are shown here.

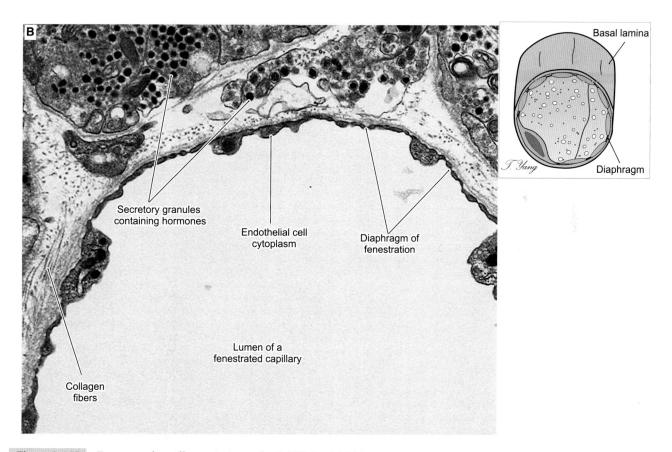

Figure 9-15B. Fenestrated capillary, pituitary gland. TEM, ×14,000

The wall of this **fenestrated capillary** consists of a thin layer of cytoplasm interrupted at frequent intervals by circular pores, termed **fenestrations**, of fairly consistent diameter (~70 nm). This permits freer movement than occurs in continuous capillaries for some molecules such as **peptide hormones**. In order to pass between the vascular compartment and the interstitial tissue compartment, dissolved molecules still must pass through the **diaphragms** that bridge the pores, and the **endothelial cells** still produce a complete basal lamina at the interface with the surrounding tissue. Fenestrated capillaries are found in the gastrointestinal tract, the kidney, and in endocrine glands. The vessel shown here is located in the anterior pituitary.

DISCONTINUOUS CAPILLARIES

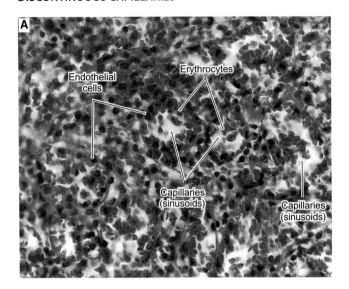

Figure 9-16A. Discontinuous capillaries, spleen. H&E, ×274

Discontinuous capillaries, also called **sinusoidal capillaries** (or **sinuses**), are characterized by **large pores,** which perforate the cytoplasm of endothelial cells, and incomplete or missing **basal laminae.** In addition, the sinusoids have large **intercellular clefts** (gaps between endothelial cells). These structures permit free movement of proteins, plasma constituents, and other materials. In some cases, even cells can pass through the capillary wall. This type of capillary has a large diameter (30–60 µm) and may have an irregular shape due to an incomplete basal lamina, spindle-shaped endothelial cells, and fenestrated structures. Discontinuous capillaries can be found in the liver, spleen, bone marrow, and lymph nodes.

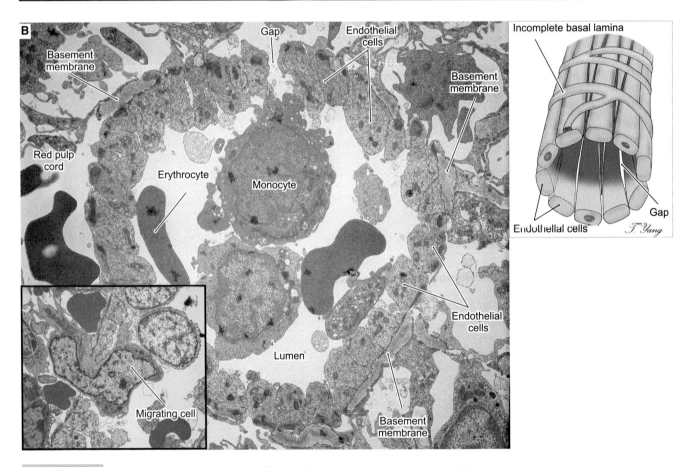

Figure 9-16B. Discontinuous (sinusoidal) capillary, spleen. TEM, ×5,200; inset ×3,400

Sinusoidal capillaries vary greatly in appearance, but they all have as common features, lumens of large diameter and gaps or potential gaps between and sometimes even within endothelial cells. Objects as large as cells can pass through these discontinuities. The sinusoidal capillary shown here is located in the red pulp of the spleen, and it is termed a **red pulp sinusoid.** The endothelial cells are elongated with the long axis parallel to the long axis of the vessel. In cross section, as seen here, the endothelial cells are nearly circular in shape. There are **gaps** between cells, such as the one seen at the top edge of this example, but many neighboring endothelial cells are in close contact. Nevertheless, as seen in the *inset*, motile blood cells and macrophages can pass readily between adjacent endothelial cells because of sparseness of intercellular junctions and the **incomplete basement membrane.**

Venous System

VENULES AND SMALL VEINS

A   **Venule**   **Small vein**

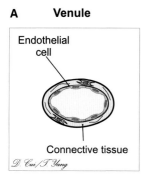
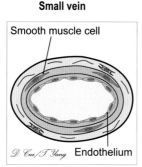

Figure 9-17A.   Representation of a venule and small vein.

The **venous system** is composed of **venules, small veins, medium veins**, and **large veins**. These vessels carry blood from capillaries in the tissues back to the heart. Small veins and venules are very similar in structure and are sometimes difficult to distinguish from one another. In general, *small veins* have larger lumens and more visible smooth muscle cells than venules. *Venules*, the smallest veins, receive blood from the capillary network. Venules have small lumens and very thin walls, with only a single layer of endothelium and a small amount of underlying connective tissue (like large capillaries). They may have a few scattered smooth muscle cells in the vessel walls. Venules gradually increase in size to form small veins. They can be categorized as **postcapillary venules** (10–30 μm in diameter), **collecting venules** (30–50 μm), and **muscular venules** (50–100 μm). *Postcapillary venules* connect directly to capillaries and drain blood into the collecting venules. *Muscular venules* often accompany arterioles.

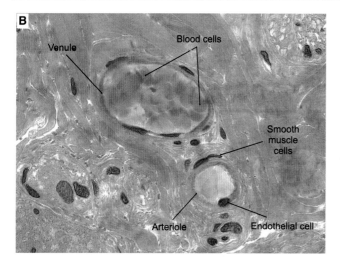

Figure 9-17B.   Venule and arteriole, colon. H&E, ×680

This **venule** (**muscular venule**) and companion **arteriole** were taken from the colon of the large intestine. Venules have larger lumens than arterioles. In histological sections, they often have blood cells remaining inside the lumen. Venules are the smallest veins; they drain blood from capillaries into the small veins. They are also involved in exchange of metabolites with tissues and allow blood cells to migrate from the vessels into the tissues (**diapedesis**). The **postcapillary venules** are the primary sites involved in the inflammatory response; they allow leukocytes (white blood cells) to migrate into the affected tissues in cases of inflammation or infection. Note that the companion artery has a small, round lumen and a single layer of **smooth muscle cells**. There are fewer or no **blood cells** in the lumen of an arteriole specimen, because of the higher pressure and stronger contraction of the arteriole wall.

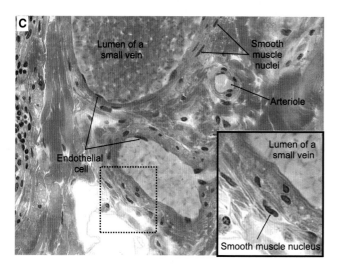

Figure 9-17C.   Small vein, colon. H&E, ×272; inset ×527

Small veins have one to three layers of isolated **smooth muscle cells** in the walls. The tunica adventitia of small veins is a little thicker than that of venules. Small veins have a thinner wall and less distinguishable **smooth muscle** layers than do small arteries. Small veins gradually increase in size to become medium veins. **Microvessels** include **arterioles, capillaries**, and **venules** and play a key role in the response to inflammation. During infection or tissue injury, immune cells (such as mast cells and basophils) release histamine and heparin. In response, the endothelium of microvessels allows fluid leakage (**edema**) and relaxation of smooth muscle cells, leading to vessel dilation (redness and heat).

Exudation is the escape of blood fluid and protein from the lumen of the vessel into the interstitial tissue when the cell-to-cell junctions of the endothelium loosen. **Transudation** is movement, due to hydrostatic imbalance, of the blood plasma fluid from the lumen to the interstitial tissue, with large protein and cells filtered out by the normal endothelial wall.

MEDIUM VEINS

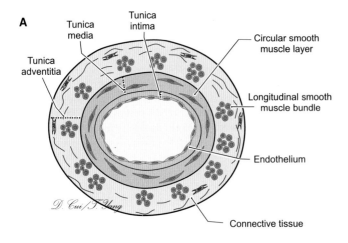

A

Tunica media
Tunica intima
Tunica adventitia
Circular smooth muscle layer
Longitudinal smooth muscle bundle
Endothelium
Connective tissue

D. Cui/T. Yang

Figure 9-18A. **Representation of a medium vein.**

In general, the **tunica media** of veins is thinner than the **tunica adventitia**, and smooth muscle cells in this layer are not as well organized as in arteries. The **tunica adventitia** of **medium veins** is more prominent and much thicker than the tunica media. Medium veins have various sizes and structural features depending on their location. The **tunica intima** consists of an **endothelium** and a thin **subendothelial layer**. The tunica media contains a few layers of circularly arranged smooth muscle cells, which usually do not form a distinct sheet. In some areas, large-sized medium veins have a structure like that of large veins. Their tunica intima is thinner, and the tunica adventitia contains fewer bundles of **longitudinal smooth muscle** than large veins. However, this characteristic is not prominent in small segments of the medium veins. Valves are prominent in medium veins, especially in the extremities of the body.

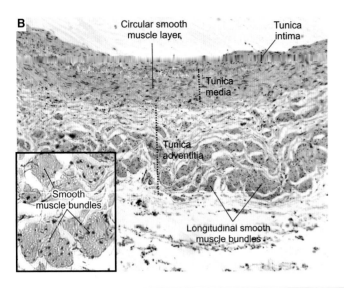

B

Circular smooth muscle layer
Tunica intima
Tunica media
Tunica adventitia
Smooth muscle bundles
Longitudinal smooth muscle bundles

Figure 9-18B. **Medium vein, large segment of medium vein.** H&E, ×68; inset ×182

This sample of a large segment of **medium vein** has a similar structure to a large vein but has fewer longitudinal smooth muscle bundles in the tunica adventitia. The **tunica intima** is thinner than in the large veins, and the **tunica media** contains several layers of circular smooth muscle. The **tunica adventitia** is the thickest and the most prominent layer in most medium veins. There are some **longitudinal smooth muscle bundles** (*inset*) and connective tissue in the tunica adventitia. In the extremities, such as the legs and arms, there are many valves at varying intervals in the innermost layer of veins. They prevent blood backflow against gravity. Veins carry blood toward the heart under lower pressure than arteries and have a great capacity for housing blood (~65% of blood is in the venous system); for this reason, they are sometimes called **capacitance vessels.**

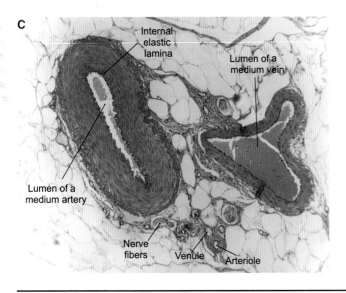

C

Internal elastic lamina
Lumen of a medium vein
Lumen of a medium artery
Nerve fibers
Venule
Arteriole

Figure 9-18C. **Medium vein, small segment of medium vein.** H&E, ×68

Veins accompanying companion **arteries** are often found in the tissues and organs. Structurally, medium arteries have relatively smaller lumens, thicker walls, and more prominent **IEL** than medium veins. The IEL is usually absent in medium veins. In this example, a small segment of a medium vein with a companion medium artery, the vein has a larger **lumen** and a thinner wall than a companion artery. This medium vein does not show the prominent tunica adventitia or the longitudinal smooth muscle bundles usually seen in medium veins.

LARGE VEINS

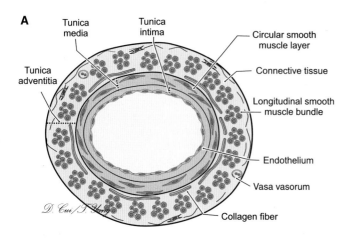

A

Tunica media

Tunica intima

Tunica adventitia

Circular smooth muscle layer

Connective tissue

Longitudinal smooth muscle bundle

Endothelium

Vasa vasorum

Collagen fiber

D. Cui/T. Yang

Figure 9-19A. Representation of a large vein.

The **vena cava** and **pulmonary veins** are the largest veins in the **venous system**. They connect directly to the heart. The **tunica adventitia** is the most prominent and distinct layer in large veins; it contains numerous longitudinally arranged **smooth muscle bundles** and some connective tissues (mostly **collagen fibers**). The **vasa vasorum** are also present in the tunica adventitia; they provide blood and nutrient supply to the wall of the large vein. The **tunica media** contains a few layers of smooth muscle cells that are loosely arranged and do not form a distinct sheath. Contraction of the circularly arranged smooth muscle cells in the tunica media and the longitudinally arranged smooth muscle bundles in the tunica adventitia help to push blood toward the heart.

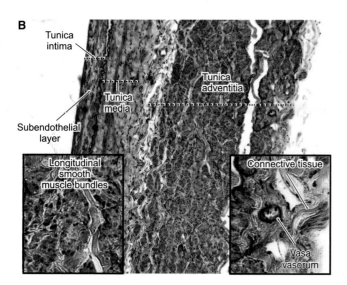

B

Tunica intima

Subendothelial layer

Tunica media

Tunica adventitia

Longitudinal smooth muscle bundles

Connective tissue

Vasa vasorum

Figure 9-19B. Large vein, vena cava. H&E, ×68; insets ×185

The **tunica intima** of the **vena cava** consists of an endothelial layer, a thick subendothelial layer (connective tissue), and an IEL. In general, the IEL is not well developed in veins. Although it is not commonly seen in veins, it may still be present in some large veins. The **tunica media** contains a few layers of loosely organized smooth muscle cells; the tunica media is much thinner compared to its tunica adventitia. There are densely arranged **smooth muscle bundles** in the **tunica adventitia**, which give the large vein a distinct appearance. There is a thin layer of connective tissue (mainly collagen fibers) between the circular smooth muscle and the longitudinal smooth muscle bundles in the tunica adventitia. A **vasa vasorum** is shown on the right, and a cross section of longitudinal smooth muscle bundles is shown on the left.

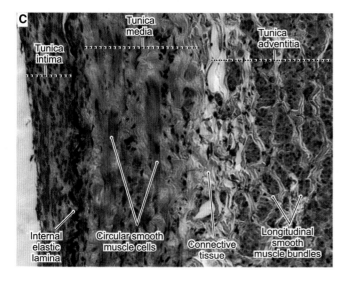

C

Tunica intima

Tunica media

Tunica adventitia

Internal elastic lamina

Circular smooth muscle cells

Connective tissue

Longitudinal smooth muscle bundles

Figure 9-19C. Large vein, vena cava. H&E, ×186

A high-power view of a **large vein** with smooth muscle cells in the circular **smooth muscle layer** in the **tunica media**. The **longitudinal smooth muscle bundles** are surrounded by collagen fibers in the **tunica adventitia**. There are some connective tissues (mainly collagen bundles) between circular smooth muscle and longitudinal smooth layers. The **IEL** is clearly visible here between the tunica intima and the tunica media. However, the IEL is not usually present in the veins.

TABLE 9-1   Blood Vessels

Types of Arteries and Veins	Tunica Intima	Tunica Media	Tunica Adventitia	Size (Diameter)	Main Functions
Arterial System					
Large/elastic (conducting) arteries	Endothelium; subendothelial layer (connective tissue); IEL	Abundant fenestrated elastic membranes; interspersed smooth muscle cells; EEL	Thinner than its tunica media (connective tissue); vasa vasorum present	>10 mm	Conducting blood flow from the heart to the arterial system; being able to recoil (elastic membranes) to buffer pressure against arterial wall and conserve energy to force the blood forward, even while the ventricle is relaxing
Medium/ muscular (distributing) arteries	Endothelium; subendothelial layer (connective tissue); prominent complete IEL	Abundant, thick layer of smooth muscle cells (6–40 layers of muscle cells); prominent EEL in larger-sized medium arteries	Thinner than its tunica media (connective tissue); vasa vasorum not prominent	10–0.5 mm	Distributing blood flow to small arteries in various parts of body; adjusting the rate of blood flow by vasoconstriction and vasodilation
Small arteries	Endothelium; thin subendothelial layer; thin IEL	3–6 layers of smooth muscle cells; EEL absent	Thinner than its tunica media (loose connective tissue); no vasa vasorum	500–100 μm	Distributing blood to arterioles and to capillaries; participating in vasoconstriction and vasodilation to adjust the blood flow
Arterioles	Endothelium; no subendothelial layer; IEL not prominent	1–2 layers of smooth muscle cells; no EEL	Very thin; a sheath of loose connective tissue	100–30 μm	Leading blood to the capillary beds; regulating resistance; controlling blood flow to capillaries
Venous System					
Venules (postcapillary, collecting, and muscular venules)	Endothelium; no subendothelial layer; no valves	Very thin; smooth muscle cells not prominent	Very thin; layer of collagen fibers	10–100 μm	Draining exchanged blood from capillaries to the small veins; promoting leukocyte migration from bloodstream to inflamed tissue; primary sites for inflammatory response
Small veins	Endothelium; subendothelial layer; few valves	Thin; 1–3 layers isolated smooth muscle cells	Thin; connective tissue layer	0.1–1 mm	Collecting blood flow from venules to the medium veins
Medium veins	Endothelium; subendothelial layer; increased number of valves	Thicker than small vein; a few layers of smooth muscle cells that usually do not form a distinct sheath	Thicker than its tunica media; variable number and size of longitudinal bundles of smooth muscle mixed with connective tissue	1–10 mm	Carrying blood to large veins leading toward the heart; preventing blood from backflow
Large veins	Endothelium; thick subendothelial layer; large valves; IEL may be present	Thinner than its tunica adventitia layer; several layers of circularly arranged smooth muscle cells but do not form a distinct sheath; some collagen fibers	Thickest layer in large veins; composed of many large bundles of longitudinal smooth muscle; cardiac muscle may be present near the atria	>10 mm	Transporting blood from the venous system back to the heart; forcing blood toward the heart by constriction of circular and longitudinal smooth muscle

Lymphatic Vascular System

SMALL LYMPHATIC VESSELS

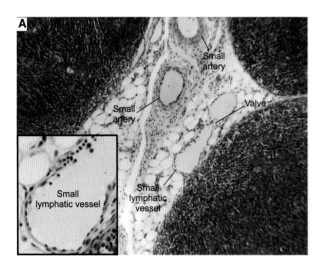

Figure 9-20A. Small lymphatic vessels, lymph node. H&E, ×272; inset ×767

The **lymphatic vascular system** is composed of **lymphatic capillaries**, **lymphatic vessels**, and **lymphatic ducts**, which collect and drain interstitial fluid from the tissue into the large veins (for subclavian veins, see Chapter 10, "Lymphoid System"). **Lymph** (fluid in the lymphatic system) contains lymphocytes, immunoglobulins, plasma, foreign antigens, and other substances. *Lymphatic vessels* carry lymph through the **lymph nodes** along the lymphatic vessels. *Lymph nodes* filter lymph and expose lymphocytes to antigens as part of the immune response (see Chapter 10, "Lymphoid System"). After filtration, the lymph is transported via large lymphatic vessels to lymphatic ducts (the thoracic right lymphatic ducts) and finally enters the subclavian veins and becomes part of the blood plasma. An example of **small lymphatic vessels** is shown in the hilus of a lymph node. Small lymphatic vessels have large lumens and very thin walls, which are composed of a layer of endothelium and a little connective tissue with a few smooth muscle cells.

LARGE LYMPHATIC VESSELS

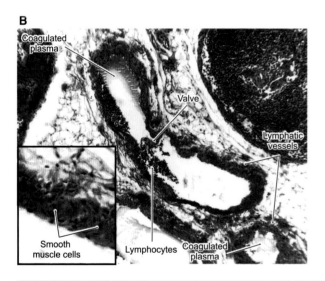

Figure 9-20B. Large lymphatic vessels, lymph node. H&E, ×136; inset ×422

Large lymphatic vessels have thicker walls than small lymphatic vessels. Large lymphatic vessels are composed of connective tissues and multiple layers of **smooth muscle cells**. Contraction of smooth muscle cells helps to move the lymph forward. Large lymphatic vessels are structurally similar to small veins, except they have larger lumens and prominent **valves**. Valves are present in all sizes of lymphatic vessels. They prevent lymph from flowing backward. Lymphatic vessels are often distinguished by lumens that contain clusters of lymphocytes and **coagulated plasma**. Lymphatic vessels can be found in most of the tissues of the body but not in the central nervous system, the bone marrow, or the hard tissues.

CLINICAL CORRELATION

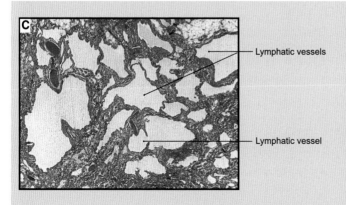

Figure 9-20C. Lymphangioma, Skin. H&E, ×44

Lymphangioma is a congenital malformation of the lymphatic system that involves the skin and subcutaneous tissues. It occurs most often in the head and the neck. It is characterized by multiple clusters of translucent vesicles that contain lymph fluid varying from clear to pink to dark red. These vesicles are separated from the normal network of lymphatic vessels but have communications with the superficial lymph vesicles through vertical and dilated lymph channels. Skin lesions range from minute vesicles to cystic and cavernous spaces. Clinically, it appears as a raised, soft, spongy, and pinkish white lesion. Surgical excision may be chosen if vital structures are involved or for cosmetic correction, but it has a high recurrence rate after surgery.

From Histology to Pathology

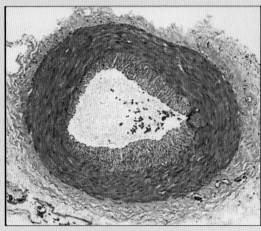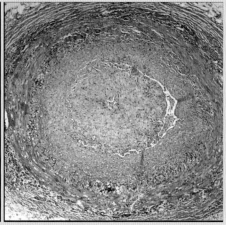

Figure 9-21.   Normal temporal artery and temporal arteritis. H&E, ×40

Normal medium-sized artery on the *left*. **Temporal arteritis** on the *right* is a granulomatous vasculitis of medium-sized arteries, usually in the head and neck region. Histologic changes include intimal thickening, often with thrombosis, fragmentation of the *internal elastic lamina*, and an inflammatory infiltrate including *lymphocytes* and *giant cells* (cells formed by the fusion of epithelioid cells derived from macrophages). This process may involve the ophthalmic artery with resultant visual symptoms, such as diplopia (double vision).

Clinical Vignette Questions

1. The parents of an 11-month-old male infant with a history of asthma noticed that the baby appeared to be having difficulty breathing, and they also noted that he had a fever. The parents began giving the child breathing treatments with a nebulizer without noticeable improvement in his ability to breath. The parents subsequently brought the child to a local emergency department where he was found to be hypotensive, tachycardic (heart rate >100 beats per minute), febrile (temperature ≥100.4°F), and in respiratory distress. Despite efforts to stabilize the patient, the child dies, and an autopsy is requested. Gross examination of the heart is unremarkable, but microscopic sections show the cardiac myocytes diffusely infiltrated with inflammatory cells with evidence of myocyte necrosis. Cultures taken at autopsy return positive for a virus in the enterovirus family. The cause of death is attributed to viral myocarditis. Which of the following would be the predominant inflammatory cell type expected in the myocardium in this case?

A. Eosinophil
B. Lymphocyte
C. Macrophage
D. Mast cell
E. Neutrophil

2. A 45-year-old woman with a history of substernal chest pain presented to the emergency department with complaints of shortness of breath (dyspnea) that has progressively worsened over the last several weeks. The patient reports waking up at night "gasping for air" (paroxysmal nocturnal dyspnea). Physical exam reveals a diastolic murmur consistent with mitral stenosis. A chest radiograph reveals possible atrial enlargement with tracheal deviation. Echocardiogram reveals an intracardiac mass that is ~6.5 cm in its greatest dimension. The mass is resected and diagnosed as a myxoma. In which location do most of these lesions arise?

A. Aortic arch
B. Left atrium
C. Left ventricle
D. Right atrium
E. Right ventricle

3. A previously asymptomatic and physically active 59-year-old woman presents to the emergency department after developing retrosternal chest pain radiating to her neck and left arm. She began experiencing chest pain associated with exertion 2 months ago, and upon cessation of activity, the pain subsided. On this occasion, however, the pain is unremitting and severe. She has a history of diabetes and dyslipidemia and a family history of coronary artery disease. An electrocardiogram (ECG) shows T-wave inversion in leads V3 to V6 with dynamic ST-segment deviation. Vital signs show tachycardia and a blood pressure of 140/92 mm Hg. An initial high sensitivity troponin T assay is elevated above the reference interval, and a repeat test 6 hours later is higher than the initial test. This clinical scenario most likely demonstrates which of the following diagnoses?

A. Aortic dissection
B. Gastroesophageal reflux
C. Acute coronary syndrome
D. Cardiac tamponade

10 Lymphoid System

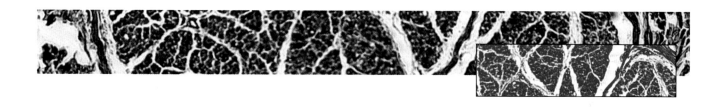

Introduction and Key Concepts for the Lymphoid System

Cells in the Lymphoid System
B Lymphocytes
T Lymphocytes
Null Cells
Plasma Cells
Antigen-Presenting Cells

Lymphatic Tissues and Lymphoid Organs
Mucosa-Associated Lymphatic Tissues
Lymph Nodes
Thymus
Spleen

Introduction and Key Concepts for the Lymphoid System

The **lymphoid system** is composed of **lymphocytes, lymphoid organs,** and **lymphatic vessels.** The structure of lymphatic vessels is discussed in Chapter 9, "Circulatory System." Lymphoid organs include the **bone marrow** (see Chapter 8, "Blood and Hemopoiesis"), **lymph nodes, thymus, spleen,** and **mucosa-associated lymphatic tissue (MALT),** such as tonsils and Peyer patches. Most lymphoid organs contain lymphatic nodules or diffuse lymphatic tissues and play an important role in providing sites for lymphocytes to come into contact with antigens; promote proliferation and maturation of lymphocytes; and promote B lymphocytes to become plasma cells, which produce antibodies. Lymphoid organs can be divided into two groups: (1) **Primary lymphoid organs,** also called **central lymphoid organs,** are the sites where lymphocytes differentiate and develop the ability to recognize foreign antigens and distinguish nonself from self. Primary lymphoid organs include the *bone marrow* for B lymphocytes and the *thymus* for T lymphocytes. (2) **Secondary lymphoid organs,** also called **peripheral lymphoid organs,** are where mature lymphocytes (both B and T cells) encounter foreign antigens and the immune response takes place. Secondary lymphoid organs include *MALT, lymph nodes,* and the *spleen.*

Cells in the Lymphoid System

Lymphocytes can be classified into three major types based on their immunologic functions: **B lymphocytes (B cells), T lymphocytes (T cells),** and **null cells.** B cells and T cells are the two main cell types found in lymphoid organs. Lymphocytes originate in the bone marrow and develop and mature in primary lymphoid organs. B-cell antigen recognition is mediated by Ig molecules in their surface membranes, whereas T-cell antigen recognition is mediated by the T-cell receptor (TCR), and activation requires presentation of the antigen in association with a major histocompatibility complex (MHC) molecule on the surface of another cell. MHC molecules are genetic materials and contain glycoproteins, which allow T lymphocytes to recognize epitopes of antigens and discriminate self from nonself. There are two types of MHC: MHC class I and MHC class II. All nucleated cells express MHC class I; the MHC class II is expressed by antigen-presenting cells. Exposure to foreign antigens initiates the immune response in secondary lymphoid organs. It is impossible to distinguish between the T and B cells in routine tissue preparation without using immunohistochemical stains. However, they have a tendency to reside in certain regions of the lymphoid organs. For example, most B cells reside in lymphatic nodules of the secondary lymphoid organs, whereas T cells reside in the thymus, paracortex of the lymph nodes, and periarterial lymphatic sheath (PALS) of the spleen. *B cells* participate in the **humoral immune response,** and *T cells* are involved with the **cell-mediated immune responses.** Other cells in the lymphoid organs include **plasma cells** and **antigen-presenting cells.**

B Lymphocytes

B lymphocytes originate from precursor cells in the **bone marrow** and become **naive (virgin) B cells** in the bone marrow. These B cells develop their **surface antibody (Ig),** which enables them to recognize **non–self-antigens.** If B cells recognize self-antigens during the maturation process, these B cells will undergo **apoptosis** (negative selection). Naive B cells migrate from the bone marrow to the **secondary lymphoid organs** through the blood circulation. If naive B cells do not meet a specific foreign antigen, they will die in a short time. If they encounter such an antigen, recognizing and binding to the antigen will allow them to survive and become **active B cells.** Activated B cells undergo cell division and differentiate into **plasma cells** and **memory B cells.** Memory B cells have a long life and can live for decades in circulating blood in an inactive state. They can differentiate into plasma cells, which produce antibodies to participate in the humoral immune response.

T Lymphocytes

T lymphocytes also originate from precursor cells in the bone marrow, but they do not mature in the bone marrow. **Pro-T lymphocytes** enter the blood circulation and travel to their **primary lymphoid organ (thymus)** to finish their maturation. They develop into **thymocytes** in the cortex of the thymus and undergo a differentiation process to become **naive (virgin) T cells.** Naive T cells have surface markers on their cytoplasmic membrane and have a short life as do naive B cells. They will die if they do not meet an antigen. Naive T cells migrate from the thymus to secondary lymphoid organs where they encounter foreign antigens and become **active T cells.** Once T cells are activated, they can boost the action of cytotoxic T cells and macrophages and help to expedite proliferation of B lymphocytes, which increase the production of antibodies. Activated T cells undergo cell division to become **memory T cells** or **effector T cells.**

MEMORY T CELLS have a much longer life than **naive (virgin) T cells.** They can survive for a long period in an inactive state and can differentiate into effector T cells to participate in a stronger and faster secondary immune response when they encounter the same antigen for the second time. Memory T cells include **central memory T cells** and **effector memory T cells.** *Central memory T cells* express **CCR7 (chemokine receptor)** surface molecules and secrete **interleukin-2 (IL-2)** that stimulates B cells to proliferate. They reside in secondary lymphoid organs, such as the paracortex of the lymph nodes, and are capable of differentiating into effector memory T cells. *Effector memory T cells* do not express CCR7 surface molecules but secrete **IL-4** (to stimulate B cells and increase **immunoglobulin G [IgG]** and **IgM).** They often migrate to an inflammatory site and develop into effector T cells.

EFFECTOR T CELLS include **helper T cells, cytotoxic T cells,** and **regulatory (suppressor) T cells.** (1) *Helper T cells* have the surface marker **CD4,** which restricts activation to antigens only if it is presented by another cell in association with **MHC class II.** Helper T cells include **Th0, Th1,** and **Th2 cells.** *Th0 cells* can differentiate into Th1 and Th2 cells; *Th1 cells* secrete **IL-2, interferon-γ,** and **tumor necrosis factor** and down-regulate Th2 cells' response; *Th2 cells* secrete IL-4, IL-5, IL-6, and IL-10, which help promote antibody production, stimulate proliferation of eosinophil and mast cells, and down-regulate Th1 cells' response. Helper T cells do not directly kill infected cells or pathogens but function indirectly to promote and activate other immune cells. (2) *Cytotoxic (CD8) T cells* have the **CD8** surface marker, which restricts activation to antigen only if it is presented by another cell in association with **MHC class I.** They kill target cells, such as virus-infected cells, tumor cells, and transplanted cells (grafts). (3) *Regulatory T cells* are also called **suppressor T cells.** They *suppress* the humoral and cellular immune responses and are involved with immunological tolerance.

Null Cells

Null cells resemble lymphocytes but do not have surface markers, which B and T cells have. They include **pluripotential hemopoietic stem cells (PHSCs)** and **natural killer (NK) cells.** *PHSCs* function as stem cells and can give rise to various types of blood cells. *NK cells* do not require exposure to antigens to become activated. They function similarly to cytotoxic T cells but do not have the surface markers CD8 or CD4. They kill invading target cells, such as virus-infected cells and tumor cells.

Plasma Cells

Plasma cells differentiate from B cells. These activated large cells have clock-face nuclei, abundant rough endoplasmic reticulum, and a Golgi apparatus in the cytoplasm. They actively produce antibodies known as **immunoglobulins (Igs),** which are specific for each type of antigen.

Antigen-Presenting Cells

These cells process and present **antigens** to lymphocytes. Most of them are MHC-II class, which have surface membrane molecules MHC-II (histocompatibility complex). These cells present antigen to T cells. Antigen-presenting cells include **macrophages, dendritic cells, Langerhans cells,** and **B cells.** In general, B cells are both antigen-presenting and antigen-receiving cells. They present antigens to T cells and also receive antigens by either binding antigen to their receptors or through antigen-presenting cells (**follicle dendritic cells**). Lymphocytes are activated after receiving an antigen.

Lymphatic Tissues and Lymphoid Organs

Mucosa-Associated Lymphatic Tissues

Diffuse lymphatic tissues or nodules are often located in the connective tissue, which support the epithelial membranes of the body mucosae. The lymphatic tissues found in the mucosa of the digestive, respiratory, and genitourinary tracts are called **mucosa-associated lymphatic tissues (MALT).** They can be subdivided into **gut-associated lymphatic tissue (GALT)** and **bronchus-associated lymphatic tissue (BALT),** according to their locations. *GALT* is found in the digestive tract, such as **Peyer patches** in the ileum and lymphatic nodules in the appendix and large intestine. *BALT* is found in the respiratory tracts, mostly in bronchi and bronchioles (see Chapter 11, "Respiratory System"). Tonsils are covered by epithelium and have an incomplete capsule. Most tonsils contain lymphatic nodules but some of them have diffuse lymphatic tissues. Tonsils are located in the oral cavity and posterior roof of the nasopharynx. Tonsils include **lingual tonsils, palatine tonsils,** and a **pharyngeal tonsil;** they are classified as MALT. MALT traps bacteria and viruses, defends against infection, and provides sites where lymphocytes meet antigens. **Lymphatic nodules** occur in most of the

secondary lymphoid organs (MALT, lymph nodes, and spleen). Lymphatic nodules with a germinal center are called **secondary nodules.** The germinal center is evidence of proliferation of lymphocytes after they encounter antigen and become activated. Lymphatic nodules contain various stages of B cells, and most are **lymphoblasts** (enlarged and proliferated lymphocytes). The **mantle zone** (peripheral to the germinal center) of the lymphatic nodule contains tightly packed small lymphocytes. The outside of the nodules is usually surrounded by T cells. A lymphatic nodule without a germinal center is called a **primary nodule,** and it contains mostly inactivated (small) B cells.

Lymph Nodes

Lymph nodes are bean-shaped organs that are covered by a layer of connective tissue (**capsule**). They are distributed throughout the body. The regions that are associated with rich clusters of lymph nodes include the neck (cervical nodes and pericranial ring), axilla (axillary nodes), thorax (tracheal nodes), abdomen (deep nodes), groin (inguinal nodes), and femoral triangle (inguinal nodes) regions. They play important roles in circulating and filtering lymph, defending against microbial invasion, and providing a place for lymphocytes to meet antigens. Each lymph node has several **afferent lymphatic vessels** and an **efferent lymphatic vessel.** Lymph enters a lymph node through *afferent vessels* and flows into subcapsular sinuses and peritrabecular sinuses and then into the medullary sinuses and exits the lymph node through an *efferent lymphatic vessel.* In general, a lymph node can be divided into three regions: **cortex, paracortex,** and **medulla.** (1) The *cortex* contains a row of **lymphatic nodules;** most of these nodules are secondary nodules. (2) The *paracortex* is located between the cortex and the medulla. Most T cells are hosted here. **High endothelial venules (HEVs)** are found in this region. HEVs are postcapillary venules, which have a cuboidal cell lining instead of the common, flat endothelial cell lining. They are specialized venules, which allow lymphocytes to pass through their walls to enter the lymphatic tissue. HEVs can also be found in other lymphatic organs such as tonsils. (3) The *medulla* is composed of **medullary cords** and **medullary sinuses.** *Medullary cords* are like small islands that are surrounded by lymphatic channels (medullary sinuses). Medullary cords contain lymphocytes, plasma cells, macrophages, and dendritic cells. *Medullary sinuses* are lymphatic sinuses. Bacteria and antigens are trapped and engulfed by antigen-presenting cells (macrophages and dendritic cells) in the medulla. Reticular fibers form meshwork to provide a structure support and allow lymphocytes move around in the lymph nodes.

Thymus

The **thymus** is the primary lymphoid organ for maturation of T cells. It is located in the superior mediastinum. The thymus continues to grow until puberty and then gradually atrophies. In elderly individuals, a large portion of the thymus tissue is replaced by adipose tissue. The thymus is covered by a thin layer of connective tissue (**capsule**) and has two lobes. Each lobe is composed of many lobules, and the lobules can be divided into a **cortex** and **medulla.** Unlike other lymphatic organs, the thymus does not have lymphatic nodules. Its stroma is composed of a framework of epithelial reticular cells derived from the endoderm. (1) The *cortex* contains **thymocytes** (developing T cells), macrophages, dendritic cells, and **epithelial reticular cells.** T-cell maturation occurs in the cortex. (2) The *medulla* contains virgin T cells, which have developed and migrated from thymocytes in the cortex. The medulla also contains a large number of epithelial reticular cells. **Hassall corpuscles (thymic corpuscles)**, which are formed by concentrically arranged **type VI epithelial reticular cells**, are found in the medulla. There are several types of epithelial reticular cells in the thymus: *Types I* to *type III epithelial reticular cells* are located in the cortex, *type IV* in the junction of the cortex and medulla, and *types V* and *VI epithelial reticular cells* in the medulla.

Spleen

The **spleen** is a large and highly vascularized lymphoid organ, located in the superior left quadrant of the abdomen. It is covered by a thick layer of dense connective tissue (**capsule**). The spleen does not have a cortex and medulla; it is organized into two regions: **white pulp** and **red pulp**. (1) The *white pulp* is an immune component in the spleen, composed of **nodules, central arteries**, and a **periarterial lymphatic sheath** (**PALS**). *Lymphatic nodules* are often secondary nodules, which have germinal centers and are often called **splenic nodules**. *Central arteries* pass through the white pulp and give rise to sinuses in the marginal zone (peripheral region of the nodule). The central artery also gives rise to the penicillar arterioles in the red pulp. The *PALS* is a sheath of concentrated T cells surrounding a central artery. (2) The *red pulp* is the main region; it filters antigens and particulate materials, engulfs aged erythrocytes, and serves as reservoir for erythrocytes and platelets. It is composed of **splenic sinuses** and **splenic cords (Billroth cords)**. *Splenic sinuses* are venous sinuses (discontinuous capillaries) that have large lumens and large gaps between endothelial cells, which permit large proteins and cells to pass through the walls of sinuses. *Splenic cords* are formed by a framework of reticular tissue, which contains lymphocytes, plasma cells, macrophages, and other blood cells.

Lymphocytes

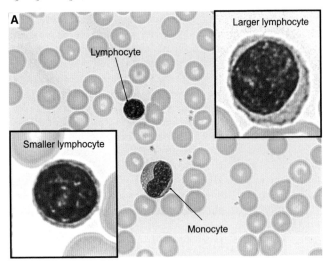

Figure 10-1A. Lymphocytes. H&E, ×702; inset, ×2,176

Lymphocytes can be found in blood and lymph circulation as well as in lymphoid organs. There are many types and subtypes of lymphocytes, which can be classified into three major types based on their immunologic functions: **B lymphocytes (B cells)**, **T lymphocytes (T cells)**, and **null cells**. Their sizes vary, but they are morphologically similar to each other. B and T cells cannot be distinguished from each other in routine H&E stain. Shown here is an example of lymphocytes in a blood smear. Lymphocytes have relatively large and round nuclei with a small rim of cytoplasm surrounding the nucleus. The two *insets* in the same magnification show the size variation of the lymphocytes. A **monocyte** is also seen in this specimen. Monocytes differentiate into tissue macrophages or special forms of **macrophages**, such as Kupffer cells in the liver, microglia in the nervous tissue, and osteoclasts in the bone tissue.

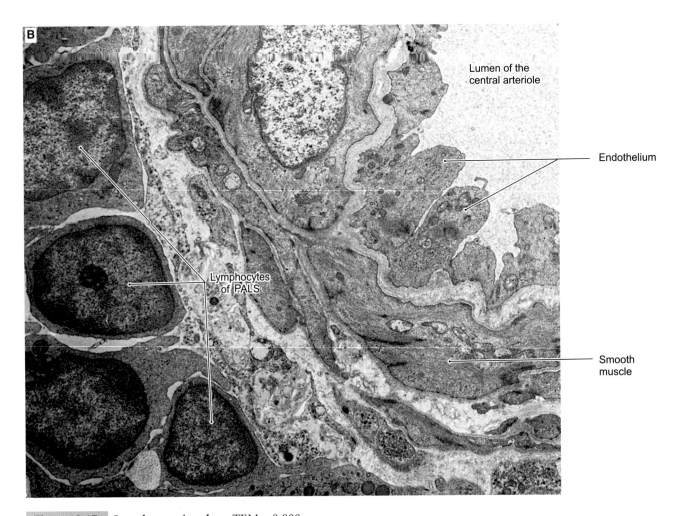

Figure 10-1B. Lymphocytes in spleen. TEM, ×8,800

The **lymphocytes** on the *left* part of this field are part of the **PALS** that surround a **central arteriole**. Part of the wall of the arteriole occupies the central part of the field, and a portion of its **lumen** is on the *right*. The lymphocytes here appear to be inactive, judging from the scant amount of cytoplasm and the small nuclei containing little **euchromatin**. However, one of the lymphocytes does display a small nucleolus, suggesting at least a basal level of protein synthesis. Although T and B lymphocytes are not distinguishable morphologically, the location of these lymphocytes in the PALS indicates that they are T lymphocytes.

Type of Lymphocytes

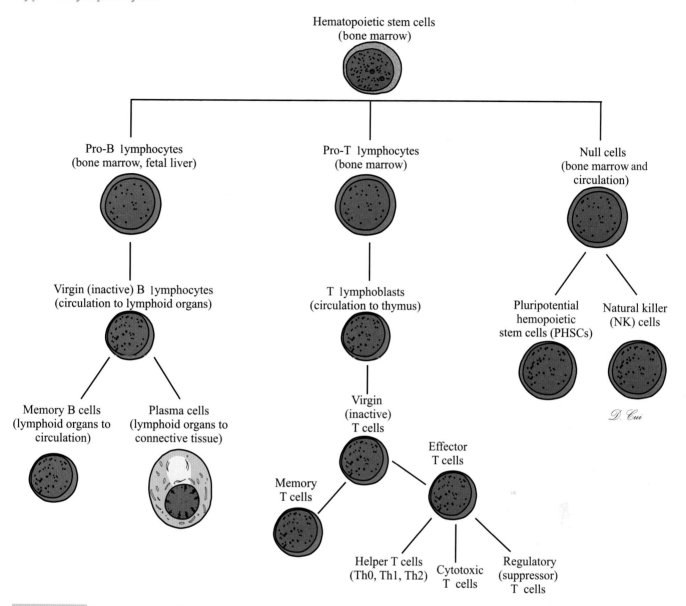

Figure 10-2.   Representation of types of lymphocytes.

B lymphocytes (B cells), **T lymphocytes (T cells)**, and **null cells** are three major cell types in the immune system. Each of these cells originates from precursor cells in the bone marrow. B and T lymphocytes are the main cell types located in lymphoid organs. (1) *B cells* mature and become **naive** (**virgin**) B cells (immunocompetent cells that have not been previously exposed to foreign antigen) in the bone marrow; they migrate to secondary lymph organs and may meet with antigens. B cells that become activated by exposure to antigens differentiate into memory B cells and effector B cells (plasma cells). (2) *T cells* differentiate from pro-T lymphocytes, which have migrated from the bone marrow into the thymus through the circulatory system. **Thymocytes** (developing lymphocytes) differentiate to **naive** (**virgin**) T cells in the thymus and then migrate to secondary lymphoid organs where they may be activated by exposure to foreign antigens. Activated T cells can differentiate into both **memory T cells** and **effector T cells**. Effector T cells include **helper T cells, cytotoxic T cells**, and **regulatory** (**suppressor**) **T cells**. B and T cells share some common features. Each B and T cell is programmed to respond to a particular antigenic determinant. Each naive B cell or T cell is relatively short lived unless it becomes activated by contact with the antigen it recognizes. Both types give rise to both memory cells and effector cells if they interact with an antigen ("antigen dependent"). Both B and T cells reside in specific regions in secondary lymphoid organs. However, there are some important differences between B and T cells. B-cell antigen recognition is mediated by Ig molecules in their surface membranes, whereas T-cell antigen recognition is mediated by the **T-cell receptor** (**TCR**), and activation requires presentation of the antigen in association with an **MHC** molecule on the surface of another cell. Finally, activated B cells function by differentiating into antibody-secreting plasma cells (humoral immune response), whereas activated T cells can differentiate into several functional forms: helper T cells, cytotoxic T cells, or suppressor T cells (cell-mediated immune responses). (3) *Null cells* are described in detail in the introduction.

B-LYMPHOCYTE MATURATION

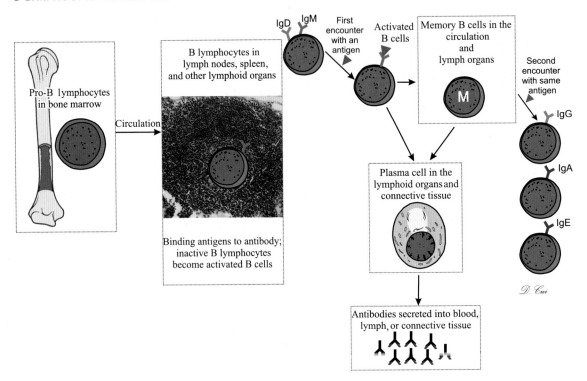

Figure 10-3.   Representation of B-lymphocyte maturation. H&E, ×83

B lymphocytes (B cells) originate and mature in the bone marrow. Because **naive (virgin) B lymphocytes** differentiate from **precursor cells (pro-B lymphocytes)**, they become randomly programmed to recognize a **specific antigenic determinant**. During the B-cell maturation process, they are subjected to **negative selection**, through which those B cells that happen to recognize self-antigens are induced to undergo **apoptosis**. Naive B lymphocytes are **immunocompetent cells** with specific **antibodies (Igs)** inserted into their plasma membrane as receptors. Each B lymphocyte has the ability to recognize and respond to a particular **antigen**. After newly matured B lymphocytes leave the bone marrow, they use the vasculature and their own motility to recirculate through the peripheral lymphoid organs (lymph nodes, spleen, MALT, etc.). This continual wandering increases the likelihood that a lymphocyte will encounter its antigen if the antigen has gained entry into the body. Naive B cells die in a few days or weeks if they do not meet their antigen, but those that encounter their specific antigen under favorable conditions will become activated. B cells that are activated by an encounter with antigens undergo cell division and differentiation. Some descendants of an activated B cell become **memory B cells**; others differentiate into **effector B cells**, that is, **plasma cells**, which are able to produce and secrete **antibodies**. Antibodies secreted by plasma cells become widely distributed throughout the body so that foreign antigens are unlikely to evade binding by antibodies and the defense mechanisms that are triggered by antibody binding. Memory B cells have a much longer life than naive B cells; they enter the blood circulation in an inactive state and may live and recirculate for decades. If there is a subsequent encounter with the same antigen, memory B cells rapidly divide and differentiate into plasma cells that secrete antibodies in great quantity, thereby producing a much quicker and more powerful **secondary immune response**.

SYNOPSIS 10-1 Characteristics of Types of Immunoglobulins

There are five types of Igs classified by their heavy chains:
- *IgG:* This is the most abundant type of Ig in blood serum and the only one that is able to cross the placenta. It is a major Ig during the secondary immune response and has high antigen-binding specificity.
- *IgA:* This is the major type of Ig in external secretions (milk, saliva, tears, sweat, and mucus) of epithelial cells, including gland epithelial cells. Its main function is to protect mucosal (epithelial) surfaces. It includes subclasses IgA1 and IgA2.
- *IgM:* This is the principal Ig in the primary immune response; it is most effective in activating a complement but with lower antigen-binding specificity. It activates macrophages and serves as an antigen receptor on the B-cell surfaces.
- *IgE:* This is found only in small amounts in blood serum; it binds to Fc receptors of the mast cells and basophils and plays an important role in allergic reactions and parasitic infections (see mast cell).
- *IgD:* This has a low concentration in blood serum; it serves along with IgM as an antigen receptor on the membranes of mature B cells.

T-LYMPHOCYTE MATURATION

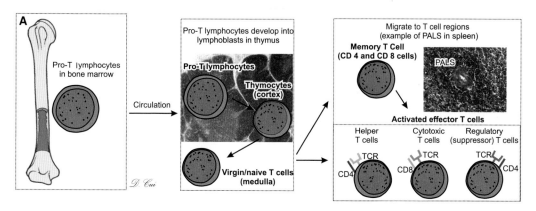

Figure 10-4A. Representation of T-lymphocyte maturation. H&E, ×19 (thymus); ×200 (spleen)

T cells are derived from **pro-T lymphocytes**, which migrate from the bone marrow to the thymus where they undergo cell division to generate a large number of developing lymphocytes (**thymocytes**). As thymocytes undergo the differentiation process, they begin to express **TCR** and other cell-surface proteins. Some of the maturation markers of T cells help them to recognize and interact with **MHC** molecules. In order to survive and mature, thymocytes must negotiate both **positive** and **negative selection processes**. *Positive selection* involves promoting survival of only those thymocytes that are able to interact at an appropriate level with **self-MHC molecules**, a capacity essential to their ability to mount effective immune responses. *Negative selection* involves destruction of thymocytes that have too strong an interaction with **self-MHC molecules**; these cells have the potential to contribute to autoimmune disease, and they are removed by macrophages. Positive selection occurs in the cortex of the thymus and negative selection mainly in the medulla. It has been estimated that only 1% to 2% of thymocytes survive these selection processes and complete differentiation to become immunocompetent T cells (naive T cells). Naive T cells leave the medulla of the thymus through the circulation and migrate to the specific regions of the secondary lymphoid organs where they may encounter the **foreign antigen** that they are programmed to recognize. If antigen stimulation occurs, virgin T cells become active, undergo cell division, and give rise to clones composed of both **memory T cells** and **effector T cells**. Memory T cells can be found in the paracortex of the lymph nodes and may migrate to inflammatory sites and give rise to effector T cells. Effector cells include **helper T cells, cytotoxic T cells**, and **regulatory (suppressor) T cells**. Each effector cell has either **CD4** or **CD8** as a surface marker. Effector cells participate in **cell-mediated immune responses**.

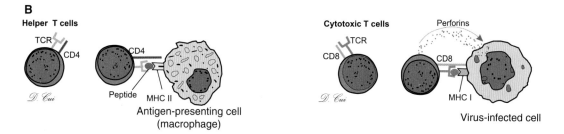

Figure 10-4B. Representation of helper T-cell and cytotoxic T-cell maturation markers.

Each **T lymphocyte** has in its plasmalemma numerous **TCRs**, each with the same antigen recognition site. Each T cell also has either **CD4** or **CD8 molecules** that act as essential **coreceptors** with the TCR. In the early stages of T-cell development, each thymocyte has both CD4+ and CD8+ markers, and mature T cells have either CD4 or CD8 markers, but not both. **CD8+ cells** have the capacity to recognize and react to their specific antigen only if it is presented by another cell in association with MHC class I. All nucleated cells of the body express MHC class I and present fragments of internally synthesized peptides on their surface MHC class I molecules. If any cell in the body becomes infected by a virus and synthesizes viral proteins, fragments of these viral proteins are presented as foreign antigens by the cell's surface MHC class I molecules. If such a virus-infected cell is encountered by a cytotoxic T cell (CD8+ cells) that bears TCRs that recognize one of the viral antigens, the cytotoxic T cell will become activated and destroy the virus-infected cell. **CD4+ cells** recognize their specific antigen only if it is presented by another cell in association with MHC class II. MHC class II is expressed by antigen-presenting cells. If an antigen-presenting cell presents antigen to a CD4+ (helper T cell) that recognizes the antigen, the helper T cell will become activated to provide signals that promote activation of other lymphocytes. The illustration on the *left* shows helper T cells with TCR and surface marker CD4. TCR is an antigen receptor that is specific to the peptide that is attached to the groove of the MHC II molecule on the macrophage. This peptide presents a foreign antigen to helper T cells. The illustration on the right shows TCR and CD8 markers on the cytotoxic T cells' surface. TCR of the cytotoxic T cell responds to antigen presented in association with MHC I molecules of the infected cells. Once a cytotoxic T cell recognizes a non–self-antigen, it releases **perforins** and **enzymes** from granules to kill the infected cells as well as some tumor cells, grafted cells, and virus-infected cells.

HELPER T-LYMPHOCYTE ACTIVATION

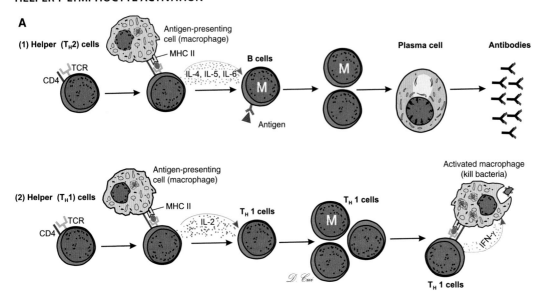

Figure 10-5A. Representation of helper T-lymphocyte activation.

The **CD4** surface marker on a **helper T cell** recognizes **MHC II** surface proteins on the **antigen-presenting cell**. The **TCR** binds with the peptide-MHC complex on the surface of the macrophage (or other types of antigen-presenting cells); therefore, antigens are presented to helper T cells. The activating signals (secreted proteins, cytokines) are exchanged between the helper T cells and the macrophages. There are two main types of helper T cells: (1) Activated **helper (T_H2) cells** release a variety of **interleukins/cytokines** that stimulate **B cells** to proliferate and increase the population of plasma cells, thereby increasing production of **antibodies**. (2) Activated helper (T_H1) cells release and bind with **IL-2**, stimulating proliferation and activation of T_H1 cells and greatly increasing their own numbers. Activated T_H1 cells provide signals that promote proliferation of **cytotoxic T cells** (CD8+ cells) and activation of **macrophages**. In turn, activated macrophages kill bacteria by a variety of mechanisms and stimulate additional inflammatory processes.

CLINICAL CORRELATION

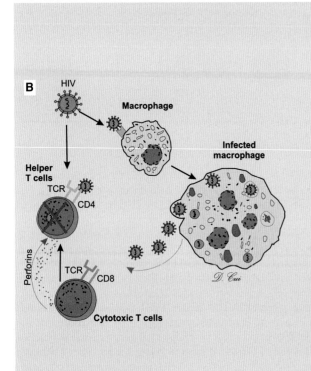

Figure 10-5B. **Human Immunodeficiency Virus Infection.**

Infection by the **retrovirus HIV** leads to **acquired immunodeficiency syndrome (AIDS)**. Infection may be transferred from an infected individual through exposure to body fluids including blood, semen, and breast milk. It is associated with a progressive **decline** in **CD4+ T cell** numbers. The stage of infection can be determined by measuring the patient's CD4+ T cell number and the level of HIV in the blood. HIV primarily infects CD4+ helper T cells, macrophages, and dendritic cells (antigen-presenting cells). The low level of CD4+ T cells in the blood of HIV-infected patients may be because of (1) the HIV virus killing infected CD4+ T cells directly, (2) increased rates of apoptosis in infected CD4+ T cells, or (3) CD8+ cytotoxic lymphocytes recognizing and killing CD4+ T cells after the virus has infected them. The HIV virus enters macrophages (CD4+ T cells as well), replicates in the host cells, and the new viruses are released from the host cells. Greatly reduced numbers of CD4+ T cells result in the loss of cell-mediated immunity. Without stimulation from CD4+ T helper cells, humoral immunity function is compromised. AIDS patients are vulnerable to opportunistic infections; common diseases include *Pneumocystis jirovecii pneumonia*, **toxoplasmosis**, and **thrush**. Histologically, lymph nodes in the early stage of HIV infection reveal large, irregular lymphatic nodules and an increased number of macrophages in the germinal centers.

Lymphoid Tissues and Lymphoid Organs

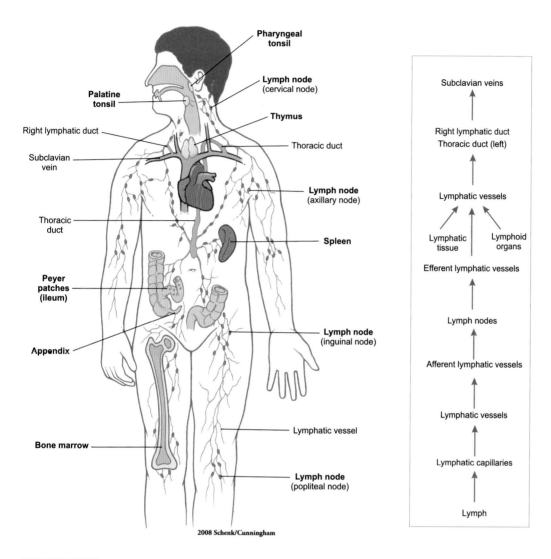

Figure 10-6. Overview of the lymphoid organs.

Locations of the principal lymphoid organs and vessels are shown on the *left*; the route of lymph drainage is shown on the *right*.

Structures of the Lymphoid Tissues and Organs

I. **Mucosa-associated lymphoid tissue**
   A. **Gut-associated lymphoid tissue:** Lymphatic tissue in the mucosa of the digestive tract, such as Peyer patches in ileum and nodules in the appendix.

   B. **Bronchus-associated lymphoid tissue:** Lymphatic tissue in the mucosa of the respiratory tract, such as lymphatic tissue in bronchi, bronchioles.

   C. **Tonsils**
      1. Palatine tonsils
      2. Pharyngeal tonsils
      3. Lingual tonsils

II. **Lymphoid organs**
   A. **Bone marrow** (see Chapter 9, "Circulatory System")
   B. **Thymus**
      1. Cortex
      2. Medulla
   C. **Lymph nodes**
      1. Afferent lymphatic vessels
      2. Efferent lymphatic vessels
      3. Cortex
      4. Paracortex
      5. Medulla
   D. **Spleen**
      1. White pulp
      2. Red pulp

Figures and Images Orientation

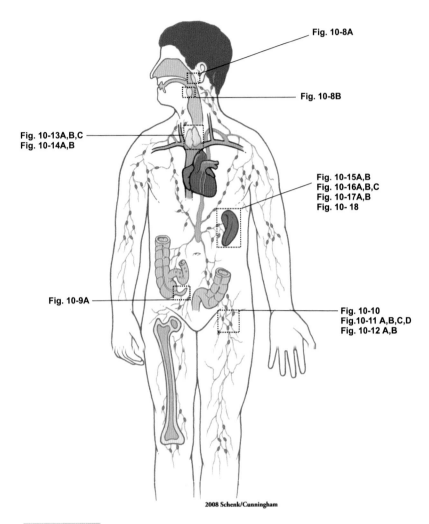

Fig. 10-8A

Fig. 10-8B

Fig. 10-13A,B,C
Fig. 10-14A,B

Fig. 10-15A,B
Fig. 10-16A,B,C
Fig. 10-17A,B
Fig. 10- 18

Fig. 10-9A

Fig. 10-10
Fig.10-11 A,B,C,D
Fig. 10-12 A,B

2008 Schenk/Cunningham

Figure 10-7.   Orientation of detailed lymphoid organ illustrations.

Structures of Lymphoid Organs with Figure Numbers

Pharyngeal tonsil
Figure 10-8A

Palatine tonsil
Figure 10-8B

Appendix
Figure 10-9A

Lymph node
Figure 10-9B
Figure 10-9C
Figure 10-10
Figure 10-11A
Figure 10-11B
Figure 10-11C
Figure 10-11D
Figure 10-12A

Figure 10-12B
Figure 10-12C

Thymus
Figure 10-13A
Figure 10-13B
Figure 10-13C
Figure 10-14A
Figure 10-14B

Spleen
Figure 10-15A
Figure 10-15B
Figure 10-16A
Figure 10-16B
Figure 10-16C
Figure 10-17A
Figure 10-17B
Figure 10-18

Mucosa-Associated Lymphoid Tissue (MALT)

PHARYNGEAL TONSIL

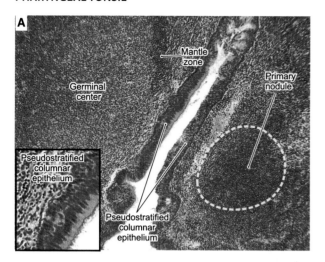

Figure 10-8A. **Pharyngeal tonsil, MALT.** H&E, ×76; inset ×184

MALT refers to diffuse lymphatic tissues or aggregate lymphatic nodules in the mucosa of the digestive, respiratory, and genitourinary tracts. Comparable tissue is **GALT** in the gut and **BALT** in the respiratory system. Tonsils are composed of aggregate lymphatic nodules and belong to MALT. Tonsils include **pharyngeal, palatine,** and **lingual tonsils.** The pharyngeal tonsil is located in the roof of the nasopharynx. It has epithelial invaginations, but no crypts, and is covered by **pseudostratified columnar epithelium.** The pharyngeal tonsil traps bacteria and viruses and is one of the lymphoid organs that provides an environment for lymphocytes to meet antigens. It mostly consists of secondary nodules and a few primary nodules. A secondary nodule is composed of a **germinal center** and **mantle zone.** Activated B cells are found mainly in the germinal centers of secondary nodules and inactivated B cells primarily in primary nodules.

PALATINE TONSIL

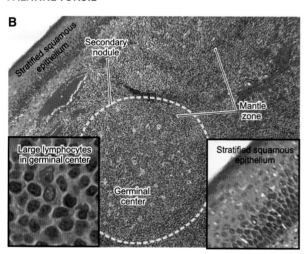

Figure 10-8B. **Palatine tonsil, MALT.** H&E, ×83; inset ×750 (*left*); 197 (*right*)

Palatine tonsils are paired and are located in the posterior and lateral portions of the oral cavity. They have 10 to 20 crypts and the portion facing the oral cavity is covered by **stratified squamous epithelium.** The nodules usually lie as a row beneath the epithelium and surround each crypt. They safeguard the entrance of the respiratory and digestive tracts against microbe invasion. They also function in the recirculation of lymphocytes and provide sites for the lymphocyte to interact with antigens. The **germinal center** of a nodule contains large-sized B cells and antigen-presenting cells where B cells encounter antigens and continue to proliferate and develop into plasma cells. The **mantle zone** of the nodule contains mostly small inactive B cells. The peripheral region of the nodule contains mostly T cells.

Palatine tonsils are common sites for infection, such as **acute tonsillitis,** recurrent **tonsillitis,** or **tonsillar hypertrophy** due to lymphoid hyperplasia. **Tonsillectomy** may be a choice in some children with recurrent tonsillitis.

TABLE 10-1 Tonsils

Name	Location	Epithelial Covering	Crypts	Capsule	Lymphatic Nodules (Follicles)
Palatine tonsils (2)	Posterolateral walls of the oral cavity	Stratified squamous epithelium (nonkeratinized)	Yes, deep and branched crypts divide tonsil into lobules	Thick, incomplete connective tissue capsule; partially covered by epithelium	Each lobule contains numerous lymphatic nodules, most having a germinal center
Pharyngeal (adenoid) tonsil (1)	Posterior roof of the nasopharynx	Pseudostratified ciliated columnar epithelium	No, only epithelial invagination	Thin, incomplete connective capsule; partially covered by epithelium	Mostly diffuse lymphoid tissues and some lymphatic nodules
Lingual tonsils (2)	Posterior floor of the mouth (surface of the posterior third of the tongue)	Stratified squamous epithelium (nonkeratinized)	Yes, wide nonbranched crypt; duct of mucous gland opens into the crypt	No capsule; partially covered by epithelium	Rows of lymphatic nodules supported by connective tissue septa

APPENDIX

A

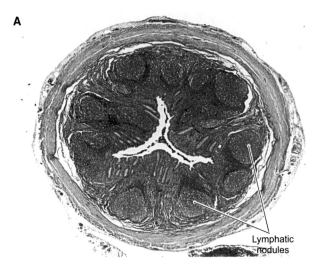

Lymphatic nodules

Figure 10-9A. Appendix, MALT. H&E, ×18

The **appendix** and **Peyer patches** in the ileum of the digestive system are **GALT**. The **appendix** is a small, blind tube that extends from the cecum in the lower right quadrant of the abdomen. It contains large numbers of **lymphatic nodules** in its lamina propria. Most of the nodules are secondary nodules with germinal centers. The secondary nodules often penetrate into the submucosa.

Appendicitis is a common disease. It is usually triggered by bacterial and viral infections that result in hyperplasia of lymphatic nodules and obstruction of the lumen of the appendix. Patients may experience abdominal pain, which most likely will be localized at the **McBurney point** (one third of the distance between the anterior superior iliac spine and the umbilicus on the right side) as the disease progresses. Fever, nausea, and vomiting are the common symptoms. Emergency **appendectomy** is the first treatment choice for most cases.

CLINICAL CORRELATIONS

B

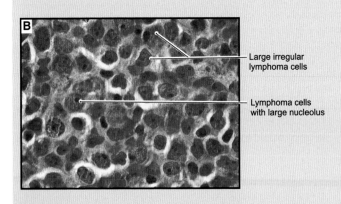

Large irregular lymphoma cells

Lymphoma cells with large nucleolus

Figure 10-9B. Diffuse Large B-Cell Lymphoma. H&E, ×1,000

Diffuse large B-cell lymphoma (DLBCL) is the most common type of **non-Hodgkin lymphoma** (25% of all lymphomas), characterized by a fast-growing and often symptomatic mass at a nodal or extranodal site. The most common extranodal site is the gastrointestinal tract, but other sites include skin, soft tissue, **Waldeyer ring**, lung, spleen, and kidneys. Patients may experience fever, weight loss, and drenching night sweats. Histologically, tumor cells are large with **large nuclei, open chromatin**, and **prominent nucleoli**. The tumor grows in a diffuse pattern. Treatment for DLBCL includes intensive combination chemotherapy with possible radiotherapy to the involved tumor site.

C

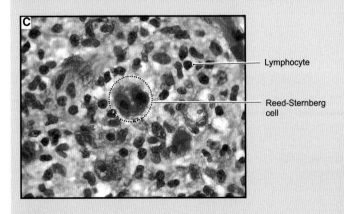

Lymphocyte

Reed-Sternberg cell

Figure 10-9C. Hodgkin Lymphoma. H&E, ×824

Hodgkin lymphoma, also known as **Hodgkin disease,** is one of the two major categories of malignant lymphoid cancers, characterized by painless enlargement of lymph nodes, spleen, and liver. Patients often experience fever, night sweats, unexpected weight loss, and fatigue. The cancer cells are transformed from normal lymphoid cells, which reside predominantly in lymphoid tissues. Characteristic **Reed-Sternberg cells,** of B-cell origin, can be found in affected lymphoid tissues. These cells are large (20–50 μm) and contain abundant, **amphophilic,** and finely granular/homogeneous cytoplasm with two mirror-image nuclei ("owl's eyes"), each with an eosinophilic nucleolus and a thick nuclear membrane. Radiotherapy and chemotherapy are both effective in treatment of Hodgkin lymphoma. The 5-year survival rate is ~90% when the disease is detected and treated early.

Lymph Nodes

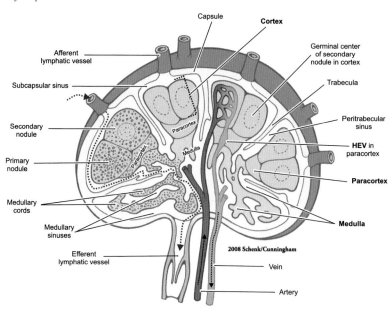

Figure 10-10. Overview of the lymph node.

This is a representation of a **lymph node**. It is covered by a capsule consisting of a layer of connective tissue, which extends into the substance of the node to form trabeculae. The lymph node is divided into three regions: **cortex, paracortex,** and **medulla.** (1) The *cortex* is composed of a row of lymphatic nodules; the majority are **secondary nodules** with **germinal centers.** Occasionally, primary nodules (without germinal centers) may be found in the cortex region. (2) The *paracortex* lies between the cortex and medulla; most T cells reside in this region. **HEVs** are located in paracortex and are the sites where circulating lymphocytes enter the node. (3) The *medulla* is composed of **medullary cords** and **medullary sinuses.** Lymph enters the lymph node through **afferent lymphatic vessels;** courses through the **subcapsular, peritrabecular,** and **medullary sinuses;** and exits the lymph node through the **efferent lymphatic vessel** (follow the *dotted magenta line*). The artery and vein enter and exit by passing through the hilum of the lymph node.

Comparison of Lymph and Blood Flow

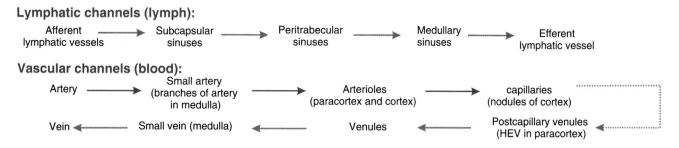

SYNOPSIS 10-2 Lymphoid Organs

■ In *primary lymphatic organs*, lymphocytes differentiate and mature; B cells' primary lymphoid organ is bone marrow; T cells' primary lymphoid organ is the thymus.
■ In *secondary lymphatic organs*, lymphocytes encounter and respond to foreign antigens; secondary lymphoid organs include MALT, lymph nodes, and spleen.
■ *Lymphatic nodules* are spherical structures that contain accumulated lymphocytes. They include primary nodules and secondary nodules.
■ *Primary nodules* contain mostly small (inactivated) B cells and do not have a germinal center.
■ *Secondary nodules* contain mostly large (activated) B cells and have a germinal center (light area in the center).
■ *Lymphatic nodules* contain mostly B cells.
■ The *thymus, paracortex* of the lymph node, and *PALS* in the spleen contain mostly T cells.

CORTEX AND MEDULLA OF LYMPH NODE

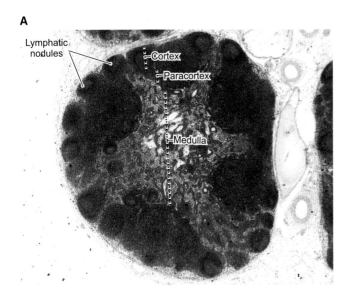

A

Lymphatic nodules — Cortex — Paracortex — Medulla

Figure 10-11A. Lymph node. H&E, ×43

Lymph nodes are bean shaped and are the only lymphoid organs that have afferent lymphatic vessels. This is a cross section of a lymph node. (1) The **cortex** is the peripheral region of the lymph node and consists of a row of nodules. (2) The **medulla** stains lighter and is located at the center area; it is composed of medullary sinuses and medullary cords. (3) The **paracortex** lies between the cortex and the medulla. Lymph nodes are the major sites to filter incoming lymph and are the sites for lymphocytes to meet antigens.

Figure 10-11B. Lymph node. H&E, ×100

The **subcapsular sinus** carries lymph from **afferent lymphatic vessels** into the node by passing through **peritrabecular sinuses** to the **medullary sinuses**. The nodules in the cortex consist of a **germinal center** (loosely packed large B cells) and a **mantle zone** (containing tightly packed small B cells). T cells mainly reside in the **paracortex** region where they interact with antigen-presenting cells; lymphocytes enter the lymph node through HEVs in the paracortex region.

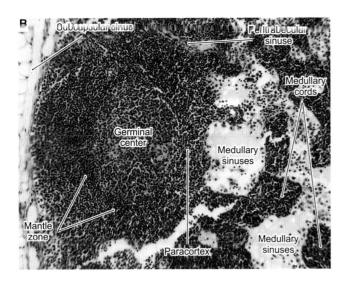

B

Subcapsular sinus — Peritrabecular sinuse — Medullary cords — Germinal center — Medullary sinuses — Mantle zone — Paracortex — Medullary sinuses

Figure 10-11C. Germinal center, lymph node. H&E, ×658

The **germinal center** is composed of activated B cells in various stages of maturation. Cell size and nuclear shape are varied. The large immature cells with round nucleus and dispersed euchromatin are **lymphoblasts** and **plasmablasts**. They differentiate into memory B cells and plasma cells. The germinal center also contains **follicular dendritic (antigen-presenting) cells**, which help pass antigens to B cells. They are difficult to recognize in H&E stain.

Figure 10-11D. Medullary sinuses and cords, lymph node. H&E, ×658

A **medullary sinus** surrounded by a **medullary cord** is shown here. *Medullary sinuses* carry lymph to where antigens are removed by **macrophages** from slow-flowing lymph. The *medullary cords* contain B cells, plasma cells, dendritic cells, and macrophages held within a network of reticular fibers.

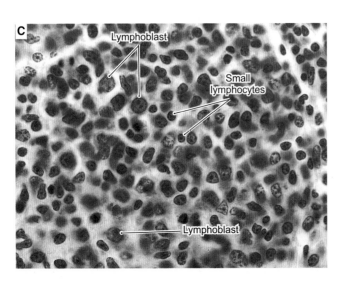

C

Lymphoblast — Small lymphocytes — Lymphoblast

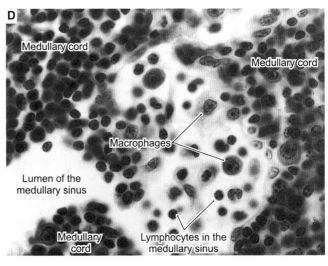

D

Medullary cord — Medullary cord — Macrophages — Lumen of the medullary sinus — Medullary cord — Lymphocytes in the medullary sinus

HIGH ENDOTHELIAL VENULES IN PARACORTEX

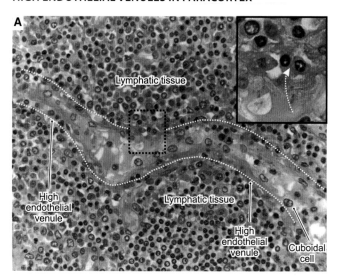

Figure 10-12A. High endothelial venules (HEVs), paracortex of lymph node. H&E, ×272; inset ×720

Arteries that serve a lymph node enter the hilum and give rise to branches that pass through the medulla and reach the cortex where they form a network of capillaries in the nodule (follicle) region. Postcapillary venules (in the paracortex region) carry blood from the capillary bed back to the venule system and out of the lymph node at the hilum. HEVs are specialized postcapillary veins, which are lined by **cuboidal cells** instead of squamous endothelial cells. The apical surfaces of these cuboidal cells contain rich glycoproteins that attract lectinlike receptors (L selectin) on the surface of the lymphocytes, which helps lymphocytes stop and attach to the HEVs. Lymphocytes pass through HEVs by way of **diapedesis** and enter the lymph node from blood circulation. The *inset* shows a lymphocyte escaping from a HEV into the lymphatic tissue.

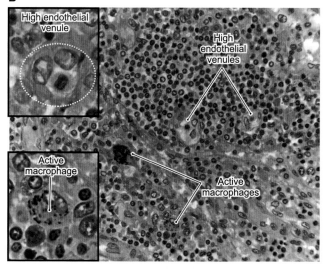

Figure 10-12B. High endothelial venules, paracortex of lymph node. H&E, ×281; insets ×725

HEVs can be found in all of the secondary lymphoid organs except the spleen. They are the major sites for both **naive B** and **T lymphocytes** that have migrated from circulation into the lymphatic tissue. After they enter the lymph node, *B cells* migrate to the cortex region where they differentiate in the **germinal center.** Most *T cells* remain in the **paracortex** region where they interact with **antigen-presenting cells (macrophages).** Once T cells acquire antigens, they release cytokine (IL-4, IL-5, and IL-6), which stimulates B cells' division and maturation to become memory B cells and plasma cells with the consequent production of antibodies. Endothelial cells of HEVs are cuboidal cells and have large round or oval nuclei with pale chromatin. The *insets* show a lymphocyte in the cross section of a **HEV** (*upper*) and an **active macrophage** in the paracortex region (*lower*).

CLINICAL CORRELATION

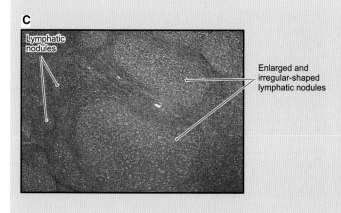

Figure 10-12C. Lymph Node, HIV Infection. H&E, ×40

HIV infection is associated with a progressive decline in helper T lymphocytes, resulting in immunosuppression. Patients with acute HIV infection may experience fever, **lymphadenopathy, pharyngitis, rash,** and **myalgia.** The chronic phase of HIV infection may last from months to years with patients exhibiting few symptoms. During the final crisis phase, patients are at increased risk of opportunistic infections and neoplasms. **Lymph nodes** in the early stage of HIV infection show marked follicular **lymphoid hyperplasia** with enlarged, irregularly shaped follicles (lymphatic nodules) and increased numbers of **macrophages** in the **germinal center.** The enlarged lymph nodes may be found first in the upper body, then around the lungs, and finally around the bowel. Patients with compromised immunity are highly likely to be infected by bacteria and other microbes. Anti-HIV drugs include four major classes: **reverse transcriptase inhibitors, protease inhibitors, entry** and **fusion inhibitors,** and **integrase inhibitors.**

Thymus

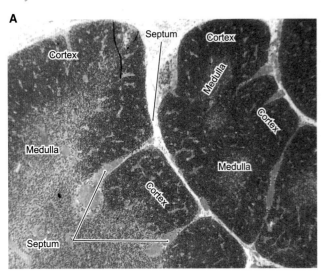

Figure 10-13A.   Thymus. H&E, ×46

The **thymus** is a primary lymphoid organ in which T-cell matura-tion takes place. The thymus is large in children and gradually atro-phies to be replaced by fat after puberty. The thymus is located in the superior mediastinum and is divided into smaller units called **lobules** by connective tissue **septae**, which extend inward from the surface of the organ. The thymus does not have lymphatic nodules; it is organized into **cortex** (peripheral) and **medulla** (center). There are no afferent lymphatic vessels; its efferent lymphatic vessels arise from the corticomedullary junction and medulla and leave the thy-mus in company with the blood vessels. **Thymocytes** (developing T cells) are concentrated in the cortex region, and as they undergo dif-ferentiation, they move down to the medulla. The blood vessels pass through the interlobular septa and enter the thymus at the junction of the cortex and medulla. Thymic capillaries are continuous cap-illaries with thick basement membranes. They are surrounded by epithelial reticular cells and form an effective thymic-blood barrier, which prevents foreign antigens from entering the thymus.

THYMIC CORTEX

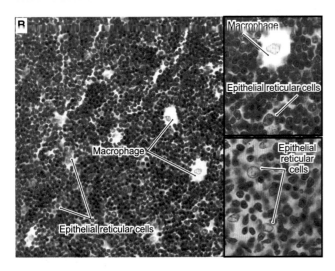

Figure 10-13B.   Thymus, cortex. H&E, ×278; insets ×510

The **cortex region** contains **thymocytes, macrophages, dendritic cells,** and **epithelial reticular cells.** The *macrophages* and *dendritic cells* are antigen-presenting cells; they present self-antigens to *thy-mocytes.* Only 1% to 2% of thymocytes survive and continue to develop. *Epithelial reticular cells* are derived from endoderm (lym-phocytes are derived from mesoderm). They are interconnected with each other to form a framework to hold T lymphocytes together. They have large, ovoid nuclei and long processes and make contact with each other by desmosomes. They contain secre-tory granules and produce thymosin, serum thymic factor, and thy-mopoietin hormone. These hormones play an important role in T-cell maturation. The epithelial reticular cells can be classified into six types based on their functions and locations. Types I to III are located in the cortex region, and type IV in the corticomedullary junction. Types V and VI are located in the medulla of the thymus.

THYMIC MEDULLA

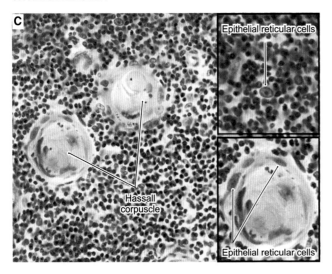

Figure 10-13C.   Thymus, medulla. H&E, ×624; insets ×843

The **medulla region** contains **naive (virgin) T cells, macrophages,** and **types V and VI epithelial reticular cells.** The *naive T cells* are immunocompetent cells. They mature from thymocytes in the cortex and migrate from the medulla to secondary organs where they become effective or memory T cells if they meet with spe-cific foreign antigen. The medulla of the thymus is also the place where T cells are selectively removed by *macrophages.* Both *types V* and *VI epithelial reticular cells* are located in the medulla. The type VI epithelial reticular cells show various degrees of keratini-zation and are arranged into concentric layers forming a spheri-cal structure called a **Hassall corpuscle.** Although the function of Hassall corpuscles is not fully understood, their numbers are increased in older individuals. Hassall corpuscles can be used as one of the unique features to distinguish the thymus from other lymphatic organs during the histological slide examination.

EPITHELIAL RETICULAR CELLS

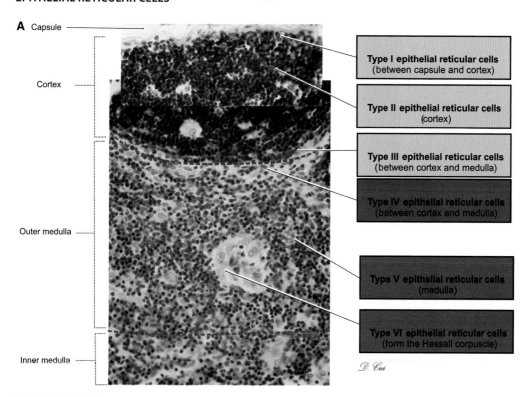

A Capsule

Cortex

Outer medulla

Inner medulla

Type I epithelial reticular cells
(between capsule and cortex)

Type II epithelial reticular cells
(cortex)

Type III epithelial reticular cells
(between cortex and medulla)

Type IV epithelial reticular cells
(between cortex and medulla)

Type V epithelial reticular cells
(medulla)

Type VI epithelial reticular cells
(form the Hassall corpuscle)

D. Cui

Figure 10-14A. Types of epithelial reticular cells. H&E, ×400

Epithelial reticular cells are derived from endoderm. They often have long processes and form a meshwork to support and protect thymocytes. They are also called thymic epithelial cells and can be divided into six types. (1) **Type I epithelial reticular cells** are found between the cortex of the thymus and the capsule and the trabecular region. Tight junctions exist between type I epithelial reticular cells and between type I cells and the endothelial cells lining the cortical vessels to form the thymic-blood barrier that prevents foreign antigens from entering the thymus. (2) **Type II epithelial reticular cells**, which have long processes and desmosomal junctions, are found within the cortex. Each cell has a large, pale cytoplasm, which is filled with tonofilaments (keratin intermediate filaments). Type II cells produce thymic hormones (thymosin, thymopoietin, and thymulin) and promote T-cell maturation. (3) **Type III epithelial reticular cells** are located between the cortex and the medulla. They are interconnected with each other by tight junctions, and they form a border between the cortex and the medulla. (4) **Type IV epithelial reticular cells** are found between the cortex and the medulla and assist the type III epithelial reticular cells to form the corticomedullary junction. (5) **Type V epithelial reticular cells** are located in the medulla. They are similar to type II epithelial reticular cells as they are interconnected with each other by desmosome junctions, but type V cells form a meshwork in the medulla. (6) **Type VI epithelial reticular cells** are large and show various degrees of keratinization. They are arranged in concentric layers to form Hassall corpuscles (thymic corpuscles).

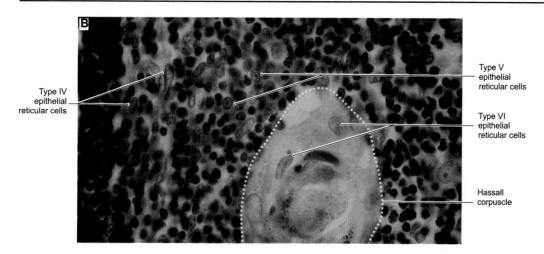

B

Type IV
epithelial
reticular cells

Type V
epithelial
reticular cells

Type VI
epithelial
reticular cells

Hassall
corpuscle

Figure 10-14B. Types V and VI epithelial reticular cells, thymus medulla. H&E, ×1,000

Anatomy of the Spleen

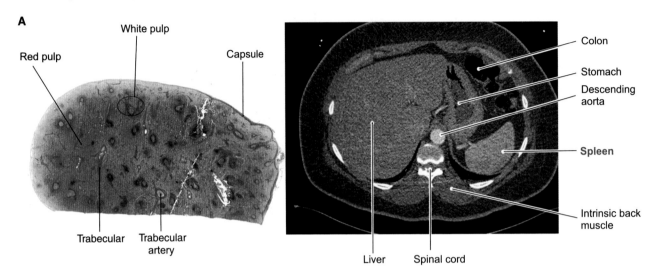

Figure 10-15A. Overview of anatomy of the spleen. H&E (*left*); computed tomography angiography (*right*)

The spleen is the largest of the lymphoid organs, weighing about 7 oz. It measures 1 × 3 × 5 in, and it is about the size of a clenched fist. It lies under the diaphragm on the left side of the abdomen, adjacent to ribs 9 to 11. The spleen has a rich blood supply from the splenic artery, which branches out from the **celiac trunk**. Veins accompany the arteries and unite to form the splenic vein, which drains into the **hepatic portal vein**. Lymph from the spleen drains into several nodes lying at the hilum and then drains to the celiac lymph nodes via the **pancreaticosplenic nodes**. The spleen is covered by a thick layer of capsule, and it contains many lymphoid nodules (**splenic nodules**) and **splenic arteries, veins,** and **splenic sinuses (venous sinuses).** The spleen serves as a **hematopoietic organ**, forming blood cells during the prenatal stage of the infant. In the adult, it serves as a lymphoid organ and a reservoir for **erythrocytes** and **platelets**.

A ruptured spleen may happen due to trauma, such as in a car accident. Patients may have left upper quadrant pain, left chest pain, and hypotension. Active hemorrhage and sudden loss of a large amount of blood may become a life-threatening situation. An emergency surgical procedure involving spleen removal (splenectomy) to stop bleeding is required.

CLINICAL CORRELATION

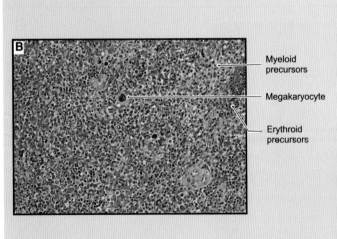

Myeloid precursors

Megakaryocyte

Erythroid precursors

Figure 10-15B Extramedullary Hematopoiesis. H&E, ×200

Extramedullary hematopoiesis (EMH, or EH) refers to hematopoiesis outside of the bone marrow medullary space, a process that may be physiologic or pathologic. Physiologic EH includes **primitive hematopoiesis** in the yolk sac and later definitive **hematopoiesis** in the liver and spleen during fetal development, after which hematopoiesis occurs in the bone marrow cavity. Pathologic EH may occur in many conditions, including severe **anemia, bone diseases** like **osteopetrosis** and **Paget disease,** and myeloproliferative disorders like **chronic myelogenous leukemia (CML), polycythemia vera,** and **myelofibrosis.** Pathologic EH occurs most commonly in the spleen and liver, but it may occur in other organs and tissues including the lymph nodes, heart, skin, lungs, retroperitoneum, and others. In the spleen, EH occurs primarily in the **red pulp,** and it may cause organ enlargement (**splenomegaly**). Therapy includes treatment of the underlying disease and surgical removal of the spleen (**splenectomy**).

Spleen

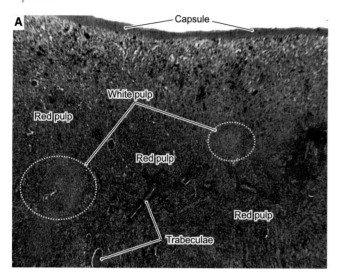

Figure 10-16A. Spleen. H&E, ×60

The **spleen** is a large lymphoid organ (about 140–180 g in humans) located in the left superior quadrant of the abdomen. It is covered by a thick, **dense connective tissue** (**capsule**), which extends into the organ to form trabeculae. **Trabeculae** provide structural support for arteries and veins, which supply the compartments (white and red pulp) of the spleen. The spleen is not organized into a cortex and medulla as are lymph nodes and the thymus but is divided into **white pulp** associated with a central artery and **red pulp** associated with a vein and venous sinusoids. Functions of the spleen include (1) an immune component (white pulp) to activate lymphocytes and promote antibody production by plasma cells, (2) filtration of blood and destruction of aged erythrocytes in red pulp, and (3) serving as reservoir for erythrocytes and platelets.

WHITE PULP

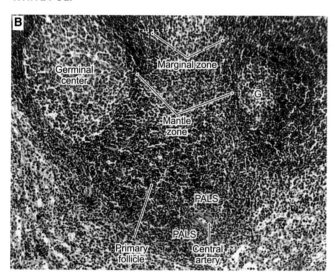

Figure 10-16B. White pulp, spleen. H&E, ×194; inset ×748

White pulp and **red pulp** are the two basic components of the spleen. **White pulp** is composed of a **central artery**, a periarterial lymphatic sheath (**PALS**), and a **lymphatic nodule**. The nodules with **germinal centers** are secondary nodules (follicles) where B cells actively differentiate into large cells (**lymphoblasts** and **lymphocytes**). The dark ring region around the germinal center is the **mantle zone** where small inactive B cells are hosted. The mantle zone stains dark because of densely packed lymphocytes. The nodules without the germinal centers are primary nodules, which contain most of the inactive B cells. The region that surrounds the white pulp is the **marginal zone**, which contains marginal sinuses. (G, germinal center.)

RED PULP

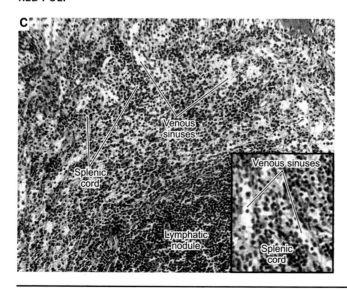

Figure 10-16C. Red pulp, spleen. H&E, ×256; inset ×385

Red pulp (red because it is rich in blood) stains light and contains **splenic cords** and **venous sinuses** that are filled with blood. Venous sinuses are discontinuous capillaries, which have large lumens, incomplete basal laminae, and gaps between endothelial cells. These special features allow blood cells to pass through the capillary wall. The **splenic cord** is a framework of reticular tissue that contains B cells, T cells, plasma cells, macrophages, and other blood cells. **Macrophages** in the splenic cord often extend their processes into the lumen of the sinuses to reach and engulf foreign substances, microbes, and aged erythrocytes. The red pulp of the spleen also serves as a reservoir for platelets.

SPLENIC CIRCULATION

A

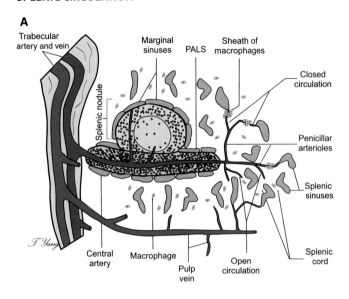

Figure 10-17A. Splenic circulation.

The **splenic artery** enters the spleen at the hilum and branches into **trabecular arteries**, which follow the trabeculae into the white pulp where they become the **central artery**. Lymphatic tissue that immediately surrounds the central artery is called the **PALS**. The central artery passes through the white pulp and gives rise to two routes of capillaries: (1) those which supply sinuses (**marginal sinuses**) around the lymphatic nodule and (2) those which supply sinuses in the red pulp. The central artery leaves the white pulp and forms several **penicillar arterioles** (not surrounded by PALS). The branches of the penicillar arterioles are called **terminal arterial capillaries**, which either give rise directly to the **splenic sinuses** (**closed circulation**) or terminate as open-ended vessels within the splenic cord of the red pulp (**open circulation**). Open circulation allows blood passing through the splenic cord to be filtered by macrophages before the blood cells enter the sinuses. The aggregation of the macrophages surrounding the terminal arterial capillaries is called the **sheath of macrophages** or the **Schweigger-Seidel sheath**.

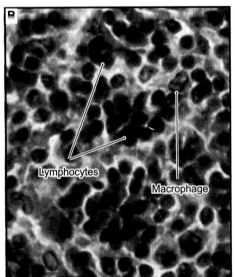

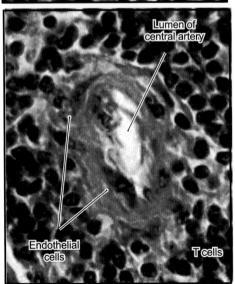

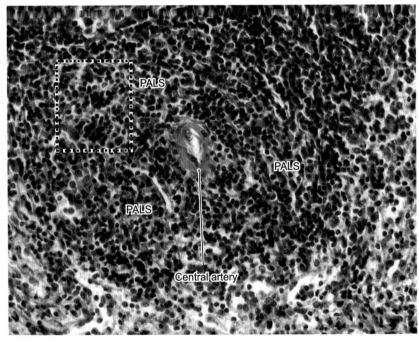

Figure 10-17B. Periarterial lymphatic sheath (PALS), spleen. H&E stain, ×564; insets ×1,727

The **central artery**, which helps to maintain the **lymphatic sheath**, continues through the white pulp and branches before supplying the **marginal sinuses** (capillaries). Its distal branches supply the red pulp. The central artery carries lymphocytes into the marginal sinuses in the **marginal zone**, where B cells encounter antigens. Naive B cells become memory B cells and plasma cells, which produce antibodies. **T cells** migrate to the central artery region and form multiple layers that surround that artery to form the **PALS**. T cells interact with antigen-presenting cells (*inset* shows a **macrophage**) and receive antigens. Active T cells undergo proliferation to increase their population.

RED PULP SINUSOID OF SPLEEN

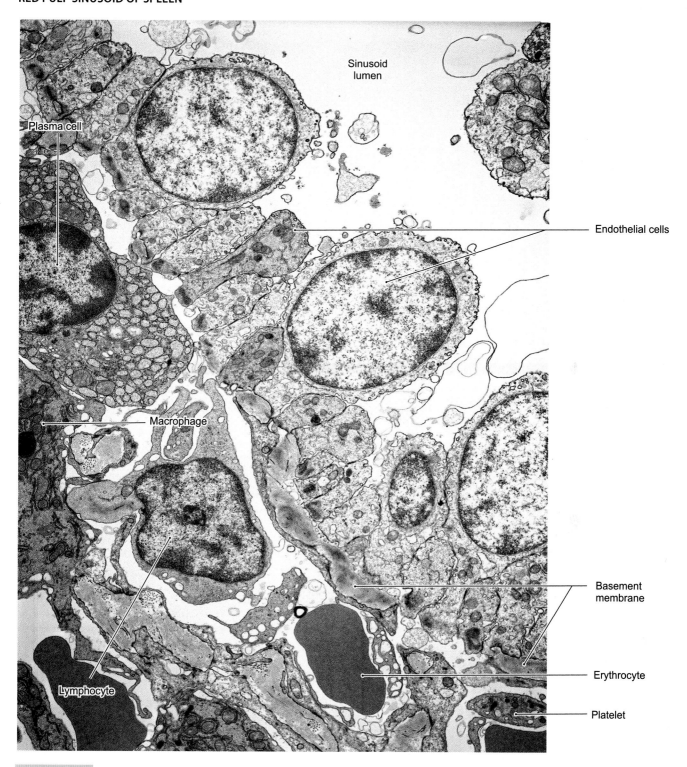

Figure 10-18. **Red pulp of the spleen.** TEM, ×7,100

Part of the wall and lumen of a **red pulp sinusoid** is shown here along with some adjacent **red pulp cord** (**cord of Billroth**) on the left. The plane of section through the sinusoid appears to be transverse to its long axis as indicated by the varying shapes and sizes of the many profiles of **endothelial cells** that make up this part of its wall. These cells have a fusiform three-dimensional shape, and their long axis parallels that of the vessel. A few endothelial cells are cut through the nucleus, but many more show only small pro-files of cytoplasm. The basement membrane of the endothelium is incomplete, and only a couple of pieces are visible here. In life, the formed elements of blood squeeze between endothelial cells to move into and out of the red pulp cords. **Macrophages, plasma cells,** and all types of **blood cells** and **platelets** are suspended in the reticular framework of the red pulp cord tissue.

TABLE 10-2 Lymphoid Organs

Organ	Epithelium/ Capsule Covering	Cortex and Medulla	Cords and Sinuses	B-Cell Main Region	T-Cell Main Region	Special Features (1) and Functions (2)
Tonsils	Incomplete epithelium and capsule	No	No	Primary and secondary nodules	Outside of the lymphatic nodules	1. Epithelial covering 2. Promotes B cells to proliferate and to produce IgA; immune defense against upper respiratory infections, where B and T cells encounter foreign antigens and initiate immune response
Lymph nodes	Capsule (thin)	Cortex, paracortex, and medulla	Medullary cords and medullary sinuses	Primary and secondary nodules (most nodules are secondary); medullary cords	Paracortex	1. Afferent lymphatic vessels and subcapsular sinuses 2. Filter lymph and recirculate both B and T cells; provide place for lymphocytes to meet antigens and start immune response
Thymus	Capsule (thin)	Cortex (without lymphatic nodules); medulla (with Hassall corpuscles)	No	No	Cortex and medulla	1. Epithelial reticular cells and Hassall corpuscles; no lymphatic nodules 2. Development and maturation of T cells
Spleen	Capsule (thick)	No, arranged in white pulp and red pulp	Splenic cords and venous sinuses	Secondary nodules (splenic nodules)	PALS	1. Central arteries and PALS 2. Red pulp filters blood, removes aged erythrocytes, and acts as a reservoir for erythrocytes and platelets; the white pulp hosts B and T lymphocytes, where they meet antigens, mature and proliferate, and initiate immune response

---

SYNOPSIS 10-3 Pathological and Clinical Terms for the Lymphoid System

- Lymphadenopathy: Enlarged lymph nodes due to a variety of causes including lymphoma, infection, autoimmune disease, medications, and metastatic disease.
- Myalgia: Muscle pain that may be caused by a variety of conditions including exercise, autoimmune disease, medications, infections, and neoplasms.
- Lymphoid hyperplasia: A reactive proliferative process of lymphoid tissues, particularly lymph nodes, characterized by enlarged follicles with abundant macrophages within the germinal center.
- Reed-Sternberg cell: Characteristic cell of classical Hodgkin lymphoma containing two nuclei or nuclear lobes, each with a prominent nucleolus.
- Waldeyer ring: Lymphoid tissues of the nasopharynx including the palatine tonsils and pharyngeal tonsils (adenoids) that may be an extranodal site of lymphoma development.

From Histology to Pathology

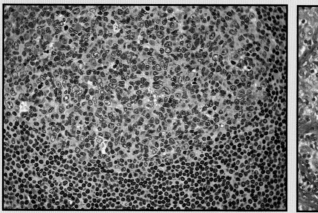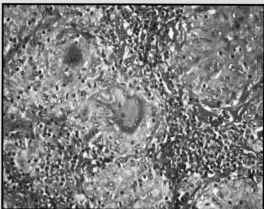

Figure 10-19. Normal lymphoid nodule and noncaseating granulomas. H&E, ×400

Normal lymphoid nodule with a germinal center on the *left*. **Noncaseating granulomas** from **sarcoidosis** on the *right*. Nongranulomas show aggregates of epithelioid histiocytes, which are modified macrophages with multinucleated giant cells. A rim of lymphocytes is displayed around caseating the central epithelioid histiocytes. Patients often present with hypercalcemia and elevated angiotensin-converting enzyme (ACE) levels.

Clinical Vignette Questions

1. A 26-year-old female presents with fever, pharyngitis (sore throat), a rash, and myalgia (muscle ache). She was diagnosed with human immunodeficiency virus (HIV) infection 6 months ago. Physical exam shows enlarged cervical lymph nodes. A laboratory test is done. Which of the following is most likely to show in her lab test?

A. Decreased CD4 helper T-cell numbers
B. Decreased erythrocyte (red blood cell) numbers
C. Increased B-lymphocyte numbers
D. Increased neutrophil numbers

2. A 28-year-old African American woman complains of progressive fatigue and shortness of breath (dyspnea). Physical exam is unremarkable, but laboratory studies show an increased serum calcium level. A chest radiograph reveals enlarged lymph nodes (lymphadenopathy) in the hilar areas of both lungs and nodular densities within the lung fields. Biopsy of the hilar lymph nodes is obtained and processed by touch preparation (lymph node tissue is lightly touched against a glass slide and stained). Pathologic exam reveals lymphocytes and many histiocytes, some of which appear in clusters. A portion of tissue biopsy is submitted for mycobacterial and fungal cultures, which ultimately show no growth. Microscopic sections of the lymph node show numerous granulomas with occasional giant cells. No necrosis is identified. Which of the following is the most likely diagnosis in this case?

A. Cryptococcosis
B. Foreign body reaction
C. Rosai-Dorfman disease
D. Sarcoidosis
E. Tuberculosis

3. A 19-year-old male with β-thalassemia complains of easy fatigability and a "racing heart." Physical exam reveals tachycardia (rapid heartbeat), pale conjunctivae, and a palpable spleen. An ultrasound reveals splenomegaly (28 cm). Laboratory studies show a hemoglobin of 3.6 g/dL (13.5–17.5 g/dL), indicating severe anemia. Which of the following is the most likely cause for this patient's splenomegaly?

A. Extramedullary hematopoiesis
B. Littoral cell angioma
C. Marginal zone lymphoma
D. Metastatic malignancy to the spleen

11 Respiratory System

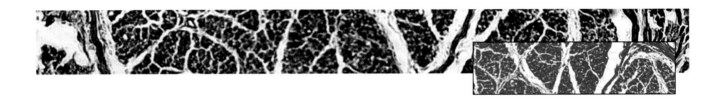

Introduction and Key Concepts for the Respiratory System

Conducting Portion
Upper Respiratory Airway
Lower Respiratory Airway

Respiratory Portion
Respiratory Bronchioles
Alveolar Ducts and Alveoli

Introduction and Key Concepts for the Respiratory System

The primary function of the **respiratory system** is to supply the body's need for oxygen and to give off carbon dioxide. Other functions include maintaining homeostasis and a normal pH and participating in the body's immune defense against bacterial and viral infections. Anatomically, the respiratory system can be divided into an **upper respiratory airway** and a **lower respiratory airway**. Functionally, the respiratory system can be divided into a **conducting portion** for the transportation of gases and a **respiratory portion** for gas exchange. The *conducting portion* includes the *upper respiratory airway* and the *lower respiratory airway*. These conducting airways include the **nasal cavity, pharynx, larynx, trachea, extrapulmonary** and **intrapulmonary bronchi, bronchioles,** and **terminal bronchioles.** The *respiratory portion* includes the **respiratory bronchioles, alveolar ducts, alveolar sacs,** and **alveoli.** The respiratory muscles (skeletal muscles: external intercostal muscle and the diaphragm) play an important role in producing the movement of air into and out of the lungs. The sympathetic and parasympathetic nervous systems innervate the smooth muscle of the bronchial tree as well as the mucous membranes and blood vessels in the lungs. Sympathetic fibers cause **bronchodilation** (relaxation of bronchial smooth muscles), whereas parasympathetic fibers cause **bronchoconstriction** (contraction of bronchial smooth muscles).

Conducting Portion

Upper Respiratory Airway

The **upper respiratory airway** functions as a part of the **conducting portion**; it consists of the **nasal cavity, nasopharynx, oropharynx,** and **larynx.** In general, the conducting airway is composed of bone, cartilage, and fibrous tissue and is lined with stratified squamous and ciliated pseudostratified columnar epithelia moistened with mucus and other glandular secretions. Cilia on the surface of the pseudostratified columnar epithelia sweep particles out of the respiratory airway.

NASAL CAVITY is the first portion of the upper respiratory airway. It can be divided into three regions based on the types of epithelial coverings. (1) The **nasal vestibule** is the most anterior part of the nasal cavity and is covered by a keratinized stratified squamous epithelium and **vibrissae** (stiff hairs); it is continuous with a mucosa of nonkeratinized stratified squamous epithelium. (2) The **nasal mucosa region** is covered by pseudostratified ciliated epithelium (respiratory epithelium), which contains ciliated columnar cells, goblet cells, basal cells, and, occasionally, neuroendocrine cells. The goblet cells manufacture **mucus**, which traps particles of dust and bacteria and moves them out of the nasal fossa, sinuses, and the nasopharynx, with the help of the ciliary action of the epithelium. Nasal mucosa filters, warms, and moistens the inhaled air. Mucus serves as a protective mechanism for preventing pathogens and irritants from entering the respiratory airway. There is a special vascular arrangement in the lamina propria of the nasal conchae called **swell bodies (venous plexuses)**, which alternately fill with blood from the small arteries directly into the venous plexuses on each side of the nasal cavity to help reduce air flow and increase air contact with nasal mucosa. (3) The **olfactory mucosa region** is located in the roof of the nasal cavity and is covered by pseudostratified columnar epithelium, which is composed of ciliated olfactory cells (olfactory receptor neurons), nonciliated columnar cells, and basal cells. It functions as a site for odorant chemoreception.

NASOPHARYNX AND OROPHARYNX conduct air from the nasal cavity and oral cavity to the larynx. The **oropharynx** is lined by stratified squamous epithelium, and the **nasopharynx** is lined by respiratory (pseudostratified columnar) epithelium (Table 11-1). The nasopharynx contains seromucous glands in the lamina propria. The **pharyngeal tonsil**, an unencapsulated patch of lymphoid tissue, is located in the posterior aspect of the nasopharynx. The **palatine tonsils** are located at the junction of the oral cavity and the oral pharynx, between the palatoglossal and the palatopharyngeal folds, which indicate the posterior boundary of the oral cavity. Tonsils, rich in lymphoid tissue, are the first line of defense against many airborne pathogens and irritants. Streptococcal pharyngitis is the most frequent bacterial upper respiratory infection in children.

LARYNX conducts air from the pharynx to the trachea. It is supported by a set of cartilages of complex shape and covered by a ciliated, pseudostratified respiratory epithelium. This mucosa continues from that of the pharynx and extends to the trachea. The larynx contains several structures, including the **epiglottis**, **vocal cords**, and nine pieces of cartilage located in its wall. The *epiglottis* is a thin leaflike plate structure; its central cord contains a large piece of **elastic cartilage**. This cartilage is attached to the root of the tongue and projects obliquely upward behind the tongue and the hyoid body. The epiglottis stands in front of the laryngeal inlet and bends posteriorly to cover the inlet of the larynx when food is swallowed. The upper anterior surface of the epiglottis is covered by nonkeratinized stratified squamous epithelium. In children, the epiglottis will occasionally become infected with *Haemophilus*. In elderly individuals, the elastic cartilage of the epiglottis is often reduced in size and is replaced by adipose tissue. The *vocal cords (folds)*, which contain striated skeletal muscle and ligaments (mainly elastic fibers), are lined by thin nonkeratinized stratified squamous epithelium, which is firmly attached to the underlying vocal ligaments. The stratified squamous epithelium protects the vocal cords from mechanical stress. The main functions of the vocal cords are to control airflow and facilitate speaking.

Lower Respiratory Airway

The **lower respiratory airway** includes the **trachea, bronchi, bronchioles**, and **terminal bronchioles**. Each portion of the lower respiratory airway has unique tissue components, which facilitate oxygen delivery, gas exchange, and immune defense mechanisms. Individual airways decrease in diameter as they continue branching.

TRACHEA is a tube formed of cartilage and fibromuscular membrane, 10 to 12 cm long, with a diameter of 2 to 2.5 cm. It extends from the larynx, at the cricoid cartilage, to the bifurcation of the bronchi. The trachea is lined by pseudostratified ciliated columnar epithelium and reinforced by 10 to 12 C-shaped hyaline cartilage rings. A band of smooth muscle is located between the two ends of the C-shaped cartilage. The epithelium is composed of several cell types including **goblet cells, ciliated columnar cells, basal cells**, and, occasionally, **neuroendocrine cells**, which are also called **diffuse neuroendocrine system (DNES)** cells. Chronic irritation of the epithelium will lead to an increase in goblet cells and a transformation to a stratified squamous epithelium, known as **squamous metaplasia**.

EXTRAPULMONARY BRONCHI are the **primary bronchi**, which begin at the bifurcation of the trachea and lead to the right and left lungs. They are called "extrapulmonary" bronchi because they are positioned outside the lungs. They are structurally similar to the trachea, are lined by respiratory epithelium (pseudostratified columnar epithelium), and have C-shaped hyaline cartilage. The *left primary bronchus* is narrower and less vertical than the right one and gives rise to two secondary (lobar) bronchi. The *right primary bronchus* is wider and shorter and more vertical than the left one; it gives rise to three secondary (lobar) bronchi. That is the reason foreign body aspiration occurs more often to the right lung.

INTRAPULMONARY BRONCHI are secondary and tertiary bronchi. As the primary (extrapulmonary) bronchi enter the hiluses of the lungs, they become the **secondary (lobar) bronchi**, which eventually divide into the **tertiary (segmental) bronchi**. They are lined by respiratory epithelium, and the **bronchial glands (seromucous glands)** are found in the submucosa. A band of spiral smooth muscle separates the lamina propria and submucosa of the intrapulmonary bronchi. The skeletal support for each intrapulmonary bronchus is provided by several hyaline cartilage plates instead of C-shaped cartilage rings. As the bronchi continue branching, there is a decrease in airway diameter and in the amount of cartilage in their walls. The number of goblet cells, glands, and the height of epithelial cells also decrease. However, the airways tend to have increased amounts of smooth muscle and elastic tissues. Smooth muscle in the bronchi is innervated by the sympathetic and parasympathetic nervous systems. In patients with asthma, this smooth muscle thickens with **hyperplasia** and **hypertrophy** and undergoes extensive and prolonged contraction causing reduction in airway luminal diameter and difficulty in exhaling and inhaling. Bronchial branches are accompanied by branches of the pulmonary arteries, pulmonary veins, nerves, and lymph vessels. These structures usually travel in intersegmental and interlobar layers of connective tissue.

BRONCHIOLES are smaller airways deriving from tertiary bronchi, which continue to branch into **terminal bronchioles**.

Bronchioles have no cartilage in their walls. Large bronchioles are lined with ciliated columnar epithelial cells and a gradually decreasing number of goblet cells. Small bronchioles are covered with ciliated cuboidal epithelial cells and with **Clara cells**. The number of Clara cells is greatly increased in the terminal bronchioles. Terminal bronchioles are the smallest and last of the conducting portion of the respiratory system and they have no gas exchange function. Terminal bronchioles give rise to **respiratory bronchioles**, which connect to the **alveolar ducts**, **alveolar sacs**, and **alveoli**.

Respiratory Portion

The **respiratory portion** of the lungs includes the **respiratory bronchioles**, **alveolar ducts**, **alveolar sacs**, and **alveoli**. This portion of the respiratory system does not have cartilage and has gradually increasing numbers of alveoli.

Respiratory Bronchioles

Respiratory bronchioles are lined by cuboidal epithelium and are interrupted by pouchlike, thin-walled structures called **alveoli**. Alveoli function in gas exchange. Respiratory bronchioles continue to branch to become alveolar ducts.

Alveolar Ducts and Alveoli

Alveolar ducts arise from respiratory bronchioles. They have more alveoli and some cuboidal epithelium on the walls as compared to respiratory bronchioles. They terminate as blind pouches with clusters of **alveolar sacs**. An alveolar sac is composed of two or more **alveoli** that share a common opening. Alveolar ducts and alveoli are rich in capillaries, which make gas exchange more efficient. Alveoli are thin-walled pouches, which provide the respiratory surface area for gas exchange. The wall of the alveolus is formed by a delicate layer of connective tissue with reticular and elastic fibers covered by **type I** and **type II pneumocytes**. The type I pneumocytes lie on a basal lamina, which is fused with the basal lamina surrounding the adjacent capillaries to form a **blood-air barrier**. The blood-air barrier is an important structure for oxygen and carbon dioxide exchange. The neighboring alveoli are separated by **alveolar septa**, which contain elastic connective tissue and may have capillaries within them. The lumina of the neighboring alveoli may be connected to each other by small **alveolar pores**.

TYPE I PNEUMOCYTES are also called **type I alveolar cells**. These cells cover 95% to 97% of the alveolar surface, whereas type II pneumocytes cover the rest of the surface. Type I pneumocytes are squamous cells with a flat, dark, oval nucleus. **Tight junctions** between type I pneumocytes help prevent movement of extracellular fluid into the alveolar sacs. Type I pneumocytes are unable to divide; however, they can be regenerated from type II pneumocytes.

TYPE II PNEUMOCYTES cover about 3% to 5% of the alveolar surface and form tight junctions with type I pneumocytes. Their cytoplasm contains numerous characteristic secretory **lamellar bodies**, which are mainly composed of **phospholipids** and **proteins**. These components can be released by exocytosis into the alveolar lumen to form a thin film of **pulmonary surfactant**. The function of the pulmonary surfactant is to increase pulmonary compliance and decrease surface tension of the alveoli to prevent them from collapsing. Type II pneumocytes can undergo mitosis to regenerate and also can form type I pneumocytes. The pulmonary surfactant is recycled by type II pneumocytes or cleared by alveolar macrophages.

ALVEOLAR MACROPHAGES are also called **dust cells**. They originate in bone marrow and circulate in blood as monocytes. They become mature and migrate into the connective tissue of the alveolar septa and into the lumina of the alveoli from blood capillaries. They move around on the epithelial surfaces and help to clear particles, as well as excessive surfactant, out of the respiratory spaces.

Anatomy of the Sinuses

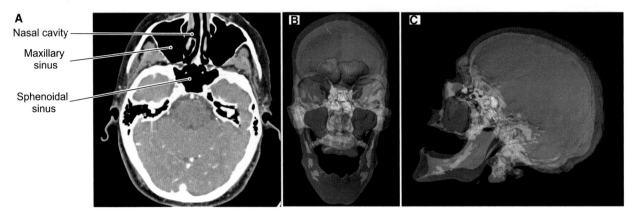

A
Nasal cavity
Maxillary sinus
Sphenoidal sinus

Figure 11-1. Overview of the paranasal sinuses. (A) Computed tomography (CT) image; (B) 3D stereoscopic model image, anterior view; (C) 3D stereoscopic model image, left lateral view.

The **paranasal sinuses** are hollow air-filled spaces within the skull. They surround and connect to the nasal cavity. The sinuses are covered by a membranous layer of mucosa that produces mucus. They aid in lightening the skull and assist with vocal sounds. There are four pairs: **maxillary, sphenoidal, ethmoidal,** and **frontal sinuses.** The **maxillary sinuses** are the largest sinuses located within the maxillae, above the maxillary teeth, and near the **zygomatic** (cheek) **bone.** The **sphenoidal sinuses** are located within the sphenoid bone and separated by a septum. The **ethmoidal sinuses,** which are anterior to the sphenoidal sinuses, are located within the ethmoid bone between the eyes. The **fontal sinuses** are located near to the center of the forehead within the frontal bone. Maxillary sinuses (*blue*), sphenoidal sinuses (*yellow*), ethmoidal sinuses (*green*), and frontal sinuses (*red*) are visible in the stereoscopic model images.

Chronic sinusitis is a persistent inflammation of the paranasal sinuses and the linings of the nasal passages that last 12 weeks or longer. Patients may present with nasal congestion, sinus fullness, nasal mucopurulent drainage, facial pain, headache, and reduction or loss of sense of smell. Histologic changes include edematous mucous membranes, a paucity of submucosal glands and stromal fibrosis, and mononuclear cell and eosinophil infiltrations. Eosinophils predominate in the mucous membranes. CT imaging is characterized by bilateral mucosal thickening, and polyps may be present.

Anatomy of the Lungs

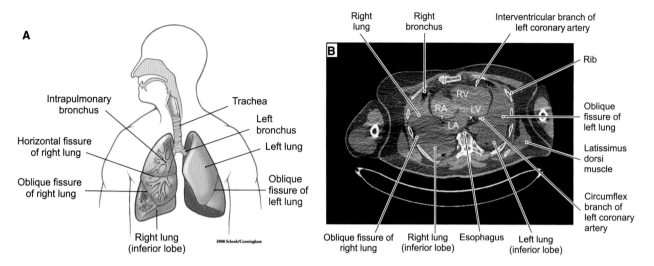

Figure 11-2A,B.   Overview of the lungs (*left*). Computed tomography angiography (CTA) image (*right*).

The **lungs** are situated on the lateral side of the **mediastinum** in the thorax. They are conical in shape, attached to the **mediastinum** by their roots. Each lung is covered by a layer of **visceral pleura,** and the thoracic wall is lined by a layer of **parietal pleura.** Between the layers of parietal and visceral pleurae, there is a potential space called the **pleural cavity** around each lung. There is a thin layer of lubricant known as **pleural fluid** in each pleural cavity. Anteriorly, the apex of the lung projects superiorly above the level of the **clavicle**; posteriorly, it lies level with the **seventh cervical vertebra.** The inferior surfaces of the lungs rest on the **diaphragm.** The right lung has **two fissures** and **three lobes,** and the left lung has one fissure and two lobes. The root of the lung, which contains the **pulmonary arteries, pulmonary veins,** and **bronchi,** connects the lung to the **heart** and the **trachea** in the mediastinum. The chambers of the heart are depicted and labeled with their abbreviations in the CTA image above. (RV, right ventricle; LV, left ventricle; RA, right atrium; LA, left atrium.)

In **pneumothorax**, air leaks into the **pleural space.** It can be categorized into **primary spontaneous, secondary spontaneous,** and **traumatic pneumothorax. Primary spontaneous pneumothorax** is not caused by any obvious external event or known clinical lung disease, whereas **secondary spontaneous pneumothorax** presents as a complication of underlying lung disease. Cigarette smoking and genetic predispositions, including **human leukocyte antigen (HLA) haplotype A2B40,** alpha-1 antitrypsin **(M1M2) mutations,** and **fibrillin 1 (FBN1) mutations,** may increase the risk of **pneumothorax.** Patients who present with **acute dyspnea** (shortness of breath) and **chest pain,** especially in those with an underlying lung disease and trauma, need to be assessed for potential pneumothorax.

CLINICAL CORRELATION

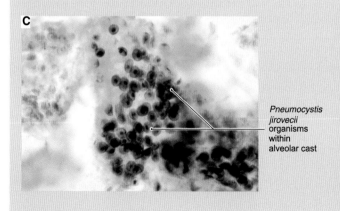

Figure 11-2C.   **Pneumocystis.** Grocott methenamine silver stain (GMS), ×600

Pneumocystis pneumonia is caused by a fungal organism, *Pneumocystis jirovecii,* formerly called *Pneumocystis carinii.* This fungus is an opportunistic organism primarily affecting immunosuppressed individuals including those with **acquired immunodeficiency syndrome (AIDS)** or patients on immunosuppressive therapies. Tissue diagnosis can be obtained from a variety of specimens including bronchial wash and **bronchoalveolar lavage specimens,** which tend to be higher yield in terms of demonstrating the organisms. The classic cytologic feature consists of **foamy alveolar casts** that contain the organisms. Several stains, including silver stain, can be used to elucidate the fungal organisms. Treatment of *P. jirovecii* pneumonia includes oxygen, antibiotics, and steroids if the patient is hypoxic.

Respiratory System

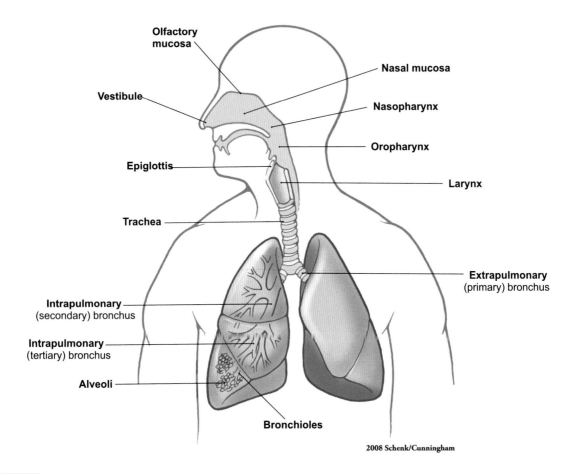

Figure 11-3. Overview of the respiratory system.

The **respiratory system** plays the essential role of supplying oxygen to the body. It can be divided into the **upper respiratory airway** and **lower respiratory airway**; functionally, the respiratory system can also be divided into a **conducting portion** and **respiratory portion**. Upper respiratory airway infection is a common term in clinical diagnosis. The *upper respiratory airway* consists of the **nasal cavity, nasopharynx, oropharynx,** and **larynx**. There are three regions in the nasal cavity classified according to types of epithelial covering: the **nasal vestibule** (stratified squamous epithelium), the **nasal mucosa** (ciliated pseudostratified columnar epithelium), and the **olfactory mucosa** (specialized olfactory epithelium). The nasopharynx is continuous with the oropharynx and extends to the larynx. The larynx is composed of the **epiglottis, vocal cords (folds),** and a set of **cartilages** of complex shape. The *lower respiratory airway* consists of the **trachea, bronchi, bronchioles,** and **alveoli** in the lungs. The skeletal support changes from **C-shaped hyaline cartilage** in the trachea and primary bronchi to **cartilage plates** in secondary and tertiary bronchi. Bronchioles have no cartilage support. Terminal bronchioles give rise to respiratory bronchioles, which have the function of gas exchange along with the alveoli.

Structures of the Respiratory System

I. Conducting portion
  A. Upper respiratory airway
    1. Nasal cavity
      a. Nasal vestibule
      b. Nasal mucosa
      c. Olfactory mucosa
    2. Nasopharynx
    3. Oropharynx
    4. Larynx
      a. Epiglottis
      b. Vocal cords (folds)

  B. Lower respiratory airway
    1. Trachea
    2. Extrapulmonary bronchi (primary bronchi)
    3. Intrapulmonary bronchi
      a. Secondary bronchi
      b. Tertiary (segmental) bronchi
      c. Bronchioles
      d. Terminal bronchioles
II. Respiratory portion
  A. **Respiratory bronchiole** (respiratory portion begins)
  B. **Alveolar ducts and alveoli**
  C. **Types I and II pneumocytes**
  D. **Alveolar macrophages**

Figures and Images Orientation

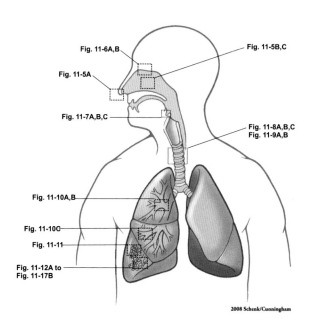

Figure 11-4. Orientation of detailed respiratory system illustrations.

Structures of the Respiratory System with Figure Numbers

Nasal vestibule

Figure 11-5A

Nasal mucosa

Figure 11-5B
Figure 11-5C

Olfactory mucosa

Figure 11-6A
Figure 11-6B

Epiglottis

Figure 11-7A
Figure 11-7B
Figure 11-7C

Trachea

Figure 11-8A
Figure 11-8B
Figure 11-8C
Figure 11-9A
Figure 11-9B

Bronchi

Figure 11-10A
Figure 11-10B
Figure 11-10C

Small bronchus and bronchioles

Figure 11-11A
Figure 11-11B
Figure 11-11C

Overview of bronchioles and alveoli

Figure 11-12A

Terminal bronchioles

Figure 11-13A
Figure 11-13B

Respiratory bronchioles

Figure 11-13C

Alveoli, type I and II pneumocytes, and macrophages

Figure 11-14A
Figure 11-14B
Figure 11-15A
Figure 11-15B
Figure 11-16A
Figure 11-16B
Figure 11-17A
Figure 11-17B
Figure 11-18A
Figure 11-18B

Kartagener syndrome is a genetic disorder characterized by the triad of **chronic sinusitis, bronchiectasis,** and **situs inversus** (major visceral organs are reversed or mirrored from their normal positions). This disorder is also known as **primary ciliary dyskinesia.** Patients generally present with recurrent upper and lower respiratory tract infections because of **abnormal microtubules** (disabling of dynein) in the **cilia,** which cause ineffective **mucociliary clearance.** It can also cause impaired cilia motility in the lining of the **fallopian tubes,** leading to infertility. For males, the moveable tails, or flagella, of sperm can also be affected by this disorder, resulting in abnormal sperm motility and infertility.

Conducting Portion: Upper Respiratory Airway

NASAL VESTIBULE AND MUCOSA

A

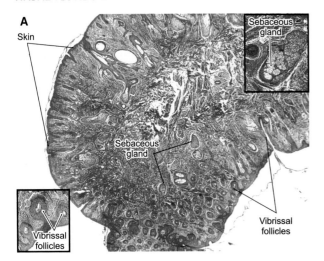

Skin

Sebaceous gland

Sebaceous gland

Vibrissal follicles

Vibrissal follicles

Figure 11-5A. Nasal vestibule, nose. H&E, ×12; insets ×42 (*left*); 334 (*right*)

The nasal cavity contains pairs of chambers separated by the nasal septum; the air passing through these chambers is moistened and warmed before it enters the lungs. There are three types of epithelia lining the nasal cavity in different regions: (1) the **vestibule region** is lined by stratified squamous epithelium; (2) the **nasal mucosa region** is lined by respiratory epithelium, which occupies most of the area in the nasal cavity, such as the **conchae** and nasal cavity wall; and (3) the **olfactory mucosae** are covered by a specialized olfactory epithelium and are concerned with the sense of smell. The external surface of the **nasal vestibule** is covered by the skin and its internal surface is covered by stratified squamous epithelium with numbers of **vibrissae** (stiff hairs) that entrap dust particles and prevent them from entering the lungs. The vibrissae are greater in number at the anterior end and gradually decrease at the posterior end of the vestibule. **Sebaceous glands** are found around the roots of the **vibrissal follicles**.

B

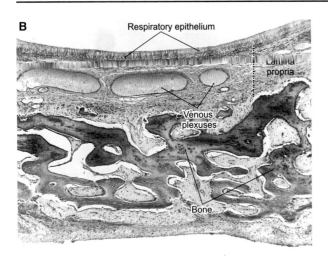

Respiratory epithelium

Lamina propria

Venous plexuses

Bone

Figure 11-5B. Nasal mucosa, nose. H&E, ×42

Nasal mucosa lines most of the nasal cavity. It is made up of **respiratory epithelium** (a layer of ciliated pseudostratified columnar epithelium) and a layer of connective tissue beneath the **lamina propria**. The nasal mucosa is attached to the bone for skeletal support. Respiratory epithelium is composed of ciliated cells, goblet cells, and basal cells as well as rarer cell types such as endocrine cells. This type of epithelium lines most regions of the respiratory system. There are many blood vessels (**venous plexuses**) in the lamina propria of the nasal mucosa; these small veins provide a rich blood flow, which warms the air passing through the nasal cavity before air enters the lungs. The large venous plexuses within the lamina propria of the nasal conchae are called **swell bodies**. Small arteries empty blood directly into the venous plexuses within the conchae; this causes the lamina propria to swell, reducing airflow through the nasal cavity and increasing air contact with the nasal mucosa.

C

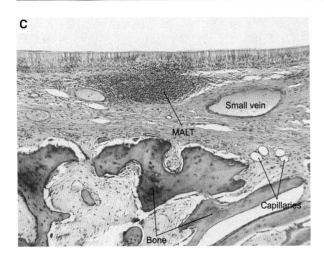

Small vein

MALT

Capillaries

Bone

Figure 11-5C. Nasal mucosa, nose. H&E, ×70

Lymph nodules or diffuse lymphocytes are often found in the lamina propria of the nasal mucosa, bronchi, and bronchioles. They are called **mucosa-associated lymphatic tissue (MALT)** and are usually located in the connective tissue where they can infiltrate the epithelium (see *inset*). The lymphoid tissues immunologically support the wet epithelial membranes of the body's mucosae and can be found in mucosae of other organs, such as the appendix and the ileum of the digestive tract (see Chapter 10, "Lymphoid System" and Chapter 15, "Digestive Tract"). Mucous and mixed mucoserous glands may be found in the lamina propria in some specimens.

In response to upper respiratory airway infection or allergic reaction, the nasal mucosa may become swollen (especially the inferior concha) and inflamed, blocking air passage through the nasal cavity. This condition is called **rhinitis**. Symptoms may include a stuffy or runny nose; common treatments are antihistamine and decongestant pills and sprays, etc.

OLFACTORY MUCOSA

A

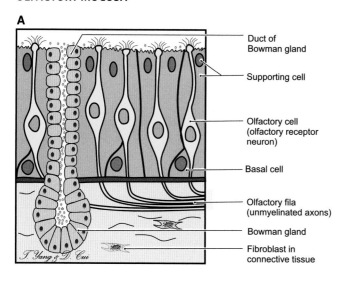

Duct of Bowman gland

Supporting cell

Olfactory cell (olfactory receptor neuron)

Basal cell

Olfactory fila (unmyelinated axons)

Bowman gland

Fibroblast in connective tissue

T. Yang & D. Cui

Figure 11-6A. Representation of olfactory mucosa.

The **olfactory mucosa** is located in the roof of the nasal cavity; it is composed of **olfactory cells** (olfactory receptor neurons), **supporting cells**, and **basal cells** in the epithelium, and of **olfactory fila** (unmyelinated axons) and **Bowman glands** in the lamina propria. Bowman glands release their product onto the surface of the epithelium via ducts. The main function of the olfactory mucosa is to detect odor. Odorant molecules come into contact with the surface of the olfactory epithelium in the nasal cavity and bind to receptors on the cilia of the olfactory cells. Olfactory cells transmit signals through the olfactory fila to the olfactory bulb and to the olfactory centers of the central nervous system. Olfactory neurons are able to proliferate after being damaged.

Clinically, loss of smell is called **anosmia**, and decreased sensitivity to odorants is called **hyposmia**. These symptoms are often associated with upper airway infections.

B

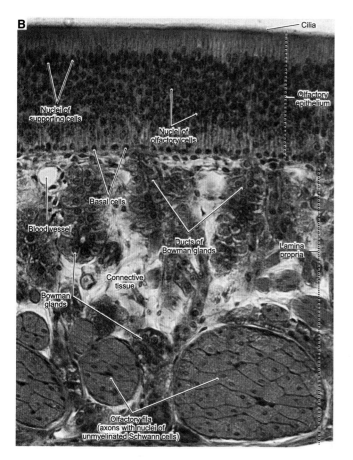

Cilia

Nuclei of supporting cells

Nuclei of olfactory cells

Olfactory epithelium

Basal cells

Blood vessel

Ducts of Bowman glands

Lamina propria

Connective tissue

Bowman glands

Olfactory fila (axons with nuclei of unmyelinated Schwann cells)

Figure 11-6B. Olfactory mucosa, nose. H&E, ×326

Olfactory mucosa is composed of specialized epithelium (**olfactory epithelium**) and **lamina propria** with **Bowman glands**, nerve axons (**olfactory fila**), and **blood vessels**. The olfactory epithelium looks like other pseudostratified columnar epithelium but contains different types of cells: **olfactory cells** (**receptor neurons**), **supporting** (**sustentacular**) **cells**, and **basal cells**. Olfactory receptor neurons are bipolar cells with long, nonmotile cilia, which function as receptors for odorants. Supporting cells are columnar shaped; their nuclei are dark and ovoid and are positioned in the apical region of the cells. Microvilli and a terminal web of the supporting cells may be seen at the electron microscopy level. The function of the supporting cells is to provide mechanical support; they may also be involved in binding or inactivation of odorant molecules. Basal cells are short cells with round nuclei. They lie in a single layer at the basal region of the epithelium, serve as stem cells, and are capable of regenerating into the other types of cells in the epithelium. The lamina propria of the olfactory mucosa contains Bowman glands, **olfactory fila** (collective unmyelinated axons), and blood vessels. Bowman glands are serous glands, which release a watery secretion onto the surface of the epithelium. These watery secretions (containing water-soluble proteins) serve to bathe the surface of the olfactory epithelium and help trap and dissolve odorant molecules. The olfactory fila are axons of the olfactory receptor neurons.

EPIGLOTTIS

A

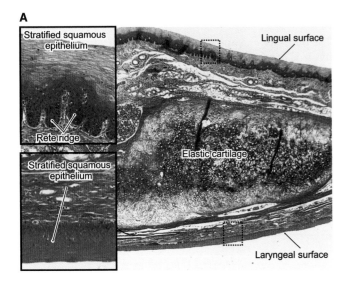

Stratified squamous epithelium

Rete ridge

Stratified squamous epithelium

Lingual surface

Elastic cartilage

Laryngeal surface

Figure 11-7A. Epiglottis, larynx. H&E, ×18; inset ×99

The **larynx** is the short passage that connects the pharynx with the trachea; its main function is to produce sound and prevent food or liquid from entering the trachea. Laryngeal structures include the **epiglottis, vocal cords,** and nine pieces of **cartilage** located in its wall (including the thyroid cartilage—"Adam's apple"). The **epiglottis** is a flattened, leaf-shaped structure with elastic cartilage support. Classically, the epiglottis is covered by two types of epithelia: **stratified squamous** on the lingual surface facing the oropharynx and **respiratory epithelium** on the laryngeal surface facing the larynx. However, this normal condition is rarely found, because of **squamous metaplasia,** resulting from aging and irritation (even in young individuals). The stratified squamous epithelium on the lingual surface has the distinguishing feature of **rete ridges** on its basal region, whereas the stratified squamous epithelium (squamous metaplasia) on the laryngeal surface is flattened on its basal region.

B

Mixed (mucous and serous) gland

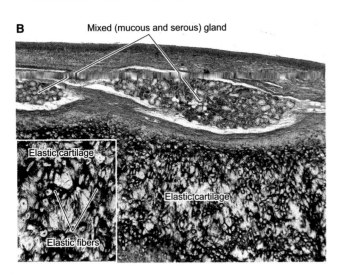

Elastic cartilage

Elastic fibers

Elastic cartilage

Figure 11-7B. Epiglottis, larynx. Elastic fiber stain, ×35; inset ×105

This sample of **epiglottis** tissue was stained with an elastic fiber stain. The **elastic fibers** are visible in *black*. Chondrocytes are embedded with the elastic fibers in the cartilage matrix. Elastic cartilage has different properties than hyaline cartilage; it forms the framework and provides a firm and elastic support for the epiglottis. There are some **mixed glands** (most are mucous) in the lamina propria. These glands produce mucin and a watery fluid on the surface of the epiglottis. The inferior portion of the epiglottis is attached to the rim of the thyroid cartilage and hyoid bone. The superior portion is free to move up when making sounds and to move down to close the airway while food and fluid are passing through the pharynx. The main functions of the epiglottis are to prevent food and fluid from entering the trachea and to cooperate with the vocal cords to produce sound.

CLINICAL CORRELATION

C

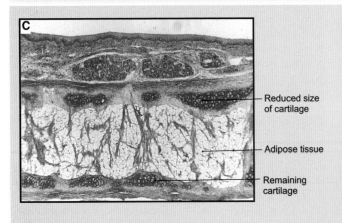

Reduced size of cartilage

Adipose tissue

Remaining cartilage

Figure 11-7C. Age Impact on the Epiglottis. H&E, ×21

The integrity of the **epiglottis** is affected by age and other factors. Structurally, variations include not only the change from pseudostratified columnar epithelium to stratified squamous epithelium (**squamous metaplasia**) but also **reduction in cartilage size** due to replacement of the central portion of the cartilage by a large amount of **adipose tissue.** Loss of elastic cartilage is associated with loss of elastic fibers in the epiglottis. These changes result in a reduction of the elasticity and stiffness of the epiglottis. Epiglottis abnormalities, such as the **hypoplastic, bifid epiglottis** associated with **cleft palate** in children, can cause episodic choking during food or fluid intake. Recurrent foreign substances entering the respiratory tract can cause chronic inflammation of the respiratory tract. Nasogastric tube feeding and surgical repair of the deformed epiglottis may be necessary in severe cases.

Conducting Portion: Lower Respiratory Airway
TRACHEA

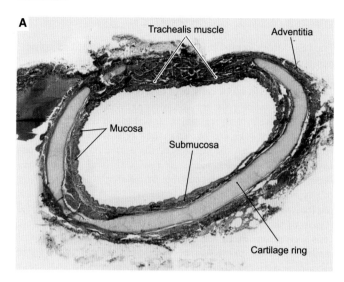

A

Trachealis muscle

Adventitia

Mucosa

Submucosa

Cartilage ring

Figure 11-8A. Trachea. H&E, ×7

The **trachea** is a flexible tube that connects the larynx to the primary bronchi. It is about 10 to 12 cm long, 2 to 2.5 cm in diameter, and is located immediately anterior to the esophagus. It is composed of **mucosa, submucosa, hyaline cartilage**, and **adventitia**. (1) The *mucosa* covers the inner surface of the trachea and contains respiratory epithelium and the lamina propria. (2) The *submucosa* contains connective tissue, which is denser than the lamina propria. (3) *Hyaline cartilage* has a unique C shape (some animals, e.g., the rat, may have O-shaped cartilage), and there are about 16 to 20 rings in the trachea. (4) The *adventitia* is composed of connective tissue, which covers the outer surface of the cartilage and connects the trachea to the adjacent structures. There are some elastic connective tissues and smooth muscles (**trachealis muscle**) in the opening between the two ends of the cartilage; this stabilizes the opening.

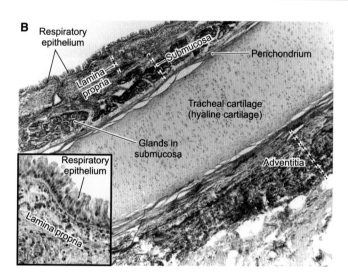

B

Respiratory epithelium

Lamina propria

Submucosa

Perichondrium

Tracheal cartilage (hyaline cartilage)

Glands in submucosa

Adventitia

Respiratory epithelium

Lamina propria

Figure 11-8B. Trachea. H&E, ×35; inset ×146

The luminal surface of the **trachea** is covered by **ciliated pseudostratified columnar epithelium**, also called **respiratory epithelium**. The epithelium plus the **lamina propria** constitute the **mucosa**. The lamina propria is a layer of loose connective tissue beneath the epithelium. The **submucosa** is a layer of dense connective tissue located between the lamina propria and cartilage; it contains many **trachealis glands (seromucous glands)**. Mucin and watery secretions from tracheal glands are delivered through their ducts to the surface of the epithelium. The C-shaped hyaline cartilage rings (**tracheal cartilages**) provide support for the trachea. They are covered by **perichondrium** and many chondrocytes are embedded in their matrix.

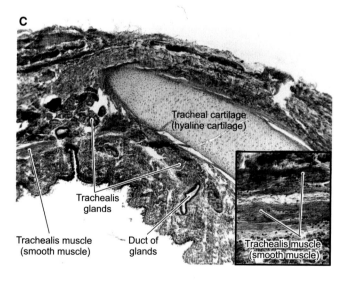

C

Tracheal cartilage (hyaline cartilage)

Trachealis glands

Trachealis muscle (smooth muscle)

Duct of glands

Trachealis muscle (smooth muscle)

Figure 11-8C. Trachealis muscle, trachea. H&E, ×35; inset ×100

The **trachealis muscle** is a smooth muscle located between the open ends of the C-shaped cartilage rings. Trachealis muscle fibers attach directly to the perichondrium of the cartilage together with connective tissue, which stabilizes the cartilage's open ends. The contraction and expansion of smooth muscle help to adjust the airflow through the trachea.

If a foreign object enters the airway, smooth muscle in the trachea and bronchi contracts, narrowing the lumina, helping to induce coughing. (**Cough reflex**: cooperation among the epiglottis, vocal cords, trachea, bronchi, lungs, respiratory muscles, and the autonomic nervous system.) In **asthma**, the smaller airways (bronchi and bronchioles) are narrowed because of excessive contraction of the smooth muscle of the lower airway in response to histamine released in an allergic reaction.

RESPIRATORY EPITHELIUM

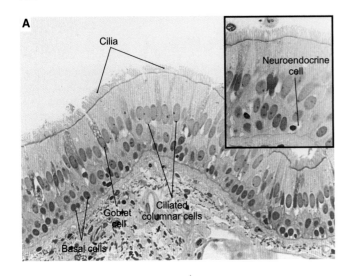

A

Cilia

Neuroendocrine cell

Goblet cell

Ciliated columnar cells

Basal cells

Figure 11-9A. Respiratory epithelium, trachea. H&E, ×284; inset ×403

The **respiratory epithelium** is a **ciliated pseudostratified columnar epithelium** that lines the inner surface of the respiratory tract. It is composed of several types of cells: **ciliated columnar cells, goblet cells, basal cells,** and **neuroendocrine cells (DNES).** *Ciliated columnar cells* are tall and have long, actively motile cilia, which help to move mucus and trapped dust toward the mouth. *Goblet cells* are goblet-shaped cells without cilia; they secrete mucus onto the surface of the epithelium. The mucus captures dust particles when air passes through the trachea. *Basal cells* are short cells capable of differentiating into other cell types in the epithelium. *DNES cells* have a round, dark nucleus with clear cytoplasm and contain granules at the basal region of the cytoplasm facing the basement membrane. These cells secrete serotonin and peptide hormones that act as local mediators. This may affect nerve endings as well as regulate mucous secretion and ciliary beating of nearby cells.

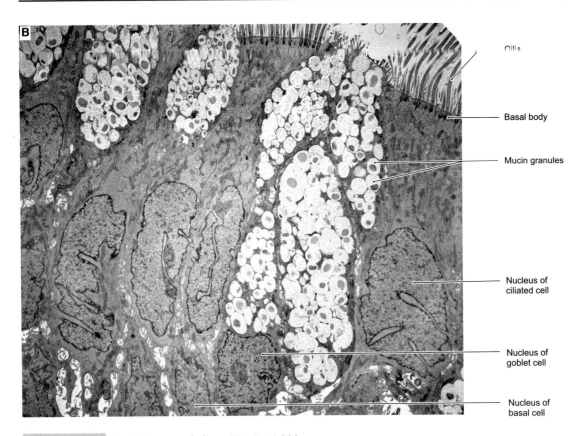

B

Cilia

Basal body

Mucin granules

Nucleus of ciliated cell

Nucleus of goblet cell

Nucleus of basal cell

Figure 11-9B. Respiratory epithelium. TEM, ×4,200

The epithelium that lines the nasal cavities, trachea, bronchi, and larger bronchioles has a characteristic composition of cell types arranged as **pseudostratified columnar epithelium. Ciliated cells** and **goblet cells** are the most prominent cell types, and they function together to generate a mechanism called the **mucociliary escalator,** which functions to entrap airborne debris in mucus and transport it along the surface toward the oral cavity. The numerous cilia projecting from the apical surface of the ciliated cells (most abundant cell type) beat in a coordinated fashion to move material toward the oropharynx. Parts of **basal cells** are visible at the bottom of the field; these serve as stem cells for replacement of the other cell types. Not visible here are two other cell types that occur in lower numbers in respiratory epithelium. **Brush cells** are columnar cells with microvilli at the apical surface. These cells are contacted by nerve endings, indicating a sensory function. **DNES** are the fifth cell type; they are short basal cells with small cytoplasmic granules that contain signaling molecules.

BRONCHI

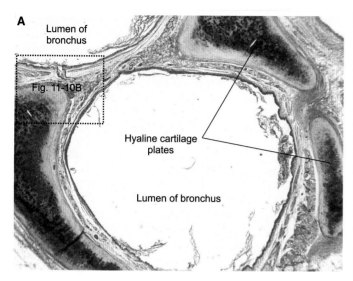

A
Lumen of bronchus

Fig. 11-10B

Hyaline cartilage plates

Lumen of bronchus

Figure 11-10A. Bronchus, secondary bronchus. H&E, ×11

The trachea bifurcates to give rise to two main bronchi (**primary bronchi**), which are also called **extrapulmonary bronchi** because they have not yet entered the lungs. Primary bronchi give rise to **secondary bronchi** and continue to divide into **tertiary bronchi**. The extrapulmonary bronchi have a similar structure to the trachea; the cartilage is still C shaped and lined with ciliated pseudostratified columnar epithelium. Bronchi that enter the lung tissue are called **intrapulmonary bronchi**; they include the **secondary bronchi** and **tertiary (segmental) bronchi**. Here is an example of a secondary bronchus, which has bifurcated from a primary bronchus at the hilus just above the entry to the lung. Large plates of **hyaline cartilage**, no longer C shaped, provide support for the secondary bronchi. Bronchi are also covered by respiratory epithelium.

The right primary bronchus is wider and shorter and more vertical than the left one; **foreign body aspiration** happens more often to the right lung than to the left lung.

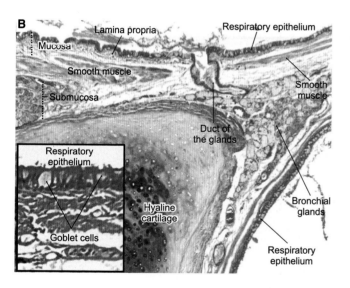

B
Lamina propria   Respiratory epithelium
Mucosa
Smooth muscle
Submucosa
Smooth muscle
Duct of the glands
Respiratory epithelium
Hyaline cartilage
Bronchial glands
Goblet cells
Respiratory epithelium

Figure 11-10B. Bronchus, secondary bronchus. H&E, ×37; inset ×198

Secondary bronchi are also called **lobar bronchi**. The right lung has three lobar bronchi, and the left lung has two lobar bronchi. The epithelial lining of secondary bronchi is similar to that of the trachea and primary bronchi. **Goblet cells** can be seen in this figure interspersed in the ciliated pseudostratified columnar epithelium. There is a band of **smooth muscle** that is arranged in a spiral fashion between the **mucosa** and **submucosa** that surround the lumen of the bronchi. This smooth muscle is controlled by the **sympathetic** and **parasympathetic nervous systems**. *Sympathetic fibers* cause **relaxation** of the smooth muscle; *parasympathetic fibers* cause smooth muscle to **contract**, reducing the diameter of the lumen of the bronchi. **Bronchial glands** (**seromucous glands**) located in the submucosa, and the **ducts** of these glands, are visible in this specimen.

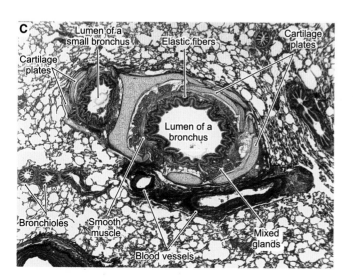

C
Lumen of a small bronchus   Elastic fibers   Cartilage plates
Cartilage plates
Lumen of a bronchus
Bronchioles   Smooth muscle   Blood vessels   Mixed glands

Figure 11-10C. Bronchus, tertiary bronchus. H&E, ×17

Secondary bronchi divide into **tertiary bronchi**, also known as **segmental bronchi**. These decrease in size as they branch distally within the lung. Two tertiary bronchi are shown here. The luminal surfaces of the tertiary bronchi are covered with respiratory epithelium; **smooth muscle** and submucosal glands are also present. **Elastic fibers** are prominent in the lamina propria and are stained red in this example. The **cartilage plates** of the tertiary bronchi are smaller than the plates in the secondary bronchi. As the tertiary bronchi continues to branch, their diameters gradually decrease; as the cartilage plates become smaller and fewer, the bronchial glands and goblet cells decrease in number as well.

SMALL BRONCHUS AND BRONCHIOLES

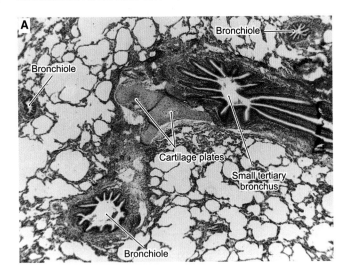

Figure 11-11A. Small tertiary bronchus and bronchioles, lung. H&E, ×25

A **small tertiary bronchus** and several different sizes of **bronchioles** are shown here. Small tertiary bronchi have much smaller diameters than large tertiary bronchi. Its hyaline cartilage is reduced to a few plates and the epithelial lining has decreased numbers of goblet cells and glands in the submucosal layer. These submucosal glands gradually disappear as the airways become smaller. Small tertiary bronchi give rise to smaller airways called **bronchioles**, which, because of the random branching pattern of the airway, appear at various places in the section. The glands and the cartilage plates of the bronchioles have completely disappeared at this level. Bronchioles continue to branch and decrease in size and give rise to **terminal bronchioles.**

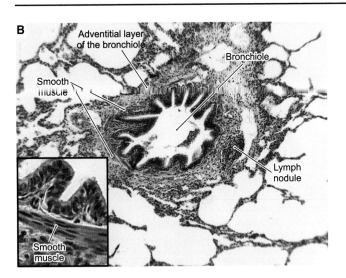

Figure 11-11B. Bronchioles, lung. H&E, ×71; inset ×612

The **bronchioles** are lined by ciliated columnar or cuboidal epithelium with decreased numbers of **goblet cells** and increased numbers of **Clara cells.** *Goblet cells* occasionally can be found in larger bronchioles. *Clara cells* are present in small bronchioles, and their numbers are greatly increased in **terminal bronchioles.** There are many elastic fibers in the lamina propria, which are not easy to see here with H&E stain. A layer of **smooth muscle** on the bronchiole wall is shown in the *inset*. The **connective tissue (adventitial) layer** is attached to the surrounding alveoli. **Lymph nodules** or diffuse lymphocytes are occasionally found in the connective tissue layer. The epithelium lining the bronchioles changes from columnar to cuboidal cells. Each bronchiole gives rise to several terminal bronchioles as it branches distally in the lung.

CLINICAL CORRELATION

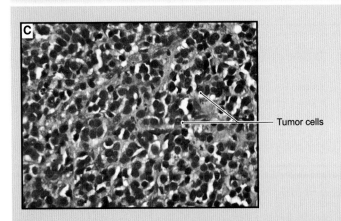

Figure 11-11C. Small Cell Neuroendocrine Carcinoma. H&E, ×213

Small cell neuroendocrine carcinoma is a highly malignant lung tumor characterized by its origin from the epithelium of the central airways, rapid growth, infiltration, gradual obstruction of the airways, and early metastases. It is associated with **genetic mutations, air pollution,** and **cigarette smoking.** Patients will likely present with large hilar lymph nodes with prominent mediastinal adenopathy in computed tomography or other radioimaging. Symptoms include weight loss, cough, chest pain, and dyspnea. The liver, adrenals, bones, bone marrow, and brain are the common sites of metastasis. The **tumor cells** are round, small, and spindle shaped with spare cytoplasm, ill-defined cell borders, prominent nuclear molding, and finely dispersed chromatin without distinct nucleoli. The tumor cells are about twice the size of lymphocytes and have characteristic "blue" cell features. Small cell carcinoma is initially very sensitive to chemotherapy and radiotherapy but loses its sensitivity within months. Treatment also includes surgery if the cancer is discovered at an early stage.

A

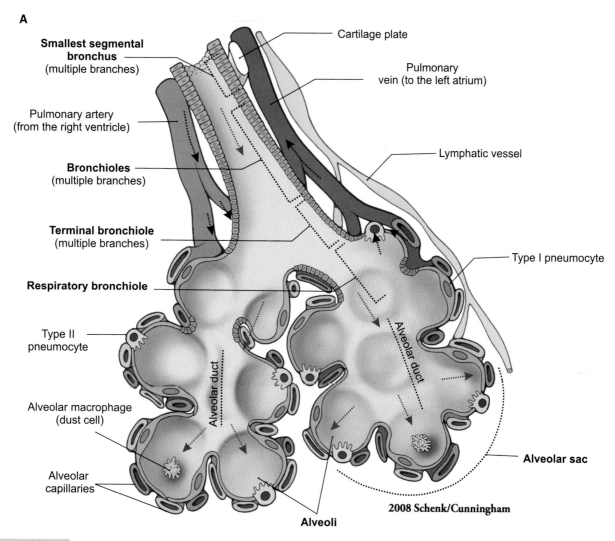

Smallest segmental bronchus
(multiple branches)

Pulmonary artery
(from the right ventricle)

Bronchioles
(multiple branches)

Terminal bronchiole
(multiple branches)

Respiratory bronchiole

Type II
pneumocyte

Alveolar macrophage
(dust cell)

Alveolar
capillaries

Cartilage plate

Pulmonary
vein (to the left atrium)

Lymphatic vessel

Type I pneumocyte

Alveolar duct

Alveolar duct

Alveolar sac

Alveoli

2008 Schenk/Cunningham

Figure 11-12A. ■ Overview of the bronchioles and alveoli.

This is a representation of the **bronchioles** and **alveoli**; the length of the different types of bronchioles is not drawn to scale. **Segmental bronchi** bifurcate into **bronchioles**, which give rise to many branches as they move distally within the lung. Bronchioles have no cartilage and continue to divide into smaller bronchioles. **Terminal bronchioles** are the final parts of the conducting airway. They extend into alveolar sacs to give rise to **respiratory bronchioles**, which connect to the alveolar ducts. Respiratory bronchioles are small in diameter, are lined by cuboidal cells, and contain increased numbers of alveoli. Respiratory bronchioles mark the transition from the conducting portion to the respiratory portion in which gas exchange occurs. An **alveolar duct** is a hallway that connects the respiratory bronchiole to an alveolar sac. Alveolar ducts are lined by squamous alveolar epithelium and knobs of cuboidal epithelium lying on the smooth muscle cells. An **alveolar sac** is the blind end of an alveolar duct and includes a common opening for two or more alveoli. Alveoli have very thin walls lined by alveolar epithelium that contains **type I and II pneumocytes (alveolar cells)**. The basement membrane of the type I pneumocytes and endothelial cells of the capillaries are fused together to form the **air-blood barrier**. Type I pneumocytes are squamous cells that line the alveoli. Type II pneumocytes are **pulmonary surfactant–producing cells** that are important for reducing the surface tension of the alveoli. **Alveolar macrophages**, also called **dust cells**, lying free on the alveolar wall, are shown here and can also be found in the septa of the alveoli. Dust cells move around on the alveolar surface like vacuum cleaners to clear dust particles and other debris on the surface of the alveoli and also help remove excess surfactant.

CLINICAL CORRELATION

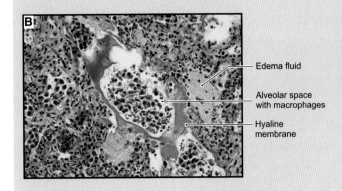

Edema fluid

Alveolar space
with macrophages

Hyaline
membrane

Figure 11-12B. | **Diffuse Alveolar Damage.** H&E stain, ×200

Diffuse alveolar damage (DAD) represents the spectrum of histologic features seen in cases of acute lung injury, including **acute respiratory distress syndrome (ARDS).** Clinical features of ARDS include **dyspnea** and **tachypnea** followed by **cyanosis, hypoxemia,** and **respiratory failure.** ARDS may result from diverse conditions including those that cause direct lung injury like **pneumonia, toxic inhalation,** and lung contusion to indirect lung injury including sepsis, drug toxicity, massive transfusion, and trauma. **Viral infections,** including **COVID-19,** may lead to ARDS and diffuse alveolar damage. Endothelial activation and damage to **type II pneumocytes** lead to the accumulation of **intra-alveolar fluid** and ultimately the formation of **hyaline membranes** composed of protein and necrotic debris. Aside from addressing the underlying cause, treatment of ARDS includes supportive measures like oxygen therapy, prone positioning, ventilator support, sedation, fluid management, and extracorporeal membrane oxygenation (ECMO).

TERMINAL BRONCHIOLES

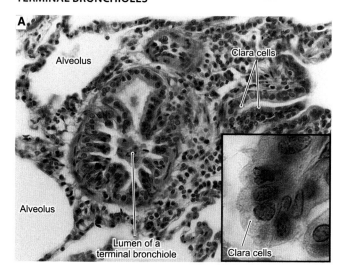

Figure 11-13A. Clara cells, terminal bronchioles. H&E, ×284; inset ×1,181

Clara cells are secretory cells scattered among ciliated cells and often project into the lumen of the bronchioles. They are **dome-shaped cells** without cilia and contain apical granules (visible only with a special stain); they are more abundant in terminal bronchioles. The substances (including **glycosaminoglycans** and **secretory proteins**) produced by Clara cells help to form the lining of the bronchiole. Clara cells play a role in **immunomodulatory** and **anti-inflammatory** activities, thereby helping to protect the bronchiolar epithelium. They also function as progenitor cells that can differentiate into other epithelial cell types, especially in epithelial repair after airway injury.

Research has shown that in heavy **smokers, Clara cells** are greatly decreased, and **goblet (mucus-producing) cells** are greatly increased in the epithelium of the bronchioles. These changes are caused by directly inhaled irritants and chronic exposure to harmful substances.

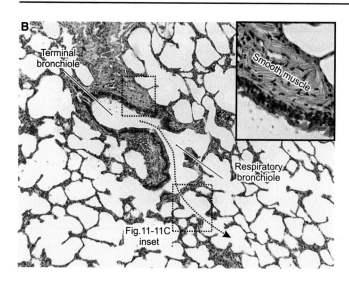

Figure 11-13B. Terminal bronchiole, lung. H&E, ×70; inset ×179

The **terminal bronchioles** are the last segment (most distal) of the conducting portion of the respiratory system. They are lined by simple cuboidal cells consisting mainly of Clara cells, with some ciliated cells and a few basal cells. Gradually, as the bronchioles proceed distally in the lung, the epithelium changes from columnar to cuboidal cells. The terminal bronchioles contain large amounts of **smooth muscle** in the airway wall. This smooth muscle is controlled by the sympathetic and parasympathetic nervous systems. At this point, cartilage and submucosal glands are absent from all bronchioles.

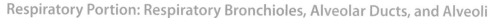

Respiratory Portion: Respiratory Bronchioles, Alveolar Ducts, and Alveoli

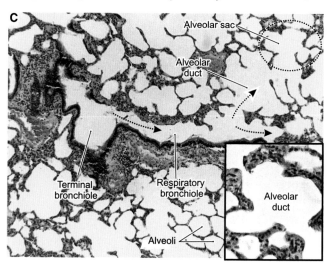

Figure 11-13C. Respiratory bronchioles, lung. H&E, ×71; inset ×179

The **terminal bronchioles** give rise to **respiratory bronchioles**. Respiratory bronchioles are the first airways that function in gas exchange. They are lined by cuboidal cells and have gradually increasing numbers of alveoli. Respiratory bronchioles connect to alveolar ducts. **Alveolar ducts** are lined by squamous alveolar cells (type I pneumocytes) and knobs of cuboidal epithelium lying on the smooth muscle cells. Each alveolar duct functions structurally as a corridor, which connects to several alveoli. Each **alveolar sac** is composed of two or more alveoli that share a common opening. The arrows indicate the direction of the airflow, from the terminal bronchiole to the respiratory bronchiole, then to the alveolar duct and, eventually, into the alveolar sac.

GAS EXCHANGE AND BLOOD-AIR BARRIER

A

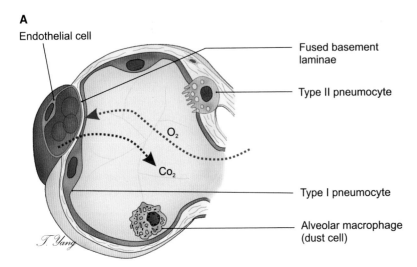

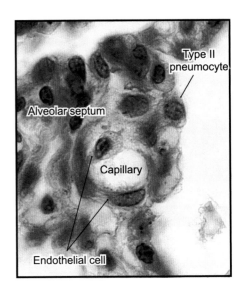

Figure 11-14A. Alveolus and gas exchange. H&E, ×1,077

An alveolus is the terminal unit of the respiratory system. It functions as a primary site for gas exchange. Its wall is composed of **type I and II pneumocytes**. *Type I pneumocytes* are primary cells, which form the structure of alveolar walls and are in contact with the capillary walls. *Type II pneumocytes* are septal cells, which are located in the connective tissue of the septal junction. They produce a surfactant, which reduces surface tension of the alveolus. Gas exchange occurs between the alveolus and capillary wall in a structure called the **blood-air barrier**. The blood-air barrier is composed of **type I pneumocytes**, the **endothelial cells of the capillary**, and the **fused basement laminae** of these cells. The exchange of O_2 and CO_2 occurs by passive diffusion across the thin blood-air barrier. The difference in O_2 and CO_2 tensions across the membrane determines the driving pressure for diffusion of the gases. In normal conditions, at sea level, air has a high O_2 and a low CO_2, concentration, whereas blood in the pulmonary capillaries has a low O_2 and a high CO_2 concentration. The net driving pressure will force CO_2 out of the blood into the alveolar space and O_2 into the blood from the alveoli.

B

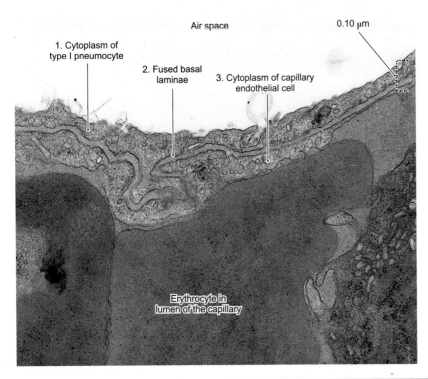

Figure 11-14B. Blood-air barrier. TEM, ×27,000

Three elements separate the air in alveoli from the blood in the underlying capillaries: (1) Air first passes through the highly flattened **type I pneumocyte** with its coating of **surfactant**. The cytoplasm can be even thinner (25 nm) than the segment highlighted in this view. (2) The middle element is the **fused basal laminae** of the type I cell and the underlying endothelial cell. (3) The **endothelial cell** lining the alveolar capillary, like the type I cell, has an extremely thin cytoplasm, so that the total thickness of the blood-air barrier can be as little as 0.1 μm.

TYPE I PNEUMOCYTES

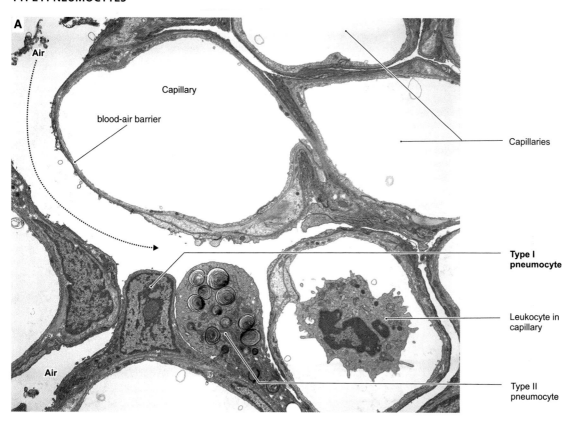

Air

Capillary

blood-air barrier

Capillaries

Type I
pneumocyte

Leukocyte in
capillary

Air

Type II
pneumocyte

Figure 11-15A. Type I pneumocytes, lung. H&E, ×725; inset ×1,145

Type I pneumocytes are squamous cells and make up 95% to 97% of the alveolar wall. A small percentage of the alveolar wall is covered by **type II pneumocytes**. Each type I pneumocyte has a flat, dark oval nucleus and very thin cytoplasm. These cells form the **blood-air barrier** together with the endothelial cells of the capillaries. They connect with each other by **tight junctions** to prevent leakage of fluid into the airspace. Type I pneumocytes are not able to divide; if they are damaged, type II pneumocytes will differentiate to replace the damaged type I cells. There are delicate connective tissues (including fibroblasts, elastic, and reticular fibers) and capillaries between the alveoli, forming the **alveolar septa**. Alveolar septa contain a blood-air barrier where gas exchange occurs. It is not easy to distinguish between type I pneumocytes and endothelial cells, because they are both squamous cells.

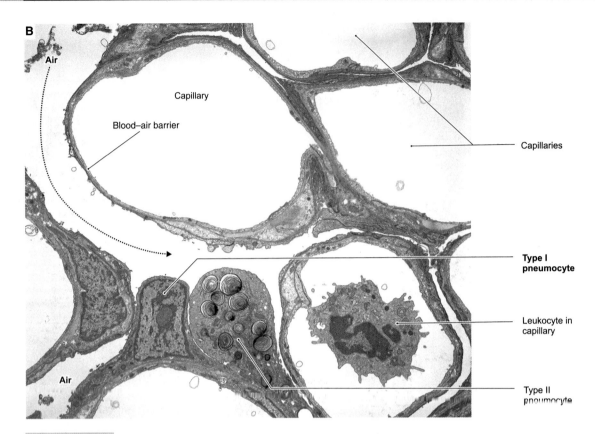

B

Air

Capillary

Blood–air barrier

Capillaries

Type I
pneumocyte

Leukocyte in
capillary

Air

Type II
pneumocyte

Figure 11-15B.   Type I pneumocytes and other constituents of alveoli. EM, ×5,250

The open spaces in this view are a mixture of air-filled spaces (**alveoli**) and the lumens of capillaries that were emptied of blood in the preparation of the specimen. The distinction between the air spaces and the blood spaces is not obvious because of the similarity in ultrastructural appearance of the **endothelial cells** lining the capillaries and the **type I pneumocytes** lining most of the alveolar surfaces. Both cell types are extremely flattened to produce thin sheets of cytoplasm. The type I pneumocyte (squamous alveolar cell) provides the covering of most (about 97%) of the surface of alveoli. **Type II cells** cover the remaining small fraction, and the single type II cell provides an important clue in distinguishing the capillaries from the alveoli here. Adjacent to the type II cell is the nucleus of a type I cell. This is the only part of the type I cell that is not extremely flattened. The various cells and structures in the field provide some context for appreciating the thinness of the **blood-air barrier**.

TYPE II PNEUMOCYTES

A

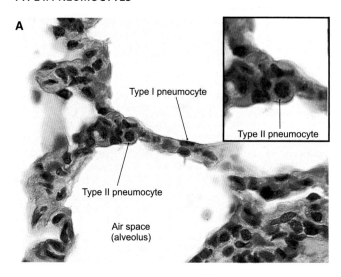

Figure 11-16A. Type II pneumocytes, lung. H&E, ×725; inset ×1,253

Type II pneumocytes are also called **septal cells** or **type II alveolar cells**. These are large polygonal cells (or cuboidal cells) with a large round nucleus. They bulge into the air space, often sit at the corner of the alveoli (**alveolar septa**) and make up 3% to 5% of the alveolar wall. Type II pneumocytes have **microvilli** in their apical surfaces and contain **lamellar bodies** in the cytoplasm. Type II pneumocytes can divide and also regenerate both type I and II pneumocytes. They produce a **pulmonary surfactant** (**phospholipids** and **proteins**), which is important in reducing the surface tension of the alveoli, thereby preventing lung collapse.

An example of lack of surfactant is **respiratory distress syndrome (RDS)** in premature infants. These infants' lungs are not sufficiently well developed to produce adequate surfactant. They have difficulty breathing and **apnea** (pauses in breathing). Treatment with surfactant and the use of a mechanical respirator are necessary to assure their survival.

B

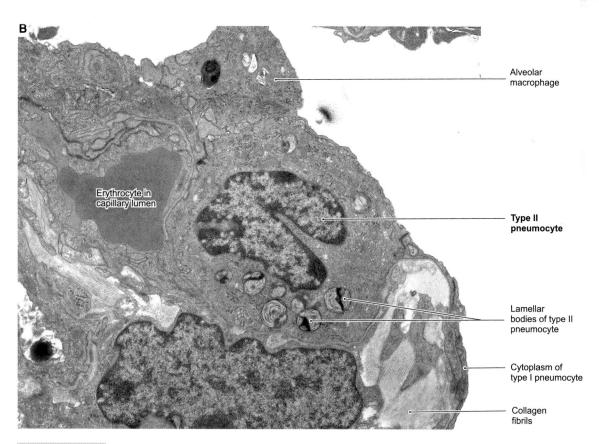

Figure 11-16B. Type II pneumocyte. EM, ×10,900

Type II pneumocytes are easy to identify in transmission electron micrographs, owing to the presence in their cytoplasm of **lamellar bodies** with their distinctive concentric lamellae. Unlike type I cells, the type II cells are compact in shape, either oval or cuboidal. They have two main functions: They are precursors of type I cells, and they secrete **surfactant**, an essential complex of lipids and proteins that serves to reduce surface tension, thereby preventing collapse of the alveoli. Type II pneumocytes are connected to their neighboring type I pneumocytes by junctional complexes. Part of an **alveolar macrophage** is visible in this field.

ALVEOLAR MACROPHAGES

A

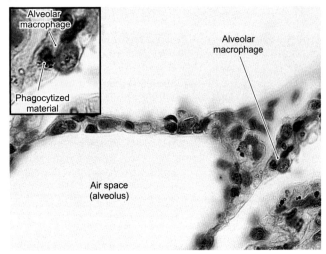

Figure 11-17A. Alveolar macrophages, lung. H&E, ×725; inset ×1,465

Alveolar macrophages are also called **dust cells**; they can be found on the surface of the alveoli and in the connective tissue of the septa. They are derived from blood monocytes and migrate out of the capillaries to enter alveoli. Alveolar macrophages are irregular in shape and have round nuclei; they often contain **phagocytized material** (*brown* in color) in the cytoplasm of active cells. Their function is to remove dust particles, debris, and bacteria on the surface of the alveoli, and they may also play an important role in initiating and maintaining chronic inflammatory processes and regulating tissue repair and remodeling in the lung.

Clinically, **alveolar macrophages** may also be called "heart failure cells." During **heart failure**, the heart is unable to pump blood at an adequate volume, and the backup of blood causes increased pressure in the alveolar capillaries. Red blood cells (erythrocytes) then leak into the alveoli. Alveolar macrophages engulf these erythrocytes. Pathologically, heart failure cells (alveolar macrophages) are identified by a positive stain for iron pigment (hemosiderin).

B

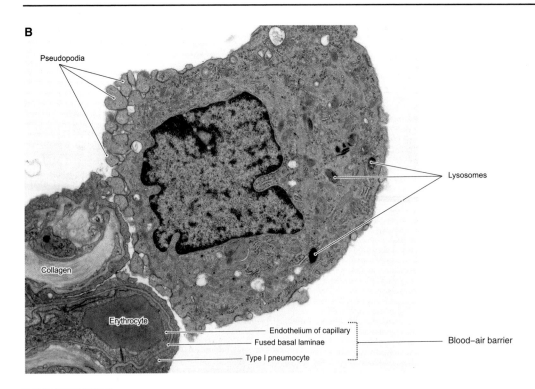

Figure 11-17B. Alveolar macrophage. EM, ×12,000

The surfaces of alveoli are continually swept by **alveolar macrophages**. In common with macrophages elsewhere, these cells are derived from **monocytes** that have left the circulation, in this case through the walls of pulmonary capillaries. These cells phagocytose any particles that have escaped capture in the conducting portion of the respiratory system. They also have a role in turnover of **surfactant** produced by type II pneumocytes. As expected in a macrophage, the cytoplasm contains **lysosomes**, most of which appear to be primary lysosomes in the cell shown here. Evidence of the cell's motility is seen here as extensions of cytoplasmic processes (**pseudopodia** or **filopodia**) extending from the surface of the cell that faces the surface of the alveolus. A view of the **blood-air barrier** can also be seen.

CLINICAL CORRELATIONS

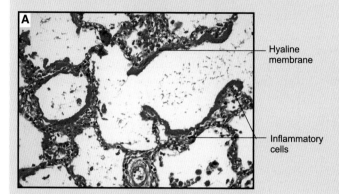

Hyaline membrane

Inflammatory cells

Figure 11-18A. Acute Respiratory Distress Syndrome. H&E, ×1,079

Acute respiratory distress syndrome (ARDS) is a clinical term describing acute lung injury, correlating with the pathologic entity of **diffuse alveolar damage.** ARDS is a respiratory emergency, characterized by an acute onset of shortness of breath (developing in 4–48 hours), which progresses to respiratory failure. It is caused by a broad spectrum of diseases such as **pneumonia,** severe injury to the lungs, severe trauma, burns, **sepsis,** medications, and shock. ARDS is not a specific lung disease, but a spectrum of clinical and pathological changes due to acute lung injury. Pathologic findings depend on the stage of the condition and include (1) excess fluid in the interstitium and alveoli with rupture of the alveolar structures; (2) proliferation of type II pneumocytes and squamous metaplasia and myofibroblasts infiltration; and (3) hyaline membranes. **Hyaline membranes** consist of fibrin and remnants of necrotic pneumocytes that line the alveolar spaces, as seen in the photomicrograph. Treatment includes using mechanical ventilation and treating the underlying disease.

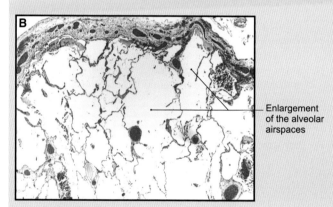

Enlargement of the alveolar airspaces

Figure 11-18B. Emphysema. H&E, ×27

Chronic obstructive pulmonary disease (COPD) includes **emphysema** and **chronic bronchitis.** Emphysema is characterized by the permanent destruction of alveolar structures, **enlargement of the alveolar airspaces** distal to the terminal bronchioles, and loss of elasticity of the lung tissue without obvious fibrosis. Cigarette smoking is the primary cause of the disease. Signs and symptoms include **pursed-lip breathing, central cyanosis, finger clubbing,** and shortness of breath (**dyspnea**), hyperventilation, "barrel chest," and recurring respiratory infections. Treatments include cessation of smoking, bronchodilating agents, supplemental oxygen, and antibiotics for respiratory infections.

SYNOPSIS 11-1 Pathologic and Clinical Terms for the Respiratory System

- *Hyaline membrane:* A histological feature of diffuse alveolar damage in early ARDS. It is a proteinaceous alveolar exudate at the periphery of the alveolar space; also seen in hyaline membrane disease (RDS) of neonates.
- *Dyspnea:* Shortness of breath; may be due to a myriad of causes including congestive heart failure (pulmonary edema), pulmonary embolus, asthma, and COPD.
- *Finger clubbing:* Also called "hypertrophic osteoarthropathy," it represents enlargement of the distal aspect of the digits due to proliferation of connective tissue and bone changes caused by many conditions including pulmonary diseases such as COPD, infection, and malignancy.
- *Asthma:* A chronic inflammatory disease of airways that manifests as paroxysmal contraction of airway smooth muscle, which causes narrowing of the airway lumens in response to exposure to a variety of triggers including allergens, infection, and exercise; airway narrowing results in shortness of breath.
- *Squamous metaplasia:* A reversible change from mature cell types to squamous epithelium, such as occurs in ciliated pseudostratified columnar respiratory mucosa when exposed to environmental changes such as cigarette smoke.

TABLE 11-1 Respiratory System

Tract			Epithelium	Glands	Skeletal Support	Muscle	Special Features and Main Functions
Concucting portion	Nasal cavity	*Upper Airway*					
		Nasal vestibule	Stratified squamous epithelium	Sebaceous and sweat glands	Hyaline cartilage	None	Vibrissae present; block large particles and small insects
		Nasal mucosa	Respiratory epithelium	Mixed mucoserous glands	Bone and hyaline cartilage	None	Venous plexuses warm air to body temperature
		Olfactory mucosa	Specialized olfactory epithelium	Serous (Bowman) glands	Bone	None	Olfactory receptor neurons in epithelium detect smell and odorants
		Nasopharynx and oropharynx	Respiratory and stratified squamous epithelium	Seromucous (mixed) glands	Bone	Skeletal muscle	Pharyngeal and palatine tonsils; first-line immunological defense
	Larynx	Epiglottis and vocal cords	Stratified squamous and respiratory epithelium	Mostly mucous glands and some serous or mixed glands	Hyaline and elastic cartilage	Skeletal (vocalis) muscle	Vocal cords control airflow and speaking; epiglottis prevents food and fluid from entering trachea
		Lower Airway					
		Trachea	Respiratory epithelium	Mostly mucous glands and some serous or mixed glands	C-shaped hyaline cartilage rings	Smooth (trachealis) muscle	Trachealis muscle bridges opening ends of cartilage
		Extrapulmonary (primary) bronchi	Respiratory epithelium	Mucous and serous (mixed glands)	C-shaped hyaline cartilage rings	Smooth muscle	Two primary bronchi outside each lung bifurcate from trachea; C-shaped cartilage
		Intrapulmonary bronchi	Respiratory epithelium	Mucous and serous (mixed glands)	Large and small plates of hyaline cartilage	Prominent spiral band of smooth muscle	Secondary and tertiary bronchi branch repeatedly; spiral smooth muscle band lies between lamina propria and submucosa
		Bronchioles	Simple ciliated columnar to cuboidal; Clara cells present	Occasional goblet cells in large bronchioles, but not in small bronchioles	No cartilage	Smooth muscle	Clara cells are present
		Terminal bronchioles	Simple ciliated cuboidal; numerous Clara cells	No goblet cells in normal cases	None	Some smooth muscle	Numerous Clara cells are present in these smallest conducting airways
Respiratory portion		Respiratory bronchioles	Simple cuboidal cells with few cilia; a few Clara cells; some type I and II pneumocytes	No goblet cells	None	Few smooth muscle cells	Alveoli interrupt simple cuboidal epithelium; gas exchange begins here
		Alveolar ducts/ alveolar sacs	Rarified simple cuboidal epithelium between alveoli; no Clara cells	No goblet cells	None	Few smooth muscle cells	Air passes into alveoli for gas exchange
		Alveoli	Type I and II pneumocytes	No goblet cells	None	None	Blood-air barrier is the primary site for gas exchange

SYNOPSIS 11-2 Structural Differences (from Upper to Lower Airway) in the Respiratory System

- ■ *Epithelium* changes from keratinized to nonkeratinized stratified squamous and then to respiratory epithelium.
- ■ *Respiratory epithelium* changes from simple columnar to cuboidal and then to simple squamous (alveolar cells).
- ■ *Glands* gradually decrease in numbers and disappear in bronchioles as airways become smaller.
- ■ *Skeletal support* changes from bone to cartilage to none at all.
- ■ *Cartilage* changes from C-shaped rings to large irregular plates to small plates and disappears in bronchioles and levels below.
- ■ *Muscle* changes from skeletal to smooth muscle; numbers of smooth muscle cells decrease.

From Histology to Pathology

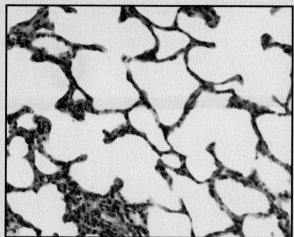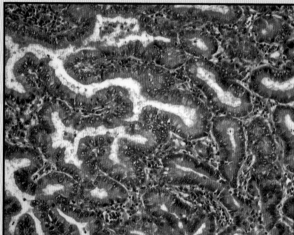

Figure 11-19.   Normal lung tissue and lung adenocarcinoma. H&E, ×100

Normal lung tissue on the *left*. **Lung adenocarcinoma** on the *right*. Lung adenocarcinoma is one of the primary malignant lung neoplasms commonly called "lung cancer." Histologically, these tumors range from well-differentiated, recapitulating, well-formed glandular structures to poorly differentiated structures in which sheets of malignant cells predominate with scarce evidence of glandular expression. The onset of symptoms is gradual, and the symptoms include cough, weight loss, chest pain, anorexia, and hemoptysis (coughing blood).

Clinical Vignette Questions

1. A 72-year-old nursing home resident initially experiences fever and cough, followed by dyspnea (shortness of breath) the next day. The patient's respiratory status declines further, and the patient is taken to the emergency department, where a nasopharyngeal swab sample is submitted for COVID-19 testing by real-time reverse transcription polymerase chain reaction (RT-PCR). The patient is admitted to the medical intensive care unit where the patient is intubated and given supplemental oxygen. A chest CT scan reveals bilateral pulmonary ground glass opacities and areas of consolidation. The COVID-19 test returns as positive. The patient becomes severely hypoxemic, and despite all efforts, dies. An autopsy is performed and shows bilateral pleural effusions with heavy, stiff lungs. Histologic sections of the lungs are likely to show which of the following histologic features?

A. Interstitial fibrosis
B. Hyaline membranes
C. Thickened bronchial walls with hyperplastic glands
D. Caseating granulomatous inflammation

2. A 32-year-old male with acquired immunodeficiency syndrome (AIDS) and a history of poor compliance with his antiretroviral pharmacologic regimen has been experiencing increased difficulty breathing and shortness of breath (dyspnea). He awoke in extreme respiratory difficulty and called emergency medical services. Once in the emergency room, he received oxygen, which improved his respiratory status. A pulmonology consult was ordered, with subsequent bronchoscopy yielding a bronchoalveolar lavage (BAL) specimen for cytopathologic examination. The fluid specimen revealed numerous foamy alveolar casts with no significant inflammatory cell component identified. Within the foamy casts, a silver stain revealed round, darkly staining organisms that were oval, often cup shaped, ~4 to 8 μm in diameter, and containing a central dark dot. Which of the following is the most likely causative organism?

A. Aspergillus fumigatus
B. Candida albicans
C. Cryptococcus neoformans
D. Pneumocystis jirovecii
E. Streptococcus pneumoniae

3. A 55-year-old man with a 2-month history of progressive dry cough, malaise, and intermittent chest pain experienced an episode of hemoptysis (coughing up blood) while taking a hot shower. He has a 20 pack-year history of smoking. Alarmed, he presented to the emergency department of a local hospital where physical examination was essentially unremarkable. A chest radiograph, however, revealed a 3.9-cm solid mass in the periphery of the superior lobe of his right lung. Review of a chest x-ray from 2 years ago revealed no abnormalities. The patient is scheduled for a right upper lobectomy. The lung specimen was grossly examined by pathology and showed a tan, solid mass within the parenchyma of the lung, abutting the pleural surface. Based on this information, which of the following is the most appropriate diagnosis in this patient?

A. Adenocarcinoma
B. Carcinoid tumor
C. Large cell carcinoma
D. Small cell carcinoma
E. Squamous cell carcinoma

12 Urinary System

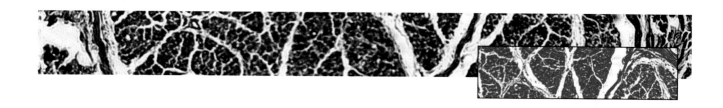

Introduction and Key Concepts for the Urinary System
Kidneys
Ureters
Urinary Bladder
Urethra
Production and Drainage of Urine

Introduction and Key Concepts for the Urinary System

The **urinary system** is composed of two **kidneys**, two **ureters**, the **bladder**, and the **urethra**. The *kidneys* produce urine, the *ureters* transport urine to the bladder, and the *bladder* temporarily stores and empties urine through the *urethra* to outside of the body. The urinary system functions to (1) filter blood and reabsorb nutrients; (2) control the water, ion, and salt balance of the body; (3) maintain the acid-base balance of the blood; (4) excrete metabolic wastes (urea and uric acid), toxins, and drug components; (5) secrete hormones, such as renin and erythropoietin; and (6) produce calcitriol (an active form of vitamin D) to help the body absorb dietary calcium into the blood.

Kidneys

The **kidneys** are bean-shaped organs located in the posterior abdominal region on each side of the vertebral column.

The kidney can be divided into the **renal cortex**, the **renal medulla**, and the **hilum**. The *renal cortex* is composed of renal corpuscles and various cortical tubules, which include the proximal convoluted tubules, the distal convoluted tubules, and the cortical collecting tubules. The *renal medulla* is located deep to the cortex, and its tubules extend as **medullary rays** into the cortex region. The medulla comprises 10 to 18 renal pyramids; each pyramid contains the **loops of Henle, collecting ducts, and papillary ducts**. The apical projection of a renal pyramid is called the **renal papilla**. The papillary ducts empty urine at the tip of a renal papilla onto its surface, which is called the **area cribrosa** (perforated area). Each renal papilla is surrounded by a space, the minor calyx; several minor calices unite to form a major calyx. There are two or three major calyces for each kidney. The major calices unite to form the renal pelvis, which funnels urine into the ureter. The *hilum* is the region in the medial portion of the kidney where the renal artery, the renal vein, and the ureter enter and exit the kidney. Functionally and structurally, the kidney can be divided into the **nephron** and the collecting system. The *nephron* produces urine. The *collecting system* adjusts the composition of urine and transports urine to the calyces.

NEPHRON comprises a **renal corpuscle**, a **proximal convoluted tubule**, a **loop of Henle**, and a **distal convoluted tubule.**

Renal corpuscle is composed of a **glomerulus** and a **Bowman capsule.** (1) A *glomerulus* consists of a spherical knot of capillaries, which is fed by an afferent arteriole and drained by an efferent arteriole at the vascular pole. (2) A *Bowman capsule* consists of a **visceral layer** and a **parietal layer.** The *visceral layer* is composed of podocytes, which cover the capillaries of a glomerulus. These cells have long, interdigitating cellular processes and play an important role in blood filtration. The interstitial tissues surrounding the glomerular capillaries contain cells called **intraglomerular mesangial cells.** The *parietal layer* of the Bowman capsule is a hollow spherical structure lined by simple squamous epithelium. The space between the visceral and the parietal layers of the Bowman capsule is called the **Bowman space.** Blood flows through the glomerular capillaries, and its plasma passes through the glomerular filtration barrier (the fused basal laminae of the endothelial cells and the podocytes); the filtrate is collected in the Bowman space. Thus, the renal corpuscle, as a whole, forms a blood-filtering unit, which allows water, metabolic wastes, ions, and small molecules to pass through the capillary wall but prevents circulating cells and large plasma proteins from leaving the blood.

Proximal convoluted tubules are long tubes that follow a serpentine course as they drain the filtrate from the renal corpuscles into the loop of Henle. Each is lined by a simple cuboidal epithelium with abundant long microvilli (brush border) bordering the lumen. Each proximal convoluted tubule connects to a renal corpuscle at its **urinary pole.** The relatively large epithelial cells of the proximal convoluted tubule contain many mitochondria, which render their cytoplasm brightly acidophilic (pink). The lateral boundaries between the cells interdigitate, so that the boundaries between adjacent cells are unclear in light microscopy. Their long microvilli appear to fill much of the space within the lumen. The combined structural features of the proximal convoluted tubules contribute to their functions of actively transporting ions and reabsorbing water, glucose, amino acids, proteins, and vitamins from the filtrate.

Loop of Henle is a continuation of the proximal convoluted tubule. It is a U-shaped structure that includes a **descending limb** and an **ascending limb.** The *descending limb* consists of a **thick descending limb** (proximal straight tubule) and a **thin descending limb** (descending thin segment). The *ascending limb* contains a **thin ascending limb** (ascending thin segment) and a **thick ascending limb** (distal straight tubule). The loop of Henle plays a crucial role in generating a high sodium concentration gradient in the interstitium of the renal medulla. This permits water to move passively from collecting ducts into the interstitium. Some physiology textbooks do not include the thick descending limb (proximal straight tubule) as a part of the loop of Henle proper because it does not significantly contribute to its physiological function. The proximal straight tubules are similar in structure to the proximal convoluted tubules. The

descending and ascending thin segment tubules are lined by squamous cells and are structurally similar to each other. The *descending limb* is permeable to water, Cl^-, and Na^+. The tubules of the descending limb reabsorb water and salts and reduce the volume of the filtrate that has passed through the proximal convoluted tubules. The *ascending limb* is very active physiologically. It is impermeable to water, and it actively pumps Cl^- and Na^+ from the lumen into the medullary interstitium.

Distal convoluted tubules are lined by small, simple cuboidal epithelial cells, which have no brush border. They may show a few short, irregular microvilli on their apical surfaces and plasma membrane infoldings on their basal region at the EM level. Their lumens appear clearer and wider than those of proximal tubules. The distal convoluted tubules are located in the cortex of the kidney and are closely associated with the renal corpuscles. At the junction between the distal straight and the convoluted tubules, there is an important specialized sensory structure, the **macula densa**, which senses and monitors ionic content and water volume of the filtrate. The macula densa is composed of cells that are taller and more tightly packed than other cells of the distal tubule. This portion of the distal tubule is positioned between afferent and efferent arterioles at the vascular pole of the renal corpuscle. The distal convoluted tubules remove Na^+ and add K^+ to the filtrate if aldosterone stimulation is present; they also reabsorb bicarbonate ions and secrete ammonium to adjust the pH balance. The distal convoluted tubules connect distal straight tubules (thick ascending limb of the loop of Henle) to the collecting tubules. The distal convoluted and straight tubules are structurally similar to each other, differing mainly in their locations and courses.

COLLECTING SYSTEM consists of **cortical collecting tubules, collecting ducts,** and **papillary ducts.** The *collecting tubules* are small and lined by cuboidal cells. They are located in the renal cortex, so they are also called **cortical collecting tubules.** They drain the filtrate from distal convoluted tubules into the **collecting ducts** of the medullary rays, which, in turn, drain into larger collecting ducts in the medulla. *Collecting ducts* have larger lumens than collecting tubules, and they are lined by taller cuboidal or columnar cells. Both collecting tubules and ducts have clear cytoplasm and distinct cell-to-cell boundaries. These tubules become highly permeable to water under the influence of antidiuretic hormone (ADH). Depending on ADH levels, the tubules passively diffuse a variable volume of water from their lumens into the medullary interstitium, thus increasing the concentration of urine. The collecting ducts are the last components of the kidney that process and determine the final urine composition. *Papillary ducts*, also called **ducts of Bellini**, are continuations of the collecting ducts. They are located in the papilla of the renal medulla. Several collecting ducts merge into a single papillary duct, which empties urine into the minor calyx at the tip of the renal papilla.

VASCULAR SUPPLY TO THE KIDNEY comes from the renal artery, which enters the kidney at the hilum; segmental branches of the renal artery give rise to the **interlobar arteries.** These pass through the renal columns between the renal pyramids and give rise to **arcuate arteries.** The arcuate arteries run along the junction between the cortex and the medulla of the kidney and give rise to the **interlobular arteries**, which extend into the cortex to supply the **afferent arterioles** of renal corpuscles. Each afferent arteriole supplies a glomerulus of capillaries from which blood is drained by an **efferent arteriole** at the **vascular pole**. The efferent arterioles of corpuscles in the outer cortex feed into the **peritubular capillary network**, which supplies the cortical tissue surrounding the cortical tubules. These peritubular capillaries provide for gas and material exchange and also receive renal interstitial fluid, which is reabsorbed out of the tubules and goes back into the vascular bed. Venules carry blood to the **interlobular veins** and to the **arcuate veins** in the renal corticomedullary junction. The efferent arterioles of deeper (juxtamedullary) corpuscles extend into the medulla where they give rise to capillaries called **vasa recta**, which receive interstitial fluid (reabsorbed from filtrate) in the medulla and send it back to the circulation. The vasa rectae take a hairpin course in the medulla following the loop of Henle. They return to the corticomedullary junction to join the interlobular veins and then drain into the arcuate veins. The arcuate veins drain blood into the interlobar veins, which then merge to form the branches of the segmental renal veins, which in turn finally merge into the renal vein.

Ureters

The two **ureters** lie in the extraperitoneal connective tissue, laterally positioned on each side of the vertebral column. The ureters are long, relatively small tubules lined by **transitional epithelium** and surrounded by a thin layer of smooth muscle and connective tissue. Superiorly, they drain the funnel-shaped **renal pelvis**, and inferiorly, they empty into the bladder by penetrating its posterior wall. The ureters have a much thinner wall than the bladder. Like most tubular organs, the wall of the ureter is composed of several layers of tissues: **mucosa, muscularis, and adventitia**.

Urinary Bladder

The **urinary bladder**, a distensible sac-shaped organ located in the pelvic cavity, temporarily stores urine. The wall of the bladder has three openings, two of them for ureters to enter and one for emptying urine into the urethra. Like the ureter, the urinary bladder wall consists of **mucosal, muscularis, and adventitial** layers, but the bladder wall is much thicker, having three substantial layers of smooth muscle in the muscularis. (1) The *mucosa* consists of a transitional epithelium lining and a layer of connective tissue (lamina propria) containing blood vessels and nerve fibers. (2) The *muscularis* contains the three layers of smooth muscle: inner longitudinal smooth muscle, middle circular smooth muscle, and outer longitudinal smooth muscle. The muscularis contracts in different directions to enable the urinary bladder to empty urine. (3) The outer portion of the bladder is protected by both a **serosa** and an **adventitia** depending on whether it projects into the peritoneal cavity. The superior surface of the bladder is covered by *serosa*, which is a layer of connective tissue covered by mesothelium; the inferior surface of the bladder is covered by *adventitia*, which is a layer of connective tissue without a mesothelial covering.

Urethra

The **urethra** is structurally different in the male and female. The proximal end of the *male urethra* is surrounded by an internal urethral sphincter (smooth muscle) that functions mainly to prevent seminal fluids from entering the bladder during ejaculation. The male urethra is about 20 cm long, and it is composed of three segments: **prostatic, membranous, and penile (spongy) urethra**. The *prostatic portion* is surrounded by the prostate gland and is lined by transitional epithelium. The *membranous portion* is a short segment surrounded by the skeletal muscle of the external sphincter (urogenital diaphragm) and is lined by pseudostratified columnar epithelium. The *penile (spongy) urethra* (also called the **cavernous urethra**) is surrounded by the corpus spongiosum of the penis, and its epithelial lining changes from pseudostratified columnar to stratified squamous. In this region, there are many small mucous glands called the **glands of Littré**, which secrete mucus to coat and protect the lining of the urethra.

The *female urethra* is short, about 4 to 5 cm. It is lined chiefly by stratified squamous epithelium and, in a few places, may have patches of pseudostratified columnar epithelium. Glands of Littré are also present in the female urethra. The proximal end of female urethra is surrounded by skeletal muscle (external sphincter) where it penetrates the urogenital diaphragm. The external sphincter muscle in both male and female is innervated by the pudendal nerves; it functions to control retention or release of the urine from the urinary bladder through the urethra and helps maintain urinary continence. A female does not have an internal sphincter.

Production and Drainage of Urine

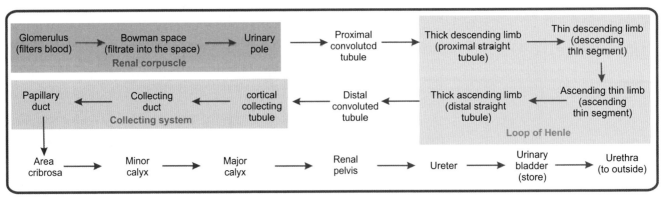

Urinary System

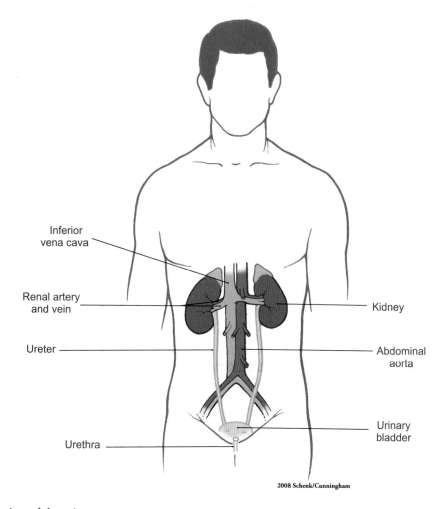

Inferior
vena cava

Renal artery
and vein

Ureter

Urethra

Kidney

Abdominal
aorta

Urinary
bladder

2008 Schenk/Cunningham

Figure 12-1. Overview of the urinary system.

The **urinary system** plays an important role in eliminating the body's metabolic wastes and toxins; controlling water and ion balance and regulating blood pressure; maintaining the acid-base (pH) balance of the blood; and in reabsorbing and conserving nutrients. The urinary system achieves these goals by filtering the blood and producing urine. The complex tubule system in the kidney helps to reabsorb and readjust water and ion content and to excrete urine. The urinary system consists of two **kidneys**, two **ureters**, the **urinary bladder**, and the **urethra**. The **kidneys** are the organs that produce urine and accomplish the essential functions listed above. After urine is produced, it passes through the ureters to the bladder for temporary storage, finally exiting the body through the urethra.

Structures of the Kidney

General structure of the kidney:
I. **Renal cortex**
   A. Renal corpuscles
   B. Proximal convoluted tubules
   C. Distal convoluted tubules
   D. Cortical collecting tubules
II. **Renal medulla (renal pyramids)**
   A. Outer medulla
   B. Inner medulla
   C. Renal papillae
III. **Renal hilum**
   A. Minor calyx
   B. Major calyx
   C. Renal pelvis

Functional and histological unit of the kidney:
I. **Nephron**
   A. Renal corpuscle
   B. Proximal convoluted tubule
   C. Loop of Henle
     1. Descending limb
       a. Thick descending limb (proximal straight tubule)
       b. Thin descending limb (descending thin segment)
     2. Ascending limb
       a. Thin ascending limb (ascending thin segment)
       b. Thick ascending limb (distal straight tubule)
   D. Distal convoluted tubules
II. **Collecting system**
   A. Cortical collecting tubule
   B. Collecting ducts
   C. Papillary ducts

Anatomy of the Kidney

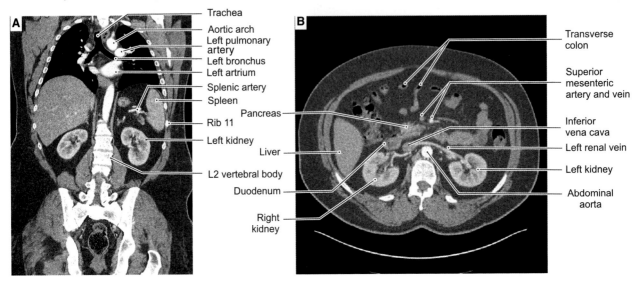

Figure 12-2A,B. **Kidney.** Computed tomography angiography, coronal view (*left*), transverse, or axial, view (*right*).

The kidneys are two "**bean-shaped**" organs lying along either side of the vertebral column in **the retroperitoneal space**. They are between rib 11 and lumbar 2 vertebral levels. In adults, the average size of the kidneys is about 10 to 13 cm long, 5 to 7.5 cm wide, and 3 to 4 cm thick. The kidneys are important organs that regulate fluid in the body by filtering plasma and removing impurities from the blood. The kidneys have a rich blood supply from the renal arteries, which branch off the **abdominal aorta**. The **renal veins** drain into the **inferior vena cava**. The filtered fluid and waste products enter the **renal pelvis**, flow through **the ureters** to the **urinary bladder**, and pass out of the body as urine. Many conditions can affect the kidneys, such as **kidney stones** and **kidney cysts**. Severe dehydration, sepsis, hemorrhage can cause blood pressure and blood circulation changes and lead to inadequate **renal perfusion** and **kidney failure**.

Cysts of the kidney may be **congenital** or **acquired. Congenital cystic renal diseases** include, but are not limited to, **multicystic renal dysplasia, autosomal-dominant** (adult) **polycystic kidney disease,** and **autosomal recessive** (childhood) **polycystic kidney disease. Acquired renal cystic diseases** include **simple cysts** and **dialysis-associated cystic renal disease. Multicystic renal dysplasia** may be unilateral or bilateral, and it is characterized by variably sized cysts giving the kidney an irregular appearance. Histologically, the affected kidney shows cysts, mesenchyme, and cartilage with a haphazard arrangement of nephrons and tubules. **Autosomal-dominant** (adult) **polycystic kidney disease** is characterized by multiple cysts involving both kidneys due to mutations in the *PKD1* or *PKD2* genes. The kidneys may grow to massive proportions as patients slowly develop renal insufficiency. Importantly, affected individuals are at risk for extrarenal manifestations, such as **cerebral berry aneurysms** in the circle of Willis that may lead to life-threatening subarachnoid hemorrhage upon rupture.

CLINICAL CORRELATION

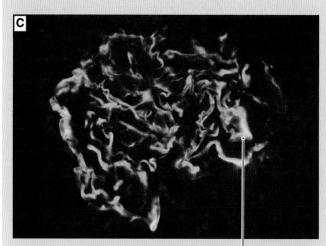

Immunofluorescence for IgG showing linear pattern
due to antibodies to type IV collagen in the
glomerular capillary basement membranes

Figure 12-2C. Goodpasture Syndrome. Immunofluorescence for IgG, ×400

Goodpasture syndrome, also called **anti–glomerular basement membrane disease (anti-GMB disease)**, involves the kidneys and lungs. It is rare, and it is characterized by circulating antibodies to domains of **type IV collagen** in **renal** and **alveolar basement membranes**. It is more common in Caucasian populations, and it tends to show a bimodal distribution with individuals in the third and sixth decades of life. The etiology of the syndrome is uncertain, but it tends to occur more often in individuals with a genetic susceptibility and subsequent environmental trigger, such as smoking tobacco, hydrocarbon exposure, and infection. Patients may present with **concurrent renal** and **pulmonary symptoms**, as in this case. **Renal failure** may take a rapidly progressive course. Kidney biopsy typically shows **glomerular cellular crescents** with **linear IgG deposits** in **glomerular capillaries** on immunofluorescence studies.

Kidney and Vascular Supply

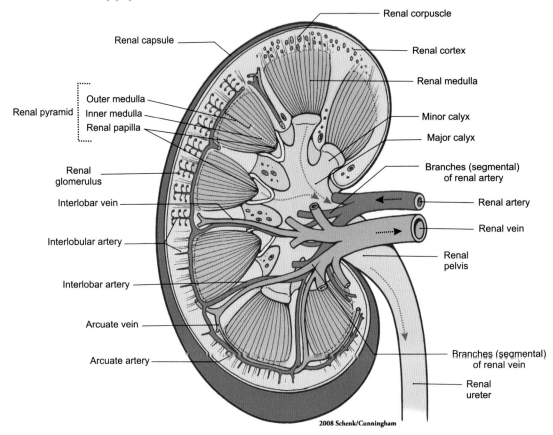

Figure 12-3. Overview of the kidney.

The kidney can be divided into three regions: the **renal cortex**, the **renal medulla**, and the **hilum**. The *renal cortex* is composed of renal corpuscles, proximal and **distal convoluted tubules**, **cortical collecting tubules**, and the blood vessels supplying the renal cortex. The *renal medulla* is made up of **renal pyramids**. The renal pyramids can be divided into three zones: the **outer medulla**, the **inner medulla**, and the **renal papillae**. The renal medulla is composed of several types of tubules oriented parallel to one another: the **descending limb of the loop of Henle** (thick descending and thin descending limbs), the **ascending limb of the loop of Henle** (thin ascending and thick ascending limbs), the **cortical collecting tubules**, the **collecting ducts**, and the **papillary ducts**. The papillary ducts drain urine into the **minor calices** and then to the **major calices**; the major calices merge into the **renal pelvis**, which drains urine into the **renal ureter**. The blood vessels supplying the kidneys include the **renal artery and vein**, branches of the renal artery and vein (**segmental arteries and veins**), **interlobar arteries and veins**, **arcuate arteries and veins**, **interlobular arteries and veins**, and **afferent and efferent arteries**. The microvasculature consists of the **glomeruli** of the renal corpuscle, the peritubular capillaries, and the vasa recta.

Vascular Supply of the Kidney

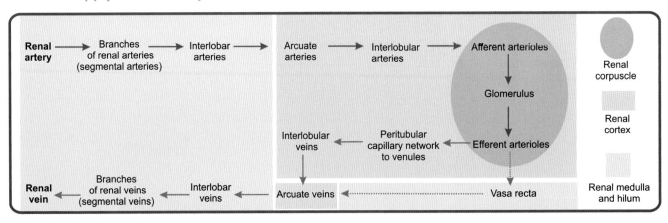

Figures and Images Orientation

Renal cortex and medulla, kidney. H&E, ×11

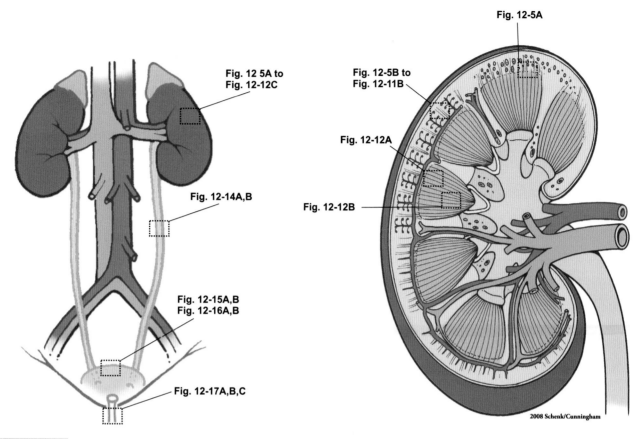

Fig. 12 5A to
Fig. 12-12C

Fig. 12-14A,B

Fig. 12-15A,B
Fig. 12-16A,B

Fig. 12-17A,B,C

Fig. 12-5A

Fig. 12-5B to
Fig. 12-11B

Fig. 12-12A

Fig. 12-12B

2008 Schenk/Cunningham

Figure 12-4. Orientation of detailed urinary system illustrations.

Structures of the Urinary System with Figure Numbers

Kidney

Renal cortex and medulla
  Figure 12-5A
  Figure 12-5B
  Figure 12-5C

Renal corpuscles
  Figure 12-6A
  Figure 12-6B

Glomerulus and filtration barrier
  Figure 12-7A
  Figure 12-7B
  Figure 12-8

Medullary ray and urinary tubules
  Figure 12-9A
  Figure 12-9B

Proximal tubules
  Figure 12-10A
  Figure 12-10B

Distal tubules
  Figure 12-11A
  Figure 12-11B

Medullary tubules
  Figure 12-12A
  Figure 12-12B
  Figure 12-12C
  Figure 12-12D
  Figure 12-13A

Ureter
  Figure 12-14A
  Figure 12-14B
  Figure 12-14C

Urinary bladder
  Figure 12-15A
  Figure 12-15B
  Figure 12-15C
  Figure 12-16A
  Figure 12-16B

Male and female urethrae
  Figure 12-17A
  Figure 12-17B
  Figure 12-17C

RENAL CORTEX AND MEDULLA

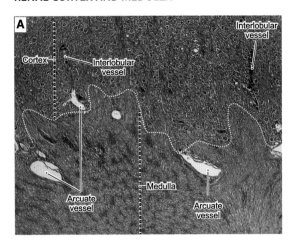

Figure 12-5A. Renal cortex and medulla, kidney. H&E, ×11

This section shows the **renal cortex** and the **medulla**. The *dashed white line* indicates the junction between the cortex and the medulla. The difference in appearance between the cortex and the medulla is due to the arrangement of the **uriniferous tubules** (**nephrons** and **collecting ducts**). The *renal cortex* is stained darker than the renal medulla. There are numerous renal corpuscles and various convoluted tubules in the cortex region. Both the cortex and the medulla have a rich blood supply. The arcuate vessels (arteries and veins) are visible at the border of the **corticomedullary junction**. The **interlobular vessels** (arteries and veins) arise from **arcuate vessels** and course upward (arteries) or downward (veins) in the renal cortex. The *renal medulla* is composed of 10 to 18 renal pyramids. Each pyramid contains numerous medullary tubules (**loops of Henle, collecting ducts, and papillary ducts**). Each papillary duct opens at the surface of the renal papilla (called the **area cribrosa**) where it empties urine into the minor calyx. The renal medulla can be divided into inner and outer zones based on differences in the types of tubules residing in the two regions.

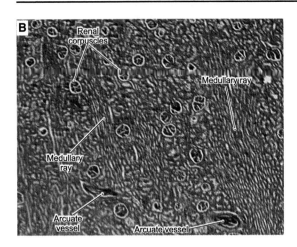

Figure 12-5B. Renal cortex, kidney. H&E, ×32

The **renal cortex** is composed of the **renal corpuscles**, the **proximal convoluted tubules**, the **distal convoluted tubules**, and the **cortical collecting tubules**. The renal corpuscles look like small balls interspersed among a tangle of tubules (**cortical labyrinth**) in the cortex region. The cortical labyrinth (with its corpuscles) is subdivided into columns by groups of parallel tubules called **medullary rays**. The medullary rays belong to the renal medulla proper; however, they extend into the cortex region. The renal cortex contains various convoluted tubules and is supplied by **interlobular arteries**, which give rise to afferent arteries. The afferent arterioles supply the glomeruli of renal corpuscles; blood exits the glomeruli through **efferent arterioles**. The cortical tubules are supplied by a peritubular capillary network, which arises from efferent arterioles that exit renal corpuscles located in the outer cortex. The renal medulla is supplied by the **vasa recta**, which arise from efferent arteries that exit renal corpuscles in the inner (juxtamedullary) cortex. The vasa recta follow the loop of Henle downward into the medulla and loop back toward the cortex. Both the **peritubular capillaries** and **vasa recta** converge into the **interlobular vein** and then drain into the **arcuate vein** at the corticomedullary junction.

CLINICAL CORRELATION

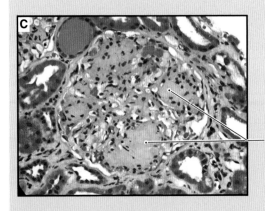

Figure 12-5C. Glomerular Disorders: Diabetic Nephropathy. H&E, ×216

Diabetic nephropathy, a complication of both type 1 and type 2 diabetes mellitus, may result in chronic renal failure and is the leading cause of end-stage renal disease in the United States and other Western countries. Major histologic changes in the glomeruli in diabetic nephropathy include **thickening of the glomerular basement membrane, diffuse glomerulosclerosis, and nodular glomerulosclerosis,** also called **Kimmelstiel-Wilson disease.** As the disease progresses, edema (swelling), hypertension, foamy urine, fatigue, headache, and nausea and vomiting may occur. Tight control of blood glucose levels tends to delay the onset of development. Treatment includes dialysis and renal transplantation. Shown here is a renal glomerulus with nodular glomerulosclerosis, or Kimmelstiel-Wilson disease.

RENAL CORPUSCLE

A

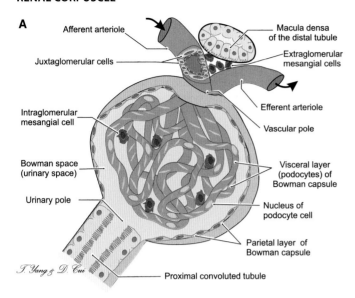

Afferent arteriole
Juxtaglomerular cells
Intraglomerular mesangial cell
Bowman space (urinary space)
Urinary pole
T. Yang & D. Cui
Macula densa of the distal tubule
Extraglomerular mesangial cells
Efferent arteriole
Vascular pole
Visceral layer (podocytes) of Bowman capsule
Nucleus of podocyte cell
Parietal layer of Bowman capsule
Proximal convoluted tubule

Figure 12-6A. Renal corpuscle, renal cortex.

The **renal corpuscle** is the site of blood filtration and initial production of urine. The main components of a renal corpuscle are a tuft of capillaries called the **glomerulus** and a surrounding sac, the **Bowman capsule.** The area of the renal corpuscle through which the arterioles pass into and out of the glomerulus is called the **vascular pole.** The surfaces of the capillaries of the glomerulus are covered by podocytes, which make up the **visceral layer** of the Bowman capsule. The outer wall of the renal corpuscle is a simple squamous epithelium called the **parietal layer** of the Bowman capsule. Fluid is filtered from the blood in glomerular capillaries into the space between the two layers, the **Bowman space.** Fluid exits through the **urinary pole** to enter the **proximal convoluted tubule.** There are phagocytic cells called **mesangial cells** (or **intraglomerular mesangial cells**) in the interstitial tissue between the glomerular capillaries. Similar cells are called **extraglomerular mesangial cells** when located at the vascular pole of the corpuscle. **Juxtaglomerular cells** in the walls of afferent arteriole are modified smooth muscle cells that secrete **renin** in order to regulate blood pressure. The **macula densa** of the distal tubule is located between the afferent and the efferent arteries.

B

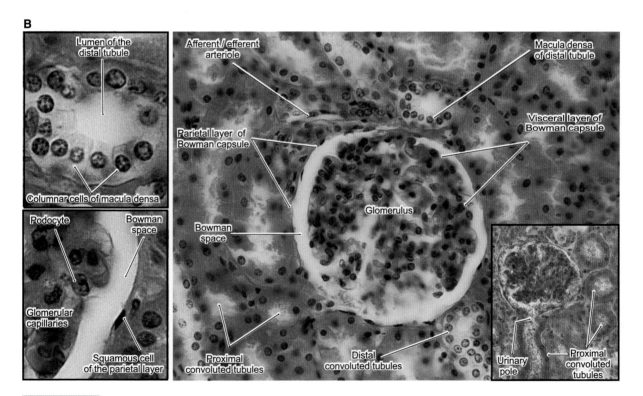

Lumen of the distal tubule
Columnar cells of macula densa
Podocyte
Bowman space
Glomerular capillaries
Squamous cell of the parietal layer
Afferent / efferent arteriole
Parietal layer of Bowman capsule
Bowman space
Proximal convoluted tubules
Distal convoluted tubules
Macula densa of distal tubule
Visceral layer of Bowman capsule
Glomerulus
Urinary pole
Proximal convoluted tubules

Figure 12-6B. Renal corpuscle, glomerulus and Bowman capsule. H&E, ×402; insets *(left)* ×921; insets *(lower right)* ×183

A **glomerulus** housed within the **Bowman capsule** is shown here. The lighter space between these two structures is the **Bowman space.** The *upper left small inset* shows the **macula densa,** a row of columnar cells that are densely packed together. This is a special sensory structure of the distal tubule as it passes close to the afferent and efferent arterioles at the vascular pole. The macula densa plays a role in monitoring ionic content and volume of the filtrate. The *lower left small inset* shows the Bowman space between the glomerulus and the parietal layer of the Bowman capsule. The *lower right inset* shows the **urinary pole.**

GLOMERULUS AND FILTRATION BARRIER

A

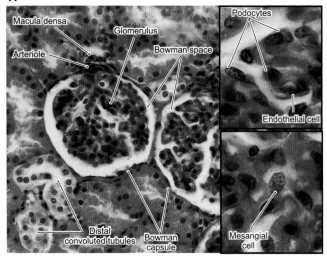

Figure 12-7A. Glomerulus, renal cortex. H&E, ×310; insets ×841

Each **glomerulus** is formed by a tuft of capillaries that is fed by the **afferent arteriole** and drains into the **efferent arteriole**. Pressure in the glomerulus due to resistance of the efferent artery provides the force for filtration into the **Bowman space**. The glomerular capillaries are fenestrated capillaries lined by endothelial cells with gaps (**fenestrae**) that lack the usual diaphragms. These capillaries are covered by processes of **podocytes**. The endothelial cells, basal lamina, and podocytes combine to form a **glomerular filtration barrier**. Intraglomerular mesangial cells within the glomerulus provide structural support as well as phagocytosis of debris and large molecules, thereby preventing material from accumulating on the filtration barrier. They also have a contractile capability, which may function in regulating glomerular blood flow.

B

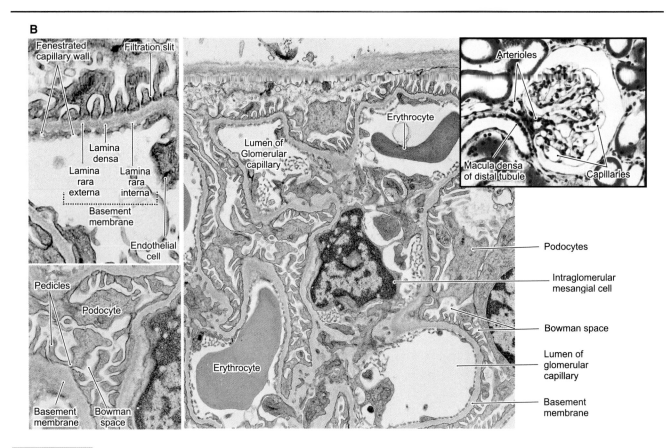

Figure 12-7B. Glomerulus and filtration barrier. EM, ×16,667; insets, *lower left* ×29,206; *upper left* ×41,818; *upper right* (color), H&E × 219

The central part of a renal corpuscle is composed of a bed of capillaries, the **glomerulus**, and the cells and structures associated with the glomerulus. In addition to the endothelial cells of the capillaries are two other cell types, **podocytes** and the **intraglomerular mesangial cells**. The endothelial cells of the fenestrated glomerular capillaries coproduce and share a common basal lamina with the terminal **podocyte processes** (**pedicles, foot processes**) that cover them. As blood flows through the capillaries, a filtrate of plasma is formed as it passes through several layers (fenestrations of the capillary, trilayered basal lamina, and filtration slits between podocytes) to enter the **Bowman space** (**urinary space**). **Intraglomerular mesangial cells**, lodged among the podocytes and endothelial cells, serve an incompletely understood maintenance function. The *upper left inset* shows the **basement membrane** of the glomerulus, **pedicles** (**small podocyte processes**), and cytoplasm of the **endothelial cell**, which together form a **filtration barrier** that selectively allows water, ions, and small molecules to pass through but not large molecules and blood cells. The *lower left inset* shows foot processes of the **podocyte** resting on the **basement membrane** of the glomerulus. The *upper right color inset* indicates the afferent and efferent arterioles.

GLOMERULUS AND PODOCYTE

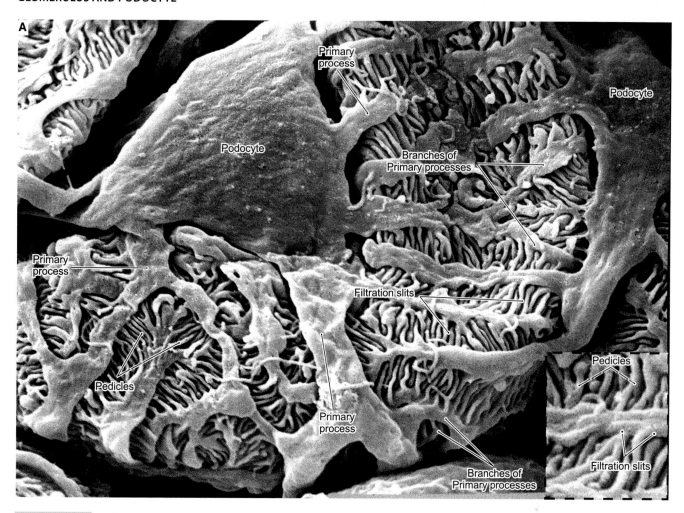

Figure 12-8A. Glomerulus and podocyte. SEM, ×9,677

This scanning electron microscopy (SEM) image shows that the surface of the **glomerulus** is entirely covered by **podocytes** and their **processes**. Each **podocyte** is composed of a cell body (with nucleus) and several **branching processes**. The small terminal branches that cover the capillaries are called **foot processes** or **pedicles**. The pedicles from two podocytes interdigitate with each other. The gaps between adjacent pedicles are referred to as **filtration slits**, which are bridged by **filtration slit diaphragms**. The inner core of the pedicles is supported by actin filaments. The inner core of the primary processes is supported mainly by microtubules and intermediate filaments. The podocytes and their unique arrangement are important components in establishing the glomerular filtration barrier.

CLINICAL CORRELATION

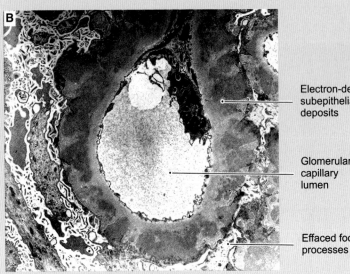

Electron-dense subepithelial deposits

Glomerular capillary lumen

Effaced foot processes

Figure 12-8B. Membranous Glomerulonephritis. TEM, ×16,000

Membranous glomerulonephritis, also called **membranous glomerulopathy** or **membranous nephropathy**, is one type of glomerulonephritis that is characterized by the accumulation of **immune-complex deposits** on the outer aspect of the glomerular basement membrane. Deposited immune complexes cause an immune reaction and **thickening of the basement membrane**. This disease is the most common cause of the adult-onset **nephrotic syndrome**. This electron photomicrograph shows the thickening of the glomerular capillary basement membrane with **subepithelial dense deposits** consisting of immune complexes. In addition, the foot processes of the podocytes show diffuse effacement.

MEDULLARY RAY AND COLLECTING SYSTEM

A

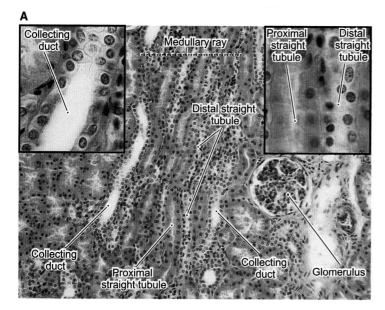

Figure 12-9A. Medullary ray, renal cortex. H&E, ×142; insets ×448

Each **medullary ray** is composed of **proximal straight tubules**, **distal straight tubules**, and **collecting ducts**. These tubules run parallel to each other within a medullary ray, which separates the glomeruli into groups. Although medullary rays are located in the renal cortex region, they are an extension of the renal medulla. The *proximal straight tubules* are lined by cuboidal cells with acidophilic cytoplasm and long microvilli. The *distal straight tubules* and *collecting ducts* are lined by cuboidal cells with clear cytoplasm. However, the collecting ducts have a larger lumen and more distinct cell-to-cell borders than do distal straight tubules. The proximal straight tubules convey filtrate from the proximal convoluted tubules into the thin segment tubules. The distal straight tubules convey the filtrate into the distal convoluted tubules, from which it drains into the collecting tubules and ducts (see below).

B

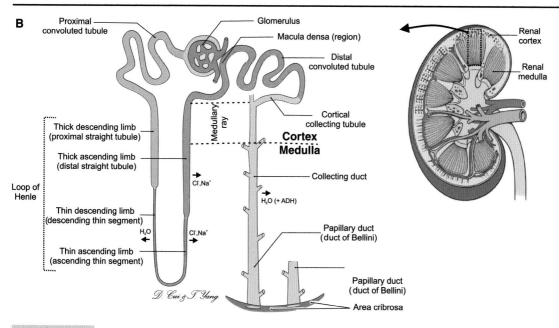

Figure 12-9B. Nephron and collecting system of the kidney.

The kidney is composed of **nephrons** and a **collecting system**. Each *nephron* comprises a **renal corpuscle**, a **proximal convoluted tubule**, a **loop of Henle**, and a **distal convoluted tubule**. The U-shaped *loop of Henle* connects the *proximal convoluted tubules* to the *distal convoluted tubules*. The loop of Henle creates a high concentration of solutes in the interstitium of the medulla, which is essential in controlling the concentration of urine. The *collecting system (yellow)* includes **cortical collecting tubules, collecting ducts**, and **papillary ducts**. The *dashed lines* indicate the junction between the cortex and the medulla and the medullary ray region in the cortex. When the blood pressure in the glomerular capillaries is within certain limits, water and some solutes of the blood plasma are forced through the **filtration barrier** into the **Bowman space** and then into the **proximal convoluted tubules**. Most glucose and amino acids and a large volume of water and salt are reabsorbed by the **proximal convoluted** and **straight tubules** before the filtrate enters the descending thin segment of the **loop of Henle**. The thin descending segment is highly permeable to water and less permeable to salt, so water passes from the lumen to the interstitium of the medulla and returns back to the blood circulation via the vasa recta. The thin ascending limb is impermeable to water but permeable to salt, and the thick ascending segment, which is also impermeable to water, actively pumps salt into the interstitium. As a result, the concentration of solutes increases to about four times the normal amount in the interstitium of the deep medulla. This hyperosmotic environment drives the movement of water from the lumens of the collecting ducts, therefore, increasing the concentration of the urine. The permeability to water in the cortical collecting tubules and collecting ducts (and, therefore, the final concentration of urine) is controlled by the level of **ADH** released by pituitary glands. The reabsorption of various ions by the distal convoluted tubule is controlled by hormones, primarily **aldosterone**. The final urine is collected by papillary ducts and emptied at the **area cribrosa** into the minor calyx.

PROXIMAL TUBULES

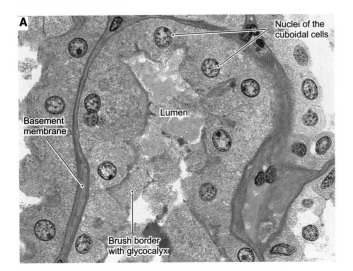

Figure 12-10A.   Proximal tubules, renal cortex. H&E, ×754

Both **proximal convoluted** and **straight tubules** have a similar structure and function. They are lined by large **acidophilic cuboidal cells** with **brush borders** formed by numerous **long microvilli**. The brush border extends into the **lumen**, which, in conjunction with postmortem changes, makes the lumen appear smaller and filled with acidophilic material (**brush border** and **glycocalyx**). The proximal tubules have a substantial reabsorption function. About 65% of the water and sodium and more than 90% of glucose, amino acids, and bicarbonate are reabsorbed by the proximal convoluted tubules. The proximal convoluted tubules are located in the cortical labyrinth and are connected to the renal corpuscle at the urinary pole. The proximal straight tubules are part of the loop of Henle.

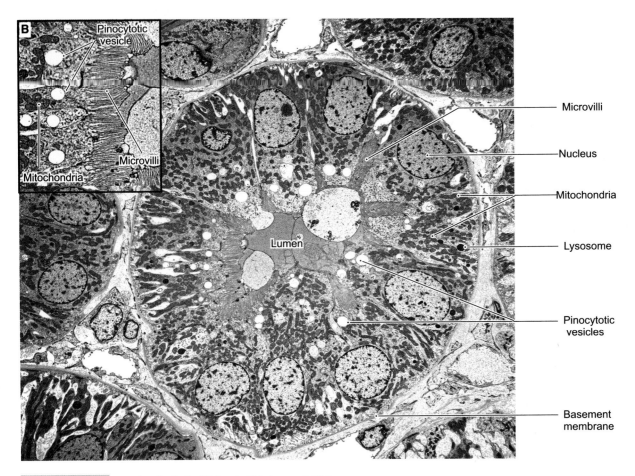

Figure 12-10B.   Proximal tubule. EM, ×4,606; inset ×9,208

This is a cross section of a **proximal tubule.** It is lined by cuboidal and low columnar cells with apical **microvilli**, which form a **brush border**, a feature that is associated with reabsorption function. The numerous **mitochondria** are more concentrated at the basolateral surface where they support the energy requirements of sodium pumps located in the expanded plasmalemma. The apical regions of the cells contain **pinocytotic vesicles**, which reflect the uptake of proteins that evaded the filtration barrier in the renal corpuscle and entered the filtrate. The *inset* shows long microvilli and pinocytotic vesicles in the apical surface of the cells.

DISTAL TUBULES

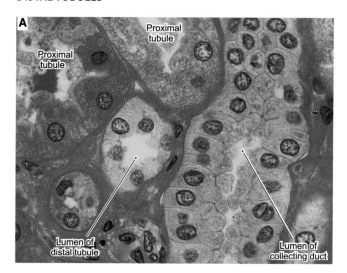

Figure 12-11A. Distal tubules. H&E, ×739

The **distal tubules** are lined by small cuboidal cells with faintly eosinophilic or clear cytoplasm. The lateral boundaries between cells are not as distinguishable as those of the collecting duct. The distal convoluted and straight tubules are similar in structure. The distal straight tubule exits the medullary ray and approaches the vascular pole of the renal corpuscle of the same nephron to which the distal tubule belongs. As the distal tubule passes adjacent to the afferent and efferent arterioles, part of its wall becomes modified as a sensory structure, **macula densa**, which monitors ionic content and water volume of the filtrate. The macula densa is considered to mark the transition from the distal straight to the distal convoluted tubule. This figure shows the distal convoluted tubules in the renal cortex. Distal tubules function mainly to remove sodium and add potassium ions to the filtrate when stimulated by **aldosterone**, a hormone produced by the adrenal gland.

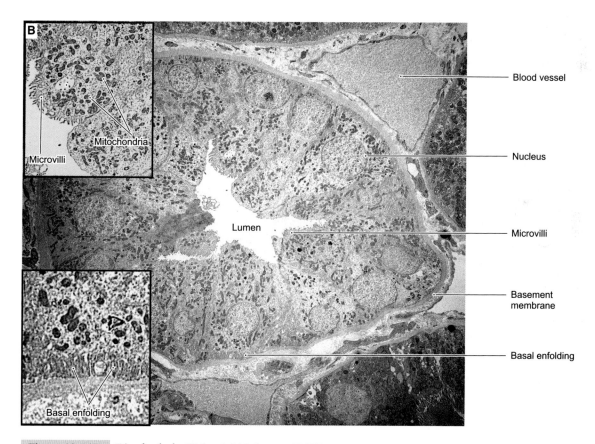

Figure 12-11B. Distal tubule. EM, ×4,441; insets ×7,377

A cross section of a **distal tubule**, which is lined by cuboidal and columnar cells, is shown. In contrast to the extravagant brush border of cells lining the proximal tubule, these cells have just a few, short **microvilli**. These cells have basally located nuclei and tightly interdigitated lateral walls. In distal tubules, there are many **mitochondria** in the cytoplasm as there are in the proximal tubules. The *upper left inset* shows short and irregular microvilli bulging into the **lumen** and many mitochondria beneath them. The *lower left inset* shows a **nucleus** and **basal enfolding** (basal plasma membrane enfolding) of the cell. The basal enfolding is due to corrugation of the cell membrane in the basal region of the cell. This increases the surface area of the cell and is closely associated with mitochondria, which produce adenosine triphosphate for active transport of ions.

MEDULLARY TUBULES

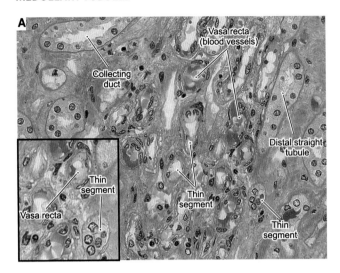

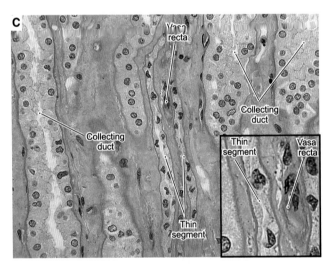

Figure 12-12A. Medullary tubules, outer zone of the medulla. H&E, ×296; inset ×435

The **renal medulla** is composed of the **loop of Henle**, the **collecting ducts**, and the **papillary ducts** (**ducts of Bellini**). It can be divided into an outer zone and an inner zone. The **thin segment tubules** and **distal straight tubules** of the loop of Henle and **collecting ducts** of the outer zone are shown here. The inner zone contains only thin segments and collecting ducts, along with the **vasa recta**. Blood vessels (vasa recta) are found throughout the medulla.

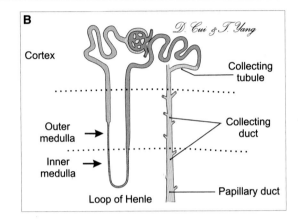

Figure 12-12B. Orientation of the kidney tubules in the cortex and medulla.

This illustration shows the orientation of the kidney **tubules** in the **cortex** and **medulla**. The outer zone and inner zone of the medulla indicate the levels of Figures 12-12A and 12-12C.

Figure 12-12C. Medullary tubules, inner zone of the medulla. H&E, ×296; inset ×726

This figure shows the inner zone of the medulla. The **collecting ducts** gradually increase in size. The **thin segment tubules** and the **vasa recta** (blood vessels) are seen here.

CLINICAL CORRELATION

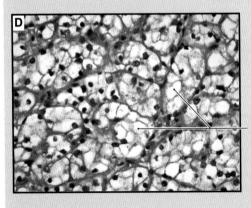

Clear cells (tumor cells)

Figure 12-12D. Renal Cell Carcinoma (Clear Cell Type). H&E, ×216

Renal cell carcinoma, which arises from the **renal tubular epithelium**, is the most common renal cancer in adults. Risk factors for development of renal cell carcinoma include **smoking**, exposure to **toxic substances, chronic renal failure,** and **acquired cystic disease** of the kidney as well as **genetic predisposition** in various familial syndromes. Renal carcinoma presents clinically with hematuria, abdominal mass, or flank pain. Renal cell carcinoma tends to metastasize early, especially to the lungs and bones. On gross examination, renal cell carcinoma is well circumscribed, lobulated, and yellow, with areas of hemorrhage and necrosis. The most common renal cell carcinoma is the **clear cell type,** the cells of which may be arranged in cords, nests, or tubules. The cells are large and polygonal with clear or granular cytoplasm. Other types of renal cell carcinoma include papillary carcinoma, chromophobe carcinoma, and collecting duct carcinoma. Treatment is primarily surgical removal, with lesser roles for immunotherapy and chemotherapy.

CLINICAL CORRELATIONS

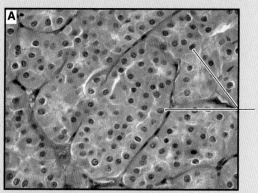
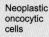

Neoplastic oncocytic cells

Figure 12-13A. Renal Oncocytoma. H&E, ×216

Renal oncocytoma is a benign and less common neoplasm of the kidney and originates from the epithelium of the proximal tubules. It is typically a solid, encapsulated mass with homogeneous enhancement in radiographic imaging. Gross examination shows a spherical mass with a mahogany cut surface and a tan, fleshy central scar. Histologically, the tumor cells are large with abundant eosinophilic cytoplasm due to the presence of numerous mitochondria. The cells are arranged in sheets or in a tubulocystic pattern. It is usually asymptomatic and detected as an incidental renal mass on imaging. Treatment options include surgical excision of the kidney (**nephrectomy**) or removal of a portion of the kidney (partial nephrectomy).

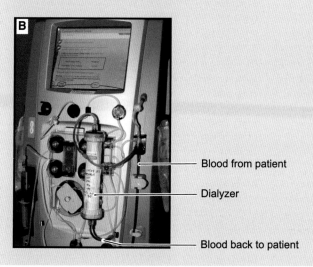

Blood from patient

Dialyzer

Blood back to patient

Figure 12-13B. Hemodialysis.

Hemodialysis is a common treatment for end-stage kidney disease. The **dialyzer** is a canister containing thousands of small fibers through which blood is passed. The fibers are made up of semipermeable membranes with small pores allowing wastes and extra fluids to pass from the blood into a solution. A cleansing fluid called **dialysate** is pumped around the fibers. Solute and extra fluids are cleared from the blood compartment by either diffusion or ultrafiltration, depending on the concentration gradient and pressure difference between the blood and the dialysate. The cleansed blood is returned via the circuit back to the body. Hemodialysis is usually given three times a week and can be done in a dialysis center or at home. The model illustrated here is commonly used in critical care units.

SYNOPSIS 12-1 Pathologic and Clinical Terms for the Urinary System

■ *Glomerulonephritis:* Refers to primary glomerular disease not related to infection of the kidneys themselves. The causes of glomerulonephritis are heterogeneous, such as viral or bacterial infection; drugs; and malignancy, resulting in many distinct clinical entities including focal and segmental glomerulonephritis and membranous nephropathy. The causes are often not identified (idiopathic glomerulonephritis).

■ *Glomerulopathy:* Refers to secondary glomerular injury as a result of systemic diseases, such as diabetes mellitus and systemic lupus erythematosus.

■ *Glomerulosclerosis:* Scarring or sclerosis of the renal glomeruli in diseases such as diabetic nephropathy and focal segmental glomerulosclerosis.

■ *Dysuria:* Pain or burning upon urination, most often caused by a urinary tract infection affecting the bladder (cystitis) or urethra (urethritis).

■ *Frequency:* The need to urinate more often than normal without an increase in total urine output; common causes include lower urinary tract infection and benign prostatic hyperplasia; other less common causes include tumors and extrinsic bladder compression.

■ *Hematuria:* The presence of blood in the urine, causes of which include trauma, infection, tumors of the urinary system, kidney stones, and hyperplasia of the prostate gland; hematuria may be microscopic or "macroscopic," meaning visible to the unaided eye.

■ *Lithotripsy:* Extracorporeal shock wave lithotripsy is a procedure for treating kidney and ureteral stones using focused high-energy shock waves that pass through the body and break stones into small pieces that can then pass into the urine and be eliminated.

■ *Urgency:* A strong urge to urinate, most often caused by a lower urinary tract infection or other causes of bladder irritation such as interstitial cystitis, which mainly affects females.

TABLE 12-1   Kidneys

Structure	Epithelial Lining of the Tubules	Characteristics of the Tubules	Main Locations	Main Functions
Nephron				
Renal corpuscle	Simple squamous epithelium	Composed of glomerulus (blood vessels covered by podocytes) and Bowman capsule	Renal cortex	Filters blood and forms urine
Proximal convoluted tubule	Simple cuboidal epithelium with long microvilli (brush border)	Long and highly convoluted tubule; relatively small lumen and acidophilic cytoplasm; abundant mitochondria; numerous basolateral plasma membrane enfoldings	Renal cortex	Drains fluid from the renal corpuscle to the loop of Henle; reabsorbs 70%–80% Na$^+$ and Cl$^-$ and water; also reabsorbs glucose, amino acids, and proteins and produces calcitriol (active form vitamin D)
The loop of Henle — Thick descending limb (*proximal straight tubule*)	Simple cuboidal epithelium with long microvilli (brush border)	Similar to proximal convoluted tubule but shorter and straight; small mitochondria; no basolateral plasma membrane enfoldings	Medullary ray and outer zone of the renal medulla	Absorptive function is similar to proximal convoluted tubule but less significant
The loop of Henle — Thin descending limb (*descending thin segment*)	Simple squamous epithelium	Thin, small tubule; epithelial cells may reveal basolateral enfoldings and small microvilli	Partial outer zone and most of the inner zone of the renal medulla	Highly permeable to water (loss of water from lumen to interstitium); less permeable to salt (keeps or may gain some Na$^+$ and Cl$^-$ in the lumen)
The loop of Henle — Thin ascending limb (*ascending thin segment*)	Simple squamous epithelium	Similar to descending thin segment; may have basolateral enfoldings and small microvilli	Inner zone of the renal medulla	Impermeable to water (retains water); highly permeable to salt (loss of Na$^+$ and Cl$^-$ from the lumen to the interstitium)
The loop of Henle — Thick ascending limb (*distal straight tubule*)	Simple cuboidal epithelium with short microvilli	Straight tubule; numerous mitochondria; less acidophilic cytoplasm; many basolateral plasma membrane enfoldings	Medullary ray and outer zone of the renal medulla	Impermeable to water (retains water); highly permeable to salt (loss of Na$^+$ and Cl$^-$ from the lumen to the interstitium)
Distal convoluted tubule	Simple cuboidal epithelium with short microvilli	Numerous mitochondria; basolateral plasma membrane enfoldings; less acidophilic cytoplasm; highly convoluted tubule	Renal cortex	Reabsorbs Na$^+$ and secretes K$^+$, if aldosterone stimulation is present; reabsorbs bicarbonate ions and secretes ammonium to adjust pH
Collecting System				
Collecting tubule	Simple cuboidal epithelium with few microvilli	Straight tubule; much less acidophilic cytoplasm; more than one cell type	Renal cortex	Highly permeable to water; loss of water from the lumen to the interstitium when ADH is present
Collecting duct	Simple cuboidal to columnar epithelium	Large straight tubule; clear cytoplasm and distinct boundaries between cells; well-developed basal enfoldings	Medullary ray and renal medulla	Highly permeable to water; loss of water from the lumen to the interstitium when ADH is present
Papillary duct	Simple columnar epithelium	Short duct; links collecting duct to the minor calyx	Bottom tip of the pyramid of the medulla	Conducts urine

Ureters

A

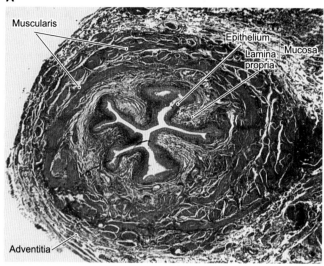

Muscularis
Epithelium
Mucosa
Lamina propria
Adventitia

Figure 12-14A. Ureter. H&E, ×61

The **ureter** is a small muscular tubule lined with transitional epithelium. It carries urine from the renal pelvis to the urinary bladder. The wall of the ureter is composed of **mucosa, muscularis,** and **adventitia.** The *mucosa* consists of transitional epithelium and loose connective tissue (**lamina propria**). The middle layer, the *muscularis,* is relatively thick and contains inner longitudinal and outer circular smooth muscle layers. These two muscle layers are often difficult to distinguish. The wall of the ureter becomes thicker as it nears the bladder. As it approaches the urinary bladder, the ureter may also contain a third layer of smooth muscle. The *adventitia* layer is composed of connective tissues, nerve fibers, and blood vessels. It provides protection, blood supply, and nervous innervation to the ureter.

B

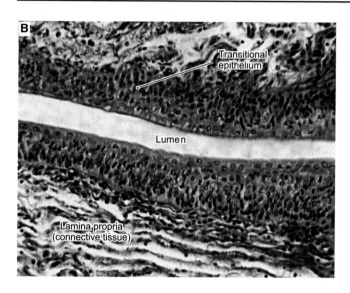

Transitional epithelium
Lumen
Lamina propria (connective tissue)

Figure 12-14B. Transitional epithelium, ureter. H&E, ×190

Transitional epithelium lines the urinary tract from the urinary calyces to the bladder. This type of epithelium can change shape as it is stretched to accommodate a change in volume. Cells on the surface layer appear round and dome shaped when the bladder is in a relaxed state. These cells become flattened, and the layers of cells are reduced in number when the epithelium is stretched. The transitional epithelium lining the urinary tract is also called **urothelium**; it has tight junctions and thick cytoplasm. The **lumen** of the ureter appears as a white space here.

CLINICAL CORRELATION

C

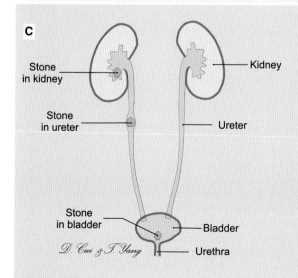

Stone in kidney
Kidney
Stone in ureter
Ureter
Stone in bladder
Bladder
Urethra

D. Cui & T. Yang

Figure 12-14C. Nephrolithiasis (Renal Stones).

Nephrolithiasis (renal stones) is common in clinical practice. Symptoms range from vague abdominal pain to renal colic and hematuria when stones pass from the renal pelvis into the narrow portion of the ureter. Most renal stones are composed of the calcium salts, calcium oxalate, or calcium phosphate. Other less common forms include uric acid, magnesium ammonium phosphate (struvite), and cystine stones. Risk factors for the development of kidney stones include dietary factors, metabolic abnormalities, abnormal urine pH, family history of renal stones, frequent upper urinary tract infections, and low fluid intake. Struvite stones are associated with urinary tract infection with urea-splitting bacteria such as *Proteus* species. Treatment varies based upon the location and size of the stones and includes analgesics, shock wave lithotripsy, ureteroscopy, and surgery.

Urinary Bladder

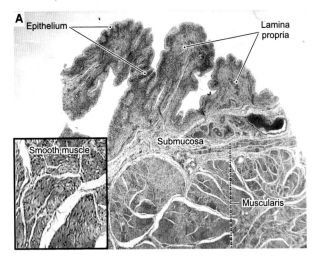

Figure 12-15A. Urinary bladder, bladder wall. H&E, ×17; inset ×82

The **urinary bladder** has three layers (**mucosa, muscularis,** and **adventitia/serosa**), similar to those in the ureter, but its wall is much thicker. Thick mucosa and muscularis layers make up the wall of the urinary bladder. The *mucosa* is composed of extensively folded **transitional epithelium** and **lamina propria**. This arrangement gives the bladder the distensibility needed to store urine. The *muscularis* consists of three **smooth muscle** layers: the inner longitudinal, middle circular, and outer longitudinal smooth muscle. These three smooth muscle layers are arranged in two different orientations to help the urinary bladder contract to empty urine efficiently. The outer layer of the bladder is mainly covered by *adventitia* (connective tissue); its superior (free) surface is covered by **serosa**, which is a layer of connective tissue with a lining of **mesothelium**.

UROTHELIUM, TRANSITIONAL EPITHELIUM

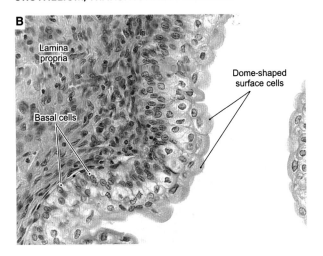

Figure 12-15B. Urothelium, bladder wall. H&E, ×278

This figure shows the **urothelium** (transitional epithelium) in a relaxed state. The urothelial lining of the urinary bladder is thicker than that of the ureter. The **basal cells** of the urothelium are cuboidal or columnar in shape, the cells in the middle layer of the urothelium are polygonal, and the surface cells are **dome shaped** and bulge into the lumen when the bladder is empty (relaxed state). When the bladder is full, the urothelium is stretched, the cells become flattened, and the thickness of the urothelium is greatly reduced.

CLINICAL CORRELATION

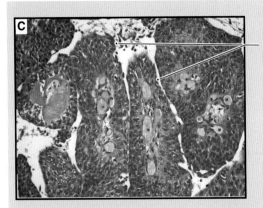

Figure 12-15C. Urothelial (Transitional) Carcinoma. H&E, ×108

Urothelial carcinoma may arise in the urinary bladder, ureters, or renal pelvis and is the most common urinary bladder carcinoma. More than 90% of bladder cancers originate from the transitional epithelium (**urothelium**) in the urinary system. Urothelial carcinoma is most prevalent in older men but may occur at any age. Risk factors include **cigarette smoking**, exposure to **arylamines** and **radiation**, long-term use of cyclophosphamide, and infection by the parasite *Schistosoma haematobium*. Infection with *S. haematobium* is also a risk factor for the development of **squamous cell carcinoma** of the urinary bladder. Symptoms include painless gross hematuria, frequency, urgency, and dysuria. Urothelial carcinomas typically display a papillary morphology and are subdivided into low and high grade depending on cytologic features and the amount of architectural disorder present. Treatment includes transurethral resection, chemotherapy, immunotherapy, and radical cystectomy. Tumors have a high recurrence rate after local excision.

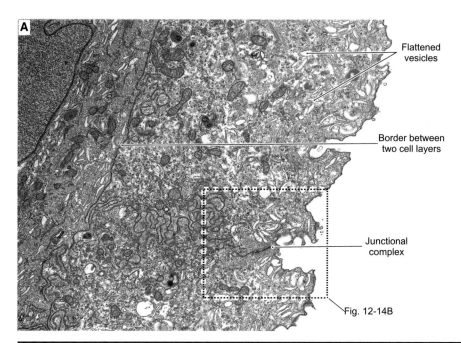

Figure 12-16A. Transitional epithelium, urinary bladder. TEM, ×7,280

This figure shows the surface of **transitional epithelium** and the border between the cells of the top layer and the underlying layer. There are many **flattened vesicles** (membrane vesicles) in the cytoplasm of these cells. The vesicles are more numerous close to the apical region of the cytoplasm. These vesicles are formed from the surface membrane when the bladder is in a relaxed state. It is important to recall that the surface of the transitional epithelium of the bladder is highly convoluted when the bladder is empty (relaxed). This may create many "pseudovesicles"; most of the vesicles disappear when the surface of the epithelium is stretched and flattened in the distended state. The *boxed area* indicates Figure 12-16B at higher magnification.

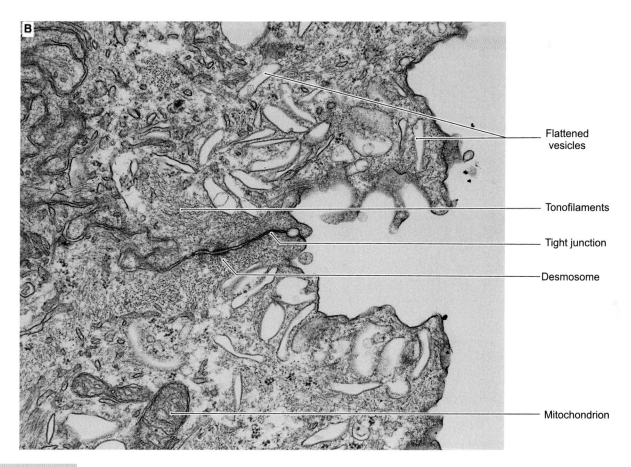

Figure 12-16B. Transitional epithelium, urinary bladder. TEM, ×35,753

A higher power view of the surface of the top layer cells in the **transitional epithelium** is shown. The **junction complex** indicates the border of neighboring cells. **Tight junctions** (**zonula occludens**) and **desmosomes** (**macula adherens**) can be observed here. The cells are filled with **flattened vesicles** and **tonofilaments**.

Urethra

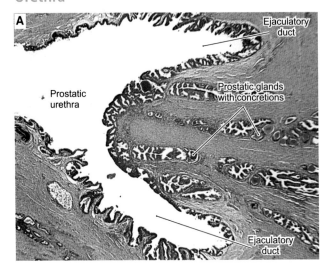

Figure 12-17A.   Prostatic urethra, male urethra. H&E, ×17

The **urethra** provides for the passage of urine from the bladder to the outside of the body. The male urethra is significantly different from that of the female. It is a long tube (18–20 cm), which passes through the prostate and penis. The male urethra can be divided into three parts: **prostatic**, **membranous**, and **penile** (**spongy**) based on its anatomical location. This figure shows a cross section of the **prostatic urethra** connecting to two **ejaculatory ducts**, surrounded by the prostate. The *prostatic urethra* is a short segment (3–4 cm), usually lined by transitional epithelium. This portion of the urethra is surrounded by prostatic glands. The *membranous urethra* is narrow and short (1–2 cm) and passes through the deep perineal pouch. It is lined by pseudostratified columnar epithelium and surrounded by an inner longitudinal smooth muscle and an outer skeletal muscle of the external urethral sphincter. The *penile (spongy) urethra* is the longest segment (12–14 cm).

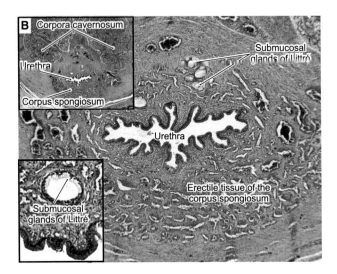

Figure 12-17B.   Penile (spongy) urethra, male urethra. H&E, ×34; inset ×6 (*upper*), ×170 (*lower*)

The **penile urethra** is also called the **spongy urethra** because it passes through the penis and is surrounded by **erectile tissue** (**corpus spongiosum**). The terms "cavernous" or "bulbous" urethra may also be used to refer to the penile urethra. The penile urethra is lined by pseudostratified columnar epithelium. Close to the tip of the penis, the lining becomes stratified squamous epithelium. This view shows the urethra in the corpus spongiosum, surrounded by spongy erectile tissue. Within the lining of pseudostratified columnar epithelium are clusters of mucus-secreting cells, the **glands of Littré**. The glands of Littré located in the epithelium are called **intraepithelial glands of Littré**; similar glands found in the submucosa are termed **submucosal** or **extraepithelial glands of Littré**. The secretions of the mucous cells of these glands protect the urethra from the effects of the urine. The *upper left inset* shows the urethra associated with the corpus spongiosum and corpora cavernosa in the penis.

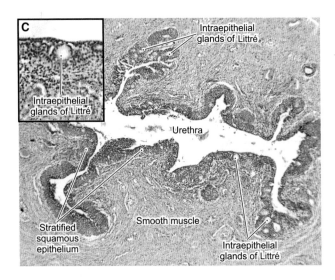

Figure 12-17C.   Urethra, female urethra. H&E, ×34; inset ×177

The **female urethra** is 4 to 5 cm long, much shorter than the male urethra. It conveys urine from the urinary bladder, passing inferiorly through the pelvic floor and exiting anterior/superior to the vaginal opening in the vestibule. The female urethra is initially lined by pseudostratified columnar epithelium, which changes to **stratified squamous epithelium** as it approaches the external opening of the urethra. It has a thick lamina propria with many elastic fibers and venous plexuses. The **glands of Littré** are also present in the female urethra. Its wall is surrounded by longitudinal **smooth muscle**. The middle portion of the wall of the urethra is surrounded by the outer layer of the **external urethral sphincter**, which has the same function as in the male urethra.

From Histology to Pathology

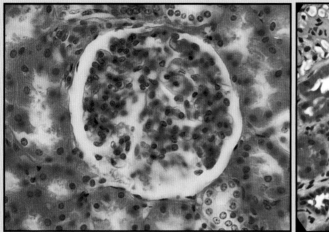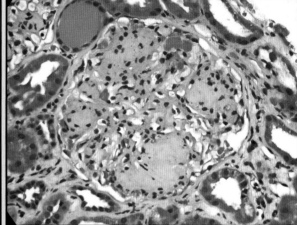

Figure 12-18.   Normal glomerulus and diabetic nephropathy. H&E, ×400

Normal glomerulus on the *left*. **Glomerular disorder of diabetic nephropathy** on the *right*. This disorder is a complication of **diabetes mellitus. Hyperglycemia** activates various inflammatory pathways, leading to podocyte injury, malfunction, **apoptosis**, and **protein** **deposition** in the extracellular matrix of the nephron, causing albumin to leak into the urine. **Kimmelstiel-Wilson nodules** and **glomerulosclerosis** can be developed. Patients may have edema, hypertension, foamy urine, fatigue, headache, nausea, and vomiting.

Clinical Vignette Questions

1. A previously healthy 24-year-old man experiences malaise shortly followed by an episode of hemoptysis (coughing up blood) and hematuria (blood in the urine). Alarmed, he presented to the emergency department where he was found to be mildly hypertensive and dyspneic (short of breath). Urinalysis revealed hematuria with red cell casts. Laboratory studies revealed elevated blood urea nitrogen and serum creatinine. Chest imaging showed changes consistent with intra-alveolar hemorrhage. A kidney biopsy is performed, and immunofluorescence studies show linear deposition of IgG antibodies in glomerular capillaries. Which of the following most likely demonstrates the clinical scenario in this patient?

A. Anti–glomerular basement membrane disease
B. Focal segmental glomerulosclerosis
C. IgA nephropathy
D. Poststreptococcal glomerulonephritis

2. A 66-year-old man with a 1-month history of painless frank hematuria comes to the physician for a check-up. He denies any history of dysuria or urethral discharge. Physical examination shows the patient is healthy without inguinal lymphadenopathy; rectal examination reveals a moderately enlarged prostate without discrete nodules. Gross blood appears in the urine sample. CT and retrograde pyelography indicate that both of the kidneys and the prostate are normal. Cystoscopy shows multiple small papillary lesions in the bladder. Biopsy of the lesions reveals urothelial cells lacking the normal cellular polarity; the cells contain large, irregular hyperchromatic nuclei with prominent nucleoli. Which of the following is the most likely diagnosis for this patient?

A. Adenocarcinoma
B. Cystitis glandularis
C. Malakoplakia
D. Squamous cell carcinoma
E. Urothelial cell carcinoma

3. A 66-year-old female with a long history of hypertension and hypercholesterolemia complains about newly developed skin rashes and edema of her face and upper eyelid. The patient has an 18-year history of type 2 diabetes mellitus, and she was diagnosed with diabetic retinopathy 5 years ago. She has been using various antihypertensive medications to control her blood pressure, and she mainly uses a low-carb diet to control her blood sugar level seldom using oral diabetes medications. Her serum creatinine levels had been around 1.7 mg/dL, but she has had several episodes of transient mild proteinuria in the past year. Laboratory results reveal a serum creatinine (female) of 2.5 mg/dL (normal: 0.5–0.95 mg/dL), C3 of 116 mg/dL (normal: 90–180 mg/dL), C4 of 45 mg/dL (normal: 16–47 mg/dL), and negative anti–glomerular basement membrane antibodies. The antinuclear antibody (ANA) titer was minimally elevated at 1:80. Assuming a kidney biopsy was performed, which of the following is the most likely finding in this patient?

A. Crescent formation, with neutrophils, macrophages, and T cells
B. Linear pattern and anti–glomerular basement membrane antibodies
C. Mesangial deposits of IgA
D. Mesangial expansion, glomerular basement membrane thickening, and glomerulosclerosis
E. Presence of numerous tubuloreticular structures in the glomerular endothelial cells

13 Integumentary System

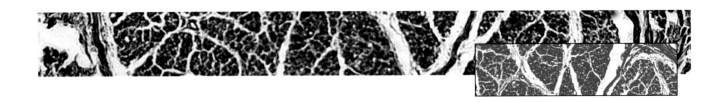

Introduction and Key Concepts for the Integumentary System
Development of the Skin
Layers of the Skin
Thick Skin Versus Thin Skin
Accessory Structures of the Skin

Clinical Vignette Questions

Introduction and Key Concepts for the Integumentary System

The skin and its accessory structures form the **integumentary system**. The skin covers the entire surface of the body and is the largest organ of the body in terms of its weight and volume. The accessory structures of the skin include hair, nails, and three types of glands: **sebaceous, eccrine sweat,** and **apocrine**. The skin is composed of several types of tissues: epithelium, connective tissue, muscles, blood vessels, and nervous tissue. The functions of skin include (1) **Protection:** The skin serves as a barrier between the internal tissues and the outside world, preventing damage to the internal tissues by physical trauma, toxic chemicals, radiation, and sunlight. (2) **Prevention of dehydration:** The skin forms a waterproof barrier, which prevents the loss of body fluids. (3) **Regulation of body temperature:** Evaporation of sweat released onto the body surface by the eccrine glands as well as dilation of the capillary network and arteriovenous anastomoses (shunts) in the skin help to regulate body temperature. (4) **Somatosensory function:** Sensory receptors in the skin transduce physical energy in an individual's surroundings into action potentials that are carried by peripheral nerves to the central nervous system where the sensations of touch, pressure, pain, warmth, cold, vibration, etc. are generated. (5) **Immunologic function:** The Langerhans cells and lymphocytes in the skin play roles in the cutaneous immune response. (6) **Production of vitamin D:** Vitamin D, an essential vitamin, is synthesized from precursors in the skin under the effects of steroids and sunlight.

Development of the Skin

The skin develops from **ectoderm** and **mesoderm**. The epithelial cells of the epidermis are *ectodermal derivatives*, whereas Langerhans cells, the dermis (connective tissue), and subcutis (hypodermis) develop from the *mesoderm*. Melanocytes and Merkel cells originate from the neural crest. The basal cells of the epidermis give rise to the accessory structures (hair follicles, nails, and glands) of the skin.

Layers of the Skin

The skin can be divided into two basic layers: **epidermis** and **dermis**. The *epidermis* is a maximally keratinized stratified squamous epithelium, which is composed of five named layers of cells called **keratinocytes**. (1) The **stratum basale** is the deepest layer of the epidermis and it borders the dermis. A single layer of cuboidal or tall cuboidal cells lies on the basement membrane. Many of these cells are **stem cells** that actively divide and give rise to the cells in the other four layers. The epidermal keratinocytes are renewed constantly, with the top layer of cells continually being shed and new cells from the stratum basale replacing them. It takes about 3 to 4 weeks for keratinocytes to finish their renewal cycle. In addition to the keratinocyte stem cells, two special types of cells, **melanocytes** and **Merkel cells** (**Merkel disks**), are found in the stratum basale. The melanocytes are melanin producing cells which are in contact with the keratinocytes that are located immediately above the stratum basale. Merkel cells (Merkel cell neurite complexes or Merkel disks) are sensory receptor cells that respond to continuous touch stimuli. (2) The **stratum spinosum** contains polyhedral keratinocytes, which become more flattened in the superficial part of this layer. The plasma membrane of neighboring cells is connected by **desmosomes** (**macula adherens**). **Langerhans cells** (modified macrophages) are an additional cell type often found in this layer. (3) The **stratum granulosum** contains keratinocytes, which are flattened cells with keratohyalin granules in their cytoplasm. These granules are basophilic in appearance in H&E-stained sections. This layer is more prominent in the thick skin than in the thin skin. (4) The **stratum lucidum** is a thin layer that is only found in the thick skin. It contains a few layers of flattened cells, which are densely packed together and lie beneath the stratum corneum. Their nuclei become pycnotic as they begin to degenerate. (5) The **stratum corneum** is the most superficial layer, which contains numerous extremely flattened cells completely filled with keratin. These cells have no nuclei or organelles and are technically dead cells. The cells on the surface are continuously shed. The *dermis* is a connective tissue layer deep to the epidermis. It contains the blood vessels, nerves, and afferent sensory receptors, including Meissner corpuscles and free nerve endings. The **hypodermis** is a transition (subcutaneous) layer below the dermis of the skin, which contains loose connective tissue, adipose tissue, nerves, arteries, and veins.

Thick Skin Versus Thin Skin

Thick skin is found in only a few places in the body, such as the palms of the hands and soles of the feet. It has a very thick epidermis. The stratum corneum is particularly prominent, being about 10 times thicker than that of thin skin. Thick skin has numerous eccrine sweat glands but has no sebaceous glands or apocrine sweat glands. In contrast, **thin skin**, which covers the rest of the body, has a thin epidermis and its stratum corneum is much thinner than that of thick skin. The epidermis of thin skin consists of only four layers; the stratum lucidum is lacking in thin skin. Thin skin contains all three types of glands.

Accessory Structures of the Skin

Accessory structures of the skin include **glands**, **hair**, and **nails**: (1) The *glands* of the skin include **sebaceous glands**, **eccrine sweat glands**, and **apocrine sweat glands**. The *sebaceous glands* secrete into hair follicles to keep the skin soft and moist and serve as a barrier to protect the skin. The *eccrine sweat glands* are important in regulating body temperature; they are found in both the thin and thick skin. The *apocrine sweat glands* are also called **sexual scent glands**; their function in humans is not clear. They may be involved in thermoregulation and are found only in some special regions of thin skin, such as the axilla, nipple, and perianal and genital areas. (2) *Hair* is found in thin skin: the scalp, pubic region, and armpit (axilla) in adults have more abundant thick hair than other surfaces of the skin on the body. Hair growth is discontinuous and is controlled by various hormones. The hair follicles produce and maintain hair growth. The cycles of hair growth include three stages (from early to late): the **anagen phase** (active growth stage, lasting 2–6 years), the **catagen phase** (regression phase, lasting about 3 weeks), and the **telogen phase** (resting stage, lasting about 3 months). The hair shaft is shed as the follicle goes through the growth cycle and a new hair replaces it. In cross section, a hair follicle looks rather like an onion, with several rings or layers. The central part is the **hair shaft**, which has a scaly surface called the **cuticle**. The hair shaft is surrounded by an **inner root sheath** (with its own cuticle) and **outer root sheath**. The outer root sheath is covered by a **connective tissue sheath**. The deep end of the hair follicle is expanded into the **hair bulb**, which is composed of a **dermal papilla** (**hair papilla**) and a **hair root** composed mostly of the hair matrix. The **hair matrix** is capable of cell division and gives rise to the hair shaft. (3) The *nail* is a translucent keratinized hard plate resting on the dorsum of the tip of each digit. The nail plate stems from the base of the nail (**nail matrix**) and grows over the nail bed toward the tip of the finger or toe. The components of the nail include the **nail root** (**nail matrix**), **nail plate**, the **eponychium** (**nail cuticle**), **perionychium** (**nail wall**), and **hyponychium**.

Structure of the Skin

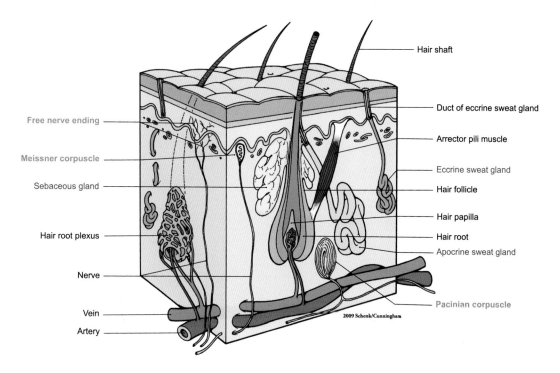

Hair shaft

Free nerve ending

Duct of eccrine sweat gland

Meissner corpuscle

Arrector pili muscle

Sebaceous gland

Eccrine sweat gland

Hair follicle

Hair papilla

Hair root plexus

Hair root

Apocrine sweat gland

Nerve

Vein

Pacinian corpuscle

Artery

2009 Schenk/Cunningham

Figure 13-1. Overview of skin structure.

The **skin** is composed of **epithelium, connective tissue, muscles, nerves, blood vessels,** and **associated structures (glands, hair follicles, and nails).** It can be divided into two basic layers: **epidermis** and **dermis.** The *epidermis* is the superficial layer of the skin. It consists of a stratified squamous epithelium. The *dermis* is a layer of connective tissue beneath the epidermis. There is a transition layer between the skin and underlying muscle called the **hypodermis** (subcutaneous layer), which, strictly speaking, is not a component of the skin but is closely associated with the skin. This layer contains loose connective tissue, adipose tissue, nerves, arteries, and veins. The skin contains several sensory structures, which respond to somatosensory stimuli. These include **free nerve endings** (pain or temperature), **Merkel disks** (continuous touch), and **Meissner corpuscles** (touch). **Pacinian corpuscles** (vibration) can be found in the subcutaneous layer (hypodermis). For the function and details of the sensory receptors, see Chapter 7, "Nervous Tissue." There are several types of glands in the skin, including **sebaceous glands, eccrine sweat glands,** and **apocrine sweat glands.**

Structures of the Skin

I. **Layers of the skin**
  A. **Epidermis**
    1. Stratum corneum
    2. Stratum lucidum
    3. Stratum granulosum
    4. Stratum spinosum
    5. Stratum basale
  B. **Dermis**
    1. Papillary layer
      a. Free nerve endings
      b. Meissner corpuscles
    2. Reticular layer
      a. Loose connective tissue
      b. Adipose tissue
      c. Arteries and veins
II. **Hypodermis (subcutaneous layer)**
    1. Loose connective tissue
    2. Adipose tissue
    3. Pacinian corpuscles
    4. Arteries and veins
    5. Nerves

III. **Accessory structures**
  A. **Glands**
    1. Sebaceous glands
    2. Eccrine sweat glands
    3. Apocrine sweat glands
  B. **Hair**
    1. Hair shaft
    2. Hair follicles
  C. **Nail**
    1. Nail bed
    2. Nail matrix
    3. Eponychium
    4. Hyponychium
  D. **Sensory receptors**
    1. Meissner corpuscles
    2. Free nerve endings
    3. Pacinian corpuscles
    4. Merkel cells (Merkel cell neurite complexes or Merkel disks)

Blood Supply to the Skin

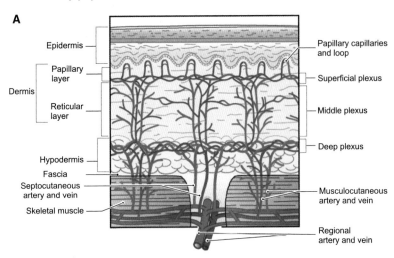

Figure 13-2A. Blood supply to the skin.

Vascular supply to the skin emerges from blood vessels traversing through and along the fasciae and superficial muscles. The arteries form a series of networks within the dermis. The capillary loops are located in the dermal papillae and drain blood into the subpapillary plexus. The vascular network associated with the skin includes: (1) the **subpapillary plexus**, the most superficial network that lies at the bases of the papillae, where the smallest arteries, arterioles, connect with capillaries and venules from which fluid and nutrients pass to nourish basal epidermal cells. (2) The **dermal plexus**, a vascular network located in the reticular layer of the dermis, contains arteriovenous anastomoses that connect arterioles directly to the venules and is important for thermoregulation. (3) The **subdermal plexus** (**deep plexus**), located between the dermis and hypodermis, provides main branches of arterial supply to the skin and drains blood back into the veins in this plexus. (4) The **subcutaneous plexus** contains **musculocutaneous, septocutaneous arteries,** and **fasciocutaneous arteries**. These arteries receive blood supply from a regional artery and drain blood from the subdermal plexus. Other capillary plexuses surround hair follicles and associated glands. Blood supply to the skin can be random or derived from a named source.

A flap is a tissue with a persistent blood supply, which does not depend on perfusion from the recipient bed to survive. It can be skin, fascia, muscle, bone, or a combination of these tissues. A flap can be removed with a single identifiable artery and vein from its original location and transferred to a new remote area while maintaining its blood supply. **Flaps** are used to fill large defects and recreate structures in reconstructive surgery. A **graft** is a piece of tissue that has been detached from its blood supply and therefore should regain a blood supply from the recipient bed to survive. Both skin grafts and skin flaps are used in reconstructive surgery.

CLINICAL CORRELATION

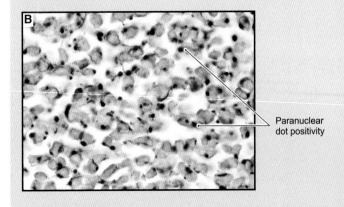

Paranuclear
dot positivity

Figure 13-2B. Merkel Cell Carcinoma. Cytokeratin 20 staining (CK 20), ×600

Merkel cell carcinoma is an aggressive **neuroendocrine carcinoma** of the skin. It is thought to arise from **Merkel cells**, which normally are scarce in the basal layer of the epidermis. Merkel cells are believed to function as touch receptors. Merkel cell carcinoma normally arises in sun-exposed areas of the head and neck in older patients. On histologic examination, Merkel cell carcinomas appear as "**small blue cell tumors**" in the dermis, and they typically do not exhibit a point of connection to the epidermis from which they originate. These tumors typically show a high mitotic rate with occasional apoptotic cells. These tumors metastasize to local lymph nodes, and distant metastases can also occur. In keeping with the neuroendocrine nature of Merkel cells, these carcinomas typically express neuroendocrine markers such as *synaptophysin*. On certain cytokeratin immunohistochemical stains, such as cytokeratin 20, a characteristic **paranuclear dotlike positivity** is observed. A pathologist must differentiate this entity from tumors that metastasize to the skin, such as small cell carcinoma of the lung.

Development of the Skin

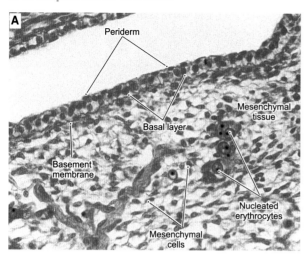

Figure 13-3A. Fetal skin (weeks 5–9). H&E, ×331

The two layers (**epidermis** and **dermis**) of the skin develop from two different embryonic tissues. The *epidermis* develops from the **ectoderm**, and the *dermis* from the **mesoderm**. About 4 weeks after conception, the human embryo is covered by a single layer of ectodermal cells, which are loosely arranged on the **basement membrane** and over the **mesenchymal tissue**. After 5 weeks, the epidermis has two layers of cells: the superficial layer (**periderm**) and **basal layers**. At 2 to 3 months, basal cells are dividing rapidly, and the epidermis becomes several cell layers thick. At the same time, the mesenchyme differentiates into a more mature connective tissue with blood vessels. By 4 months, neural crest cells migrate into the basal layer of the epidermis and differentiate into melanocytes and Merkel cells. The connective tissue layer beneath the epithelium develops into the dermis and a deeper layer, the hypodermis. At about 5 months, the appendages of the skin (hair follicles and glands) start to form. This section shows an early stage of skin development in an embryo. There are only two layers of epithelial cells in the epidermis, and fetal blood vessels are located within the mesenchyme tissue. **Nucleated erythrocytes** are shown inside the blood vessels.

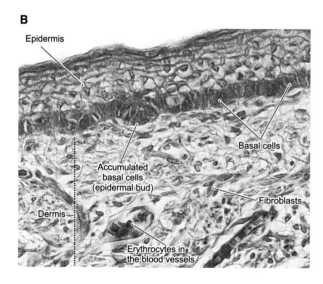

Figure 13-3B. Fetal skin (month 5). H&E, ×438

This section shows a later stage of fetal skin development. The epidermis has formed multiple cell layers, and four layers of **epidermis** can be distinguished to some extent. The **basal cells** in the stratum basale layer are highly active and appear as column-shaped cells. The underlying mesenchymal tissue has differentiated into connective tissue (**dermis**). There are many active **fibroblasts** in the dermis. An accumulation of basal cells forms a fold called an **epidermal bud**, which projects into the dermis. These accumulated cells will interact with the dermis and differentiate into **appendages** (**hair follicles** and **glands**).

SYNOPSIS 13-1 Pathologic Terms for the Integumentary System

- *Acanthosis:* Thickening of the stratum spinosum of the epidermis, typically seen in epidermal hyperplasia.
- *Hypergranulosis:* Thickening and prominence of the stratum granulosum of the epidermis, often in response to chronic mechanical irritation of the skin. Hypergranulosis may also be seen in the declivities of papillary lesions such as verruca vulgaris, or warts.
- *Hyperkeratosis:* Thickening of the stratum corneum of the epidermis. Orthokeratotic hyperkeratosis refers to hyperkeratosis without the presence of nuclei.
- *Papillomatosis:* Fingerlike projections from the epidermal surface, often with hyperkeratosis, seen in a variety of conditions including verruca vulgaris, or warts.
- *Parakeratosis:* A form of hyperkeratosis in which nuclei are retained in the stratum corneum, seen in many conditions including psoriasis.
- *Spongiosis:* Intercellular edema of the epidermis frequently seen in various etiologies of dermatitis such as allergic contact dermatitis or irritant dermatitis.
- *Ulceration:* The discontinuity of an epithelial surface including the epidermis or mucous membranes.

Layers of the Epidermis

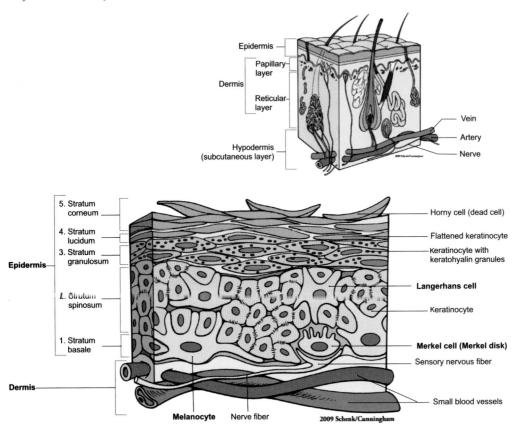

Figure 13-4. Overview of epidermis layers.

The **epidermis** is composed of five cell layers. (1) The **stratum basale** is composed of a single layer of cuboidal or tall cuboidal cells, **melanocytes** and **Merkel cells**, which are also called **Merkel cell neurite complexes** or **Merkel disks**. Many of these cells are actually **stem cells**; they divide continuously and migrate from the basal layer toward the surface and give rise to keratinocytes in the other layers. (2) The **stratum spinosum** contains polygon-shaped keratinocytes with many tonofilament bundles in their cytoplasm. These cells are interconnected with each other by desmosomes. **Langerhans cells** are often found in this layer. The stratum basale and the stratum spinosum are the only layers with mitotically active cells, and, together, they are also called the **Malpighian layer**. (3) The **stratum granulosum** contains three to five layers of **keratinocytes** with flattened nuclei. The cytoplasm of the cells is filled with basophilic keratohyalin granules from which the name derives. The cytoplasm also contains lamellar granules, which can release their contents into the intercellular spaces to help seal the skin, preventing water loss. This layer is more obvious in thick skin; only a single cell layer is visible in thin skin. (4) The **stratum lucidum** is a very thin, clear layer that contains keratinocytes with pycnotic nuclei. This layer is found only in thick skin. (5) The **stratum corneum** is the top layer of the epidermis. It contains many layers of flattened cells filled with mature keratin. These are **dead cells** with no nuclei or organelles. The cells in this layer, which are constantly replaced by cells from deeper layers, form a barrier to prevent loss of water and entry of pathogens. This layer is much thicker in thick skin than in thin skin.

SYNOPSIS 13-2 Functions of the Skin

- *Protection* of body from invasion of pathogens; prevention of tissue damage by toxic chemicals and ultraviolet light
- *Prevention* of dehydration and loss of body fluids (impermeable to water)
- *Regulation* of body temperature (production and excretion of sweat, vascular shunts)
- *Sensation* of touch, pain, temperature, pressure, and vibration; important for communication, dexterity, and injury prevention
- *Immunological function* of Langerhans cells (antigen-presenting cells) present antigens to lymphocytes in the immune responses (see Chapter 10, "Lymphoid System")
- *Production* of vitamin D from precursors under the effects of steroids and sunlight

KERATINOCYTES IN THE STRATUM CORNEUM

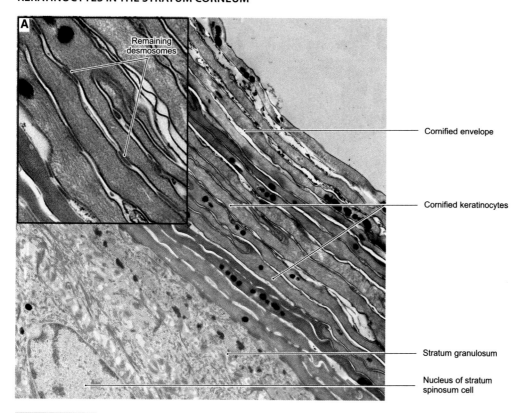

Figure 13-5A. Stratum corneum of the epidermis, thin skin. EM, ×8,065; inset ×21,889

The **stratum corneum** is the final product of the proliferation and differentiation that take place in the deeper layers of the epidermis. The dead cells (**horny cells**) of the stratum corneum have lost the usual organelles and have become filled with mature **keratin**, a tough network of keratin intermediate filaments that are cross-linked by the protein filaggrin. Keratin and the persisting **desmosomes** between cells account for the mechanical strength of the epidermis. Contributing to the relative impermeability of the stratum corneum is a coating of involucrin linked to the inner surfaces of the plasma membrane and the presence of lipid that has been secreted into the spaces between cells. In this specimen of thin skin, the **stratum granulosum** is only one cell thick, and some of its characteristic features (**keratohyalin granules** and **lamellar granules**) are not clearly discernible. Bundles of **tonofilaments, melanin granules**, and **desmosomes** can be distinguished.

CLINICAL CORRELATION

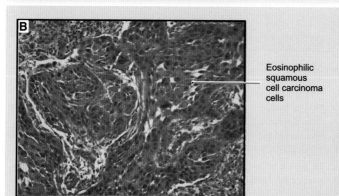

Figure 13-5B. Squamous Cell Carcinoma. H&E, ×108

Squamous cell carcinoma (SCC) is the second most common form of skin neoplasm. It originates from keratinocytes of the epidermis. This carcinoma is characterized by a slow-growing reddish or ulcerated lesion with hard, raised borders. It is often found in sun-exposed areas, with a high incidence in elderly male Caucasians. Prolonged sun exposure, chronic inflammatory lesions, and genetic factors, especially *p53 tumor suppressor gene* mutations, contribute to the development of the disease. SCCs called **actinic keratoses** commonly arise in premalignant lesions on sun-damaged skin. Carcinoma cells have enlarged and hyperchromatic nuclei with variable differentiation, some lesions producing abundant keratin. Treatment includes surgical excision, cryosurgery, electrosurgery, radiation therapy, and topical treatment.

KERATINOCYTES IN THE STRATUM SPINOSUM

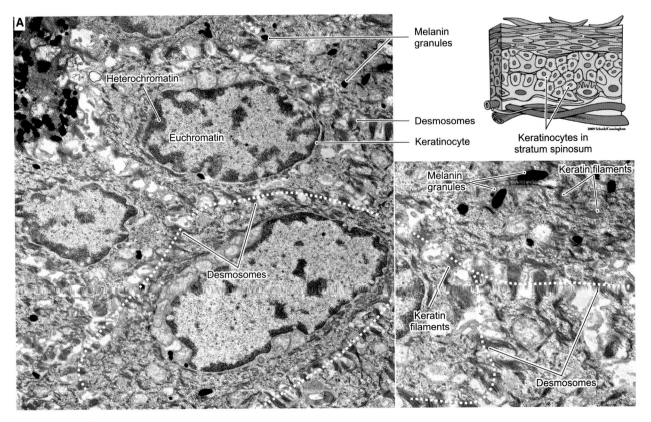

Figure 13-6A.   Keratinocytes in stratum spinosum, thin skin. EM, ×7,097 (*left*); ×12,390 (*right*)

The **stratum spinosum** gets its name from the many small processes that seem to join neighboring cells with one another. The basis for these spines is obvious in this transmission electron micrograph. Each cell is joined to its neighbors by numerous **maculae adherens (desmosomes)**, and the spines reflect the persistence of these connections after some cell shrinkage has occurred during processing of the tissue. The electron dense tuft of material evident on either side of each desmosome is a bundle of **tonofilaments** anchored into the **attachment plaques** at the cytoplasmic faces of the desmosomes. The desmosomes and tonofilament bundles are numerous and more easily seen in the higher magnification view in the right-hand panel. As indicated by the extensive **euchromatin** in the nuclei of these cells, the **keratinocytes** are actively synthesizing proteins, most prominently subunits of **keratin filaments**, which will function in establishing a tough, impermeable barrier layer at the surface of the skin.

CLINICAL CORRELATION

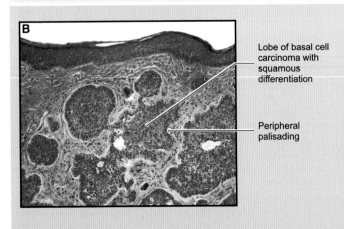

Lobe of basal cell carcinoma with squamous differentiation

Peripheral palisading

Figure 13-6B.   Basal Cell Carcinoma. H&E, ×50

Basal cell carcinoma is the most common form of malignant skin neoplasm. It originates from the basal layer of epidermis and often occurs on sun-exposed areas. Basal cell carcinoma rarely metastasizes and is usually non–life threatening if addressed early. Local invasion may damage surrounding tissues causing cosmetic concerns. Genetics and long-term exposure to ultraviolet light and arsenical compounds contribute to the disease. Clinically, basal cell carcinoma appears as pearly white nodules or waxy bumps on the face or neck with telangiectatic blood vessels. Subtypes of basal cell carcinoma include **nodular, superficial, pigmented,** and **fibrosing.** Histologic features include a **lobular growth pattern** of malignant basal cells with **peripheral palisading** and retraction of lobules from the surrounding stroma. Treatment includes surgical excision, cryosurgery, curettage, and electrodessication.

SPECIAL TYPE OF CELLS IN THE EPIDERMIS

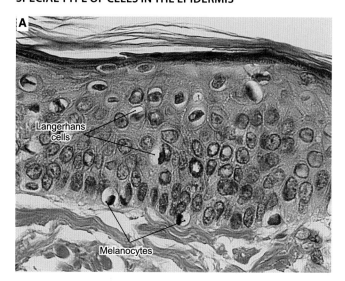

Figure 13-7A. Special types of cells in the epidermis, thin skin. H&E, ×281

Keratinocytes make up the bulk of the epidermis, but there are additional cell types: **melanocytes**, **Merkel cells**, and **Langerhans cells**. All three types of cells have clear cytoplasm and are sometimes called **clear cells**. It is difficult to distinguish among them in H&E-stained sections. Melanocytes and Merkel cells are both located in the stratum basale where they are scattered among the basal cuboidal cells. In contrast, Langerhans cells are typically found in the stratum spinosum. The functions of the three cells are quite different: (1) *Melanocytes* produce melanin granules and insert them into keratinocytes. (2) *Merkel cells* are receptor cells, which establish synaptic contacts with sensory nerve terminals; they have cytoplasmic granules, which contain neurotransmitters. (3) *Langerhans cells* are monocyte derivatives, which play an important role in capturing antigens and presenting them to lymphocytes, thereby participating in the cutaneous immune response. Langerhans cells make no desmosome junctions with neighbors; indeed, their function requires that they be motile so that they can transport any captured antigens from the epidermis to lymph nodes deep to the skin.

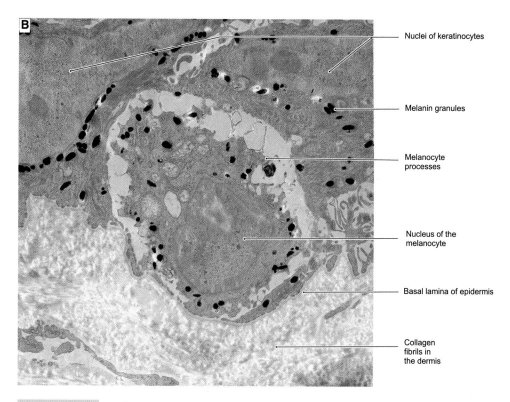

Figure 13-7B. Melanocyte. EM, ×8,129

Melanocytes, along with Merkel cells, are the two clear cell types found in the stratum basale of the epidermis. The two cells cannot be distinguished in conventionally prepared sections for light microscopy, but each has distinctive ultrastructural features. The melanocyte generates **melanin granules** and injects them into nearby **keratinocytes**. This is a continuous process because keratinocytes are constantly replaced as they differentiate and move toward the surface. The melanin protects the cells, particularly the nucleus, from the mutagenic effects of ultraviolet irradiation. As shown here, the melanocyte contacts the **basal lamina** of the epidermis, but it does not establish desmosome junctions with the keratinocytes.

MELANOCYTE AND MELANOSOME FORMATION

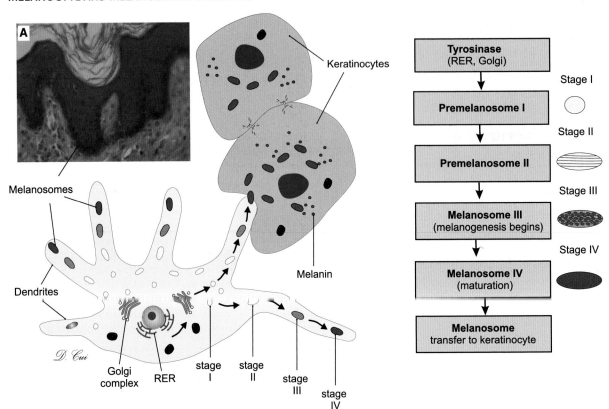

Figure 13-8A. Melanosome formation and maturation (melanogenesis).

Melanocytes are dendritic cells that differentiate from **melanoblasts**, which are derived from neural crest cells. Melanocytes are located at the **stratum basale** layer of the epidermis. Mature melanocytes are capable of producing melanosomes. Melanosomes are lysosome-related organelles that store and transfer melanin (pigments) to keratinocytes. The formation and maturation of melanosomes (melanogenesis) include four stages. (1) **Stage I (premelanosome I)**: In this initial stage, the first melanosome precursors are small, spherical, amorphous matrix–containing vesicles, which are released from the Golgi complexes of melanocytes. (2) **Stage II (premelanosome II)**: The second stage melanosome precursors are elongated vesicles with a parallel fibrillary matrix. In this stage, melanin has not yet been synthesized, but the **tyrosinase** is present. Tyrosinase is a melanocyte-specific protein important for melanin formation. Tyrosinase is synthesized in the rough endoplasmic reticulum (RER) and packaged and modified by the Golgi complex. Both melanosome precursors in stage I and II are nonpigmented and known as **premelanosomes**. (3) **Stage III (melanosome III)**: In this third stage, **melanin synthesis begins** in which the melanosomes begin producing melanin, and melanin pigments are deposited on the matrix fibrils within the large vesicles. These melanosomes appear brown in color. (4) **Stage IV (melanosome IV)**: This fourth and final stage denotes **melanosome maturation** in which melanosomes are filled with melanin pigment, and tyrosinase has lost activity at this point. Mature melanosomes appear dark brown to black in color at this stage. As soon as melanosomes become mature, the dendrites of melanocytes transfer the mature melanosomes into the cytoplasm and perinuclear region of keratinocytes. The melanin pigment granules are released from melanosomes within the keratinocytes. Melanin synthesis is ultimately stimulated by ultraviolet (UV) radiation and melanocyte-stimulating hormone secreted by keratinocytes. There are two types of melanin associated with skin: **eumelanin** and **pheomelanin**. **Eumelanin** is brown to black in color, and it determines the color of the skin. Pheomelanin is yellow to red in color and is more associated with hair color. Functions of melanin include absorption of UV radiation for protecting skin from damage by the sun and the regulation of ions for pigmentation. Basal cell and squamous cell skin cancer are associated with cumulative exposure to UV radiation.

CLINICAL CORRELATION

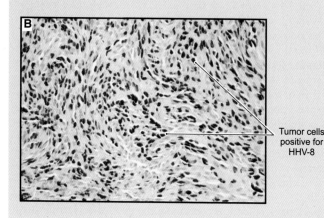

Tumor cells positive for HHV-8

Figure 13-8B. Kaposi Sarcoma. HHV-8 immunohistochemistry, ×200

Kaposi sarcoma (KS) is a vascular neoplasm that exists in four types including **classic, endemic, transplant-associated,** and **epidemic,** or those associated with **HIV infection.** Historically, KS affected older individuals in certain populations including those of Mediterranean origin, Jews, and Eastern Europeans. All types of KS are strongly associated with **human herpesvirus type 8 (HHV-8).** KS primarily affects the **skin,** but it may also affect **mucosal surfaces** and **viscera.** The clinical presentation of KS is varied, but skin lesions typically begin as **red to purple patches** that are macular (not raised above the surrounding skin), and then they form **plaques,** which become palpable as they become raised above the surrounding skin. Eventually the plaques become **large nodules.** Treatment of the HIV-associated form of KS involves **antiretroviral therapy** and **chemotherapy** or **radiotherapy** if the lesions do not regress.

Thick Skin

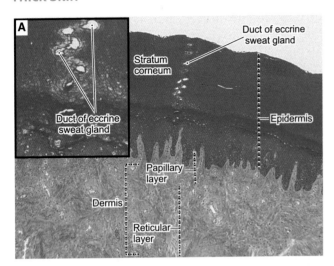

Figure 13-9A.   Thick skin, palm. H&E, ×34; inset ×116

The skin can be classified into **thick skin** and **thin skin** based on the thickness of the epidermis. *Thick skin* has a thick epidermis (400–600 μm) with five distinct cell layers. The **stratum corneum** is extremely thick in this skin. Thick skin covers the palms of the hands and soles of the feet. Thick skin has abundant eccrine sweat glands and lacks hair follicles. The epidermis is a stratified squamous epithelium. Because it is an avascular tissue (no direct blood supply), nutrients are delivered to the tissue by fluid diffusion from the dermis (connective tissue). The dermis is composed of a superficial **papillary layer**, a layer of loose connective tissue, and a deeper **reticular layer**, which is a thick layer of dense irregular connective tissue. This section shows thick epidermis containing the duct of an **eccrine sweat gland**.

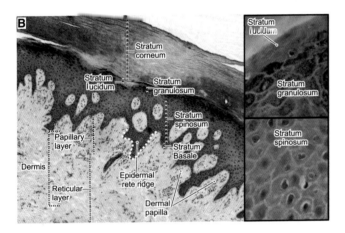

Figure 13-9B.   Layers of the epidermis, palm. H&E, ×68; insets ×422

The **epidermis** of thick skin has five layers. (1) The **stratum basale** contains a single layer of cuboidal/tall cuboidal cells (**stem cells**) and sits upon the basement membrane. This layer forms a dividing line between the epidermis and dermis (*dotted line*). (2) The **stratum spinosum** contains 5 to 10 layers of polyhedral keratinocytes, flattened toward the surface. These cells are also called **prickle cells**. (3) The **stratum granulosum** contains three to five layers of flattened keratinocytes filled with keratohyaline granules, which appear dark blue here. (4) The **stratum lucidum** is a very thin layer containing extremely flattened and tightly packed keratinocytes filled with keratin filaments. Their nuclei are beginning to be eliminated. (5) The **stratum corneum** is a layer of dead, nonnucleated cells, which form the most superficial layer of the skin. Cells in this layer are constantly sloughed off and replaced by new cells.

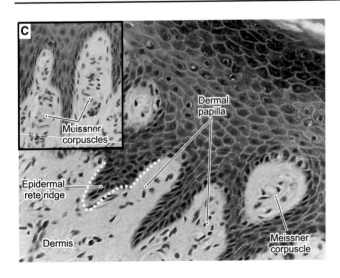

Figure 13-9C.   Dermal papilla, palm. H&E, ×272; inset ×192

The border between the epidermis and dermis (*dotted white line*) is expanded into folds. The **dermis** is a connective tissue layer, which contains **blood vessels, nerves,** and **sensory receptors** (**free nerve endings** and **Meissner corpuscles**). The portion of the epidermis that projects into the dermis is termed the **epidermal rete ridge**, and the portion of the dermis that projects into the epidermis is called the **dermal papilla**. This unique feature increases the contact area between these two layers, preventing the epidermis from detaching from the dermis. The dermal papilla contains loose connective tissue that includes many capillaries, free nerve endings, and encapsulated sensory receptors. **Meissner corpuscles** are shown here. The nerve fibers cannot be seen in H&E stains; demonstration of nerve fibers requires special stains (see Chapter 7, "Nervous Tissue"). Meissner corpuscles are responsible for discriminative touch and are more numerous in thick skin such as at the tips of the fingers. These receptors help us to distinguish between, for example, different coins by touch alone.

Thin Skin

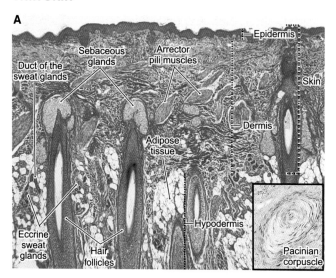

A

Duct of the sweat glands
Sebaceous glands
Arrector pili muscles
Epidermis
Skin
Dermis
Adipose tissue
Hypodermis
Eccrine sweat glands
Hair follicles
Pacinian corpuscle

Figure 13-10A. **Thin skin, scalp.** H&E, ×25; inset ×84

Thin skin covers the entire body surface except for the palms of the hands and the soles of the feet. Thin skin has a thin epidermis, largely because its stratum corneum is much reduced compared to that of thick skin. In contrast to thick skin, thin skin contains **hair follicles** and their associated **sebaceous glands**. This section shows the **epidermis** and **dermis** of the skin and a deeper layer of subcutaneous tissue called the **hypodermis**. The hypodermis is a layer of loose connective tissue, which contains **adipose tissue**, nerves, arteries, and veins. The nerves give off branches, which provide the various types of sensory and autonomic nerve endings in the dermis. **Pacinian corpuscles**, sensory receptors that respond to vibration stimuli, are found in the hypodermis of both thin and thick skin. They are found in many regions of the body but are more numerous in the tips of the fingers and toes than in other areas. The hypodermis serves as a transition layer, providing the dermis with a flexible attachment to the underlying muscles and other structures.

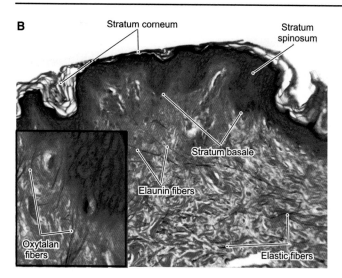

B

Stratum corneum
Stratum spinosum
Stratum basale
Elaunin fibers
Oxytalan fibers
Elastic fibers

Figure 13-10B. **Thin skin.** Elastic fiber stain, ×142; inset ×487

The epidermis of **thin skin** consists of four layers, including the **stratum basale, stratum spinosum, stratum granulosum,** and **stratum corneum.** (The stratum lucidum is absent in thin skin.) The *stratum granulosum* is very thin, often only a single cell layer, and it is not easily distinguished in thin skin. The *stratum corneum* is thin but varies in thickness from region to region. This section is stained with an elastic fiber stain, which shows the elastic fibers in the dermis. These fibers become very fine toward the epidermis. The dermis contains type I collagen fibers and elastic fibers, which give the skin flexibility and strength. The *inset* shows a few very fine fibers called **oxytalan fibers.** The elastic fibers can be classified into three types based on their **microfibril** and **elastin** content: (1) **elastic fibers,** the largest fibers, containing predominantly elastin; (2) **elaunin fibers,** intermediate in size, containing small amounts of amorphous elastin; and (3) **oxytalan fibers,** the smallest fibers, containing only microfibrils.

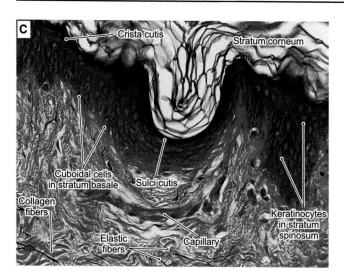

C

Crista cutis
Stratum corneum
Cuboidal cells in stratum basale
Sulci cutis
Collagen fibers
Keratinocytes in stratum spinosum
Elastic fibers
Capillary

Figure 13-10C. **Stratum corneum, thin skin.** Elastic fiber stain, ×284

Fine grooves (**sulci cutis**) and **elevated areas** (**cristae cutis**) are the basis of the varying surface contours characteristic of specific areas of both thin skin and thick skin. The orientation of the grooves varies from region to region. Fingerprints (**dermatoglyphics**) are a good example of a skin pattern, which is distinctive. The top layer of the epidermis, the **stratum corneum,** is composed of several layers of flattened and cornified keratinocytes. These cells have no nuclei and are filled with **keratin,** which helps to stabilize the cells against physical stress. This layer of cells is constantly sloughed off and replaced by differentiating cells from beneath. In this section, the extensive spaces between the dead cells of the stratum corneum are artifacts of specimen preparation. Some of the **cuboidal cells** in the **stratum basale** are stem cells capable of cell division. Some cells derived by division of the stem cells remain in the stratum basale as stem cells and some begin differentiation in the stratum spinosum. **Keratinocytes** undergo an orderly sequence of differentiation (**keratinization**) and cell death (**apoptosis**) as they move up toward the surface of the epidermis.

CLINICAL CORRELATIONS

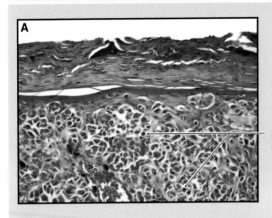

Melanoma (tumor) cells

Figure 13-11A. Malignant Melanoma. H&E, ×198

Melanoma is an aggressive malignant skin neoplasm originating from melanocytes of the skin. It is characterized by significant morphologic diversity, with skin lesions of irregular shapes and various degrees of pigmentation. Melanoma metastasizes via the lymphatic system. Malignant melanoma is less common than basal cell or SCCs, but it causes the majority of deaths from skin cancer. Genetic factors and sun exposure contribute to the development of the disease. The most common forms of melanoma include **superficial spreading melanoma** and **nodular malignant melanoma**. Melanoma cells contain large nuclei with irregular contours, often with prominent nucleoli. Treatment includes surgical excision, chemotherapy, radiation therapy, and immunotherapy.

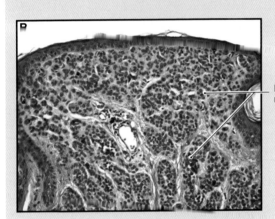

Nests of nevus cells

Figure 13-11B. Melanocytic Nevus. H&E, ×22

Melanocytic nevi, commonly referred to as "moles," may be **congenital** or acquired and are composed of melanocytes in **nests** at the dermo-epidermo junction, in the dermis, or both. If the nevus cells are restricted to the dermis, the lesion is referred to as a **dermal melanocytic nevus**. If the nevus cells are present only at the dermo-epidermo junction, the lesion is referred to as a **junctional nevus**. If the nevus cells are present in both locations, the term **compound nevus** is used. Moles typically appear as raised tan to brown soft lesions on sun-exposed or sun-restricted skin. **Dysplastic nevi**, which may transform to malignant melanoma, are typically larger than most nevi, may have irregular borders, and pigmentary variation. Microscopically, dysplastic nevi may show larger junctional nests that fuse to adjacent nests and cytologic atypia. This image shows a dermal melanocytic nevus with no evidence of dysplasia or atypia.

TABLE 13-1   Comparison of Thick and Thin Skin

Type of Skin	Epidermis	Hair/Hair Follicles	Glands	Sensory Receptors	Location/ Distribution	Special Features
Thick skin	Five layers; thick stratum corneum; thick stratum granulosum	No	Lack of sebaceous glands; more eccrine sweat glands	More receptors	Palms of the hand and soles of the feet	*Thick epidermis:* thick stratum corneum; stratum lucidum present; several cell layers of stratum granulosum
Thin skin	Four layers; no stratum lucidum; single layer of or no stratum granulosum	Present in most areas (except a few places, such as lips, labia minora, and glans penis)	Many sebaceous glands; fewer eccrine sweat glands	Fewer receptors	Entire body except thick skin areas	*Thin epidermis:* thin stratum corneum; stratum lucidum absent; one layer or no stratum granulosum

Accessory Structures

GLANDS OF THE SKIN

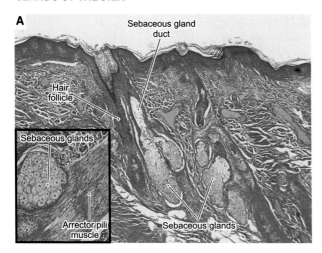

A

Sebaceous gland duct

Hair follicle

Sebaceous glands

Arrector pili muscle

Sebaceous glands

Figure 13-12A. Sebaceous gland, thin skin (scalp). H&E, ×35; inset ×66

Sebaceous glands are found in thin skin, usually associated with hair follicles. They are most numerous in the skin of the scalp and face. Sebaceous glands are classified as **simple branched acinar glands** (see Chapter 3, "Epithelium and Glands"). The secretory cells are lipid-producing cells, arranged into several acini, which open into a short duct. Usually, the ducts of sebaceous glands empty their oily secretion, called **sebum**, into a **hair follicle**; however, the ducts sometimes open directly onto the surface of the skin. Sebaceous glands release their products by **holocrine secretion**, that is, by the disintegration of entire cells. Sebum lubricates the skin and coats and protects hair shafts from becoming brittle. The *inset* shows an acinus of a sebaceous gland and a nearby **arrector pili muscle**. Arrector pili muscles are bundles of sympathetically innervated smooth muscle cells that span between hair follicles and the papillary layer of the dermis. They contract to stand the hair up in response to cold or fear.

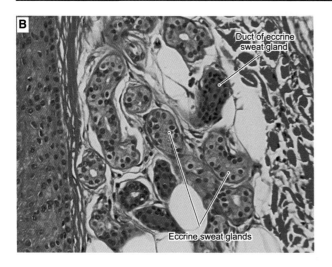

B

Duct of eccrine sweat gland

Eccrine sweat glands

Figure 13-12B. Eccrine sweat gland, thin skin (scalp). H&E, ×248

Eccrine (merocrine) sweat glands can be found in both thin and thick skin over most of the body. They are more numerous in the palms and soles. Eccrine sweat glands produce a clear watery product called **sweat**. These glands are simple glands in which the secretory cells are arranged into coiled tubules. These glands have long unbranched, but coiled, ducts, which are lined by two layers of cuboidal cells and open directly onto the surface of the skin. Sweat consists mainly of water (99%), some ions (K^+, Na^+, and Cl^-), waste, and metabolic products. Releasing sweat onto the surface of the skin helps adjust body temperature as well as aiding in the excretion of metabolic wastes. The secretory units of eccrine sweat glands contain three cell types. (1) **Dark cells** are pyramid-shaped cells containing dark secretory granules. These cells lie toward the lumen of the tubule. (2) **Clear cells** are also pyramid shaped and have no secretory granules but have ultrastructural features of ion pumping cells. They are located toward the basement membrane. (3) **Myoepithelial cells** are not secretory cells. They are spindle-shaped contractile cells, which help to push secretory products into and along the lumen.

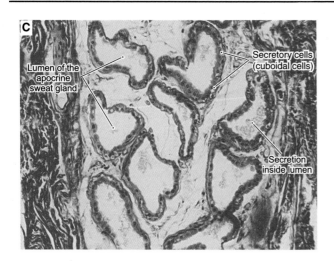

C

Lumen of the apocrine sweat gland

Secretory cells (cuboidal cells)

Secretion inside lumen

Figure 13-12C. Apocrine sweat gland, labia. H&E, ×248

Apocrine sweat glands are simple coiled tubular glands like the eccrine sweat glands, but their **lumens** are larger (about 10 times larger than those of the eccrine sweat glands) and their ducts empty into the superficial regions of the hair follicles. The **secretory cells** of the apocrine glands release their products by shedding part of their apical cytoplasm; this is called **apocrine secretion**. The tubules of the glands are lined by cuboidal or columnar epithelial cells, depending on the secretory stage. These glands are influenced by hormones and start to function at puberty. They are also called **sexual scent glands**. They are restricted in location to some specific regions of thin skin, such as the axilla, the areola (nipple), and the perianal and genital areas. Their product is a viscous, thick, milky fluid that contains protein, ammonia, lipids, and carbohydrates. These secretory fluids are odorless when they are released but may have an axillary body odor after degradation by bacteria.

HAIR FOLLICLES

A

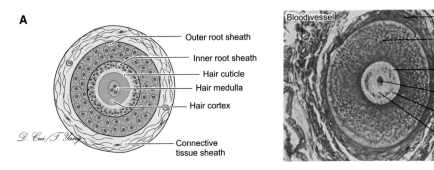

Figure 13-13A. Hair follicle. H&E, ×95

A cross section of a hair follicle is shown on the *left* and a photomicrograph of a cross section of a hair follicle from the scalp on the *right*. The structures of the hair follicle containing a hair shaft include (from inside to outside) the **hair medulla** (thin core of the hair shaft), the **hair cortex** (keratinized cells surrounding the medulla), the **hair cuticle** (outermost layer of the hair shaft), the **inner root sheath** (cellular sheath that extends from the hair bulb and surrounds and grows along with the hair), the **outer root sheath** (a cellular sheath, which is a continuation of the epidermis), and the **connective tissue sheath** (**dermal root sheath**).

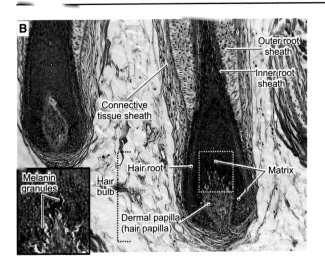

Figure 13-13B. Hair follicles, thin skin (scalp). H&E, ×78; inset ×172

Hair follicles are the structures that produce the hair and maintain hair growth. They are cellular structures extending from the epidermis into the dermis or hypodermis. The basal region of the hair follicle forms a balloon-shaped structure called the **hair bulb**, which is composed of the hair root and the dermal papilla. The **hair root** contains melanocytes and a group of epithelial cells called the **matrix** or **germinal matrix**. These cells are capable of cell division and give rise to the **inner root sheath** and to the hair. The epithelial cells form a cap around the **dermal papilla** (**hair papilla**). The dermal papilla contains capillaries and nerve fibers that supply the hair follicle. The interaction between the hair bulb and dermal papilla induces hair follicle differentiation and the growth of the hair. The photomicrograph shows a longitudinal section of hair follicles. The *inset* shows **melanin granules**, which give color to the hair. The melanin granules are produced by melanocytes in the hair bulb.

CLINICAL CORRELATION

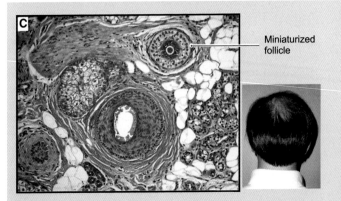

Figure 13-13C. Androgenetic Alopecia. H&E, ×50.

Androgenetic alopecia is the most common form of hair loss, affecting 30% to 40% of the adult population. Males and females have a similar incidence in developing this type of hair loss, characterized by varying degrees of partial hair thinning from the vertex and frontal areas of the scalp. In females, it rarely leads to total baldness. In males, the cause is both **genetic** and **androgen dependent**. Patients usually have higher levels of 5-alpha-reductase and androgen receptors. **5-Alpha-reductase** increases production of **dihydrotestosterone**, which binds to the androgen receptors in susceptible follicles to trigger the genes to miniaturize the follicles and weaken hair growth. Treatment options include the oral medication **finasteride** and topical solutions of minoxidil. This cross section of scalp tissue shows variation in hair follicle size with **miniaturized follicles** and the absence of inflammation.

NAILS

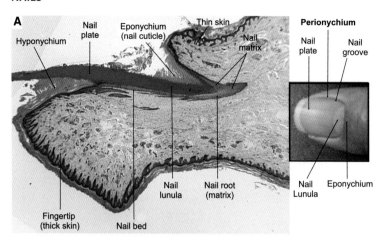

Figure 13-14A. Nail, finger. H&E, ×17

The **nail** is a translucent, hard, keratinized sheet resting on the tip of each digit. It includes many components: (1) the **nail plate**, the nail itself, which is hard keratin; (2) the **nail root**, also called the **nail matrix**, seen as the **lunula** in the living state; (3) the **nail bed**, a layer of epidermis beneath the nail plate; (4) the **eponychium**, also called the **nail cuticle**, which is the junction zone between the skin of the finger and the nail plate and which forms a protective seal; (5) the **perionychium** (**nail wall**), the skin that surrounds the edge of the nail; and (6) the **hyponychium**, the junction seal between the nail plate and the skin of the fingertip. All of the sealed areas at the edges of the nail plate protect the delicate nail matrix and nail bed from dehydration and infection.

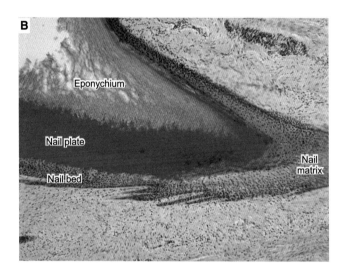

Figure 13-14B. Nail root (matrix) and nail bed. H&E, ×69

The **nail root** is a cellular layer and is also called the **matrix** or **germinal matrix**. It contains many layers of epithelial cells, which are responsible for the production of the **nail plate**. These cells proliferate and become flattened and highly keratinized and are pushed forward by newly formed cells. As they differentiate, the cells finally lose color and shape and become part of the nail plate. The nail plate is similar to the hair shaft, but the pattern of keratin formation is different. The nail bed (equivalent to the epidermis) rests under the nail plate. The nail bed extends from the nail matrix to the hyponychium.

Normally, the **nail bed** is smooth and allows for healthy nail growth and a smooth appearance. If a nail bed is infected by **bacteria** or **fungus**, the nail bed becomes rough, and an accumulation of organic waste materials can react with the nail plate and cause the nail to become thickened and distorted.

CLINICAL CORRELATION

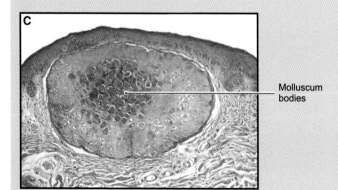

Figure 13-14C. Molluscum Contagiosum. H&E, ×53

Molluscum contagiosum is a viral skin infection, caused by the molluscum contagiosum virus, a member of the poxvirus family. The disease is characterized by flesh-colored, dome-shaped, pearly papules with a dimpled center. Lesions are typically 1 to 5 mm in diameter and common on the trunk, arms, and legs. The disease is common in childhood and usually self-limited in immunocompetent patients. In adults, the disease usually indicates cellular immunodeficiency. The papules are usually nonpainful but may itch or be complicated by secondary infection. The diagnosis is mainly based on the clinical appearance of the lesions. This slide shows lobules of keratinocytes with large eosinophilic intracytoplasmic inclusions called **molluscum bodies** within the stratum granulosum and stratum corneum. The treatment may include laser therapies, cryotherapy, or curettage, or there may be no treatment at all.

From Histology to Pathology

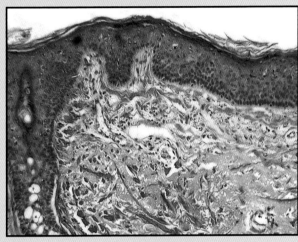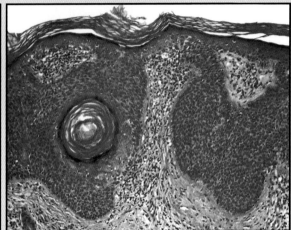

Figure 13-15. Normal thin skin and seborrheic keratosis. H&E, ×100

Normal thin skin on the *left*. Seborrheic keratosis on the *right*. This disorder is the most common benign neoplasm of the skin. Seborrheic keratosis may occur at any location, but it has a predilection for occurring in the trunk area. The lesions may be pigmented, and their histologic appearances are varied. The types include hyperkeratotic, clonal, and reticulated. These lesions may show signs of irritation with a pronounced inflammatory infiltrate. Invaginations of the surface produce horn cysts, which appear as cystic spaces containing keratin.

Clinical Vignette Questions

1. A 36-year-old man with acquired immunodeficiency syndrome (AIDS) noticed the appearance of red to purple skin lesions on his neck. The lesions are slightly raised above the surrounding skin surface. On his next appointment in the infectious disease clinic, he shows the lesions to his physician, who performs excision for pathologic examination. Histologically, the lesion consists of spindle cell proliferation and slitlike vascular spaces with surrounding hemorrhage in the dermis. These spindle cells are occasionally arranged in nodules. The pathologist performs immunohistochemistry to detect the virus associated with the vast majority of these cases. The virus in this case is most likely which of the following?

A. Cytomegalovirus
B. Epstein-Barr virus
C. Herpes simplex virus
D. Human herpesvirus type 8
E. Human papillomavirus

2. A 48-year-old Caucasian woman grew concerned about a skin lesion on her chest that had been slowly getting larger over several years, and she decided to see a dermatologist. Physical examination revealed a 0.8-cm oval, pigmented skin lesion on her right chest. The lesion appeared exophytic (raised above the skin surface) and mottled light to dark brown with discrete borders, and it appeared as though it was "stuck" on the skin. A biopsy showed inflammatory infiltrate and hyperkeratotic skin with horn cysts in the epidermis. Which of the following is the most likely diagnosis in this patient?

A. Actinic keratosis
B. Atypical nevus
C. Basal cell carcinoma
D. Malignant melanoma
E. Seborrheic keratosis

3. A 75-year-old man noticed the appearance of a red to pink skin nodule on his right temple area 2 months ago. Since that time, it has grown larger, and it is now greater than 1 cm in diameter. His dermatologist recommends complete excision of the lesion. Histologically, the lesion occupies the dermis, and it is composed of nodules of small- to medium-sized, blue-staining cells with little cytoplasm. The nuclei show fine chromatin, and numerous mitoses are identified. Multiple immunohistochemical stains were prepared, and the tumor cells are positive for neuroendocrine markers such as synaptophysin. In addition, the tumor cells are positive for cytokeratin in a paranuclear dotlike pattern. Which of the following is the most likely diagnosis of this tumor?

A. Basal cell carcinoma
B. Dermatofibrosarcoma protuberans
C. Lymphoma
D. Merkel cell carcinoma
E. Squamous cell carcinoma

14 Oral Cavity

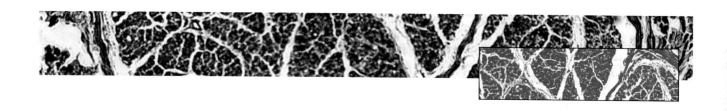

Teeth
Introduction and Key Concepts for Teeth

Oral Mucosa

Introduction and Key Concepts for Oral Mucosa

The **oral cavity** refers to the internal part of the mouth and can be divided into the **oral vestibule** and the **oral cavity proper**. The *oral vestibule* is the space between the inner lips, cheeks, and facial surface of the teeth. The *oral cavity proper* is the space between the upper and lower dental arches, extending from the inner surface of the teeth to the oropharynx. The structures inside of the oral cavity include the **lips, cheeks, tongue, teeth, gingiva, palates** (**hard** and **soft**), **salivary glands**, and **tonsils**. The tonsils are discussed in Chapter 10,

"Lymphoid System," and salivary glands are discussed in Chapter 16, "Digestive Glands and Associated Organs." The structures in the oral cavity are lined by an oral mucosa, which includes an overlying epithelium and underlying connective tissue. The oral mucosa can be divided into three types based on differences in the epithelial covering, organization of the connective tissue, and associated functions: **lining, masticatory,** and **specialized mucosa.**

LINING MUCOSA

LINING MUCOSA is covered by **non–keratinized stratified squamous epithelium** with two distinct layers: the **stratum basale** and **stratum spinosum.** The epithelium of the lining mucosa is similar to the epidermis of the skin, except that it has neither a stratum corneum nor a stratum lucidum, and the stratum granulosum is often absent (see Chapter 13, "Integumentary System"). The non–keratinized stratified epithelium is moistened by saliva. The connective tissues of the lining mucosa can be divided into the **lamina propria** and the **submucosa.** The *lamina propria* is a thin layer of loose connective tissue containing many elastic fibers and relatively few collagen fibers. This layer is equivalent to the dermis of the skin and is located beneath the epithelium. The *submucosa* is a thick layer of connective tissue, which contains minor salivary glands and is attached to the underlying muscle. The lining mucosa covers the inner oral surfaces of the lips, cheeks, soft palate, the inferior surface of the tongue, and the floor of the mouth. This type of mucosa is less exposed to abrasion than the masticatory mucosa. The lining mucosa provides a barrier against the invasion of pathogens and toxic chemicals, contains receptors for sensations, and serves immunological functions. The lining mucosa also provides lubrication and buffering by minor glands in the submucosal layer. Examples of the lining mucosa include the lip and cheek.

MASTICATORY MUCOSA

MASTICATORY MUCOSA is covered by **keratinized stratified squamous epithelium,** which is exposed to significant abrasion due to high compression and friction during chewing. The epithelium of the masticatory mucosa is composed of the **stratum basale, stratum spinosum, stratum granulosum,** and **stratum corneum.** It has a thick **lamina propria** that contains a dense network of collagen fibers and a few elastic fibers. This layer has no submucosa and is directly and firmly attached to the underlying bone. Masticatory mucosa can be found covering the oral surfaces of the gingiva (attached gingiva) and the hard palate. Injection into this area is difficult and painful because of its sensitive periosteum, high collagen density, and firm attachment to the bone.

SPECIALIZED MUCOSA

SPECIALIZED MUCOSA covers the anterior two thirds of the tongue and consists of keratinized and non–keratinized squamous epithelium and numerous papillae. These papillae can be classified into four types: **filiform, fungiform, circumvallate,** and **foliate papillae.** Most of these papillae have taste buds. The *filiform papillae* are the only papillae without taste buds; their main function is to aid in mixing food during chewing. The lamina propria (connective tissue) of the specialized mucosa is attached to the underlying skeletal muscle. These muscles produce voluntary movement of the tongue and are innervated by the hypoglossal nerve (cranial nerve [CN] XII). Lining mucosa covers the inferior surface of the tongue. The mucosa of the tongue is divided into two parts by a V-shaped groove called the **sulcus terminalis.** The anterior two thirds of the tongue is referred to as the **body of the tongue.** Its mucosa is innervated by the facial nerve (CN VII) and the trigeminal nerve (CN V). The posterior third of the tongue is the **base of the tongue.** Its taste buds and mucosa are innervated by the glossopharyngeal nerve (CN IX). The posterior third of the tongue contains the lingual tonsils.

1. *Filiform papillae* are the smallest and most numerous of the four types of papillae. They cover almost the entire superior surface of the anterior two thirds of the tongue and are packed in rows that parallel the sulcus terminalis. Each of the papillae appears cone shaped with some branching processes. Connective tissue forms the central core of each papilla. Filiform papillae have no taste buds and extend from the non–keratinized stratified squamous epithelium. The surface of the papilla is keratinized and is exposed to a great deal of abrasion.

2. *Fungiform papillae* are less numerous than the filiform papillae. They are mushroom shaped and are scattered among the filiform papillae. Fungiform papillae are located at the tip and on the two lateral edges of the tongue. They are more numerous near the tip of the tongue. Taste buds are found on the apical surfaces of fungiform papillae.

3. *Circumvallate papillae* are large and round with a flat-topped cylindrical structure. There are about 10 to 14 papillae arranged in a row along the sulcus terminalis. Each papilla is surrounded by a deep groove (moat), which forms a valley around the papilla. Taste buds are found in the lateral walls of each papilla.

4. *Foliate papillae* are leaflike folds with flat tops and have deep clefts between the papillae. They are located on the posterior lateral surface of the tongue. They are more prominent in some animals (such as rabbits) than in humans. Foliate papillae contain taste buds in the lateral walls of the papillae.

Oral Mucosa and Teeth

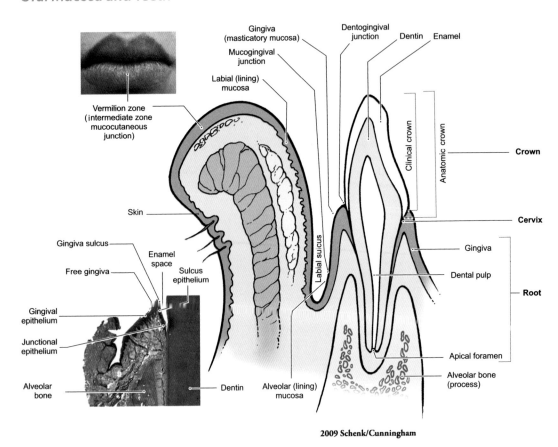

2009 Schenk/Cunningham

Figure 14-1 Overview of the oral mucosa and teeth. Lower left, H&E, ×18

The **oral cavity** is lined by oral mucosa, which can be divided into **masticatory mucosa** (gingiva, hard palate), **lining mucosa** (lips, soft palate, cheeks, inferior surface of the tongue, floor of the mouth), and **specialized mucosa** (tongue). This illustration represents the lip and a tooth and the mucosa covering these structures. The lip is covered externally with **skin** to the **vermilion zone** (**intermediate zone** or **mucocutaneous junction**); the vermilion zone continues to the **labial mucosa**, which is the lining mucosa on the internal surface of the lip. The alveolar process of the jaw (containing the tooth roots) is covered by **alveolar mucosa** (lining mucosa) and **gingiva**. The junction between the lining mucosa and attached gingiva is the **mucogingival junction**. The tooth can be divided into three parts: **crown**, **cervix**, and **root**. The crown is the part of the tooth projecting into the oral cavity and has two different definitions: The **clinical crown** is the part of the crown, which is visible in the mouth; the **anatomical crown** is the part of the tooth covered by enamel. The root is covered by the gingiva or is inside the **bony socket**. The region between the crown and root is the cervix (neck). The **gingival sulcus** is the space between the free gingiva and the enamel; it is normally 0.5 to 3.0 mm in depth.

If the depth of the **gingival sulcus** is over 3 mm, these spaces are called **gingival** or **periodontal pockets**. These pockets represent an abnormal condition. An accumulation of debris and microbes in the pockets may cause damage to the **periodontal tissue**.

Structures of the Oral Mucosa

I. **Lining mucosa** (covering of inner surface of the lips and cheeks, soft palate, inferior surface of the tongue, and floor of the mouth)
   A. **Epithelium:** non–keratinized stratified squamous epithelium
   B. **Lamina propria:** connective tissue with many elastic fibers and few collagen fibers
   C. **Submucosa: connective tissue with minor salivary glands and their ducts**
II. **Masticatory mucosa** (covering of gingiva and hard palate)
   A. **Epithelium:** keratinized stratified squamous epithelium
   B. **Lamina propria:** connective tissue with few elastic fibers and many dense collagen fibers
   C. **No submucosa**
III. **Specialized mucosa (tongue)**
   A. **Filiform papillae:** no taste buds
   B. **Fungiform papillae:** taste buds on apical surface of the papilla—sweet, sour, salty
   C. **Circumvallate papillae:** taste buds in lateral wall of the papilla—bitter
   D. **Foliate papillae:** taste buds in lateral wall of papilla

Lining Mucosa

LIP

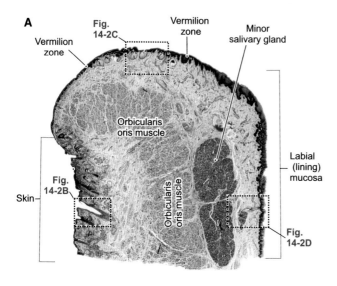

A

SKIN (EXTERNAL SURFACE) OF THE LIP

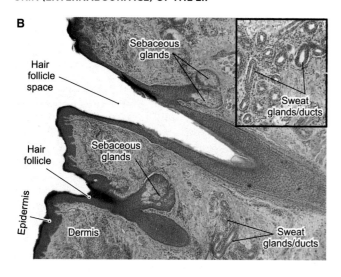

B

VERMILION (INTERMEDIATE) ZONE

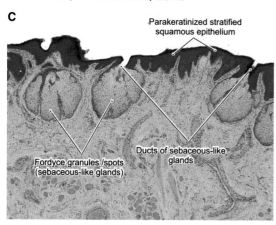

C

Figure 14-2A Overview of the lining mucosa, lip. H&E, ×7.6

Lining mucosa is a wet mucosa that covers the inside of the mouth and is lined by non–keratinized stratified squamous epithelium. The labial mucosa of the **lip** is an example of lining mucosa. The lips are soft, flexible, and movable; they play important roles in food intake, speech, and as a sensory organ (e.g., kissing). Lips can be divided into three regions: (1) **thin skin**, forming the external surface of the lip; (2) **vermilion zone**, appearing red in color, also called the **intermediate zone** or **mucocutaneous junction**; and (3) the **labial mucosa** (**lining mucosa**), the internal surface of the lip. The central core of the lip contains the orbicularis oris (skeletal) muscle, which is innervated by the facial nerve (CN VII) and contributes to lip movement and facial expressions.

Figure 14-2B Skin, lip. H&E, ×33; inset ×44

An example of the **skin** on the external surface of the **lip** is shown. It is covered by keratinized stratified squamous epithelium. The sebaceous glands in the dermis are associated with hair follicles, and sweat glands are present. The skin of the lip is like thin skin elsewhere and can be divided into epidermis and dermis.

Figure 14-2C Vermilion zone, lip. H&E, ×33

The **vermilion zone** of the **lip** is covered by parakeratinized stratified squamous epithelium. Sebaceous-like glands (**Fordyce granules** or **spots**) may be found in the connective tissue and are not associated with hair follicles. These glands have ducts that release their oily product directly onto the surface of the lip. The vermilion zone appears red because of many blood vessels near the surface of the thin and translucent epithelium. This region can become thick and forms the sucking pad in infants.

Figure 14-2D Labial mucosa (lining mucosa), lip. H&E, ×33

The **labial mucosa** of the lip is an example of **lining mucosa**, which is covered by non–keratinized stratified squamous epithelium and contains many elastic fibers; it is very flexible and can be stretched. Its submucosa layer contains many minor salivary glands (mucous glands). The minor salivary glands in the lips are often called **labial glands**.

LINING MUCOSA (INTERNAL SURFACE)

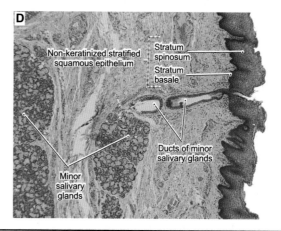

D

LINING MUCOSA, CHEEK

A

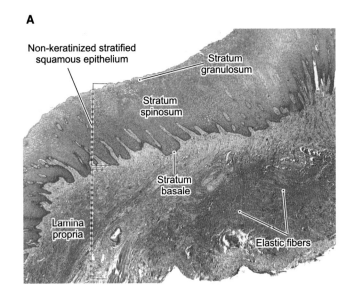

Non-keratinized stratified squamous epithelium

Stratum granulosum

Stratum spinosum

Stratum basale

Lamina propria

Elastic fibers

Figure 14-3A Buccal mucosa (lining mucosa), cheek. H&E, ×16

Each **cheek** constitutes a lateral wall of the mouth. The inner surface of the cheeks is lined by lining mucosa known as **buccal mucosa**. The buccal mucosa has a non–keratinized stratified squamous epithelium with three definite layers (stratum basale, spinosum, and granulosum) with many elastic fibers in the lamina propria and minor salivary glands (**buccal glands**) in the submucosa layer. This example shows the epithelium and lamina propria of the buccal mucosa, which has a non–keratinized stratified squamous epithelium. There are many elastic fibers in the lamina propria of the mucosa. Elastic fibers appear pink and do not readily stain with H&E stain. Fordyce spots (sebaceous-like glands) may also be found in the mucosa of the cheek. They increase with age and are more visible in elderly individuals.

The **lingual** and **inferior alveolar nerves** run through the posterior groove of the cheek (between the pterygomandibular raphe and the ramus of the mandible). This is an important landmark for local anesthesia injections in the mouth.

CLINICAL CORRELATION

B

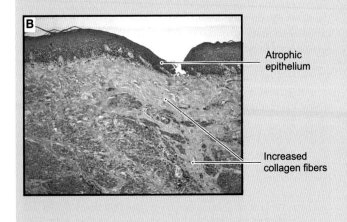

Atrophic epithelium

Increased collagen fibers

Figure 14-3B. Oral Submucous Fibrosis of the Lip. H&E, ×25

Oral submucous fibrosis is a precancerous condition characterized by a mucosal rigidity due to fibroelastic changes of the **lamina propria** and **submucosa layers** of the **lining mucosa**. This causes a progressive difficulty in opening the mouth. It affects the **buccal mucosa, lips, retromolar areas**, the **soft palate**, and even the **esophagus**. Causes of this condition include the use of **chilies** and **areca nut, collagen disorders**, and **autoimmune disorders**. Histologically, it is characterized by **atrophic** (thinned) **epithelium** and **increased collagen fiber formation** followed by the presence of dense collagen fiber bundles and different degrees of **hyalinization**. Prevention and treatments of the disease include dietary changes and having plastic surgery to improve the function of the mouth.

TABLE 14-1 COMPARISON OF LINING AND MASTICATORY MUCOSAE

Name of Mucosa	Epithelium	Lamina Propria	Submucosa	Covering Region	Special Features	Clinical Application
Lining mucosa	Non–keratinized stratified squamous epithelium	Few collagen fibers; many elastic fibers	Well-developed submucosa; attached primarily to underlying muscle rather than bone (except for alveolar mucosa)	Lips, cheeks, soft palate, inferior surface of the tongue, and floor of the mouth	Thick, soft, and loose; flexible and can be stretched	Injections are easy to make and minimally painful; if cut, a gap appears that requires suturing; infection spreads quickly
Masticatory mucosa	Keratinized stratified squamous epithelium	Dense network of collagen fibers; few elastic fibers	No submucosa present; lamina propria is directly and firmly bound to the bone	Gingiva, hard palate	Thin, stiff, dense; cannot be stretched	Injections are difficult and painful; if cut, no gap results and suturing is not necessary; infection spreads slowly

Masticatory Mucosa

GINGIVA

A

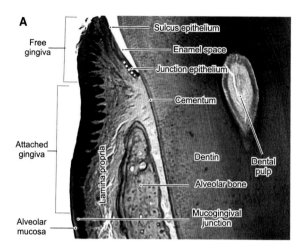

Free gingiva

Attached gingiva

Alveolar mucosa

Sulcus epithelium
Enamel space
Junction epithelium
Cementum
Lamina propria
Dentin
Dental pulp
Alveolar bone
Mucogingival junction

Figure 14-4A Masticatory mucosa, gingiva. H&E, ×22

Masticatory mucosa covers the gingiva and hard palate; it has a **keratinized stratified squamous epithelium**, which is exposed to more abrasion during chewing than the lining mucosa. Masticatory mucosa lacks a submucosa layer. The lamina propria of the masticatory mucosa consists of a dense network of collagen fibers that are firmly attached to the underlying bone. The **gingiva** (gum) surrounds the cervix of the tooth and covers the upper part of the alveolar bone at the tooth root. The gingiva can be divided into **free gingiva** and **attached gingiva**. The superior part of the gingiva is *free gingiva* and surrounds, but does not attach to, the cervix of the tooth. This nonattachment between the **sulcus epithelium** of the free gingiva and enamel creates a space called the **gingival sulcus**, or **free gingival groove** (normally 0.5–3 mm depth). The *attached gingiva* firmly attaches to the underlying hard tissues (alveolar bone, cementum, and edge of the enamel). The gingival-mucosal border is called the **mucogingival junction** (between attached gingiva and alveolar mucosa), where the epithelium changes from nonkeratinized to keratinized and the color changes from bright pink (alveolar mucosa) to pale pink (gingiva).

HARD PALATE

B

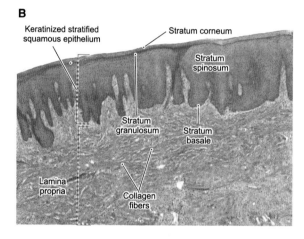

Keratinized stratified squamous epithelium
Stratum corneum
Stratum spinosum
Stratum granulosum
Stratum basale
Lamina propria
Collagen fibers

Figure 14-4B Masticatory mucosa, hard palate. H&E, ×35

The **hard palate** forms the roof of the mouth and is covered by masticatory mucosa with keratinized stratified squamous epithelium and a dense lamina propria. It has one more layer (**stratum corneum**) than the lining mucosa. The collagen fibers in the lamina are thick and dense and firmly bind to the periosteum of the underlying bone. The periosteum consists of dense connective tissue, which covers the bone and contributes to bone formation (see Chapter 5, "Cartilage and Bone"). Most of the hard palate lacks a submucosal layer. However, the posterior region near the alveolar process may present a submucosal layer that contains minor mucous glands. The hard palate significantly assists in mastication and speech.

Cleft palate is a birth defect in which there is a fissure in the hard palate that is caused by the failure of two parts of the palate to fuse during facial development. This condition impairs the quality of speech (an individual is unable to pronounce certain sounds) and also causes eating problems.

CLINICAL CORRELATION

C

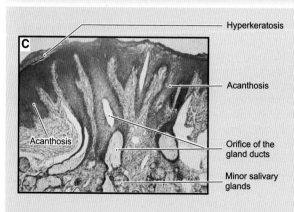

Hyperkeratosis
Acanthosis
Acanthosis
Orifice of the gland ducts
Minor salivary glands

Figure 14-4C. Nicotine Stomatitis. H&E, ×25

Nicotine stomatitis, not a precancerous condition, is characterized by a **white lesion** in the oral mucosa of the **hard palate** of the mouth. The causes of this condition are associated with long-term tobacco smoking, especially pipe smoking, and hot beverage consumption. The lesion has a white **cobblestone** or "**dried-mud**" appearance because of excessive **keratin** production. The hard palate may appear gray or white and contain many papules that are slightly elevated with red in their center. Histologically, the squamous mucosa demonstrates **hyperkeratosis** (thickening of the stratum corneum) and **acanthosis** (overgrowth of the stratum spinosum). Complete smoking cessation usually helps to diminish and resolve the condition within about 2 weeks. If the lesion persists, close monitoring may be necessary.

Specialized Mucosa

TONGUE

A

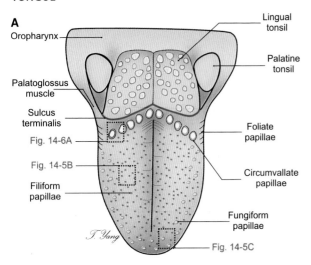

Figure 14-5A Overview of the tongue.

The inferior surface of the **tongue** and the floor of the mouth are covered by lining mucosa with a non–keratinized squamous epithelium. The superior surface of the tongue is covered by specialized mucosa with numerous projecting papillae including **filiform papillae, fungiform papillae, circumvallate papillae,** and **foliate papillae.** The specialized mucosa is attached to the underlying skeletal muscle. The tongue has a central core of skeletal muscle, which controls movements of the tongue and is innervated by the hypoglossal nerve (CN XII). The base of the tongue is attached to the floor of the mouth. The surface of the posterior third of the tongue has somatosensory receptors and taste buds that are innervated by the glossopharyngeal nerve (CN IX). The anterior two thirds of the tongue has somatosensory receptors that are innervated by the trigeminal nerve (CN V), and its taste buds are innervated by the chorda branch of the facial nerve (CN VII). The tongue plays an important role in speech, taste, and in moving and swallowing (**deglutition**) food.

FILIFORM PAPILLAE

B

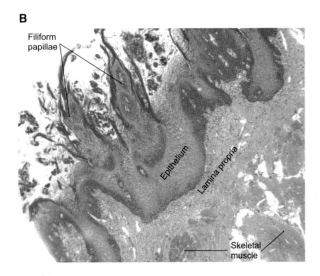

Figure 14-5B Filiform papillae, tongue. H&E, ×35

The **filiform papillae** are slender, cone-shaped papillae with keratinized outer surfaces. They are the most numerous but smallest in size of the four types of papillae. The filiform papillae are often packed in rows and cover the entire superior surface of the anterior two thirds of the tongue (anterior to the sulcus terminalis). Each filiform papilla has a central connective tissue core with several branches of small papillae. They are the only papillae that do not have taste buds. The filiform papillae's tips arc keratinized, consistent with their exposure to abrasion during chewing. Because they have no taste buds, their main functions are to help with chewing and mixing food. The submucosal layer is absent in the tongue; the mucosa of the tongue is strongly bound to the underlying skeletal muscle to allow optimum food bolus control.

FUNGIFORM PAPILLAE

C

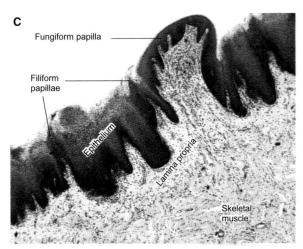

Figure 14-5C Fungiform papillae, tongue. H&E, ×44

The **fungiform papillae** are mushroom shaped and considerably more numerous than the filiform papillae. They tend to be slightly taller than the filiform papillae that surround them. Each fungiform papilla has one to five taste buds on its superior surface. These taste buds are innervated by the chorda tympani branch of the facial nerve (CN VII), which joins the lingual branch of the trigeminal nerve (CN V). The fungiform papillae are covered by non–keratinized squamous epithelium. They are distributed at the tip and two sides of the tongue. In general, the taste buds have five taste sensations: sweet, bitter, umami, salty, and sour. The salty and sour sensations are associated with ion channels; the other three taste sensations are associated with G protein–coupled receptors.

CIRCUMVALLATE PAPILLAE

A

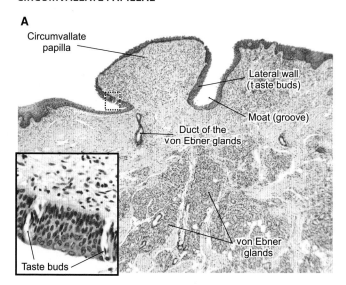

Circumvallate papilla

Lateral wall (taste buds)

Moat (groove)

Duct of the von Ebner glands

von Ebner glands

Taste buds

Figure 14-6A Circumvallate papillae, tongue. H&E, ×34; inset ×181

The **circumvallate papillae** are also called **vallate papillae.** They are arranged in a single row, which contains about 10 to 14 papillae that are located immediately anterior to the **sulcus terminalis.** Each circumvallate papilla is cylindrical in shape and is surrounded by a groove called a **moat.** The ducts of the **glands of von Ebner** (minor serous salivary glands) open and drain serous products into the groove; this helps to clear the food debris in the groove and helps in detection of taste. Most minor salivary glands in the oral cavity are mucous or mixed glands; von Ebner glands are the only ones that are pure serous glands. The taste buds of the circumvallate papillae are located on the lateral walls of the groove. These taste buds are mainly **bitter receptors** and are innervated by the glossopharyngeal nerve (CN IX).

FOLIATE PAPILLAE

B

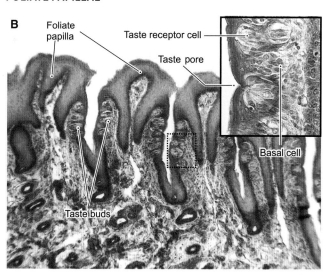

Foliate papilla

Taste receptor cell

Taste pore

Basal cell

Taste buds

Figure 14-6B Foliate papillae and taste buds, tongue. H&E, ×68; inset ×222

The **foliate papillae** are located on the posterior lateral surface of the tongue. This type of papilla is not well developed in humans but is frequently found in animals; illustrated here from rabbit tissue.

In general, **taste buds** are ovular structures embedded in non–keratinized stratified squamous epithelium of the papillae of the tongue. They also can be found in the palate of the oral cavity and in the mucosa of the oropharynx and epiglottis. Each taste bud is composed of 40 to 60 elongated **taste receptor cells** with microvilli at the apical region, which extend into the **taste pore.** The basal end of the taste bud contacts an afferent nerve fiber. The taste pore is a small opening that allows taste molecules to contact taste receptor cells. The taste receptor cells have a life span of 1 to 2 weeks, and new taste cells arise from basal cells at the basal lateral region of the taste bud. The *inset* shows taste buds.

TABLE 14-2 COMPARISON OF LINGUAL PAPILLAE

Name	Epithelial Covering	Taste Buds	Location	Main Function
Filiform papillae	Keratinized stratified squamous epithelium	No taste buds	Anterior 2/3 of tongue	Helps in chewing and mixing food
Fungiform papillae	Non–keratinized stratified squamous epithelium	Taste buds located at the apical surface of papillae	Tip and two sides of tongue	Chemoreceptor detecting taste
Circumvallate papillae	Non–keratinized stratified squamous epithelium	Taste buds located at the lateral surface of papillae	In a V-shaped row just anterior to the sulcus terminalis	Chemoreceptor detecting taste
Foliate papillae	Non–keratinized stratified squamous epithelium	Taste buds located at the lateral surface of papillae	Posterior lateral surface of the tongue	Chemoreceptor detecting taste

Teeth

Introduction and Key Concepts for Teeth

Teeth are prominent structures in the oral cavity. They can be divided into **maxillary** (upper) and **mandibular** (lower) **teeth**. The root of the tooth is surrounded by the alveolar bone (alveolar process or alveolar arch), which forms a socket to hold and support each tooth. The alveolar bone of the maxillary teeth is a part of the maxilla (upper jaw); the alveolar bone of the mandibular teeth is a part of the mandible (lower jaw). There are two sets of teeth: **primary** (baby) and **permanent teeth**. The primary teeth are eventually replaced by permanent teeth. In adults, there are 32 permanent teeth including two **incisors**, one **canine**, two **premolars**, and three **molars** on each of the four quadrants in the maxillary and mandibular arches. Each tooth can be divided into three parts: the **crown**, the **cervix** (neck), and the **root**. The *crown* of the tooth is covered by enamel and extends above the gingiva (gum); the shape of the crown is unique in different types of teeth and is adapted to their functions. The *cervix* is also called the **neck** of the tooth and is the junction between the crown and root. The region where the enamel and cementum meet is called the **cementoenamel junction (CEJ)**. The *root* of the tooth is covered by cementum and surrounded by the alveolar bone. A tooth has one or more roots; the apex is the end of the root. The **apical foramen** is a small opening where nerves and blood vessels enter and exit the dental pulp.

TOOTH DEVELOPMENT (ODONTOGENESIS) stems from two different origins: ectodermal and neural crest–derived mesenchymal tissue. The oral epithelium derives from ectodermal tissue, which gives rise to the dental lamina, and later becomes the enamel organ. The dental papilla derives from mesenchymal tissue and gives rise to the future dental pulp. The enamel organ, dental papilla, and dental sac (follicle) as a whole are described as a **tooth germ**, which eventually forms a tooth. The initiation of tooth germs occurs along the oral epithelium of the maxillary and mandibular prominences (processes). Tooth germs undergo **initiation phases** (development of the dental lamina and initiation of tooth germs), **morphogenesis phases** (cell movement and formation of the shape of the tooth), and **histogenesis phases** (formation of the hard tissue and development of the tooth root). Although tooth development is a continuous process, odontogenesis can be divided into several stages based on the shape of the tooth germ and formation of the tooth structure. These stages include **initiation, bud, cap, bell,** and **apposition (crown) stages**. When the primitive oral cavity is forming, the first pharyngeal arch gives rise to the **maxillary** and **mandibular prominences** or **processes** (developing dental arches), which lead to the future upper and lower jaws.

1. *Initiation stage*: At about 6 to 7 weeks into development, some oral epithelial cells on the surface of the maxillary and mandibular prominences increase proliferation activity, become thicker, and invaginate into the underlying mesenchymal tissue to form the **primary epithelial band**.
2. *Bud stage*: At about 8 to 9 weeks, the primary epithelial band gives rise to the **vestibular lamina** and **dental lamina**. The vestibular lamina forms a cleft that becomes the vestibule between the cheek and tooth; the dental lamina forms a U-shaped structure and develops into tooth buds (enamel organs and mesenchymal tissue), which become primary deciduous teeth. The development of permanent teeth comes from the secondary tooth buds, which sprout from the primary tooth buds.
3. *Cap stage*: At about 10 to 11 weeks, the enamel organ appears as a cap shape and the condensed mesenchymal cells beneath the enamel organ form the dental papilla.
4. *Bell stage*: At about 12 to 14 weeks, the enamel organ continues to grow into a bell shape, and cells of the enamel organ differentiate into four distinguishable cell layers: the **outer enamel epithelium, inner enamel epithelium, stellate reticulum,** and **stratum intermedium**. At the same time, the dental papilla grows and helps to form the shape of the tooth crown. Cells in the dental papilla are differentiated into outer and inner cell groups. The outer cells of the dental papilla will develop into odontoblasts that produce future dentin; the inner cells will develop into future dental pulp tissues.
5. *Apposition (crown/late bell) stage*: At about 18 to 19 weeks, beginning at the incise edge on cusp tips and progressing toward the future CEJ or cervix, cells of the tooth germ continue to differentiate; the inner enamel epithelial cells have become preameloblasts, which induce the outer cells of the dental papilla to become odontoblasts and begin to produce the dentinal matrix at the tooth crown region. This material is called **predentin** and, after undergoing calcification, will become dentin. When dentin is formed, it induces preameloblasts to differentiate and become active ameloblasts, which produce enamel. Thus, the production of both the enamel matrix and the dentin for the tooth crown has begun. When the two hard tissues, dentin and enamel, have formed and the shape of the crown is completed, the root of the tooth begins to develop. The tooth then starts to erupt into the oral cavity in order to make room for the tooth root to grow.

ENAMEL, DENTIN, AND DENTAL PULP are components of teeth. **Enamel** is the hardest tissue in the body. The basic morphological unit of enamel is the **rod**, also called the **prism**, which is composed of a head and a tail. The rods are arranged in a three-dimensional complex, perpendicular to the **dentinoenamel junction (DEJ)**. They extend from the DEJ to the surface of the enamel. Enamel provides a seal for the dentin and makes a strong surface for chewing. The crown of the tooth is covered by enamel and the root of the tooth is covered by cementum. **Dentin** surrounds and forms the walls of the dental pulp. It is composed of numerous **dentinal tubules, odontoblastic processes,** and the **dentinal matrix** and is the second hardest tissue of the body. The central core of the tooth is occupied by **dental pulp**, which is made up of loose mucous connective tissue containing blood vessels and nerve fibers.

PERIODONTIUM refers to the structures surrounding and supporting the tooth root and includes the **cementum**, the **PDL**, and the **alveolar bone**. The *cementum* is a thin layer of hard tissue that covers the root dentin. The *PDL* is the dense fibrous connective tissue that attaches the cementum to the alveolar bone. The *alveolar bone*, also called the **alveolar process**, is part of the maxilla and mandible. The alveolar bone supports and protects the tooth root. It includes the **alveolar crest**, the **alveolar bone proper**, and **supporting bone**.

Teeth

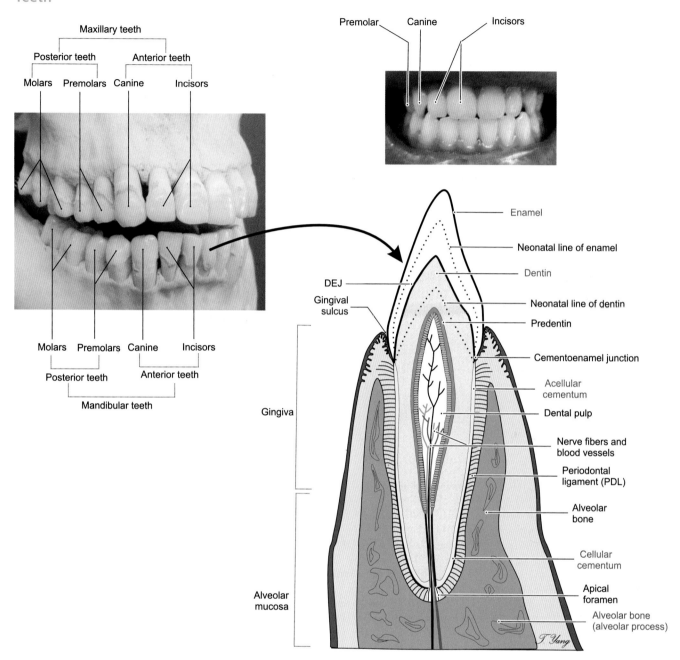

Figure 14-7 Overview of the teeth.

There are two sets of **teeth** that form during a person's lifetime: 20 **primary (baby) teeth** and the **secondary (adult) teeth**. The secondary teeth will eventually replace the primary teeth. The secondary teeth are more commonly called **permanent teeth** by dentists. There are 32 permanent teeth in an adult. Each of the four quadrants includes two **incisors**, one **canine**, two **premolars**, and three **molars** in the mandibular and maxillary dental arches (*left*). The tooth is composed of several types of hard tissues: **dentin, enamel, cementum,** and the **alveolar bone.** The central core of each tooth is a chamber containing **dental pulp** made up of mucous connective tissue with a rich supply of nerve fibers and blood vessels. Each tooth has a **crown, cervix,** and **root.** The crown of the tooth is covered by enamel, the hardest tissue found in the body; the cervix is the junction between the crown and root; and the surface of the root is covered by cementum, which connects to the alveolar bone by the **PDL.** The junction between the enamel and cementum is the **CEJ,** and the border between the dentin and enamel is the **DEJ.**

Tooth Development (Odontogenesis)

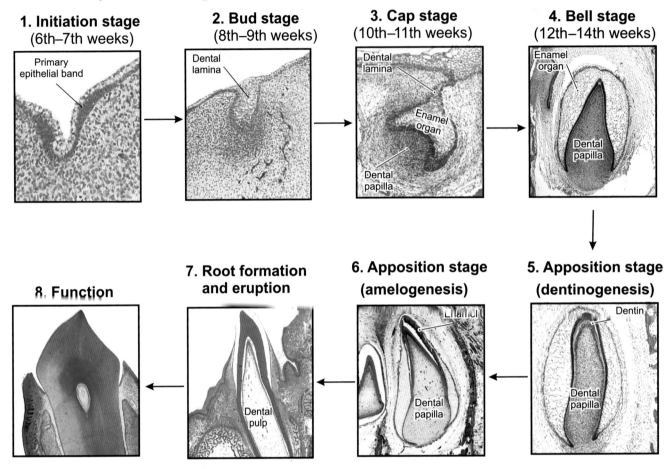

1. Initiation stage
(6th–7th weeks)

Primary epithelial band

2. Bud stage
(8th–9th weeks)

Dental lamina

3. Cap stage
(10th–11th weeks)

Dental lamina

Enamel organ

Dental papilla

4. Bell stage
(12th–14th weeks)

Enamel organ

Dental papilla

8. Function

7. Root formation and eruption

Dental pulp

6. Apposition stage
(amelogenesis)

Enamel

Dental papilla

5. Apposition stage
(dentinogenesis)

Dentin

Dental papilla

Figure 14-8   Overview of tooth development (odontogenesis). H&E, ×5 to ×128

Tooth development is also called **odontogenesis**. The tooth derives from two types of tissues: **ectoderm** (oral epithelium) and **mesenchymal** tissues, some of which originate from the neural crest. The oral epithelium forms a U-shaped structure called the **dental lamina**, which develops into an **enamel organ**. The mesenchymal tissue develops into a **dental papilla** and also forms a dental sac (follicle), which surrounds the dental papilla and enamel organ. The enamel organ, dental papilla, and dental sac (follicle) collectively are described as a **tooth germ**. Tooth development is a continuous process and can be described in several stages (like snapshots) based on the shape of the tooth germs: **initiation, bud, cap, bell,** and **apposition stages**. The illustrations represent the process of tooth development. (1) *Initiation stage*: Proliferating oral epithelial cells become thickened and form a primary epithelial band. (2) *Bud stage*: The dental lamina (derived from the primary epithelial band) forms a U-shaped structure (tooth bud). (3) *Cap stage*: The enamel organ develops into a cap-shaped structure. At the same time, mesenchymal tissue becomes condensed and forms the dental papilla. (4) *Bell stage*: The enamel organ continues to grow into a bell shape that has five distinct cell layers. (5) *Apposition stage (dentinogenesis)*: Odontoblasts begin to form dentin on the crown region. (6) *Apposition stage (amelogenesis)*: After a layer of dentin is formed at the crown of the tooth, the formation of enamel begins (produced by ameloblasts). (7) *Root formation and eruption*: When the shape of the crown and the dentin and enamel of the crown have completed, the tooth begins to develop its root structure (cementum, PDL). During this process, the tooth gradually erupts into the oral cavity. (8) *Function*: Development of the tooth root and its associated structures continues until the tooth is functional.

BUD STAGE

A

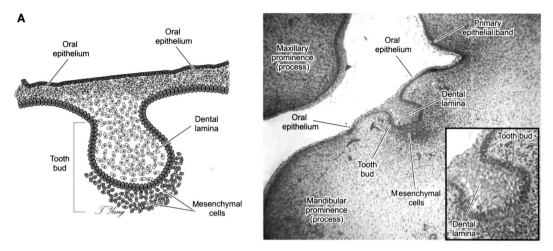

Figure 14-9A Bud stage, weeks 8–9. H&E, ×72; inset ×140

The **bud stage** is a continuation of the **initiation stage** in which the proliferating and thickening oral epithelium forms the **primary epithelial band**. In the bud stage, the tooth germ forms a budlike structure that is surrounded by proliferating and accumulating mesenchymal cells. The combination of the dental lamina and condensed mesenchymal tissues is called the **tooth bud** and develops into a primary tooth. The **maxillary** and **mandibular prominences** lead to the future upper and lower jaws.

During the bud stage, any disturbance can cause the formation of abnormal teeth, such as **microdontia** (abnormally small teeth) and **macrodontia** (abnormally large teeth).

CAP STAGE

B

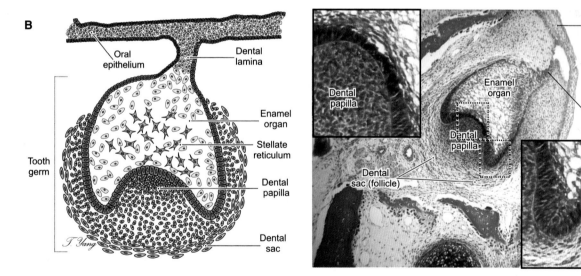

Figure 14-9B Cap stage, weeks 10–11. H&E, ×72; inset ×204

The **cap stage** is a continuation of the bud stage and results from the enlargement and unequal growth of the tooth bud. At this stage, the enamel organ is formed and attaches to the remaining dental lamina. The base of the enamel organ becomes concave and appears as a cap-shaped structure with mesenchymal cells beneath it. These mesenchymal cells are condensed, forming a **dental papilla** that will form the future dental pulp. Other mesenchymal cell layers surrounding the enamel organ and dental papilla are called the **dental sac** (**dental follicle**). At this stage, the morphogenesis and formation of the tooth germ are ongoing. The cell proliferation and movement determine the shape of the tooth.

A disturbance during the cap stage of tooth development can cause clinical tooth **fusion** (two adjacent tooth germs fuse and develop into a large macrodontic tooth) or **gemination** (one tooth germ develops into two teeth, which share a single pulp but have two crowns and **dens invaginatus** (or **dens in dente**, meaning, "tooth within a tooth").

BELL STAGE

A

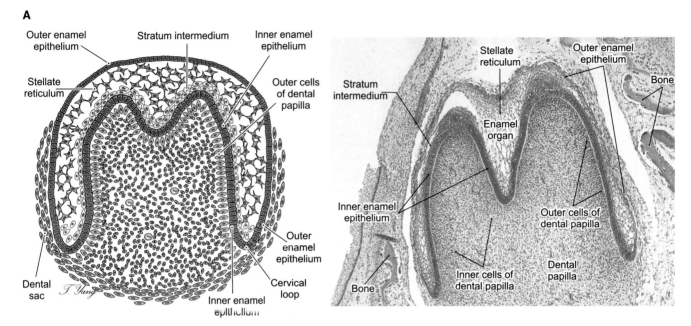

Figure 14-10A   Bell stage, weeks 12–14. H&E, ×72

The **bell stage** is a continuation of the cap stage. The tooth germ undergoes further morphogenesis, proliferation, and differentiation. At this stage, the enamel organ detaches from the dental lamina and loses connection with the oral epithelium. The dental lamina gradually degenerates. However, the enamel organ continues to differentiate and forms four cell layers: the **inner enamel epithelium, stratum intermedium, stellate reticulum,** and **outer enamel epithelium.** Some cell types may also be found in the later cap stage. The dental papilla differentiates and forms the **outer cells of the dental papilla** and the **inner cells of the dental papilla** near the base of the enamel organ. As the tooth germ continues to grow, the *outer cells* of the dental papilla will differentiate into future **odontoblasts**; the *inner cells* of the dental papilla will differentiate into future dental pulp tissues.

B

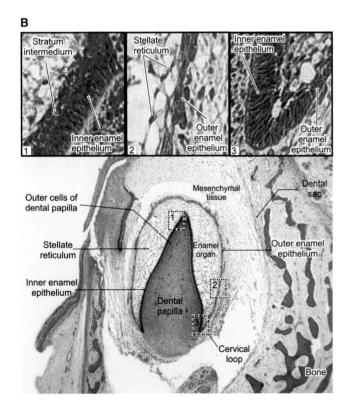

Figure 14-10B   Bell stage, cell layers. H&E, ×37; insets ×472

During the differentiation process of the enamel organ at the **bell stage,** four cell layers are distinguishable. (1) The **inner enamel epithelium** is a row of columnar cells that contain rich RNA and are much taller in the tip region where initial enamel formation will take place at the apposition stage. The inner enamel epithelium differentiates and later becomes ameloblasts. (2) The **stratum intermedium** is composed of two to three layers of squamous or cuboidal cells and is located between the stellate reticulum and inner enamel epithelium. Cells in this layer are rich in **alkaline phosphatase,** which assists in the inner enamel epithelium production of enamel. (3) The **stellate reticulum** is located within the enamel organ. It may also be present in the cap stage but is more developed in the bell stage. The cells of the stellate reticulum are star shaped and have many cellular processes interconnected with one another to form a network within the enamel organ. The extracellular spaces of the stellate reticulum are large and filled with a fluidlike, fluffy material. These cells contain **glycosaminoglycans** and **alkaline phosphatase** and have **desmosomes** and **gap junctions** between the cells. The stellate reticulum plays a role in maintaining tooth shape and protecting underlying dental tissue. (4) The **outer enamel epithelium** is composed of cuboidal cells and is the outermost layer of the enamel organ. This cell layer separates the enamel organ from the nearby mesenchymal tissues. It serves as a protective barrier and also helps maintain the shape of the enamel organ. The inner enamel epithelium and outer enamel epithelium meet to form the cervical loop.

APPOSITION STAGE

A

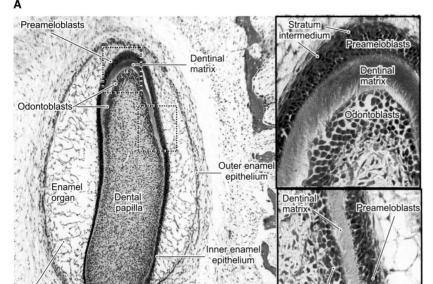

Preameloblasts

Dentinal matrix

Odontoblasts

Enamel organ

Dental papilla

Stellate reticulum

Cervical loop

Stratum intermedium

Preameloblasts

Dentinal matrix

Odontoblasts

Outer enamel epithelium

Inner enamel epithelium

Dental sac

Dentinal matrix

Preameloblasts

Odontoblasts

Figure 14-11A Apposition (crown/late bell) stage, dentinogenesis. H&E, ×76; insets ×315

During the **apposition** (**crown/late bell**) **stage**, induction occurs between the **ectodermal** (enamel organ) and **mesenchymal** (dental papilla) tissues. The inner enamel epithelium from the enamel organ has become **preameloblasts**, which induce outer cells of the dental papilla to differentiate into **odontoblasts**. When odontoblasts become mature and active, they appear columnar in shape and begin to secrete dentinal matrix (**predentin**), which is the first hard tissue formed during tooth development. The formation of dentin is called **dentinogenesis**. The crown of the tooth develops much earlier than the root of the tooth. The crown dentin is first produced as **predentin** by odontoblasts. The predentin soon becomes calcified and is called **dentin**. The cervical loop is formed by the inner enamel epithelium and the outer enamel epithelium. Along with the dental sac, the cervical loop will contribute to develop future root structures.

B

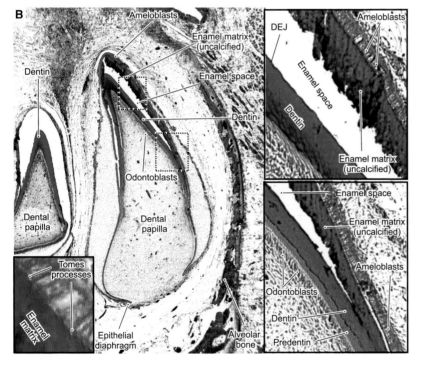

Dentin

Ameloblasts

Enamel matrix (uncalcified)

Enamel space

Dentin

Odontoblasts

Dental papilla

Dental papilla

Tomes processes

Enamel matrix

Epithelial diaphragm

Alveolar bone

DEJ

Ameloblasts

Enamel space

Dentin

Enamel matrix (uncalcified)

Enamel space

Enamel matrix (uncalcified)

Ameloblasts

Odontoblasts

Dentin

Predentin

Figure 14-11B Apposition (crown/late bell) stage, amelogenesis. H&E, ×19; insets (*right*) ×104; inset (*left*) ×354

The formation of crown dentin induces preameloblasts to differentiate and become **ameloblasts**. Active ameloblasts are columnar cells, and their nuclei are located toward the stratum intermedium. They actively secrete enamel matrix with assistance from the stratum intermedium. The newly secreted enamel matrix, in contact with the dentin matrix, forms the **DEJ**. At the same time, the ameloblasts and the odontoblasts retreat from the DEJ as deposition of the matrix proceeds. Enamel formation moves outward (toward the enamel organ), and dentin formation moves inward (toward the dental pulp). The process of enamel formation is called **amelogenesis**. During amelogenesis, conical processes, known as **Tomes processes**, are developed at the secretory (apical) surface of the ameloblasts. In the apposition stage, the two types of hard tissues (dentin and enamel) begin to form at the tooth crown. These two types of hard tissues are formed in a regular rhythm.

TOOTH ROOT DEVELOPMENT AND ERUPTION

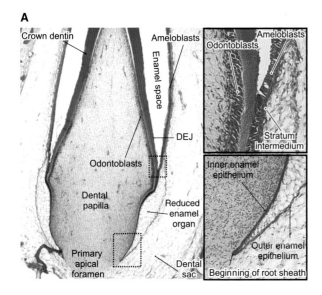

A

Crown dentin
Ameloblasts
Enamel space
Ameloblasts
Odontoblasts
DEJ
Stratum intermedium
Odontoblasts
Inner enamel epithelium
Dental papilla
Reduced enamel organ
Outer enamel epithelium
Primary apical foramen
Dental sac
Beginning of root sheath

Figure 14-12A Tooth root development. H&E, ×29; (*upper*) inset ×160; (*lower*) inset ×90

Root development begins after the shape of the crown has been completed. It involves three structures: the **epithelial root sheath**, **the dental sac (follicle)**, and the **dental papilla**. Dentin formation proceeds from the crown to the root. The formation of the root begins at the **epithelial root sheath (Hertwig epithelial root sheath)**, which develops from the cervical loop. The inner and outer enamel epithelia of the **cervical loop** extend to form the root sheath. The epithelial root sheath grows around the dental papilla. It bends at a 45-degree angle and is called the **epithelial diaphragm**. The epithelial diaphragm gradually encloses the dental papilla with the exception of the **apical foramen**. The root sheath is important in forming the shape of the root. It induces the outer cell layer of the dental papilla to differentiate into odontoblasts, which produce the root dentin. When the root dentin has formed, the mesenchymal cells from the dental sac come in contact with the surface of the root dentin and induce these cells to differentiate into cementoblasts, which produce cementum. Fibroblasts, which differentiate from the dental sac, begin to form the PDL.

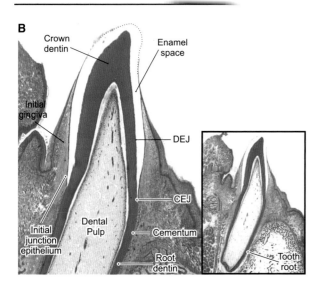

B

Crown dentin
Enamel space
Initial gingiva
DEJ
CEJ
Initial junction epithelium
Dental Pulp
Cementum
Root dentin
Tooth root

Figure 14-12B Tooth eruption. H&E, ×14; inset ×5

As root length increases, additional space is needed for root growth, and the tooth gradually moves and erupts into the oral cavity. **Tooth eruption** and root growth, therefore, occur at the same rate. The formation of the tooth root includes **root dentinogenesis** (formation of root dentin), **cementogenesis** (formation of cementum), **pulp formation**, formation of the PDL, and **alveolar bone development**. The crown of the tooth passes through the bony crypt, dental epithelium, and oral epithelium to emerge into the oral cavity. As the tooth moves vertically, the overlying bone gradually becomes absorbed by osteoclasts. The **dental epithelium** (outer enamel epithelium, stellate reticulum, stratum intermedium, and ameloblasts) is compressed into a thin layer called the **reduced enamel epithelium (REE)**. The oral epithelium fuses with the REE and gradually degenerates, enabling the tooth crown to erupt into the oral cavity. The **initial junctional epithelium** is created during tooth movement and eruption; later it becomes the **junction epithelium**, forming a seal between the gingiva and enamel. In a regular H&E stain, highly calcified enamel disappears because of the decalcification process during tissue preparation.

CLINICAL CORRELATION

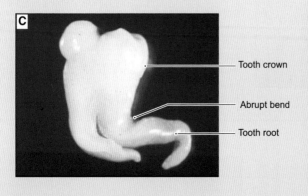

C

Tooth crown
Abrupt bend
Tooth root

Figure 14-12C. Dilaceration.

Dilaceration is a developmental anomaly of the tooth in which there is an **abrupt bend** between the crown and the root of a tooth. **Trauma** to the **primary predecessor tooth** and **developmental disturbances** to the **primary tooth germ** are the possible causes of this condition. Dilaceration can happen in any tooth, but is more common in **mandibular third molars, maxillary second premolars**, and **mandibular second molars**. Visual examination can find a crown dilaceration, but the radiograph is the most appropriate diagnostic tool to diagnose a root dilaceration. Dilacerations may be associated with some syndromes, such as **Smith-Magenis syndrome**, a chromosomal disorder that produces a set of characteristic physical, behavioral, and developmental features. Dilacerations can complicate cavity preparation, root canal preparation, and other treatments.

CLINICAL CORRELATIONS

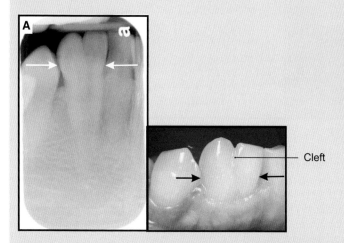

Cleft

Figure 14-13A. Gemination, Incisor.

Gemination is a variation in tooth structure that occurs when two teeth develop from the same tooth bud, resulting in a **larger than normal tooth crown**, but with a **normal number of teeth**. The gemination results from a disturbance that occurs at the **cap stage**. During the cap stage, the tooth germ is undergoing early morphogenesis and beginning to form the shape of the tooth. Gemination represents the unsuccessful division of a single tooth germ into two tooth germs. There is a deep cleft on the surface of the tooth, giving the appearance of two crowns. The radiograph at left shows two crowns (*arrows*) sharing one root. Occasionally, x-ray images may show two independent pulp chambers and root canals. The cause of gemination is unknown.

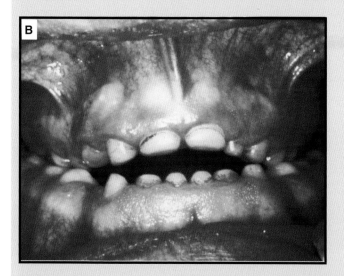

Figure 14-13B. Amelogenesis Imperfecta.

Amelogenesis imperfecta is a group of hereditary disorders that affect the **dental enamel formation** at the **apposition** and **maturation stages**. The teeth are covered with a thin, defective enamel or lack enamel covering. Mutations in different genes may affect enamel proteins, such as **amelogenin**, which is involved in enamel mineralization. The most common forms of amelogenesis imperfecta include **hypoplastic** and **hypocalcified** types. In the hypoplastic form, the teeth do not have a sufficient amount of enamel, whereas in the hypocalcified form, the quantity of enamel is normal, but it is soft and easily worn. Affected teeth are most often **yellow-brown** and **blue-gray** in color and are vulnerable to dental caries, damage, and loss. **Full crowns** will improve the appearance of the teeth and protect the teeth from damage.

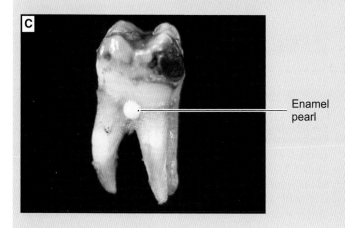

Enamel pearl

Figure 14-13C. Enamel Pearl.

Enamel pearl is an **ectopic formation** of **enamel** that is usually found close to the **CEJ** between tooth roots. Localized failure of **Hertwig epithelial root sheath** to separate from the dentin may be the cause of this anomaly. The enamel pearl results from a disturbance during the **apposition** or **maturation stages** during the tooth development. An enamel pearl may lead to **periodontal disease** because of the extension of a periodontal pocket. Histologically, enamel pearls have **reduced enamel epithelium** and are surrounded by normal **cementum**. X-rays can reveal enamel pearls. Enamel pearls cannot be removed by scaling, but they can be ground away to restore the normal shape of the tooth. An enamel pearl on a molar is shown here.

Enamel

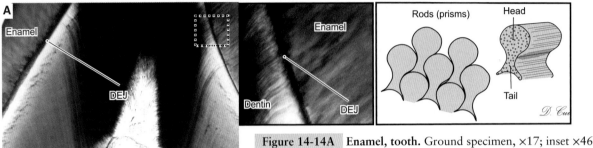

Figure 14-14A   Enamel, tooth. Ground specimen, ×17; inset ×46

Enamel is the hardest tissue in the body and is highly mineralized. It is composed of 96% inorganic material in the form of hydroxyapatite (crystalline calcium phosphate), 1% organic material, and 3% water. Enamel covers the dentin of the crown to make the tooth surface strong and suitable for chewing and to seal and protect the dentin. Enamel cannot be renewed after enamel formation has been completed, because enamel is produced by ameloblasts, which disappear after tooth eruption. However, enamel can be strengthened by fluoride. This ground specimen shows the enamel, dentin, and DEJ. The basic morphological unit of enamel is the **rod** (**prism**). Each rod has a head and tail and is tightly packed with hydroxyapatite crystals. The rods are arranged in a three-dimensional complex and are oriented generally perpendicular to the DEJ.

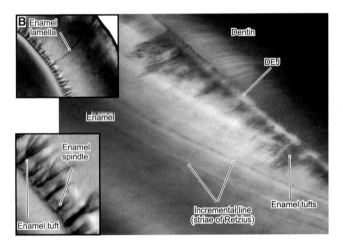

Figure 14-14B   Enamel structures, tooth. Ground specimen, ×68; inset (*upper*) ×13; inset (*lower*) ×62

The **incremental growth lines** of the **enamel**, also called the **striae of Retzius**, can be found in either cross (bands) or longitudinal sections (arcs) of the mature enamel. These patterns reflect the changes in enamel secretory rhythm. The **neonatal line** is much more prominent than the striae. It is a landmark that indicates the transition from enamel produced before birth and enamel produced after birth. This line is produced by a metabolic change that occurs at birth. There are three defects of enamel: (1) **Enamel tufts** are hypomineralized areas filled with organic material at the DEJ and toward the surface; (2) **enamel lamellae** are hypomineralized, thin, sheetlike defects that can run through the entire enamel and are commonly caused by cracks; and (3) **enamel spindles** are thin, needlelike lines extending from the DEJ to the enamel and are because of odontoblast processes trapped in the enamel during early amelogenesis.

CLINICAL CORRELATION

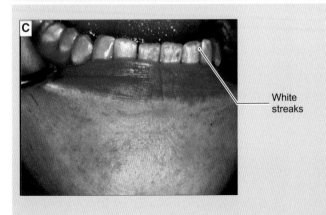

Figure 14-14C.   Enamel Fluorosis.

Enamel fluorosis is the general term for enamel changes caused by excessive **fluoride** intake during tooth development (before age 8 years). Fluoride helps to prevent and control tooth caries, but too much fluoride intake during tooth development can result in **hypomineralization** of the **enamel** surface. These changes are characterized by diffuse, opaque, and white streaks that run horizontally across the enamel. Stains with rough, irregular enamel surfaces are common. A fluoride-induced toxic effect on **ameloblasts** during enamel formation is believed to be the mechanism of the condition. Prevention is through controlling the fluoride intake, and treatments include **bleaching** and **enamel microabrasion**.

DENTIN

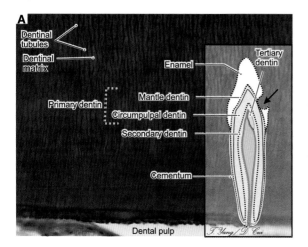

Figure 14-15A   Dentin, tooth. H&E, ×284

Dentin, which forms the bulk of the tooth, is covered by enamel on the crown and cementum on the root. It is about 70% inorganic materials (hydroxyapatite), 20% organic components (type I collagen and proteoglycans), and 10% water. Dentin is harder than bone and cementum but weaker than enamel. Dentin can be classified into three types: (1) **primary dentin,** deposited before the formation of the tooth root and tooth eruption have been completed, includes **mantle dentin** (at the DEJ) and **circumpulpal dentin;** (2) **secondary dentin,** produced after tooth eruption and root formation have been completed, is deposited very slowly and is located beneath the primary dentin; and (3) **tertiary (reparative) dentin** is produced in response to injures (caries [*arrow*], drilling, or attrition). Tertiary dentin is produced only by the odontoblasts that are directly stimulated when the tooth is injured. This type of dentin has few, mostly irregular, dentin tubules, which provide a seal to prevent bacteria and harmful molecules from invading the dental pulp. Dentin has three basic components: **dentinal tubules, dentinal matrix,** and **odontoblastic processes.**

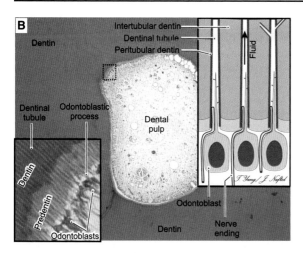

Figure 14-15B   Dentin and dentinal tubules, tooth. H&E, ×35; inset ×359

Dentin is produced by odontoblasts, and the formation of dentin is continuous throughout life. During the dentinogenesis process, the cell bodies of the odontoblasts retreat, but their cytoplasmic processes remain and are embedded in the mineralized dentinal matrix. Each odontoblastic process resides in a narrow channel, the dentinal tubule, which is lined by highly calcified peritubular dentin and traverses about half thickness of the dentin layers. The dentinal matrix, between the dentinal tubules, is called **intertubular dentin** and is less mineralized than the peritubular dentin. The dentinal tubules run from the dental pulp surface to the **DEJ.** These tubules are larger close to the pulp and more branched near the DEJ. Each dentinal tubule contains an odontoblastic process about halfway toward the DEJ; the rest of the space is filled with fluid. Nerve fibers for pain extend from the dental pulp to the inner part of the dentinal tubule.

Under certain circumstances, such as in **sensitive teeth,** the exposure of dentin to air blasts or drinking or eating cold, hot, or sweet substances will cause movement of the fluid in the dentinal tubules. This movement produces a mechanical disturbance that activates the nerve endings of pain fibers, inducing intense pain (**hydrodynamic theory**).

CLINICAL CORRELATION

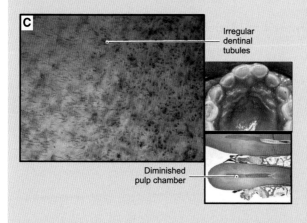

Figure 14-15C.   Dentinogenesis Imperfecta. H&E, ×329; inset (*lower*) ×2

Dentinogenesis imperfecta is an autosomal-dominant genetic disorder of tooth development caused by mutations in the **dentin sialophosphoprotein gene.** Affected teeth are often **blue-gray** or **yellow-brown** in color and **translucent.** Dentinogenesis imperfecta is classified as **types I–III.** *Type I* is associated with **osteogenesis imperfecta,** in which bones are brittle and easily fractured and pulp chambers are diminished. Type I collagen defects are also associated with type I dentinogenesis imperfecta. *Type II* is characterized by **diminished pulp chambers** and may be associated with progressive hearing loss. *Type III* has **large pulp chambers.** Patients suffer frequent **enamel fractures** and **enamel attrition.** Full crowns will improve the appearance of the teeth and protect the teeth from damage. Histologically, **dentinal tubules** are **irregular** and are **larger than normal** in diameter, and **uncalcified matrix** may be present.

CLINICAL CORRELATIONS

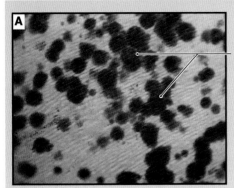

A

Calcification
defect in dentin

Figure 14-16A. Vitamin D–Resistant Rickets. H&E,
×476

Vitamin D–resistant rickets, commonly known as **X-linked hypophosphatemic rickets,** is characterized by resistance to conventional vitamin D treatment, decreased reabsorption of phosphate by the renal tubules, abnormalities in bones and teeth, **osteomalacia,** and **hypocalcemia.** It is an X-linked autosomal-dominant disorder. Patients with these rickets disorders do not respond to high-dose vitamin D treatment. Signs include rickets, short stature, bowing of lower limbs, seizures, congestive cardiac failure, and tooth defects including **calcification defects in dentin, enlarged pulp chambers, pulpitis,** and **pulp necrosis.** Treatment with 1,25-vitamin D (which is not dependent on normal hormonal mechanisms or organ systems to activate) plus controlled phosphate therapy may improve the condition.

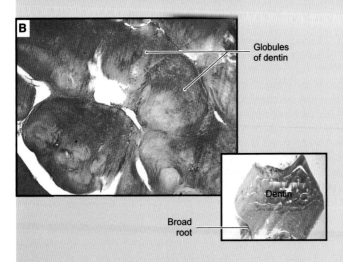

B

Globules
of dentin

Dentin

Broad
root

Figure 14-16B. Dentin Dysplasia. H&E, ×35; inset ×7

Dentin dysplasia is an autosomal-dominant tooth disorder. Teeth in this disorder are sometimes called **rootless teeth,** because they often have very short and conical roots. Dentin dysplasia can be classified into **types I** and **II.** *Type I,* also called the **radicular type,** is characterized by **short roots** and **pulp obliteration.** *Type II,* also called the **coronal type,** is characterized by a **"thistle tube" pulp.** Radiographically, extension of the pulp chamber into the root is usually observed in dentin dysplasia. Pulp stones and sudden constriction of the pulp chamber are common. Dentin dysplasia type II shares some similarities with **dentinogenesis imperfecta** type II, but in dentin dysplasia, the permanent dentition has normal color or only slight discoloration. Histologically, **globules of dentin** and **disorganized dentinal tubules** are characteristic of this condition. The *left image* shows globules of dentin; the *right image* shows a low-power photograph of a dentin dysplasia.

TABLE 14-3 DENTAL HARD TISSUE

Name of Tissue	Productive Cells	Inorganic (Mineral) %	Organic %	Water %	Sequence of Hard Tissue Formation	Sequence of Productive Cell Formation	Activity	Embryologic Origin
Dentin	Odontoblasts	70	20	10	First	Odontoblasts second	Lifetime	Dental papilla (mesoderm)
Enamel	Ameloblasts	96	3	1	Second	Ameloblasts first	Before tooth eruption	Enamel organ (ectoderm)
Cementum	Cementoblasts	65	23	12	Third	Cementoblasts third	Lifetime	Dental sac/ follicle (mesoderm)
Alveolar bone	Osteoblasts	60	25	15	—	—	Lifetime; respond to stresses and tensions	Mesoderm

Dental Pulp

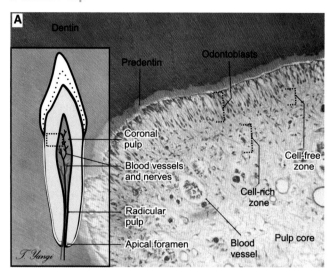

Figure 14-17A Dental pulp. H&E, ×136

Dental pulp is a specialized loose, cellular mucous connective tissue that fills the pulp chamber in the central core and root canals of the tooth. Fibroblasts are the most numerous cells in the pulp; they produce connective tissue fibers (mainly type I and III collagen, fibronectin, and elastin) and ground substance. They maintain the pulp matrix. The second most numerous cells are **odontoblasts** (producing dentin). Other defense cells, such as **macrophages** and **lymphocytes**, may be found in the pulp. **No mast cells** or **adipocytes (fat cells)** are found in a normal pulp. The pulp contains many blood vessels and nerve fibers, which enter and leave at the apical foramen. Most of the nerve fibers are afferent fibers; they are either C fibers or Aδ fibers, and both carry pain information through the trigeminal system to the brain. The efferent fibers are autonomic nerve fibers and innervate the smooth muscle of the blood vessels. Dental pulp plays an important role in producing dentin and providing nutrients and sensory input for the dentin.

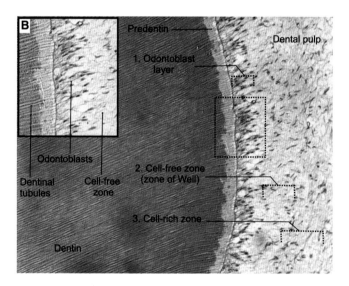

Figure 14-17B Dental pulp. H&E, ×136; inset ×190

Dental pulp is derived from mesenchymal tissue that forms the dental papilla during tooth development. The papilla becomes pulp in the mature tooth. The pulp can be divided into four zones from the periphery to the center. (1) The **odontoblast layer** forms a single cell layer along the peripheral edge of the pulp. These cells have processes extending into the dentin. (2) The **cell-free zone**, also called the **zone of Weil**, is directly under the odontoblast layer. This layer has fibers, cellular processes, axons, and capillaries running through it but contains no cell nuclei. (3) The **cell-rich zone** is beneath the cell-free zone and has many cells and nuclei of cells densely packed in rows. This layer has fibroblasts, undifferentiated mesenchymal cells, neural plexuses, and capillaries. If some odontoblasts die, the undifferentiated mesenchymal cells in this layer will differentiate into new odontoblasts. (4) The **pulp proper (pulp core)** is the central part of the pulp and contains blood vessels and nerves within the loose, mucous connective tissue. The layers of both cell-free and cell-rich zones are more visible in the **coronal** than the **radicular pulp** region.

CLINICAL CORRELATION

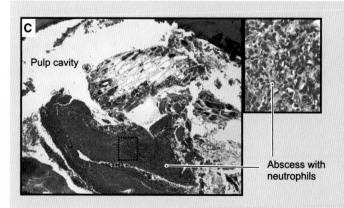

Figure 14-17C Pulp Abscess. H&E ×23; inset ×168

Pulp abscess refers to an abscess involving the pulp tissue of a tooth. Pulp abscesses are usually sequelae of dental caries, but they can also develop in teeth showing no detectable lesions. Pulp abscesses can also occur after restoration work has been performed. They are characterized by severe, intermittent pain that may intensify when a patient reclines. Periapical tissues may not be involved, and the affected tooth may not show any difference from other healthy teeth in percussion or pressure tests. Treatment includes undergoing root canals and even tooth extraction.

Periodontium

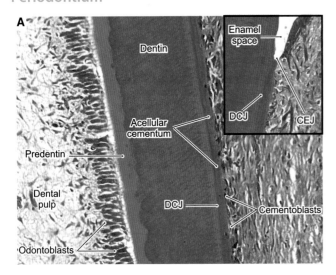

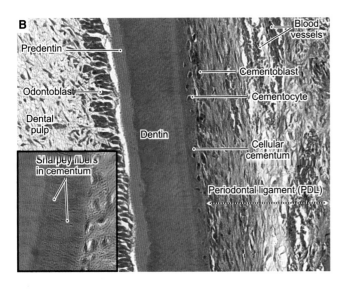

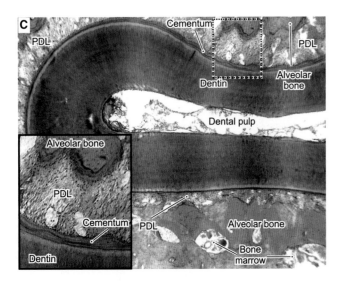

Figure 14-18A　Acellular cementum, cervical region of tooth root. H&E, ×181; inset ×158

The **periodontium** includes the **cementum**, the **PDL**, and the **alveolar bone**. These structures surround and support the tooth in the tooth socket. Cementum is a thin layer of hard tissue (calcified matrix) that does not have a direct blood supply. It covers the dentin and seals the dentinal tubules at the root region. Cementum is thicker at the root apex than at the cervix region and can be divided into **acellular** and **cellular cementum**. Acellular cementum has no cementocytes embedded within the matrix and is often found at the cervical two thirds of the root, attached to the dentin. The junction between the dentin and cementum is called the **dentinocemental junction (DCJ)**, and the junction between the cementum and enamel is the **CEJ**. There are three forms of the CEJ: (1) the cementum overlaps the enamel (60%); (2) the cementum meets the enamel end-end (30%); and (3) there is a gap between the cementum and the enamel (10%).

Figure 14-18B　Cellular cementum, apical region of tooth root. H&E, ×181; inset ×408

Cellular cementum is often found at the apical third of the tooth root and is similar to bone with a calcified intercellular matrix. During the process of formation of cementum, some cementoblasts are trapped in the matrix, and each one is surrounded by a lacuna. These **cementoblasts** then become **cementocytes**. The matrix of cellular cementum is deposited more rapidly than that of acellular cementum. **Acellular cementum** has a slower formation rate and formation continues throughout life. The slower growing cementum allows fibers (**Sharpey fibers**, *left inset*) from the PDL to become trapped in the matrix of the cementum to form the tooth attachment. Cementum is much more resistant to reabsorption than bones. This characteristic helps maintain root integrity and prevents exposure of the root dentin, which is important as teeth are moved around during orthodontic procedures.

Figure 14-18C　Periodontal ligament (PDL) and alveolar bone. H&E, ×34; inset ×72

The **PDL** is a dense fibrous connective tissue with a direct nerve and blood supply. It is located between the cementum and the alveolar bone, which surrounds the tooth root. Fibroblasts are the main cells responsible for the formation of the PDL. The PDL supports the tooth root by forming a strong attachment between the cementum and alveolar bone by **Sharpey fibers**. The functions of the PDL are to provide sensory information regarding pain and pressure, to provide signals to the alveolar bone regarding bone remodeling, and to maintain tooth position in the dental arch. The **alveolar bone** (also called the **alveolar process**) surrounds and supports the tooth root and is part of the maxilla and mandible. It is constantly remodeled and is built up by osteoblasts and absorbed by osteoclasts. Alveolar bone has the general characteristics of bones. It consists of both compact and cancellous bones (see Chapter 5, "Cartilage and Bone").

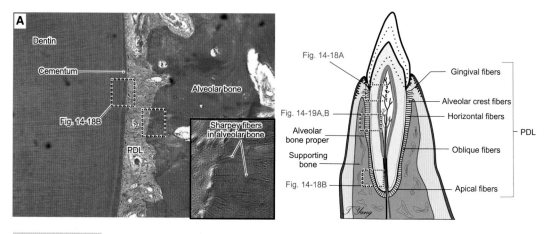

Figure 14-19A   Periodontal ligament (PDL) and alveolar bone, tooth root. H&E, ×68; inset ×408

The **cementum** and **periodontal ligament (PDL)** are derived from the dental sac. During root formation, some fibers from the PDL are trapped within the cementum and the alveolar bone. These **Sharpey fibers** bridge the space between the cementum and the alveolar bone and serve to suspend the tooth within the alveolar socket. The principal fibers of the PDL are organized in several groups based on their orientation and location: **apical, oblique, horizontal, alveolar crest, interradicular,** and **gingival fibers.** The interradicular fibers are only present between multirooted teeth. The gingival fibers attach the gingiva to the hard tissue of the tooth. The **alveolar bone** provides support and protection for the tooth root. The alveolar bone includes the **alveolar bone proper** and **supporting bone.** The *alveolar bone proper* is a thin layer of compact bone, which lines the tooth socket and has Sharpey fibers embedded in it; it is remodeled constantly to adapt to stresses and tensions. The *supporting bone* is composed of **compact bone** and **cancellous bone.** The *compact bone* forms the cortical plate, which provides surface strength. The *cancellous bone* makes up the central core of the alveolar bone and contains bone marrow.

CLINICAL CORRELATION

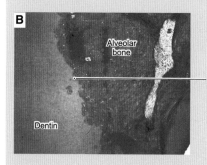

Figure 14-19B   Tooth Ankylosis. H&E, ×68

Tooth ankylosis is the fusion of a mineralized root surface to its surrounding alveolar bone. It is characterized by a typical metallic percussion sound and loss of the **PDL space** in radiographs. Periapical inflammation and subsequent tissue repair are believed to be the cause of ankylosis. Ankylosis is more common in **deciduous teeth** and usually results in **impaction** of a subjacent **permanent tooth.** Impaction of incisors is much less common than it is in the mandibular third molars. This slide shows impaction of a **central incisor** with focal loss of the PDL of the incisor.

SYNOPSIS 14-1 PATHOLOGIC AND CLINICAL TERMS FOR THE ORAL CAVITY

■ *Microdontia:* Disproportionately small teeth (disturbances occur at bud stage).
■ *Macrodontia:* Disproportionately large teeth (disturbances occur at bud stage).
■ *Dens invaginatus (dens in dente):* Developmental anomaly in tooth formation at cap stage in which the epithelium invaginates into the pulp space to form enamel and dentin, creating a "tooth within a tooth" as shown in the radiographic imaging.
■ *Misalignment:* A condition in which teeth are too crowded and incorrectly positioned.
■ *Tooth decay (caries):* Bacterial destruction of teeth, including erosion of the enamel and damage to the pulp tissue.
■ *Hypersensitivity:* A painful condition, especially to touch, sweetness, and cold drinks caused by exposed dentin.
■ *Periodontal disease:* A chronic inflammatory condition of gingival and surrounding periodontal tissues. Calculus and bacterial plaque are the major causes of the disease.
■ *Gingivitis:* Infection and inflammation of the gingival tissue.
■ *Periodontitis:* Infection and inflammation affecting the periodontium, characterized by gingivitis, destruction of the alveolar bone and periodontal ligament, and the formation of periodontal pockets.
■ *Pulpitis:* An inflammation of the pulpal tissue of a tooth.
■ *White lesions:* Lesions on the mucosa of the oral cavity that have a white coating such as leukoplakia.
■ *Red lesions:* Chronic red oral mucosal lesions in which underlying vascular structures become more visible (as in erythroplakia).

From Histology to Pathology

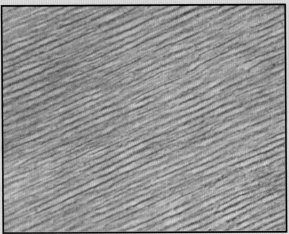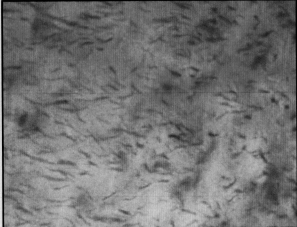

Figure 14-20. Normal dentin and dentinogenesis imperfecta. H&E, ×400.

Normal dentin on the *left*. **Dentinogenesis imperfecta** on the *right* is caused by mutations in the dentin sialophosphoprotein gene. Patients suffer frequent enamel fractures and enamel attrition. Affected teeth are often translucent and blue-gray or yellow-brown in color, and the pulp chambers are diminished. Histologically, dentinal tubules are irregular and are larger than normal in diameter, and an uncalcified matrix may be present.

Clinical Vignette Questions

1. A 9-year-old boy with poor tooth development is brought to your clinic by his mother. The history reveals that the boy had several episodes of bone fracture in the past 2 years. Physical examination reveals a well-nourished healthy boy with yellow-brown teeth, thin defective enamel, and a blue tint in his sclera. X-ray confirms some of his previous multiple fractures. Which of the following abnormalities does this boy most likely have?

A. Amelogenesis imperfecta
B. Dens invaginatus
C. Dentinogenesis imperfecta
D. Enamel fluorosis
E. Tooth ankyloses

2. A 9-year-old boy who recently emigrated from Nepal presents to your clinic for a check-up. Examination of his oral cavity reveals staining and pitting of the teeth, characterized by diffuse, opaque, and horizontal white streaks in the enamel. Which of the following is the most likely diagnosis in this case?

A. Amelogenesis imperfect
B. Enamel dysplasia
C. Enamel fluorosis
D. Enamel hypoplasia
E. Lead poisoning

3. A 45-year-old man who has a history of 26 years of cigarette smoking (1 pack per day) comes for a check-up. He complains of sore throat and cough, especially during the winter. Physical examination shows a white lesion in the oral mucosa of the hard palate. The lesion looks like cobblestone with a dried-mud appearance. Chest x-ray and other lab tests turn out to be normal. Which of the following is the most likely diagnosis for his oral lesion?

A. Histoplasmosis
B. Nicotine stomatitis
C. Oral squamous cell carcinoma
D. Palate cancer

15 Digestive Tract

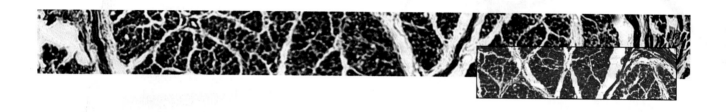

Clinical Vignette Questions

Introduction and Key Concepts for the Digestive Tract

The **digestive system** is composed of the **oral cavity**, **digestive tract**, and **digestive glands** with associated organs. The "Oral Cavity" is discussed in Chapter 14; the "Digestive Glands and Associated Organs" are discussed in Chapter 16. The digestive tract is discussed in this chapter. It includes the **esophagus**, **stomach**, **small intestine**, and **large intestine**. The digestive tract is a continuation of the oral cavity, and its main functions are to ingest food and to digest the food as it passes along the tract. In this process, nutrients and water are absorbed, and waste materials are prepared for elimination from the body. Each section of the digestive tract has its unique histologic features, which are closely associated with the function of that part of the tract, although there are some common characteristics: (1) Organs of the digestive tract are all hollow; (2) they are composed of four general tunic layers: mucosa, submucosa, muscularis externa, and adventitia or serosa; (3) they are innervated by the enteric portion of the autonomic nervous system, also known as the **enteric nervous system** (or the "second brain"); (4) they include epithelium, connective tissue, muscle, blood and lymphatic vessels, lymphatic nodules, and nerve fibers; and (5) they contain glands in the lamina propria or submucosa.

General Structure of the Digestive Tract

Based on its histologic organization, the wall of the digestive tract can be divided into four tunics.

1. *Mucosa* is the innermost layer of the digestive wall. It includes **epithelium**, **lamina propria**, and **muscularis mucosae**. The *epithelium* consists of simple columnar epithelium lining most of the tract and stratified squamous epithelium lining the two ends, the esophagus and anal canal. The *lamina propria* is a loose connective tissue that contains abundant ground substance, many fibers, and numerous connective tissue cells such as fibroblasts, macrophages, mast cells, plasma cells, and leukocytes (see Chapter 4, "Connective Tissue"). Various types of glands are found in the lamina propria depending on the region of the digestive tract. The *muscularis mucosae* is a very thin layer of smooth muscle, which is the boundary between the mucosa and the submucosa. It is usually arranged in an inner circular and outer longitudinal layer. However, the muscularis mucosae varies in different regions, and it is often difficult to distinguish between the muscle layers.
2. *Submucosa* is a thick layer of dense irregular connective tissue. This layer contains blood vessels, lymphatic vessels, and **submucosal (Meissner) plexuses**, which contain nerve fibers and neurons of the enteric nervous system. In some regions of the digestive tract, this layer is characterized by mucous glands or lymphatic nodules.
3. *Muscularis externa* is composed of two or three oblique, circular, and longitudinal muscle layers, which vary from region to region. Most of the muscularis externa consists of smooth muscle fibers, but the upper and middle esophagi contain some skeletal muscle. The **myenteric (Auerbach) plexuses** (nerve fibers and neurons of the enteric nervous system) are located between the muscle layers. They innervate and control contraction of the muscularis externa.

4. *Serosa and adventitia* are coverings of the outermost wall of the digestive tract. Most parts of the digestive tract are covered by **serosa**, a thin layer of loose connective tissue lined by **mesothelium**. The mesothelium produces a lubricating fluid that reduces friction during movement of the organs against each other (see Chapter 3, "Epithelium and Glands"). The serosa is the visceral layer of the peritoneum and covers the wall of the digestive tract where it connects to the mesentery in the peritoneal cavity (intraperitoneal organs). The **adventitia** is a layer of loose connective tissue without mesothelium that covers the upper region of the esophagus, part of the duodenum, and the lower part of the digestive tract, such as the rectum and anal canal. Adventitia covers regions of the digestive tract where it is connected to other organs or to the body wall (e.g., retroperitoneal organs).

Esophagus

The **esophagus** is the upper part of the digestive tract, connecting the oral cavity to the stomach. The major function of the esophagus is to provide passage for food from the mouth to the stomach. The luminal surface of the esophagus is lined by nonkeratinized stratified squamous epithelium. Mucous glands called **esophageal glands** are located in the submucosa of the esophagus. The muscularis externa consists of two layers of muscle: inner circular and outer longitudinal layers. Both skeletal and smooth muscle fibers are found in the muscularis externa of the esophagus. The proportions of skeletal and smooth muscle fibers are different in different regions of the esophagus. The esophagus can be divided into three regions: the **upper esophagus**, **middle esophagus**, and **lower esophagus**.

1. *The upper esophagus* connects the oropharynx to the middle esophagus. This segment contains numerous esophageal glands in the submucosa. These glands secrete mucus to lubricate the esophageal wall so that food will pass through easily. The upper esophagus contains only skeletal muscle fibers in the muscularis externa. These are voluntary muscle fibers and are innervated by the **glossopharyngeal nerve** (**cranial nerve [CN] IX**).
2. *The middle esophagus* has mucosa similar to that of the upper esophagus. The esophageal glands in the submucosa are less numerous than in the upper esophagus. The muscularis externa contains both skeletal and smooth muscles.
3. *The lower esophagus* connects the esophagus to the cardia of the stomach. This region contains large numbers of mucous glands in the lamina propria and submucosa. These are called **esophageal cardiac glands** and produce mucous secretions to protect the lower esophagus from being damaged by reflux of acidic gastric juices from the stomach. The lower esophagus contains only smooth muscle fibers in the muscularis externa. These are controlled by the enteric branches of the **vagus nerve (CN X)**.

Stomach

The **stomach** is a "J"-shaped sac (hollow) organ. It temporarily stores food, mixes food with gastric juice, and initiates the processing of food by breaking it down into simpler substances that are easier to digest. The stomach can be divided into the **cardia, fundus, body**, and **pylorus**. The inner surface of the stomach is lined by simple columnar epithelium composed mainly of surface mucous cells. The surface epithelium of the stomach is invaginated into the lamina propria to form **gastric pits**. These pits serve as ducts for the glands in the lamina propria, which vary from region to region in the stomach.

1. *The cardiac region* connects to the lower esophagus at the esophagogastric junction, which is characterized by a change from the nonkeratinized stratified squamous epithelium of the esophagus to the simple columnar epithelium of the stomach. A thickened smooth muscle ring called the **gastroesophageal sphincter** (**lower esophageal sphincter**) or **cardiac sphincter** surrounds the opening at the junction of the lower esophagus and cardiac region of the stomach. This smooth muscle contracts to prevent the acidic stomach contents from entering the esophagus. The glands in the lamina propria of the cardia are called **cardiac glands** and are branched tubular glands with coiled secretory portions. The cardiac gland contains mainly **mucus-secreting cells** and some **stem cells, enteroendocrine cells**, and, occasionally, **parietal cells**. The mucus-secreting cells mainly produce mucus and lysozymes. The mucus protects the stomach wall from acidic gastric juices; lysozymes destroy bacterial membranes, preventing bacterial infections.

2. *The fundic and body regions* form the largest portions of the stomach. Their mucosa has similar histologic characteristics, including short gastric pits and long branched tubular glands in the lamina propria. The glands are called **fundic** or **gastric glands** in both the fundus and the body regions. The gastric glands contain mainly **parietal cells** and **chief cells**, along with some **stem cells, mucous neck cells**, and **enteroendocrine cells**. Parietal cells are more numerous in the superior regions of the glands; these cells produce large quantities of **hydrochloric acid** (**HCl**), creating an acidic environment to help digestion. Parietal cells also secrete **intrinsic factor** (**IF**), which is required for the absorption of **vitamin B12**. **Chief cells** are located in the more inferior regions of the glands; they secrete precursor enzymes such as **pepsinogen**, which is activated by HCl and becomes pepsin. Pepsin helps to break down proteins (particularly protein collagen) into simpler, more absorbable compounds. Chief cells also secrete precursors of **lipases**, which help in lipid digestion.

3. *The pyloric region* is the lower end of the stomach, which connects with the duodenum. Its mucosa is similar to that of the cardia, with long gastric pits and short, coiled secretory portions. A circular smooth muscle ring called the **pylorus sphincter** (**pyloric valve**) surrounds the end of the pylorus region. This valve controls the entry of stomach contents into the duodenum. The glands in the lamina propria of the pylorus are called **pyloric glands** and contain primarily mucus-secreting cells and two special types of enteroendocrine cells: **gastrin-secreting cells** (**G cells**) and **somatostatin-secreting cells** (**D cells**). These enteroendocrine cells regulate gastric (HCl) secretion.

Small Intestine

The **small intestine** is a hollow organ of small diameter that is typically 6 to 7 m long. It is the major site for the absorption of nutrients. Important features of the small intestine are **villi** and **microvilli**, which increase surface area for absorption. Intestinal glands called **glands** (**crypts**) **of Lieberkühn** are located in the lamina propria of the small intestine. Villi project into the lumen of the intestine; the glands of Lieberkühn open into the mucosa at the base of the villi. The small intestine can be divided into three parts: the **duodenum, jejunum**, and **ileum**.

1. *The duodenum* is the shortest segment of the small intestine, about 20 to 25 cm long. It has small openings called **duodenal papillae** (*minor* and *major*), which allow pancreatic juice and bile to enter the digestive tract. It has a similar general structure to other parts of the small intestine. However, the **Brunner glands** (mucus-secreting gland) in the submucosa are a unique feature of the duodenum.

2. *The jejunum* is much longer than the duodenum, about 2.5 m long (two fifths of the rest of the small intestine). It has long villi and a somewhat increased number of goblet cells. It has neither Brunner glands nor Peyer patches.

3. *The ileum* is the longest segment, about 4 m long (three fifths of the rest of the small intestine). It has short villi with significantly increased numbers of goblet cells on the surface of the mucosa. There are clusters of lymphatic nodules in the lamina propria of the ileum; sometimes these lymphatic nodules extend into the submucosal layer. These clusters of lymphatic nodules are called **Peyer patches** and are unique to the ileum.

Large Intestine

The **large intestine** is a hollow organ with a relatively large diameter compared to the small intestine and is about 1.5 m long. It is the last region of the digestive tract and is the major site for absorption of water and salts. It also forms, stores, and eliminates feces. Most of the regions of the large intestine have tunics that are similar to those of the small intestine, but there are no villi in the mucosa. There are large numbers of **goblet cells** in the large intestine. These cells produce mucus, which helps in the formation of the feces and protects and lubricates the surface of the intestinal wall. The large intestine includes the **cecum, appendix, colon, rectum**, and **anal canal**.

1. *The cecum* is the most proximal region of the large intestine. It is a small, blind pouch of the large intestine where the ileum connects to the ascending colon. A sphincter muscle, a thickening of the muscularis mucosae, is called the **ileocecal valve** and is located at the junction of the ileum and cecum. It prevents the contents of the large intestine from backing up into the small intestine.

2. *The appendix* is a small, blind tube that attaches to the posterior-medial wall of the cecum. It has the general tunic structure of the intestine and a small irregular lumen. There are many lymphatic nodules in the lamina propria.

3. *The colon* is the longest segment of the large intestine. It includes the **ascending colon, transverse colon, descending colon**, and **sigmoid colon**. The proximal half of the colon is responsible for the majority of the absorption of water and salt; the distal half of the colon has only a small absorptive function and is predominantly for processing and storing feces. The colon does not have villi; it has a smoother surface than the small intestine. Columnar absorptive cells and goblet cells line the mucosa. The large intestinal glands, the glands (crypts) of Lieberkühn, contain primarily **goblet cells, columnar cells, enteroendocrine cells**, and **stem cells**. Lymphatic nodules may also be found in the lamina propria. The muscularis externa consists of inner circular layers of muscle; the outer longitudinal smooth muscle layer becomes three **taeniae coli**.

4. ***The rectum and anal canal*** are the last segments of the large intestine. The junction between the rectum and the anal canal is called the "anorectal junction." The mucosa of the rectum is similar to that of the colon but has fewer glands of Lieberkühn. The main function of the **rectum** is the temporary storage of feces. The sensory receptors in the rectum send signals to the brain when feces need to be evacuated. The **anal canal** is the distal end of the large intestine. Most of the anal canal is lined by stratified squamous epithelium, although simple cuboidal epithelium may be present at the anorectal junction. Sebaceous glands and hair follicles may be found at or near the anal opening. There are many veins in the lamina propria and submucosa of the anal canal. The term **hemorrhoids** refers to the condition in which these veins become chronically swollen and inflamed in the rectal and anal regions.

Anatomy of the Digestive Tract

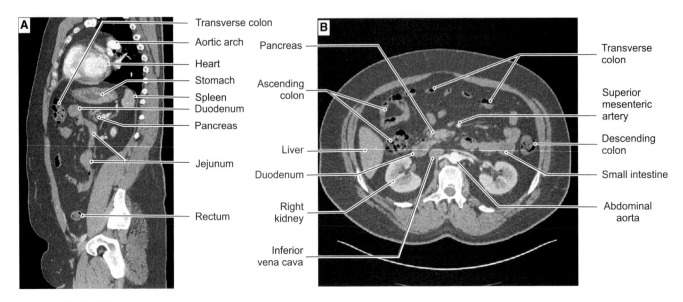

Figure 15-1A,B. **Digestive tract.** Computed tomography angiography, left (sagittal view), right (transverse, or axial, view).

The **digestive tract** can be divided into three regions: the **foregut, midgut,** and **hindgut** based on embryological development. The **foregut** includes the distal portion of the esophagus, stomach, first (superior) part of the duodenum, second (descending) part of the duodenum to the level of the major duodenal papilla (also known as the ampulla of Vater, which is the opening of the common bile duct and the main pancreatic duct into the second part of the duodenum), liver, and pancreas. The **midgut** includes the distal portion of the second part of the duodenum below the level of the major duodenal papilla, the third (horizontal) and fourth (ascending) parts of the duodenum, the jejunum, the ileum, the cecum, the ascending colon, and the proximal two thirds of the transverse colon. The **hindgut** includes the distal third of the transverse colon, the descending colon, the sigmoid colon, and the rectum. The blood supply to the digestive tract originates from the **celiac trunk, superior mesenteric artery,** and **inferior mesenteric artery,** all of which are branches of the abdominal aorta. The **foregut** mainly receives blood supply from the **celiac trunk,** the **midgut** from the **superior mesenteric artery,** and the **hindgut** from the **inferior mesenteric artery.** The digestive tract, also called the **gastrointestinal tract,** refers to the muscular structures stretching from the mouth to the anus, including the **oral cavity, esophagus, stomach, small intestine,** and **large intestine.** The digestive tract allows for the consumption of food (eating) and beverage (drinking), mastication (chewing) and processing of food, the absorption of nutrients and water, and the passage of waste products (feces) to the outside of the body through the process of defecation. The **oral cavity** helps ingest food. The salivary glands in the oral cavity help to moisturize the oral mucosa, balance the pH level of the mouth, clean the oral cavity, and control oral bacterial growth. During ingestion, the secretion of saliva increases, helping break down large pieces of food for easy digestion. The oral cavity opens into the oropharynx, a structure that is between the oral cavity and the beginning of the trachea and esophagus. The **esophagus** helps transfer food and drink to the stomach. The esophagus empties its contents into the **stomach,** which is located in the upper left part of the abdominal cavity, adjacent to the diaphragm. The stomach helps store and digest food and produce intrinsic factor that is essential for the absorption of vitamin B12 in the small intestine. The **small intestine** begins with the duodenum at the pylorus of the stomach. The **duodenum** is a C-shaped structure that can be divided into four parts: superior, descending, horizontal, and ascending. The duodenum curves around the head of the pancreas, and the common bile duct and the main pancreatic duct connect to the descending part of the duodenum, where bile and pancreatic enzymes are secreted into the small intestine to help digest food. The most distal (ascending) part of the duodenum connects to the **jejunum,** which, in turn, connects to the **ileum.** The small intestine helps digest and absorb 90% of the consumed nutrients. The **large intestine** begins at the end of the ileum and ends at the anus. It consists of the **cecum, ascending colon, transverse colon, descending colon, sigmoid colon, rectum,** and **anus.** The **appendix** attached to the cecum, can sometimes become inflamed and cause **appendicitis.** The large intestine helps reabsorb water, absorb vitamins, and store feces before defecation.

CLINICAL CORRELATION

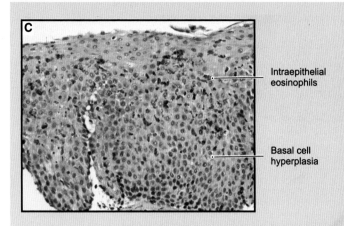

Intraepithelial
eosinophils

Basal cell
hyperplasia

Figure 15-1C. Eosinophilic Esophagitis. H&E, ×200

Eosinophilic esophagitis (EOE) is an allergic inflammatory disease of the esophagus characterized by eosinophils within the **stratified squamous epithelium (intraepithelial eosinophils)**. EOE affects children and adults, and presenting symptoms include **nausea, vomiting, pain, dysphagia (difficulty swallowing),** and **food impaction**. Infants may experience feeding difficulties. EOE tends to occur in individuals with other allergic disorders such as asthma, food allergies, and environmental allergies. Endoscopic examination of the esophagus may show **esophageal rings, furrows,** and **edema**. In severe cases, luminal stricture may occur. Histologic examination typically reveals **basal cell hyperplasia, intraepithelial eosinophils** (≥15 per high-power field), and occasional **eosinophilic microabscesses** in the upper, middle, and lower esophagus. In **gastroesophageal reflux disease (GERD)**, eosinophils are usually limited to the lower esophagus. Treatment includes allergy testing, diet modification, and topical steroids. In severe cases, systemic steroids may be required, and dilation may be required in patients with strictures.

Digestive Tract

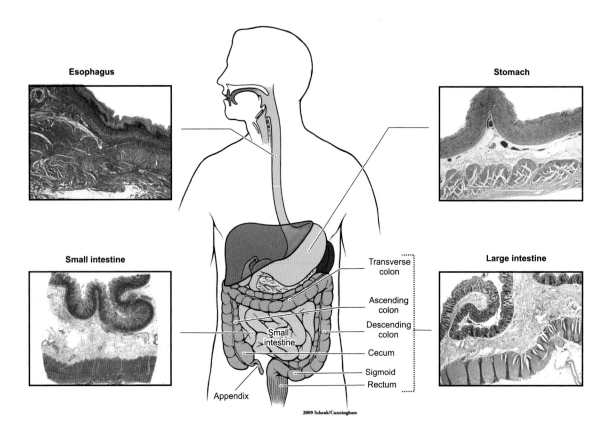

Figure 15-2. Overview of the digestive tract. H&E, ×5 to ×6

The **digestive tract**, also called the **alimentary canal**, includes the **esophagus, stomach, small intestine**, and **large intestine**. (1) The *esophagus* transports food to the stomach. Its luminal surface is lined by stratified squamous nonkeratinized epithelium and contains mucous glands in the **lamina propria**. It has both skeletal and smooth muscles in the **muscularis externa**. (2) The *stomach* temporarily stores and digests food. Its luminal surface is lined by simple columnar epithelium and contains gastric glands in the lamina propria. It has three layers of smooth muscle in the muscularis externa. (3) The *small intestine* digests and absorbs carbohydrates, proteins, and lipids. The small intestine includes the **duodenum, jejunum**, and **ileum**. The luminal surface is lined by simple columnar epithelium and contains the glands (crypts) of Lieberkühn in the lamina propria. There are two layers of smooth muscles (inner circular and outer longitudinal muscles) in the muscularis externa. (4) The *large intestine* includes the **cecum, appendix, colon, rectum**, and **anal canal**. The main functions of the large intestine are the absorption both of a large volume of the water that enters it (90%) and of electrolytes (e.g., Na^+ and Cl^-) and the formation of the feces. Most parts of the large intestine are lined by simple columnar epithelium, but stratified squamous epithelium lines the anal canal. The glands of Lieberkühn are located in the lamina propria. The muscularis externa contains an inner layer of circular smooth muscle and an outer layer of longitudinal smooth muscle, which forms three **taeniae coli**. In general, the submucosa of the digestive tract is a thick layer of connective tissue containing blood vessels, lymphatic vessels, and **submucosal (Meissner) plexuses** consisting of nerve fibers and neuron cell bodies in the **enteric nervous system**. The **myenteric (Auerbach) plexuses** located in the muscularis externa are also components of the enteric nervous system.

Digestive Tract

I. **Esophagus**
   A. Upper esophagus (skeletal muscle)
   B. Middle esophagus (mixed skeletal and smooth muscles)
   C. Lower esophagus (smooth muscle)

II. **Stomach**
   A. Cardia
   B. Fundus
   C. Body
   D. Pylorus

III. **Small Intestine**
   A. Duodenum
   B. Jejunum
   C. Ileum

IV. **Large Intestine**
   A. Cecum
   B. Appendix
   C. Colon (ascending, transverse, descending, and sigmoid)
   D. Rectum
   E. Anal canal

Figures and Images Orientation

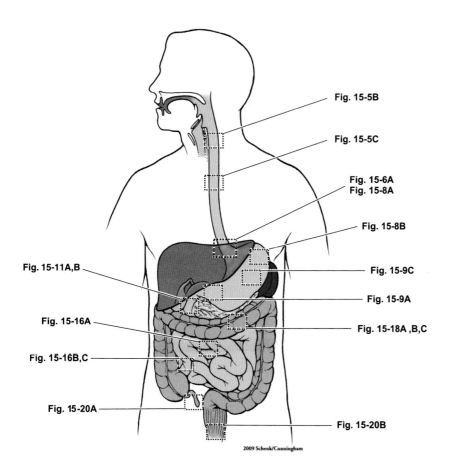

Fig. 15-5B
Fig. 15-5C
Fig. 15-6A
Fig. 15-8A
Fig. 15-8B
Fig. 15-11A,B
Fig. 15-9C
Fig. 15-9A
Fig. 15-16A
Fig. 15-18A ,B,C
Fig. 15-16B,C
Fig. 15-20A
Fig. 15-20B

2009 Schenk/Cunningham

Figure 15-3. Orientation of detailed digestive tract illustrations.

Digestive Tract with Figure Numbers

Tunics of the Digestive Tract

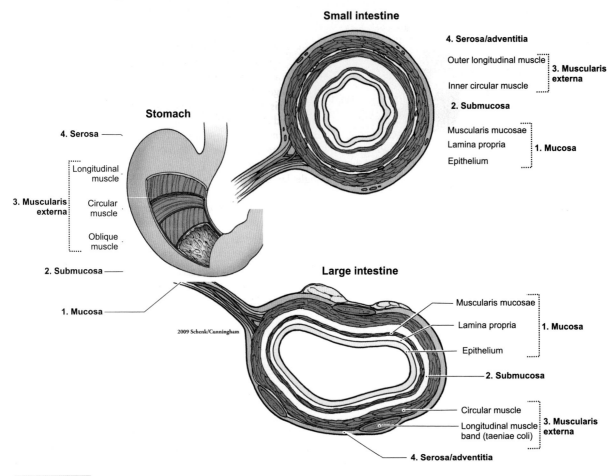

Figure 15-4. General structure of the wall of the digestive tract.

The **wall** of the **digestive tract** can be divided into several basic tunics (layers) based on histologic organization. (1) **Mucosa:** epithelium, lamina propria, and muscularis mucosae. The epithelium is composed of simple columnar cells in most of the digestive tract, except for stratified squamous cells in the esophagus and anal canal. The lamina propria is a layer of loose connective tissue beneath the epithelium. The muscularis mucosae is a thin layer of smooth muscle; it marks the boundary between the mucosa and the submucosa. (2) **Submucosa:** dense irregular connective tissue with blood vessels, lymphatic vessels, and **submucosal plexuses (Meissner plexuses)**. Mucous glands may be present in this layer. (3) **Muscularis externa:** two or three layers of smooth muscle. It may also include skeletal muscle as in the esophagus. There are blood vessels and **myenteric (Auerbach) plexuses** that lie between the muscle layers. (4) **Serosa/adventitia:** the outermost layer is called *serosa* if it is composed of loose connective tissue with blood vessels and nerves passing through and is covered by **mesothelium**. It is called *adventitia* if covered by a layer of connective tissue without mesothelium lining. The serosa covers organs within the abdominal or pelvic cavities (intraperitoneal), whereas the adventitia covers organs and serves as a capsule and attachment between the organs or between an organ and the body wall (retroperitoneal).

Tunics (Layers) of the Digestive Tract

I. **Mucosa**
   A. Epithelium
   B. Lamina propria
   C. Muscularis mucosae
II. **Submucosa**
   A. Mucous glands and lymphatic nodules may be present
III. **Muscularis Externa**
   A. Inner circular muscle layer

   B. Outer longitudinal muscle layer
   C. Oblique muscle layer (stomach)
IV. **Serosa/Adventitia**
   A. Serosa: outermost layer composed of connective tissue covered by mesothelium
   B. Adventitia: outermost layer composed of connective tissue without mesothelium covering

Esophagus

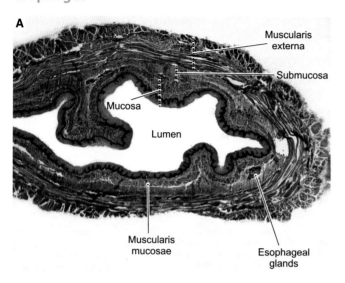

A

Muscularis externa

Submucosa

Mucosa

Lumen

Muscularis mucosae

Esophageal glands

Figure 15-5A. Overview of the esophagus. H&E, ×11

The **esophagus** can be divided into three regions: the **upper**, **middle**, and **lower esophagus**. The esophagus is a long tube that connects the oropharynx to the stomach. Like other parts of the digestive tract, the esophagus has **mucosa, submucosa, muscularis externa,** and **adventitia/serosa.** (1) The *mucosa* is composed of **epithelium, lamina propria,** and **muscularis mucosae.** The mucosa of the esophagus has folds extending into the lumen. Stratified squamous epithelium covers the inner surface of the esophagus. The **muscularis mucosae** is composed of a single layer of longitudinal smooth muscle. (2) The *submucosa* contains mucous glands called **esophageal glands,** which secrete mucus and provide lubrication that aids in swallowing. (3) The *muscularis externa* is composed of two layers of muscle organized into **inner circular** and **outer longitudinal** layers. (4) The outermost wall of the esophagus is commonly covered by *adventitia,* but the lower esophagus is covered by *serosa.*

UPPER ESOPHAGUS

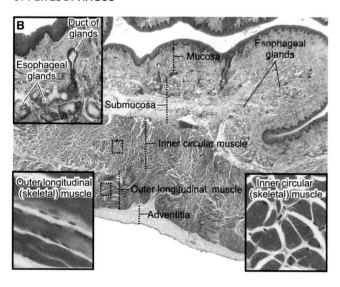

B

Duct of glands

Esophageal glands

Mucosa

Esophageal glands

Submucosa

Inner circular muscle

Outer longitudinal (skeletal) muscle

Outer longitudinal muscle

Inner circular (skeletal) muscle

Adventitia

Figure 15-5B. Upper esophagus. H&E, ×17; *(upper* inset) ×40; *(lower* insets) ×216

The **upper esophagus,** connecting to the oropharynx, is the first segment of the esophagus. The muscularis externa of the upper esophagus contains two layers of **skeletal muscle.** The skeletal muscle is a voluntary muscle that helps to initiate swallowing. This muscle is innervated by the glossopharyngeal nerve. The **muscularis externa** of the esophagus has distinguishable muscle components, which vary in different regions. The upper esophagus has skeletal muscle, the middle esophagus has mixed skeletal and smooth muscles, and the lower esophagus has only smooth muscle in the muscularis externa. The muscularis externa plays an important role in producing contractions of the esophagus that transport food from the oral cavity to the stomach. The major movement of the esophagus is **peristalsis** (waves of involuntary contraction), as in other parts of the digestive tract. The initiation of swallowing is voluntary because the upper esophagus contains only skeletal muscle fibers in the muscularis externa.

MIDDLE ESOPHAGUS

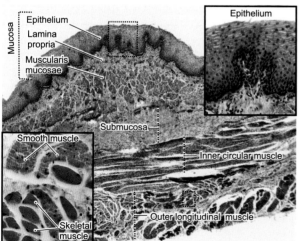

C

Mucosa

Epithelium

Lamina propria

Muscularis mucosae

Epithelium

Submucosa

Smooth muscle

Inner circular muscle

Outer longitudinal muscle

Skeletal muscle

Figure 15-5C. Middle esophagus. H&E, ×34; insets *(left)* ×208, *(right)* ×116

The **mucosa** of the esophagus is covered by a thick layer of **nonkeratinized stratified squamous epithelium,** which reflects its function in resisting abrasion and friction. The epithelium of the esophagus is continuously renewed by basal cells that migrate and differentiate from the basal layer. Most of the digestive tract is covered by **simple columnar epithelium;** only the two ends (esophagus and anal canal) are covered by stratified squamous epithelium. The **muscularis externa** of the **middle esophagus** contains mixed **skeletal** and **smooth muscle fibers,** which are organized in inner circular and outer longitudinal muscle bundles. Each skeletal muscle fiber is larger, has **multiple nuclei** positioned peripherally, and stains darker than the smooth muscle fiber. Each smooth muscle fiber has a **single nucleus** located in the center of the muscle fiber.

LOWER ESOPHAGUS (ESOPHAGOGASTRIC JUNCTIONS)

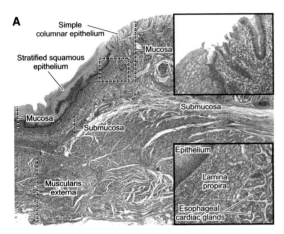

A

Simple columnar epithelium

Stratified squamous epithelium

Mucosa

Mucosa

Submucosa

Submucosa

Muscularis externa

Epithelium

Lamina propira

Esophageal cardiac glands

Figure 15-6A. Lower esophagus, esophagogastric junction (esophagus on *left*; stomach on *right* of illustration). H&E, ×11; insets (*upper*) ×57; (*lower*) ×45

The **lower esophagus** meets the stomach at the **esophagogastric junction**. The esophagus is lined by stratified squamous epithelium, and the cardiac region of the stomach is lined by simple columnar epithelium. The change in the lining epithelium reflects the change in function from a conduit for food transport to an organ of digestion. The muscularis externa of the lower esophagus is composed of two layers of smooth muscle fibers, which are controlled by the vagus nerve. Mucous glands are also found in the lamina propria of the lower esophagus (*right inset*). These glands are called **esophageal cardiac glands**. They produce mucus to protect the epithelial wall of the esophagus from the reflux of acidic gastric juices coming from the stomach.

In some patients, the epithelium of the lower esophagus (stratified squamous epithelium) changes to stomach-like epithelium (simple columnar epithelium). This pathologic change is called **metaplasia**. It is due to the long-term chemical irritation caused by **gastroesophageal reflux**.

CLINICAL CORRELATIONS

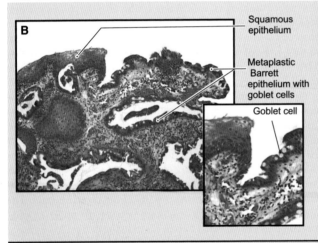

B

Squamous epithelium

Metaplastic Barrett epithelium with goblet cells

Goblet cell

Figure 15-6B. Barrett Esophagus. H&E, ×48; inset ×82

Barrett esophagus is a chronic complication of **gastroesophageal reflux disease (GERD)**, characterized by **metaplasia** of the stratified squamous epithelium of the lower esophagus into a specialized **glandular epithelium with goblet cells**. Patients with Barrett esophagus have an increased risk of developing **adenocarcinoma** (cancer of the esophagus) of the distal esophagus. Common symptoms include heartburn, trouble swallowing, and weight loss. Endoscopically, Barrett esophagus appears as salmon-colored "tongues" of mucosa extending proximally from the gastroesophageal junction. This photomicrograph shows the **metaplastic glandular epithelium with goblet cells** that have replaced the normal squamous epithelium and the inflammatory cells (mainly lymphocytes and plasma cells) infiltrating the connective tissue.

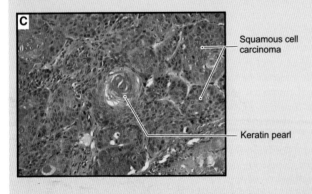

C

Squamous cell carcinoma

Keratin pearl

Figure 15-6C. Esophageal Carcinoma. H&E, ×97

Esophageal carcinoma is a **malignant neoplasm** that stems from the epithelial cells lining the inner surface of the esophagus. Worldwide, **squamous cell carcinoma** is the most common type of esophageal cancer, and it is associated with alcohol and tobacco use in the United States and Europe and with mutagenic substances and nutritional deficiencies in less well-developed parts of the world. In the United States, **adenocarcinoma** of the lower esophagus is becoming more frequent, representing about 50% of esophageal cancers. The major known risk factor for the development of adenocarcinoma is **chronic GERD** causing **Barrett esophagus**, a **metaplastic** change in the squamous mucosa of the distal esophagus to a glandular type of epithelium with goblet cells. Esophageal cancer is characterized by progressive difficulty in swallowing, loss of weight, fatigue, and chest pain. Pathological changes include **ulcerations, exophytic masses,** and thickening and narrowing of the lumen. Treatment includes surgery (**esophagectomy**) and chemotherapy. This photomicrograph shows a moderately differentiated squamous cell carcinoma with focal keratin production in the center, called a **keratin pearl**.

Stomach

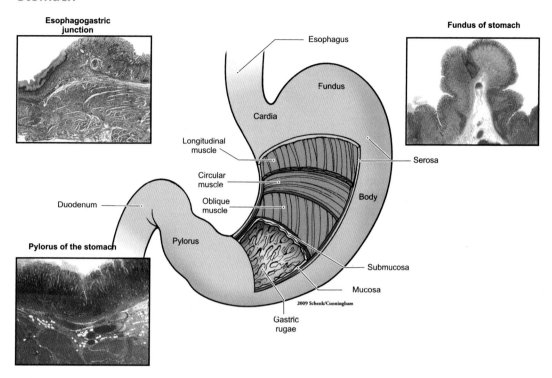

Esophagogastric junction

Fundus of stomach

Esophagus

Fundus

Cardia

Longitudinal muscle

Circular muscle

Oblique muscle

Duodenum

Pylorus

Serosa

Body

Submucosa

Mucosa

2009 Schenk/Cunningham

Gastric rugae

Pylorus of the stomach

Figure 15-7. **Overview of the stomach.** H&E, insets (*upper left*) ×5; (*lower left*) ×9; (*right*) ×7

The **stomach** is a "J"-shaped hollow organ. It connects the **esophagus** and **duodenum** of the small intestine. The stomach initiates digestion of food and temporarily stores food. It can be divided into four parts: the **cardia, fundus, body,** and **pylorus.** Histologically, stomach tissue can be distinguished by its **mucosal glands** (glands in the mucosa). (1 and 2) The *cardia* connects to the esophagus, and the *pylorus* connects to the duodenum. These two ends of the stomach have similar histologic characteristics. The mucosal glands of the cardia and pylorus are called **cardiac glands** and **pyloric glands,** respectively. Both contain many **mucus-secreting cells** and produce mucus, which is a thick, gel-like material that coats the surface of the stomach and protects it from acidic gastric fluid. Mucus-secreting cells contribute a small volume to the gastric juices. (3 and 4) The *fundus* and *body* of the stomach form the largest part of the stomach (about two thirds). The mucosal glands in this region are called **fundic (gastric) glands.** These glands are composed mainly of **parietal** and **chief cells,** which produce large volumes of gastric juices. A small number of various types of **enteroendocrine cells** are found at the base of the gastric glands. The gastric juices contain primarily **water, HCl, mucus, pepsin, IF, rennin,** and **lipase.** This is a highly acidic fluid and plays an important role in digesting food.

Stomach

I. **Cardia**
   A. Cardiac glands
   B. Mucus-secreting cells (produce mucus and lysozyme)
II. **Fundus and Body**
   A. Fundic (gastric) glands
   B. Mucous neck cells (secrete mucus)
   C. Parietal cells (secrete HCl and gastric IF)

   D. Chief cells (secrete pepsinogen, rennin, and lipase)
   E. Enteroendocrine (diffuse neuroendocrine) cells (release, e.g., gastrin, histamine, and serotonin)
III. **Pylorus**
   A. Pyloric glands
   B. Mucus-secreting cells (produce mucus and lysozyme)
   C. Enteroendocrine cells
   D. G cells (secrete gastrin)
   E. D cells (release somatostatin)

SYNOPSIS 15-1 Parietal Cells and Chief Cells

Parietal cells are located in the upper part of the fundus and body of the stomach. They are large round cell with intracellular canaliculus (secretory network) and microvilli. Parietal cells secrete gastric acid hydrogen ions (H+) and chloride ions (Cl−) to form hydrochloric acid (HCl) and gastric intrinsic factor (IF). The secretion of HCl is stimulated by **gastrin** and inhibited by **somatostatin** released from the **enteroendocrine cells.**

Chief cells are located in the lower part of the fundus and body of the stomach. They are small columnar cells with nuclei located in the base of the cells. They secrete **pepsinogen, precursors of rennin,** and **lipase.** In a low-pH environment provided by HCl, pepsinogen is converted into pepsin, which serves as the main digestive enzyme in the stomach, breaking down proteins into polypeptides.

REGIONS OF THE STOMACH

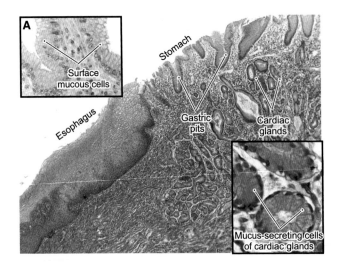

Figure 15-8A.   Cardiac region, esophagogastric junction. H&E, ×34; insets (*left*) ×192, (*right*) ×331

The inner surface of the stomach is lined by **columnar epithelium**, which forms a secretory sheath and is composed of mucus-secreting cells called **surface mucous cells**. These cells cover the entire inner surface of the stomach and also line the surface of the **gastric pits**. The gastric pits are invaginations of the epithelium and are surrounded by the lamina propria. This is an example of the **cardiac region** of the stomach at the **esophagogastric junction**. The lamina propria (loose connective tissue) contains **cardiac glands**. These glands are **branched tubular glands** and are composed of mucus-secreting cells. The secretions of the cardiac glands empty directly into the gastric pits. The cardiac glands consist of **mucous cells**, which are similar in appearance to the surface mucous cells. They have basally positioned nuclei and lightly staining cytoplasm.

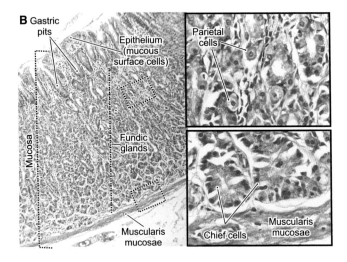

Figure 15-8B.   Fundic region of the stomach. H&E, ×51; insets ×245

The surface of the **fundus region** of the stomach is covered by **surface mucous cells**, which produce mucus to protect the epithelium from the acidic gastric juice. The fundic glands in the lamina propria are different from the cardiac glands but similar to the glands in the body of the stomach. Fundic glands contain **stem cells, mucous neck cells, parietal cells**, and **chief cells**. The **stem cells** can differentiate into other types of cells in the glands. The **parietal cells** are large, round cells with centrally positioned nuclei ("fried-egg" appearance). Their cytoplasm stains paler than that of chief cells. The parietal cells are more numerous in the superior half of the fundic glands (*upper inset*). The **chief cells** are small, columnar cells and have darkly stained cytoplasm. Their nuclei are commonly located at the base of the cells. The chief cells are more numerous in the inferior half of the fundic glands (*lower inset*).

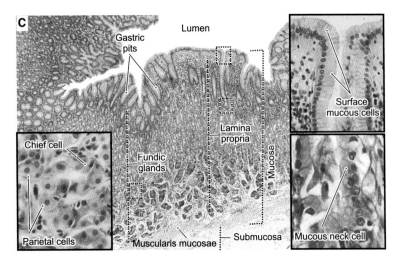

Figure 15-8C.   Body region of the stomach. H&E, ×34; insets (*left*) ×232; (*right upper*) ×164; (*right lower*) ×394

Histologically, the **body** and fundus of the stomach are similar to one another, and their glands are identical. They are called **fundic (gastric) glands**. The **mucous neck cells** are commonly found between the parietal cells at the neck region of the gastric glands. They secrete **acidic mucus**. The **parietal cells** secrete large quantities of HCl and **gastric IF**. The parietal cells are also called **oxyntic (acid-forming) cells**. The **chief cells** are often called **zymogenic** or **peptic cells**; their cytoplasm contains **zymogen granules**. They secrete **pepsinogen** and precursors of **rennin** and **lipase**. **Enteroendocrine cells** may also be found at the neck and base of the gastric glands. They release endocrine molecules (e.g., serotonin, gastrin, histamine). These cells are similar in appearance to the enteroendocrine cells in the small intestine. Stem cells may also be found at neck regions of the gastric glands.

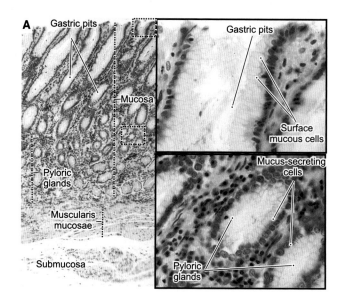

Figure 15-9A. Pyloric region of the stomach. H&E, ×68; insets ×283

The **pylorus** is the last region of the stomach and connects to the duodenum. The mucosa of the pylorus has deep **gastric pits. Pyloric glands**, composed primarily of **mucus-secreting cells**, empty their secretory products into the base of the gastric pits. These mucus-secreting cells are pale staining and have basally located nuclei, as do the cells of the cardiac glands. They produce mucus to protect the epithelium of the pylorus from acidic gastric secretions. Two types of **enteroendocrine cells** are found at the base of the pyloric glands. **G cells** release **gastrin**, which stimulates parietal cells to secrete HCl. Another type of enteroendocrine cell, called the **D cell**, releases **somatostatin**, which inhibits the release of **gastrin** by G cells. These two types of enteroendocrine cells are also found in the mucosa of the duodenum. The *upper inset* shows a **gastric pit** and **surface mucous cells** in the superior portion of the mucosa. The *lower inset* shows **pyloric glands** and **mucus-secreting cells** in an inferior portion of the mucosa. Both cell types have basally positioned nuclei and clear cytoplasm containing secretory granules.

CLINICAL CORRELATIONS

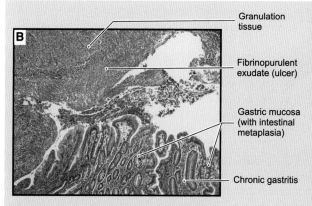

Figure 15-9B. Gastric Ulcer (Peptic Ulcer). H&E, ×19

Peptic ulcers are **chronic mucosal lesions** that occur in the gastrointestinal tract. The **duodenum** and **stomach** are the most common sites for **ulcers**. Causes of these ulcers include *Helicobacter pylori* infection, long-term use of nonsteroidal anti-inflammatory drugs and corticosteroids, and cigarette smoking. Epigastric burning or pain, bleeding, and even perforation are the common signs and symptoms of the peptic ulcers. Morphologically, peptic ulcers are usually small, round to oval in shape, less than 4 cm in diameter with well-defined margins without elevation, and have a clean, smooth base. Histologically, a thin layer of **necrotic fibrinoid debris** with **neutrophil infiltration** is seen, beneath which lies **granulation tissue**. Treatments include using H$_2$ receptor antagonists; antibiotics; proton pump inhibitors; and surgery for severe, refractory cases. Care must be taken to differentiate benign ulcers from malignant adenocarcinomas, which may appear ulcerated. This image shows the transition from gastric mucosa to ulcer, showing a **fibrinopurulent** surface with underlying **granulation** tissue. The gastric mucosa shows **chronic gastritis** with plasma cells within the lamina propria and **intestinal metaplasia** (note the goblet cells).

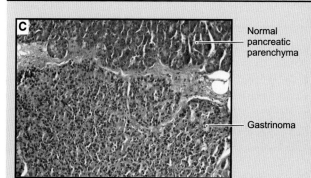

Figure 15-9C. Gastrinoma (Zollinger-Ellison Syndrome). H&E, ×97

Gastrinomas, also called **Zollinger-Ellison syndrome**, are neoplasms producing the hormone **gastrin**, which commonly arise in the **duodenum** and **pancreas**. **Hypersecretion** of **gastrin** by the tumor leads to **hypergastrinemia**, resulting in excess production of **gastric acid**. Patients have symptoms of peptic ulcers, with clinical findings, such as **epigastric tenderness**, bleeding, and perforation. Pathologic findings include **hyperplasia** of the **parietal cells** that produce gastric acid within the mucosa of the **stomach**. Tumor cells resemble pancreatic endocrine cells, are well differentiated, and contain gastrin peptides within the secretory granules. Proton pump inhibitors and surgical removal of the tumor are the first treatment choice for this syndrome. This image shows **normal pancreatic parenchyma** (*upper portion*) and a well-circumscribed **gastrinoma** (*lower portion*). Note the relatively uniform **neoplastic cells** within the gastrinoma.

Small Intestine

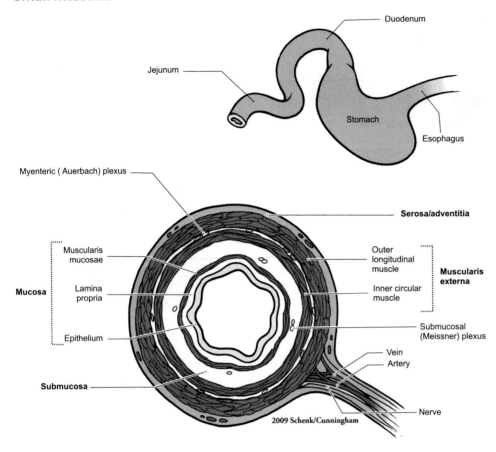

Figure 15-10. Overview of the small intestine.

The **small intestine** is a very long, tubular organ, about 6 to 7 m long, with a relatively small diameter. It connects the stomach to the large intestine and can be divided into three regions based on anatomy and function. (1) The **duodenum**, the most proximal region of the small intestine, is a short, C-shaped segment about 20 to 25 cm long. Mucous glands called **Brunner glands** are present only in the duodenum. Bile and pancreatic secretions enter the duodenum through their duct systems. (2) The **jejunum** makes up about two fifths of the rest of the small intestine. It has a larger diameter and thicker wall than the ileum. The jejunum has long villi and has neither Brunner glands nor Peyer patches. (3) The **ileum** is the most distal portion of the intestine, and it makes up about three fifths of the small intestine. The ileum has a thinner wall and fewer villi than the jejunum, and it has clusters of lymphatic nodules, called **Peyer patches**, in the lamina propria. This illustration shows the general tunics (layers) of the small intestine. Like the other parts of the digestive tract, the small intestine consists of a mucosa (epithelium, lamina propria, and muscularis mucosae), submucosa, muscularis externa, and serosa/adventitia. Several **myenteric (Auerbach) plexuses** are illustrated between the two layers of the muscularis externa; submucosal (Meissner) plexuses are located in the submucosal layer.

Small Intestine

I. **Duodenum**
   A. Mucosa
   B. Submucosa (Brunner glands)
   C. Muscularis externa
   D. Serosa/adventitia
II. **Jejunum**
   A. Mucosa
   B. Submucosa
   C. Muscularis externa
   D. Serosa

III. **Ileum**
   A. Mucosa (Peyer patches)
   B. Submucosa (Peyer patches may extend into this layer)
   C. Muscularis externa
   D. Serosa

Cell Types in the Small Intestine
Villi: columnar absorptive cells and goblet cells
Glands (crypts) of Lieberkühn: absorptive cells, goblet cells, Paneth cells, enteroendocrine cells, and stem cells

DUODENUM

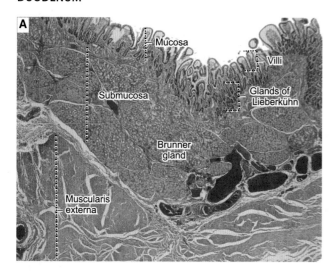

Figure 15-11A. Duodenum, small intestine. H&E, ×14

The **duodenum** connects to the stomach. The **mucosa** of the duodenum is composed of **simple columnar epithelium, lamina propria**, and **muscularis mucosae**. *Epithelial cells* lining the surface of the villi and the **glands of Lieberkühn** include absorptive cells, goblet cells, Paneth cells, enteroendocrine cells, and stem cells. The *lamina propria* is a layer of loose connective tissue, which forms the core of the villus and contains various types of connective tissue cells including fibroblasts, plasma cells, macrophages, and some leukocytes. The *muscularis mucosae* is a thin layer of smooth muscle. The **submucosa** is a layer of dense connective tissue containing mucous glands called **Brunner glands**, which produce mucus to protect the duodenal wall from acidic gastric juice from the stomach. The **muscularis externa** consists of two layers of smooth muscle: an inner circular layer and an outer longitudinal layer. The outer layer of the duodenum is mostly covered by serosa; areas where it is attached to other organs are covered by adventitia.

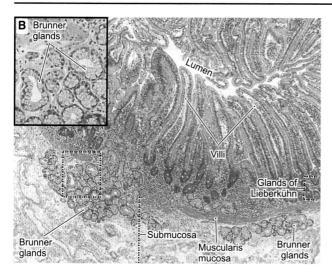

Figure 15-11B. Duodenum, small intestine. H&E, ×45; inset ×112

An example of the **mucosa** and **submucosa** of the **duodenum** is shown. A thin layer of **muscularis mucosae** lies between the lamina propria and the submucosa. Fingerlike **villi** project into the lumen. **Brunner glands** are distributed in the submucosa and extend into the lamina propria of the mucosa. Brunner glands produce mucus that protects the epithelium from **HCl** secreted in the stomach. They also secrete large numbers of **bicarbonate ions**, which neutralize acidic gastric juice from the stomach. Two types of **enteroendocrine cells** associated with the regulation of gastric secretion are also found in the glands of Lieberkühn of the duodenum: (1) **G cells** that release **gastrin**, which stimulates parietal cell secretion of HCl, and (2) **D cells** that release **somatostatin**, which inhibits gastrin release. G cells and D cells are predominantly found in the pylorus of the stomach but are also found in the duodenum.

If Brunner cells are not able to produce enough mucus and bicarbonate ions over the long term, a **duodenal (Brunner) ulcer** may develop.

CLINICAL CORRELATION

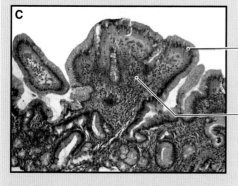

Metaplastic gastric mucosa with loss of goblet cells

Blunt, widened villus with inflammation

Figure 15-11C. Peptic Duodenitis. H&E, ×48

Peptic duodenitis is an inflammatory process caused by chronic exposure of the **duodenal mucosa** to increased levels of gastric acid and is usually found in the first portion of the duodenum, the **duodenal bulb**. Symptoms of peptic duodenitis include epigastric pain and **dyspepsia**. Histologic features include flattening, or blunting, of the normally fingerlike villi, **increased inflammatory cells** within the lamina propria, **Brunner gland hyperplasia**, **crypt hyperplasia**, and **gastric foveolar metaplasia of the epithelium**. Metaplasia to a gastric foveolar type of epithelium is an adaptive protective response to the increased levels of acid. *H. pylori* may be found in the metaplastic mucosa as seen in the stomach. In time, a duodenal ulcer may result from peptic duodenitis. This photomicrograph shows duodenal mucosa with complete replacement of the normal epithelium with goblet cells by **gastric foveolar epithelium**. Note the widened, distorted villi and increased **inflammatory cells** within the **lamina propria**.

ABSORPTION: FOLDS OF SMALL INTESTINE

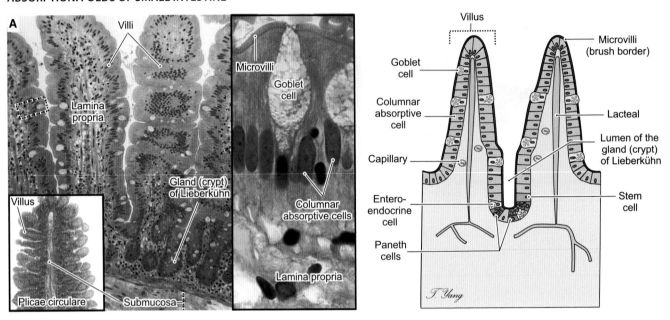

Figure 15-12A. **Plicae circulares, villi, and microvilli.** H&E, ×124; inset (*left*) ×15, (*right*) ×882

The small intestine is a long tube with three levels of folds that increase the surface area for absorption. (1) **Plicae circulares (valves of Kerckring)** are gross folds involving the mucosa and submucosa that project into the lumen (*left inset*). (2) **Villi** are smaller folds than the plicae circulares and involve only mucosa. The central core of each villus is formed by the lamina propria; the nutrients absorbed from the lumen by absorptive cells are transported into the lamina propria. The lamina propria contains a **central lacteal** (a blind-ended lymphatic vessel) and many capillaries involved in the transport of absorbed nutrients. (3) **Microvilli** are at the apical surfaces of columnar absorptive cells, increasing the surface area at the cellular level. They appear as a pink border in light microscopy and form a **brush border**. The drawing on the *right* shows various types of cells arranged in the epithelium of the mucosa. These cells include column-shaped absorptive cells (**enterocytes**), **goblet cells**, **Paneth cells**, and **enteroendocrine cells**. The **central lacteals** are also illustrated.

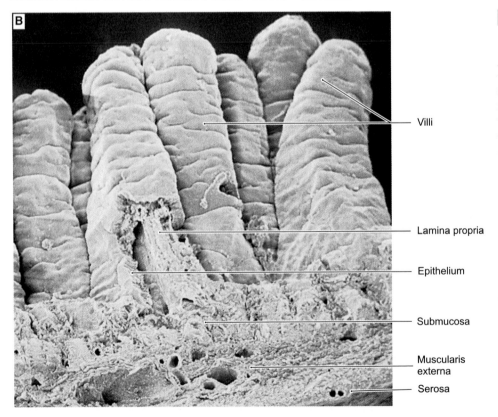

Figure 15-12B. **Villi of the small intestine.** SEM, ×170

An example of a scanning electron microscopy image showing fingerlike **villi** extending from the intestinal wall and projecting into the lumen is shown. Each villus is composed of mucosa (**epithelium** and **lamina propria**). The lamina propria (connective tissue) forms the central core of the villus. Epithelium with microvilli forms the outer layer of the villus. The villi are unique structures in the small intestine; they are found neither in the stomach nor in the large intestine. The villi are tallest in the duodenum and shortest in the ileum. They gradually reduce in height and size from the proximal regions to the distal regions of the small intestine. The **submucosa** and **muscularis externa** are also shown here. The outermost layer of the intestinal wall is **serosa**.

ABSORPTIVE CELLS AND GOBLET CELLS

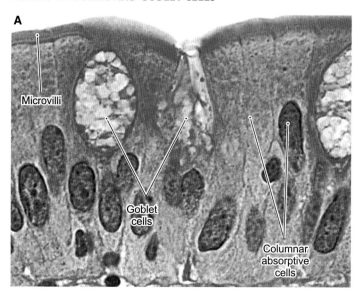

A

Microvilli

Goblet cells

Columnar absorptive cells

Figure 15-13A. Columnar absorptive and goblet cells of the small intestine. H&E, ×1,422

The **columnar absorptive cells** of the small intestine are also called **enterocytes** or **intestinal absorptive cells**. They are tall and columnar in shape; oval-shaped nuclei lie in the basal region of the cells. The columnar absorptive cells are the predominant cells in the epithelium of the small intestine. The apical surfaces of the cells are covered by **microvilli**, which are coated with **glycocalyx**. The microvilli increase the cellular surface area for absorption. **Goblet cells** are interspersed among the absorptive cells. These are **unicellular glands** with a distinctive goblet shape. The goblet cells are mucus-secreting cells, and their numbers gradually increase from the proximal (duodenum) to the distal (ileum) portions of the small intestine.

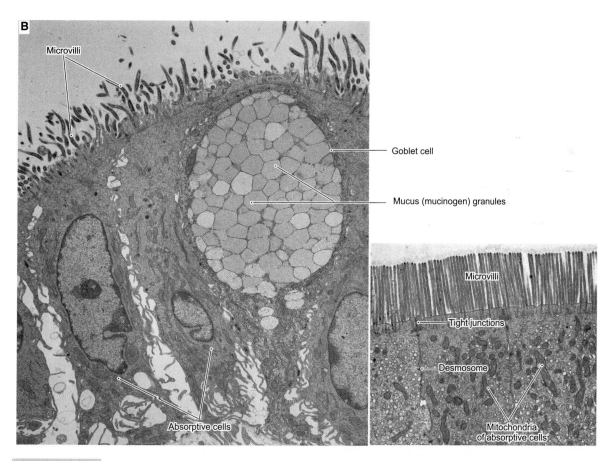

B

Microvilli

Goblet cell

Mucus (mucinogen) granules

Absorptive cells

Microvilli

Tight junctions

Desmosome

Mitochondria of absorptive cells

Figure 15-13B. Goblet cells, columnar absorptive cells, and microvilli. EM, (*left*, large intestine) ×4,831, (*right*, small intestine) ×6,906

There are numerous **mitochondria** in the apical cytoplasm of the **columnar absorptive cells**. **Junction complexes** are located between neighboring cells near the lumen, and **microvilli** are present on the apical surfaces of the **absorptive cells**. A **goblet cell** with many **mucus-secretory granules** in the cytoplasm is also shown here. These granules contain **mucinogen** and are released onto the surface of the epithelium by **exocytosis**. During exocytosis, mucinogen becomes hydrated and forms mucin, which expands greatly in volume after it is released from the goblet cell.

PANETH CELLS AND ENTEROENDOCRINE CELLS

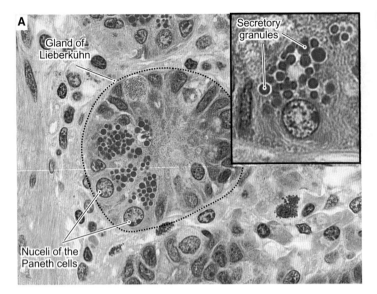

Figure 15-14A. Paneth cells, small intestine. H&E, ×702; inset ×1,488

Paneth cells have basally positioned nuclei and contain **acidophilic-secretory granules** in the apical region of the cytoplasm. These granules appear bright red in H&E stains. Paneth cells are located at the base of the **glands (crypts) of Lieberkühn.** Their secretory granules contain **lysozymes, tumor necrosis factor-α,** and **defensins (cryptidins).** These are antibacterial enzymes that help to regulate the normal bacterial flora of the intestine. Paneth cells are **protein-secretory cells** and have well-developed **rough endoplasmic reticulum (RER)** and **Golgi complexes.** Like other epithelial cells, the Paneth cells are derived from stem cells located at the base of the intestinal glands of Lieberkühn. A gland of Lieberkühn is indicated by the *dashed line* at left. Its lumen is filled with secretory material and is not easy to see.

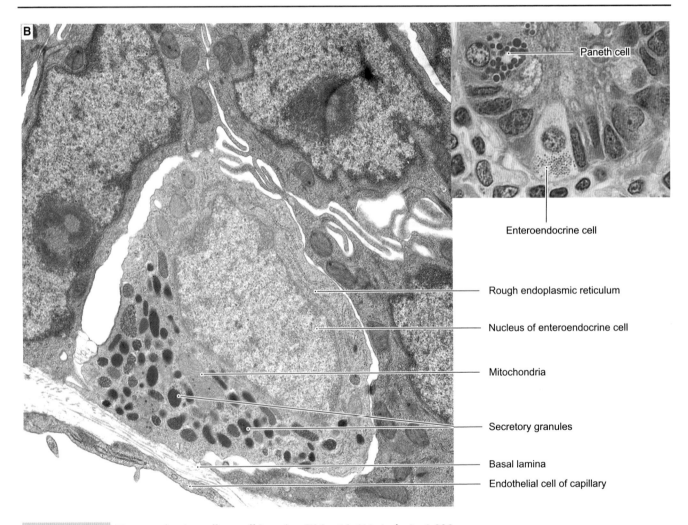

Figure 15-14B. Enteroendocrine cells, small intestine. EM, ×10,611; (color) ×1,028

There are many types of **enteroendocrine cells,** which are also called **diffuse neuroendocrine cells,** in the digestive tract. They are recognized as **hormone-releasing cells,** and the various types of enteroendocrine cells are similar in appearance. They are often found at the base of glands of Lieberkühn and have many mitochondria, abundant RER, and well-developed Golgi complexes. Their secretory granules are located at the basal cytoplasm. Each type of enteroendocrine cell releases one particular hormone.

SECOND BRAIN IN THE GUT (ENTERIC NERVOUS SYSTEM)

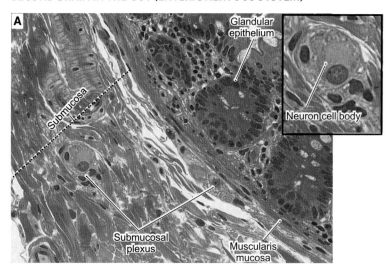

Figure 15-15A. Submucosal/Meissner plexus, small intestine. H&E, ×272; inset ×544

The enteric nervous system is able to operate independently, although it is usually influenced by the parasympathetic and sympathetic nervous systems. The two types of ganglia of the enteric nervous system are found in the wall of the digestive tract. (1) **Submucosal plexuses (Meissner plexuses)** are located in the submucosal layer. (2) **Myenteric plexuses (Auerbach plexuses)** are located between the two layers of the muscularis externa. Here is an example of a submucosal plexus in the submucosa of the wall of the small intestine. Submucosal plexuses are scattered small groups of neuron cell bodies (sensory and motor neurons and interneurons) and unmyelinated nerve fibers. The axons of the sensory neurons receive mechanical and chemical signals from the glandular epithelium; the axons of the motor neurons innervate the muscularis mucosae and glandular epithelium.

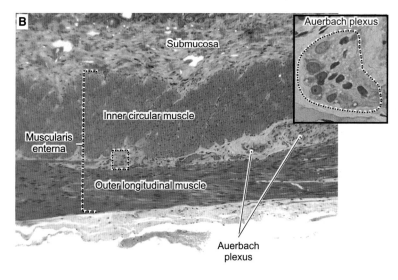

Figure 15-15B. Muscularis externa, small intestine. H&E, ×68; inset ×354

Here is an example of the **muscularis externa** of the small intestine, which contains two layers of smooth muscle. (1) **Inner circular muscle layer:** When the smooth muscle fibers in this layer contract, the diameter of lumen of the small intestine decreases. (2) **Outer longitudinal muscle layer:** This layer surrounds the inner circular muscle layer. When the smooth muscle fibers in this layer contract, the length of the intestine is reduced. These two layers of muscle work together to make successive waves of involuntary movements called **peristalsis**, which force digestive contents to move downward into the large intestine. The inner circular and outer longitudinal muscles are innervated by axons from neurons in the **myenteric/Auerbach plexuses** of the enteric nervous system.

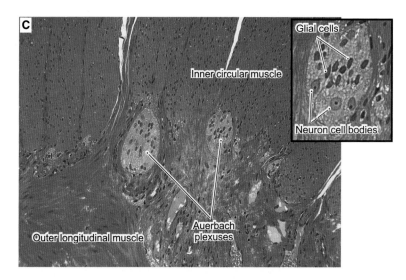

Figure 15-15C. Myenteric/Auerbach plexus, muscularis externa of the small intestine. H&E, ×136; inset ×317

Myenteric plexuses (Auerbach plexuses) are found between the inner circular muscle and the outer longitudinal muscle layers. Myenteric (Auerbach) plexuses are much larger than submucosal plexuses. The *inset* shows several **neuron cell bodies** and **enteric glial cells** surrounded by connective tissues in a myenteric plexus. Neurons in both the submucosal plexuses and the myenteric plexuses are multipolar in shape. Like submucosal plexuses, they may have little or no encapsulation and contain unmyelinated nerve fibers and ganglionic neurons mainly belonging to the enteric nervous system. The enteric nervous system coordinates peristaltic reflexes, which evoke waves of contraction and relaxation of the gut wall, moving the contents toward the anus and also regulates enteroendocrine cells.

JEJUNUM AND ILEUM

A

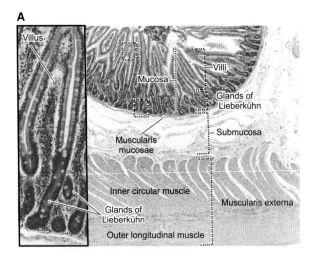

Villus
Villi
Mucosa
Glands of
Lieberkühn
Submucosa
Muscularis
mucosae
Inner circular muscle
Muscularis externa
Glands of
Lieberkühn
Outer longitudinal muscle

Figure 15-16A.　Jejunum, small intestine. H&E, ×34; inset ×103

The **jejunum** is a segment of small intestine between the duodenum and the ileum. It is similar in general structure and layers to the other regions of the small intestine. It contains **mucosa, submucosa, muscularis externa,** and **serosa.** The jejunum has neither **Brunner glands** nor **Peyer patches.** The cells of the epithelium of the mucosa are similar to those of the epithelium of other regions of the small intestine. Goblet cells steadily increase in number along the entire length of the small intestine from the duodenum to the ileum. Paneth cells are often found at the base of the **glands of Lieberkühn** (*lower inset*). The glands of Lieberkühn are intestinal glands (simple tubular glands), which extend from the spaces between the bases of the villi deep into the lamina propria.

B

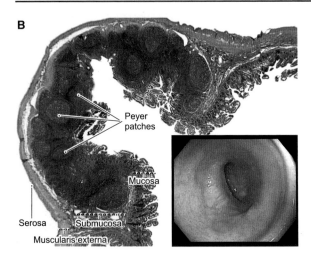

Peyer
patches
Mucosa
Serosa
Submucosa
Muscularis externa

Figure 15-16B.　Ileum with Peyer patches, small intestine. H&E, ×13

The **ileum** is the longest segment of the small intestine making up three fifths of the 6 to 7 m length of the small intestine. One of the unique features of the ileum is the presence of clusters of lymphatic nodules called **Peyer patches.** These are most numerous in the distal portion of the ileum. Some isolated lymphatic nodules may be found in other parts of the digestive tract but not in aggregations of clusters of nodules like Peyer patches. The **villi** in the ileum are shorter and smaller than in other parts of the small intestine. The numbers of **goblet cells** are greatly increased in the ileum. The *inset* shows an endoscopic image of the ileum with its relatively smooth surface.

Vitamin K is absorbed in both the jejunum and the ileum, but vitamin B12 is only absorbed in the ileum (especially the terminal ileum). The absorption of vitamin B12 requires coupling with gastric intrinsic factor, which is produced by parietal cells in the stomach; these two substances become intimately associated with the wall of the ileum. If a large portion of the stomach or ileum is surgically removed, **vitamin B12 deficiency** may result, leading to **megaloblastic anemia** and **neurologic symptoms.**

C

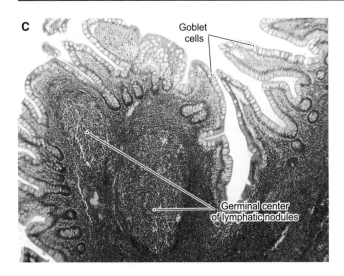

Goblet
cells
Germinal center
of lymphatic nodules

Figure 15-16C.　Mucosa of the ileum, small intestine. H&E, ×68

Here is an example of the **mucosa** of the **ileum** showing numerous **goblet cells** in the surface epithelium. In this section, two lymphatic nodules are located in the lamina propria. These lymphatic nodules have **germinal centers** and are, therefore, secondary lymphatic nodules. These nodules may extend into the submucosa. The lymphatic nodules and Peyer patches are locations where lymphocytes can interact with antigens and, therefore, play important roles in immunological function. Naive B cells (B lymphocytes) within these lymphoid patches are primed and awaiting exposure to unique epitopes. When stimulated by a specific antigen from the intestinal mucosa, they differentiate into plasma cells and memory B cells. In response, the plasma cells produce large quantities of immunoglobulins ([Ig] antibodies), especially IgA to combat mucosal infection. The memory B cells live on in the **Peyer patches** to retain immunity to a specific antigen.

Large Intestine

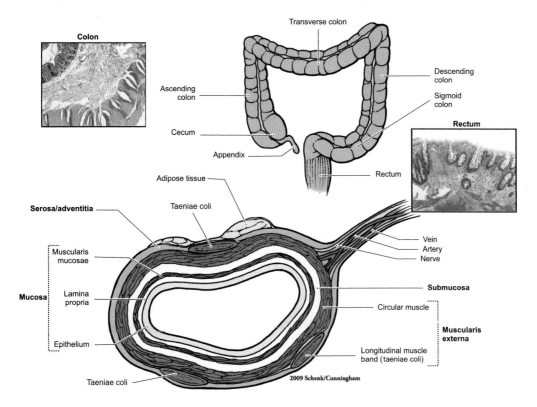

Figure 15-17. Overview of the large intestine. H&E (*left*), ×14; (*right*) ×36

The **large intestine** connects the small intestine to the anal canal. The large intestine is about 1.5 m long, much shorter than the small intestine. It consists of the **cecum, appendix, colon, rectum,** and **anal canal.** (1) The *cecum* is a small blind pouch of the large intestine, at the junction of the ileum and the ascending colon. The ileum and cecum are separated by the **ileocecal valve,** which prevents feces from backing up into the small intestine. (2) The *appendix* is a very short, small-diameter blind end tube that attaches to the posterior-medial wall of the cecum. It contains aggregates of lymphatic nodules in the lamina propria. (3) The *colon* is the longest part of the large intestine and includes ascending, transverse, descending, and sigmoid colons. (4) The *rectum* connects the sigmoid colon to the anal canal. (5) The *anal canal* is externally surrounded by a layer of skeletal muscle called the **exterior sphincter.** The junction between the rectum and the anal canal is called the **anorectal junction,** also called the **dentate line,** which marks the transitional epithelium change from simple columnar epithelium to stratified squamous epithelium. The large intestine has the same general structure of mucosa, submucosa, muscularis externa, and serosa/adventitia as the small intestine. However, the large intestine has a large lumen (excepting the appendix) and a large number of goblet cells lining the surface of the mucosa. It has crypts (intestinal glands) but no villi, and the outer longitudinal muscle layer of the muscularis externa has become three narrow bands called **taeniae coli.** Functions of the large intestine include the absorption of water and salts and the formation, storage, and elimination of feces.

Large Intestine

I. **Cecum**
  A. Mucosa (crypts/glands; no villi)
  B. Submucosa
  C. Muscularis externa (inner circular muscle; taeniae coli)
  D. Serosa

II. **Appendix**
  A. Mucosa (aggregated lymphatic nodules)
  B. Submucosa
  C. Muscularis externa (inner circular and outer longitudinal muscles)
  D. Serosa

III. **Colon: Ascending, Transverse, Descending, and Sigmoid Portions**
  A. Mucosa (crypts/glands; no villi)
  B. Submucosa
  C. Muscularis externa (inner circular muscle; taeniae)
  D. Serosa/adventitia

IV. **Rectum**
  A. Mucosa
  B. Submucosa
  C. Muscularis externa (inner circular and outer longitudinal muscles)
  D. Adventitia

V. **Anal Canal**
  A. Mucosa (stratified squamous)
  B. Submucosa
  C. Muscularis externa (internal and external sphincters)
  D. Adventitia

COLON

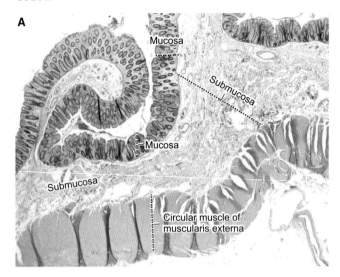

A

Mucosa

Submucosa

Mucosa

Submucosa

Circular muscle of muscularis externa

Figure 15-18A.   Colon, large intestine. H&E, ×15

The **colon** is the longest part of the large intestine. It contains an **ascending colon, transverse colon, descending colon**, and **sigmoid colon**. The colon receives digestive contents from the small intestine and absorbs a large volume of water and electrolytes from the contents. Bacteria in the colon make large quantities of vitamins K and B12, but absorption is limited. The colon also forms and stores **feces**, the waste matter leftover after the digestion process has been completed. The movement of the contents in the large intestine is slower than in the small intestine, taking 8 to 15 hours to move the **chyme** (thick, semifluid mass) from the cecum to the rectum, where feces are stored. The **mucosa** of the colon has a smooth surface (no villi) and contains glands of Lieberkühn. The **submucosa** contains blood vessels, lymphatic vessels, and nerve fibers as well as submucosal plexuses, but no glands are present. The **muscularis externa** includes the **circular muscle** (*shown here*). The longitudinal muscle is aggregated into three bands called **taeniae coli**. The myenteric (Auerbach) plexuses are located between these two muscle layers.

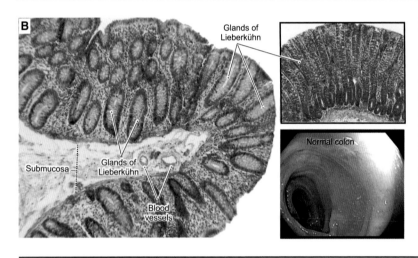

B

Glands of Lieberkühn

Normal colon

Submucosa

Glands of Lieberkühn

Blood vessels

Figure 15-18B.   Colon, large intestine. H&E, ×68 (*left*); mucous stain, ×44 (*upper right*)

The **glands of Lieberkühn** are intestinal glands that are straight tubular glands and are located in the lamina propria of the mucosa. The glands of Lieberkühn in the large intestine are similar to those of the small intestine, but they contain no Paneth cells. They are composed of great numbers of goblet cells, columnar absorptive cells, and some enteroendocrine cells. A thin layer of the muscularis mucosae is found beneath the lamina propria; it is part of the mucosa. The upper right image shows the goblet cells, which appear red because of the mucous stain.

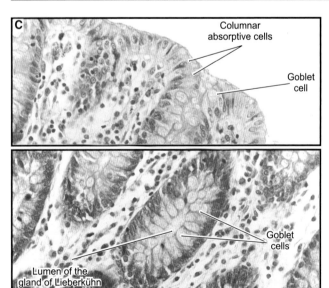

C

Columnar absorptive cells

Goblet cell

Goblet cells

Lumen of the gland of Lieberkühn

Figure 15-18C.   Mucosa of the colon, large intestine. H&E, ×272

Upper: The superior part and surface of the **mucosa** of the colon consists of **columnar absorptive cells** and **goblet cells**. These absorptive cells play an important role in the absorption of water and electrolytes. Water enters the absorptive cells entirely by diffusion. Most water absorption occurs in the colon, especially in the proximal colon. Goblet cells produce **mucus**, which protects the wall of the large intestine, glues fecal material together, and lubricates the passage. The surface of the large intestine is much smoother than the small intestine because there are **no villi**.
Lower: The inferior part of the mucosa in the colon contains straight tubular glands, **glands of Lieberkühn**, which are cut in cross section here. Most cells in these glands are goblet cells with basally positioned nuclei. The secretory (mucinogen) granules located at the apical ends of the cells appear white here. Enteroendocrine cells and stem cells also can be found. The stem cells are located at the base of the glands (crypts) of Lieberkühn and can be differentiated from other cell types of epithelia. Paneth cells are not present in the large intestine.

CLINICAL CORRELATIONS

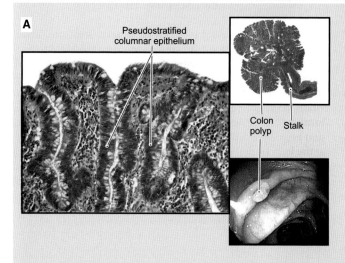

Pseudostratified columnar epithelium

Colon polyp   Stalk

Figure 15-19A.   Colon Polyps. H&E, ×97; inset (*upper*) ×1.3

Colon polyps are tissue masses that grow on the inner mucosal surface and protrude into the lumen of the colon. Polyps may contain a **stalk** or may be **sessile**, without a stalk. There are several types of polyps, the most common of which are **adenomatous** and **hyperplastic**. Adenomatous polyps are benign neoplasms, subdivided based on morphologic features into **tubular adenomas, tubulovillous adenomas,** and **villous adenomas.** Although adenomatous polyps are themselves benign, they should be considered as having malignant potential, because adenocarcinoma may arise in these polyps. **Hyperplastic polyps,** which are common in the descending colon and rectum, are considered benign with minimal risk for progression to cancer. **Pseudopolyps** may be seen in inflammatory bowel disease, particularly ulcerative colitis. Polyps may be removed during colonoscopy by endoscopic mucosal resection and sent for pathologic evaluation. These images show a large, **pedunculated tubular adenoma** (*inset*) and a higher power view of the **adenomatous epithelium** featuring **pseudostratification** of the crypt cells.

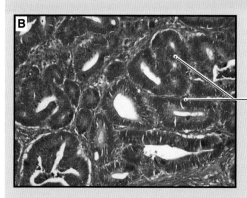

Adenocarcinoma (malignant glands)

Figure 15-19B.   Colorectal Cancer. H&E, ×97

Colorectal cancer is a **malignant neoplasm** of the colon or the rectum. Risk factors include genetics, inflammatory bowel disease—especially ulcerative colitis—adenomatous polyps, high-fat and low-fiber diets, and excessive red meat consumption. **Adenocarcinoma** is the most common type of colon cancer (98% of cases), arising from the **mucosal glandular epithelium,** often in adenomatous polyps. Colorectal carcinomas invade through the layers of the intestinal wall and metastasize predominantly through the lymphatic system. Depending on the location, colorectal cancers may be asymptomatic for years. Presenting symptoms may be a change in bowel habits due to bowel obstruction, blood in the stool, or iron deficiency anemia. Surgical resection is the first choice for early-stage cancer, although chemotherapy may be considered. This photomicrograph shows a moderately differentiated **adenocarcinoma** of the colon infiltrating the muscularis propria.

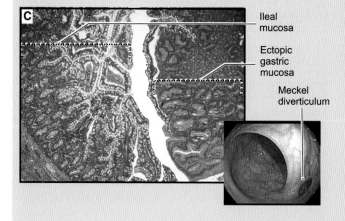

Ileal mucosa

Ectopic gastric mucosa

Meckel diverticulum

Figure 15-19C.   Meckel Diverticulum. H&E, ×19

Meckel diverticulum is a congenital abnormality characterized by an outpouching in the small bowel due to failure of the vitelline duct to close or **involute.** As a true diverticulum, it contains all three layers (mucosa, submucosa, and muscularis propria) of the normal bowel wall and is found on the antimesenteric aspect of the bowel. **Meckel diverticula** occur in 2% of the population, are usually located within 2 ft of the ileocecal valve, and are about 2 in length. Some Meckel diverticula contain **heterotopic rests** of **pancreatic** or **gastric mucosa.** Most people with a Meckel diverticulum are asymptomatic. Bleeding, inflammation, and peptic ulceration and perforation can occur, producing signs and symptoms similar to appendicitis. Surgery is the appropriate treatment for symptomatic patients. This image shows a section of a Meckel diverticulum showing normal ileal mucosa with goblet cells on the left side and **ectopic gastric mucosa** on the right side. This gastric mucosa increases the risk of perforation because of the elaboration of acid.

APPENDIX AND ANORECTAL JUNCTION

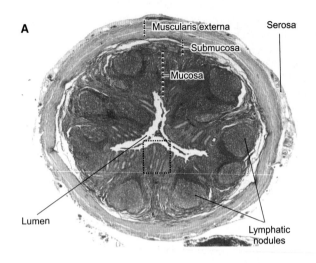

A

Muscularis externa
Submucosa
Mucosa
Serosa
Lumen
Lymphatic nodules

Figure 15-20A. Appendix and cecum. H&E, ×17

The **appendix** is a fingerlike blind-ended tubular structure, about 10 cm in length, extending from the cecum distal to the ileocecal valve. The **cecum** is the first segment of the large intestine, where it connects with the ileum. The small and large intestines are separated by the **ileocecal valve**. The appendix has a small, irregular lumen and many lymphatic nodules in the mucosa. Although its role in digestion is not clear, it may participate in immunological function and help maintain normal bacteria flora in the large intestine. The epithelium of the appendix is simple columnar epithelium, and lymphatic nodules are located in the lamina propria of the mucosa, which may extend into the submucosa. The muscularis externa contains inner circular and outer longitudinal smooth muscles.

Appendicitis usually results from a bacterial infection and may develop slowly or acutely. A cardinal sign is pain in the lower right abdominal quadrant or when pressure is applied to the **McBurney point**. The most common treatment is surgical excision of the appendix.

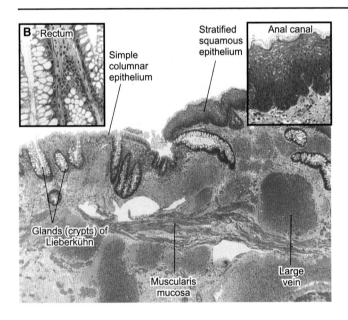

B
Rectum
Simple columnar epithelium
Stratified squamous epithelium
Anal canal
Glands (crypts) of Lieberkühn
Muscularis mucosa
Large vein

Figure 15-20B. Anorectal junction. H&E, ×34; insets (*left*) ×131, (*right*) ×87

The junction between the rectum and the anal canal is called the **anorectal junction**. The **rectum** connects the sigmoid colon to the anal canal. The rectum is the distalmost portion of the large intestine and functions mainly to store feces until elimination. The mucosa of the rectum is similar to that of the colon, but it has fewer intestinal glands of Lieberkühn. The **anal canal** is a continuation of the large intestine and has longitudinal folds (**anal columns**) in the gross view. The mucosa of the anal canal is covered by stratified squamous epithelium. The lamina propria contains many large veins (venous plexus). The muscularis mucosae is visible here. The muscularis externa contains inner circular and outer longitudinal smooth muscle layers (*not shown here*). The inner circular smooth muscle becomes thicker and forms the **internal anal sphincter**. The external anal sphincter surrounds the anal canal. It is a thick layer of skeletal muscle that voluntarily controls the elimination of feces. On the *left* in the photomicrograph is the distal end of the rectum; on the *right* is the proximal portion of the anal canal. Sebaceous glands and apocrine glands may be found in the distal end of the anal canal.

CLINICAL CORRELATION

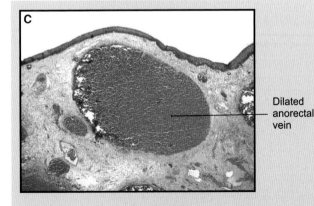

C
Dilated anorectal vein

Figure 15-20C. Hemorrhoids. H&E, ×19

Hemorrhoids are **swollen, inflamed veins** in the **anal region** deep in the anal mucosa and are classified as *internal hemorrhoids* and *external hemorrhoids*, based on whether the hemorrhoids are above (internal) or below (external) the **anorectal (line) junction** (dentate/pectinate line). Causes include repeated pregnancy, constipation, and portal hypertension. Common symptoms include bleeding, itching, and pain. Pathologically, hemorrhoids are thin-walled varicose veins that extend into the **submucosal layer**. In time, **thrombosis** (clotting) may occur with resultant infarct and fissure formation. Treatments include surgical removal of hemorrhoids, coagulation therapy, and a procedure in which a rubber band is used to tie off the hemorrhoids. This photomicrograph shows anal squamous mucosa with underlying **dilated anorectal veins**.

CLINICAL CORRELATIONS

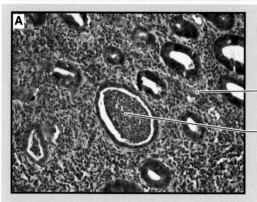

Acute and
chronic
inflammation

Crypt
abscess

Figure 15-21A. Ulcerative Colitis. H&E, ×97

Ulcerative colitis is an **inflammatory bowel disease** that causes **ulcers** in the lining of the **colon** and **rectum** characterized by intermittent exacerbations alternating with complete symptomatic remission. Major symptoms include abdominal pain, diarrhea, anemia, weight loss, bleeding from the rectum, and passage of mucus. Pathologically, the **inflammation** is predominantly confined to the **mucosa** and **submucosa** in contrast to **Crohn disease**, which is transmural. Grossly, ulcerative colitis produces shallow ulcers and **pseudopolyps**. Histologic features include **acute** and **chronic colitis, crypt abscesses, atrophy** of **glands**, and loss of mucin in **goblet cells**. Treatment includes anti-inflammatory drugs and immunosuppressants to control the symptoms and achieve remission. The risk for the development of adenocarcinoma is high in patients with ulcerative colitis, so surveillance **colonoscopy** with **biopsy** is necessary to detect early dysplasia of the glandular epithelium. Surgical removal of the colon is necessary in severe refractory cases or in cases where severe dysplasia or adenocarcinoma is detected.

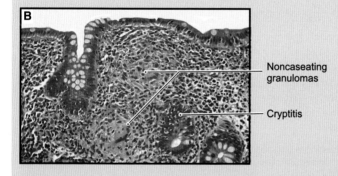

Noncaseating
granulomas

Cryptitis

Figure 15-21B. Crohn Disease. H&E, ×97

Crohn disease is a **chronic autoimmune inflammatory disease** of the **gastrointestinal tract** that may affect any location, from the oral cavity to the anus, but mostly involves the **distal small intestine** and **colon**. Crohn disease is characterized by asymmetric and segmental inflammation extending through the intestinal wall (**transmural**) from the **mucosa** to the **serosa**. Crohn disease characteristically involves areas of the bowel separated by intervening uninvolved areas or "skip" lesions. Symptoms include abdominal pain, diarrhea, vomiting, and weight loss. Pathologic changes include mucosal neutrophil and mononuclear cell infiltration, ulceration, mucosal fissures, fistulae, serosal adhesions, abscesses, **pseudopolyps**, and noncaseating granulomas. Treatment focuses on relieving symptoms through immunosuppressive agents to prevent relapse and complications. This image shows colonic mucosa with depletion of goblet cells, **noncaseating granulomas** within the lamina propria, chronic inflammation, and neutrophils invading the crypt cells.

SYNOPSIS 15-2 Pathologic and Clinical Terms for the Digestive Tract

■ *Intestinal metaplasia:* The reversible change of one mature type of epithelium to an intestinal type epithelium; may be seen in chronic gastritis when goblet cells are present within the gastric mucosa; considered a risk factor for the development of gastric adenocarcinoma.

■ *Dyspepsia:* General term for abdominal pain or indigestion associated with the intake of food.

■ *Gastric metaplasia:* The reversible change of one mature type of epithelium to a gastric type epithelium; seen in peptic duodenitis when the normal epithelial lining with goblet cells is replaced with a gastric foveolar–type mucosa in response to exposure to increased levels of stomach acid.

■ *Pseudopolyp:* Found in cases of chronic inflammatory bowel disease; consists of polypoid mounds of mucosa created by regenerating glandular epithelium; not considered true polyps, hence the name.

■ *Crypt abscess:* An aggregate of neutrophils present within a colon crypt, usually associated with inflammatory bowel disease, particularly ulcerative colitis.

■ *Cryptitis:* An indicator of acute colitis; appreciated histologically by the infiltration of neutrophils with the crypt cells of the colon.

TABLE 15-1 Digestive Tract

Regions	Mucosa (Epithelium, Lamina Propria, Muscularis Mucosae)	Submucosa (Submucosal Plexuses Present in this Layer)	Muscularis Externa (Myenteric Plexuses Present between Smooth Muscle Layers)	Serosa/ Adventitia	Main Functions
Esophagus					
Upper esophagus	Nonkeratinized stratified squamous	Esophageal glands	Inner circular and outer longitudinal skeletal muscles	Adventitia	Transport food bolus
Middle esophagus	Nonkeratinized stratified squamous	Esophageal glands	Inner circular and outer longitudinal mixed skeletal and smooth muscles	Adventitia	Transport food bolus
Lower esophagus	Nonkeratinized stratified squamous; esophageal cardiac glands in lamina propria	Esophageal glands	Inner circular and outer longitudinal smooth muscles	Serosa	Transport food bolus
Stomach (Rugae and Gastric Pits)					
Cardia	Surface mucous cells and gastric pits; mucus-secreting cells of cardiac glands in lamina propria	No glands	Inner oblique, middle circular, and outer longitudinal smooth muscles	Serosa	Add mucus and lysozyme; churn food by peristalsis
Fundus and body	Surface lining cells and gastric pits; parietal and chief cells of gastric glands in lamina propria	No glands	Inner oblique, middle circular, and outer longitudinal smooth muscles	Serosa	Same as above; add acidic gastric juice (e.g., HCl, mucus, enzymes); process food into chyme
Pylorus	Surface lining cells and gastric pits; mucus-secreting cells of pyloric glands in lamina propria	No glands	Inner oblique, middle circular, and outer longitudinal smooth muscles	Serosa	Add mucus; churn food and pass chyme to duodenum
Small Intestine (Villi and Crypts)					
Duodenum	Columnar absorptive and goblet cells; Paneth, enteroendocrine, goblet, and absorptive cells in glands (crypts) of Lieberkühn	Brunner glands	Inner circular and outer longitudinal smooth muscles	Serosa/ adventitia	Allow bile and pancreatic juice to enter small intestine; release mucus; regulate rate of emptying of stomach; absorption
Jejunum	Similar to above	No glands	Inner circular and outer longitudinal smooth muscles	Serosa	Absorption of carbohydrates, proteins, lipids, and vitamin K
Ileum	Similar to above with increased goblet cells; Peyer patches in lamina propria	Peyer patches may extend into this layer	Inner circular and outer longitudinal smooth muscles	Serosa	Similar to above; absorption of vitamins K and B12 and bile salts
Large Intestine (Crypts, No Villi)					
Cecum/ colon	Goblet cells and columnar absorptive cells; goblet, columnar, and enteroendocrine cells in glands of Lieberkühn	No glands	Inner circular smooth muscle; outer longitudinal smooth muscle layer forms three taeniae coli	Serosa/ adventitia	Absorption of water and electrolytes; formation of feces
Rectum	Similar to above; fewer glands of Lieberkühn	No glands	Inner circular and outer longitudinal smooth muscles	Adventitia	Store feces; sensory receptors signal brain of the need to evacuate
Anal canal	Nonkeratinized to keratinized stratified squamous	Sebaceous glands (distal portion); venous	Inner circular (thickened to become internal sphincter) and thin outer longitudinal smooth muscles	Adventitia	Internal sphincter and external sphincter (skeletal muscle); relax to release feces

Note: Simple columnar epithelium lines most of the digestive tract, including the stomach and the small and large intestines. It does not line the esophagus and the anal canal, however.

From Histology to Pathology

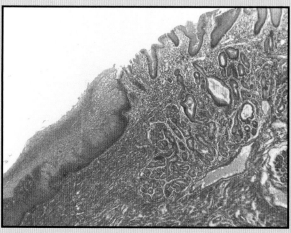
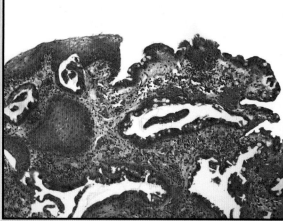

Figure 15-22. Normal esophagogastric junction and Barrett esophagus. H&E, ×100

Normal esophagogastric junction on the *left*. **Barrett esophagus** on the *right*. Barrett esophagus is a complication of **gastroesophageal reflux disease (GERD)**, characterized by metaplasia of the stratified squamous epithelium of the lower esophagus into a specialized glandular epithelium with **goblet cells**. Goblet cells are not normally present in the mucosa of the esophagus and stomach.

Clinical Vignette Questions

1. A 20-year-old woman comes to the clinic because of a several-hour history of severe lower abdominal pain. Before arriving, she had indigestion and nausea, and she vomited. She is single and not sexually active. Her temperature is 102°F (38.8°C). Physical examination showed abdominal tenderness. Laboratory investigations showed increased white blood cell count, and a diagnosis of appendicitis was made. During the surgery, the surgeon noticed her appendix is intact and without any inflammation. Which of the following is most likely associated with the patient's condition?

A. Cecum cancer
B. Colon polyp
C. Duodenal ulcer
D. Meckel diverticulum
E. Rectal abscess

2. A 15-year-old African American boy was brought to the pediatrician by his parents for chronic abdominal pain. The history revealed that symptoms included diarrhea, weight loss, and vomiting. Biopsies taken during colonoscopy shows the colon infiltrated by neutrophils and mononuclear cells, ulceration, and noncaseating granulomas. Which of the following is the most likely diagnosis for this patient?

A. Colon dysplasia
B. Colon polyp
C. Colorectal neoplasm
D. Crohn disease
E. Ulcerative colitis

3. An 8-year-old boy with a history of asthma experiences abdominal pain, nausea, vomiting, difficulty swallowing, and the feeling that food is stuck in his throat. The child's primary care provider refers him to a pediatric gastroenterologist, who performs an upper gastrointestinal endoscopy that reveals linear furrows and continuous rings from the proximal esophagus to the distal esophagus. Biopsies of the esophagus will most likely reveal which of the following histologic findings?

A. Intraepithelial eosinophils in the proximal and distal esophagus
B. Intraepithelial eosinophils in the distal esophagus only
C. Intraepithelial lymphocytes
D. Intraepithelial neutrophils with *Candida*

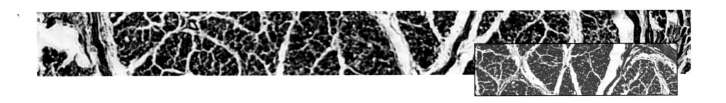

Introduction and Key Concepts for the Digestive Glands and Associated Organs
Major Salivary Glands
Pancreas
Liver
Gallbladder
Salivary Gland Duct System

Introduction and Key Concepts for the Digestive Glands and Associated Organs

Digestive glands and **associated organs** include the **major salivary glands, pancreas, liver,** and **gallbladder.** These organs are located outside the wall of the digestive tract. Their secretory products are delivered into the digestive tract via a duct system.

Major Salivary Glands

The **major salivary glands** produce saliva and empty into the oral cavity. Saliva is 99% water and contains protein, enzymes, glucose, cholesterol, urea, uric acid, ions (e.g., Na^+, K^+, Ca^{2+}, HCO_3^-), and antibacterial agents (lactoferrin, lysozyme, and IgA). Saliva is produced by both serous and mucous cells in the salivary glands. It plays important roles in aiding digestion, lubrication, protection, buffering, wound healing, maintaining the integrity of the esophagogastric epithelium, perception of taste, and in hardening of the enamel of the teeth. There are three major salivary glands: the **parotid, submandibular,** and **sublingual glands.** These are paired glands and have similar structures of secretory units (acini) and duct systems, including intralobular ducts (intercalated and striated ducts), interlobular ducts, lobar ducts, and a main duct.

1. *The parotid gland* is the largest of the three major salivary glands. This gland is surrounded by a connective tissue capsule. Its secretory unit is composed of only serous cells, which produce watery proteinaceous fluid.

2. *The submandibular gland* is the second largest salivary gland. This gland is surrounded by a connective tissue capsule. It is a mixed gland, although the majority of cells are serous cells. The secretory unit is composed of both serous and mucous cells. **Serous demilunes** (serous cell caps on the mucous cells) are present in the submandibular gland.

3. *The sublingual gland* is the smallest salivary gland. This gland is not surrounded by a connective tissue capsule. This is also a mixed gland but is predominately mucous. Acini that are completely serous are few, but serous demilunes are commonly present. Striated ducts are not as obvious as in the other two types of salivary glands.

Pancreas

The **pancreas** has **endocrine** and **exocrine** portions. The *endocrine portion* (**islets of Langerhans**) secretes blood glucose–regulating hormones (**insulin, glucagon, somatostatin, and pancreatic polypeptide**), which are released into the bloodstream (see Chapter 17, "Endocrine System"). The *exocrine portion* produces **pancreatic secretions** (**juice**), which are carried by **pancreatic ducts**. Most of these secretions go to the **main pancreatic duct**, which joins the **hepatopancreatic ampulla** (**ampulla of Vater**) and then enters the duodenum through the **major duodenal papilla** (**papilla of Vater**). The ampulla is surrounded by smooth muscle called the **sphincter of the ampulla** (**sphincter of Oddi**). A small portion of the pancreatic secretion is carried by the accessory pancreatic duct and enters the duodenum through the minor duodenal papilla. The pancreatic duct system includes intralobular ducts, interlobular ducts, and a main duct. The pancreas does not have striated ducts, and the smallest intralobular ducts are intercalated ducts. The initial portions of the intercalated ducts are lined by **centroacinar cells**. The initial pancreatic secretions (enzymes) are produced by **pancreatic acinar cells**, and a large volume of fluid (water, sodium, and bicarbonate) is added by intercalated duct cells. Pancreatic secretions contain enzymes for digesting proteins, carbohydrates, and fats. The major components include **water, sodium, bicarbonate ions, trypsinogen, chymotrypsinogen, procarboxypolypeptidase, amylase, lipase, cholesterol esterase, phospholipase, and nucleases**. The main enzymes for digesting **protein** are trypsinogen, chymotrypsinogen, and procarboxypolypeptidase; the main enzyme for digesting **carbohydrates** is amylase; and the main enzymes for digesting **fat** are lipase, cholesterol esterase, and phospholipase. The nucleases degrade nucleic acids. When the pancreatic digestive enzymes are first synthesized by the pancreatic cells, they are in an inactive stage. They become activated after they enter the duodenum and come into contact with **enterokinase** in the **glycocalyx**. The glycocalyx is an extracellular polymeric material (glycoprotein), which coats the surface of microvilli in the small intestines.

Liver

The **liver** also plays both **endocrine** and **exocrine** roles. Its *endocrine role* is in synthesizing and releasing plasma proteins, such as **fibrinogen, prothrombin, lipoproteins,** and **albumins**, into the bloodstream. Its *exocrine role* is the production of **bile**. Bile is important in emulsifying and degrading fat into smaller molecules and in carrying wastes out of the body. Bile contains **water, bile salts, bilirubin, cholesterol, fatty acids, lecithin,** and **electrolytes**. Bile is produced by **hepatocytes** and is collected by **bile canaliculi**; it drains into the hepatic duct, then into the cystic duct, and finally enters the gallbladder. Other functions of the liver include detoxification; involvement in **lipid, carbohydrate,** and **protein metabolism**; and storage of **iron, blood, glycogen, triglycerides** (lipid droplets), and **vitamins A, D, and B12**. The liver is supplied by the **portal veins** and the **hepatic arteries** at the **portal triads**. The hepatic arteries carry oxygen-rich blood, and the portal veins carry nutrient-rich blood to the **hepatic sinusoids** through their branches (hepatic arterioles and portal venules). The hepatocytes are not in direct contact with the blood stream. A small space between the hepatocyte and the endothelium of the sinusoids is called the **perisinusoidal space** or **space of Disse**. The discontinuous endothelium of the sinusoids allows proteins, nutrients, wastes, and plasma components (but not blood cells) from the hepatic sinusoids to enter the space of Disse. Hepatocytes take up nutrients and transport wastes, such as **bilirubin**, into the bile. The central veins collect the exchanged blood from sinusoids and drain into the sublobular veins and then into the large hepatic veins. The basic structure of the liver includes the **classic lobule**, the **portal lobule**, and the **liver acinus**.

Gallbladder

The **gallbladder** is a pear-shaped, saclike organ closely associated with the liver. It stores, concentrates, and releases bile. When the smooth muscle (muscularis) of the gallbladder contracts, bile is released from the gallbladder through the cystic duct into the bile duct. This joins the **hepatopancreatic ampulla** and drains into the duodenum at the **major duodenal papilla**. The wall of the gallbladder is composed of three layers: (1) **mucosa**, which includes epithelium (simple columnar epithelium) and lamina propria; (2) **muscularis**, which contains interlacing smooth muscle bundles and contracts in response to **cholecystokinin**, which is released by **enteroendocrine cells** in the small intestine (the smooth muscle of the gallbladder extends from the body into the neck where it is known as the **spiral valve of Heister** and is vital in controlling gallbladder flow); and (3) **serosa/adventitia**, a connective layer with a lining of mesothelium (serosa) or without mesothelium (adventitia). Most of the outer surface of the gallbladder is covered with **serosa**, which is continuous with the peritoneum that covers the liver. A small region of the gallbladder is covered by **adventitia**, which attaches the gallbladder to the liver.

Salivary Gland Duct System

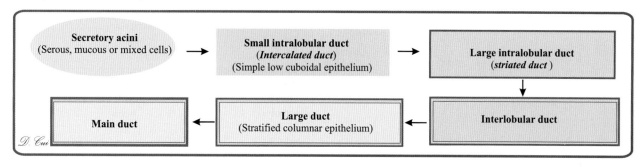

Anatomy of the Digestive Glands

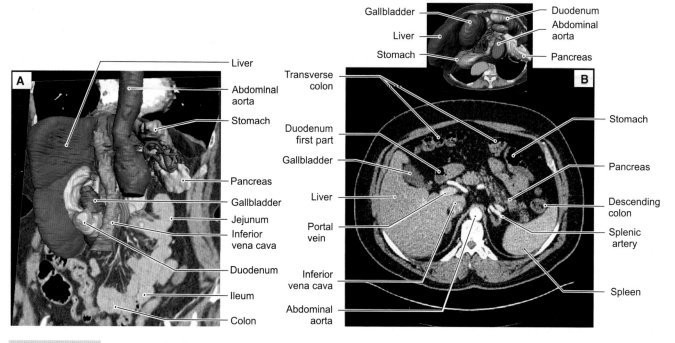

Figure 16-1A,B. **Digestive glands.** Stereoscopic model with coronal view of computed tomography angiography (CTA) image (A), transverse view (CTA) and stereoscopic model (B).

The **gastrointestinal (GI) tract** contains various glands such as the **salivary glands, gastric glands, liver, gallbladder,** and **pancreas.** The **salivary glands** include the **parotid salivary glands,** the **sublingual salivary glands,** and the **submandibular salivary glands.** The **parotid salivary glands** are located under the skin covering the lateral and posterior surface of the mandible, anterior to the ears. The **parotid ducts** empty into the vestibule of the mouth at the level of the second upper molars. The **sublingual salivary glands** are located beneath the mucous membrane of the floor of the oral cavity. The main duct of the sublingual gland either drains into the **sublingual papilla** or joins the submandibular duct. Numerous ducts of the anterior portion of the sublingual gland open into the **sublingual fold.** The submandibular glands are located on the floor of the mouth along the inner surfaces of the mandible. They empty into the mouth behind the teeth on either side of the **lingual frenulum.** The gastric glands are located in the lamina propria of the mucous membrane within the stomach, and they open into the bases of the gastric pits formed by the epithelium. The **liver** is the largest visceral organ of the human body, which lies in the right **hypochondriac** and **epigastric abdominal** areas. The **liver** can be divided into **four lobes: the left, right, caudate,** and **quadrate.** The **gallbladder** lies in a recess on the posterior surface of the right lobe. The **gallbladder** is a hollow organ that collects and stores bile. The **pancreas** lies posterior to the stomach, and the head of the pancreas is enclosed by the **duodenum,** while the tail of the **pancreas** extends to the **spleen.** The **main pancreatic duct** and the **bile duct** merge together near the **head of the pancreas** and empty into the **descending part of the duodenum.**

CLINICAL CORRELATION

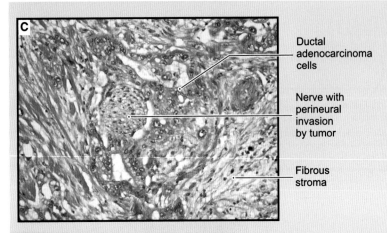

Ductal
adenocarcinoma
cells

Nerve with
perineural
invasion
by tumor

Fibrous
stroma

| Figure 16-1C. | **Pancreatic Adenocarcinoma.** H&E, ×200 |

Pancreatic adenocarcinoma (pancreatic cancer) is a malignant neoplasm of the pancreas. Exocrine pancreatic cancers are much more common than endocrine pancreatic cancers. About 95% of **exocrine cancers** are **adenocarcinomas** arising from the epithelium of pancreatic ducts. Risk factors for the development of pancreatic adenocarcinoma include **chronic pancreatitis**, smoking, **diabetes mellitus**, and **genetic predisposition** to the disease. This cancer is characterized by upper abdominal pain that radiates to the back, severe weight loss, and jaundice. In many cases, the tumor is at an advanced stage by the time symptoms appear. Pathologically, **ductal adenocarcinomas** show infiltrating small glands that are lined by **low-columnar** and **mucin-containing cells. CA19-9 antigen** is a tumor marker that is characteristically elevated in patients with pancreatic cancer. Although it is not specific to this tumor, it is valuable in both the diagnosis of pancreatic cancer and in surveillance for recurrence in patients after surgical resection. Surgical resection is the only potentially curative treatment. Use of adjuvant chemoradiotherapy may increase the survival rate.

Digestive Glands and Associated Organs

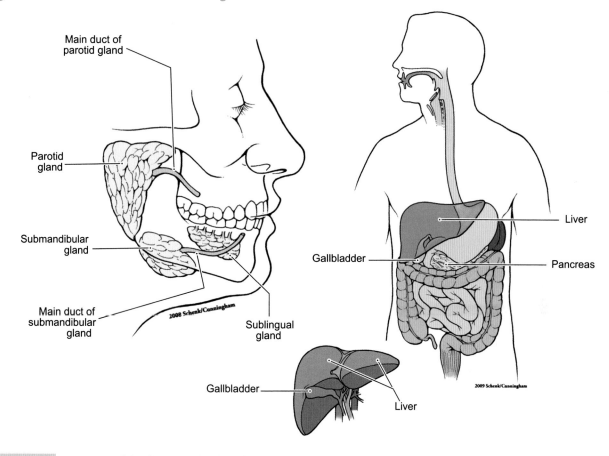

Main duct of
parotid gland

Parotid
gland

Submandibular
gland

Main duct of
submandibular
gland

2008 Schenk/Cunningham

Sublingual
gland

Liver

Gallbladder

Pancreas

Gallbladder

Liver

2009 Schenk/Cunningham

Figure 16-2. Overview of the digestive glands and associated organs.

The **major digestive glands** include the **salivary glands, pancreas,** and **liver**. Although the **gallbladder** is not a gland, it is closely associated with the liver and digestive system. The digestive glands and gallbladder are located outside of the digestive tract. Their ducts carry their products (**saliva**) into the oral cavity or into the lumen of the duodenum of the small intestine (**pancreatic secretions and bile**). The *salivary glands* include the **major salivary glands** and the **minor salivary glands**. The **parotid, submandibular,** and **sublingual glands** are the three major salivary glands. These glands are either serous glands or mixed glands (both serous and mucous). Most of the minor salivary glands are mucous or mixed glands, with only von Ebner glands being entirely serous glands. For details of classification of the glands, see Chapter 3, "Epithelium and Glands." The *pancreas* includes an **endocrine portion** (islets of Langerhans) and an **exocrine portion**. The *endocrine portion* secretes hormones into the bloodstream (see Chapter 17, "Endocrine System"), whereas the *exocrine portion* has ducts that carry enzyme products into the lumen of the duodenum. The *liver* produces **bile**, which is carried by the bile duct system into the gallbladder. The liver also aids in the metabolism of lipids, carbohydrates, and proteins; stores iron, glycogen, triglycerides, and vitamins A, D, and B12; and detoxifies certain toxic substances in the blood. The *gallbladder* stores, concentrates, and releases bile into the duodenum.

Digestive Glands and Associated Organs

I. Major Salivary Glands
   A. Parotid glands (serous)
   B. Submandibular glands (mixed, predominately serous)
   C. Sublingual glands (mixed, predominately mucous)

II. Pancreas
   A. Exocrine portion
   B. Endocrine (islets of Langerhans) portion

III. Liver
   A. Central vein
   B. Portal triad
   C. Liver lobules
      1. Classic lobule
      2. Portal lobule
      3. Hepatic acinus

IV. Gallbladder
   A. Mucosa
   B. Muscularis
   C. Serosa

Figures and Images Orientation

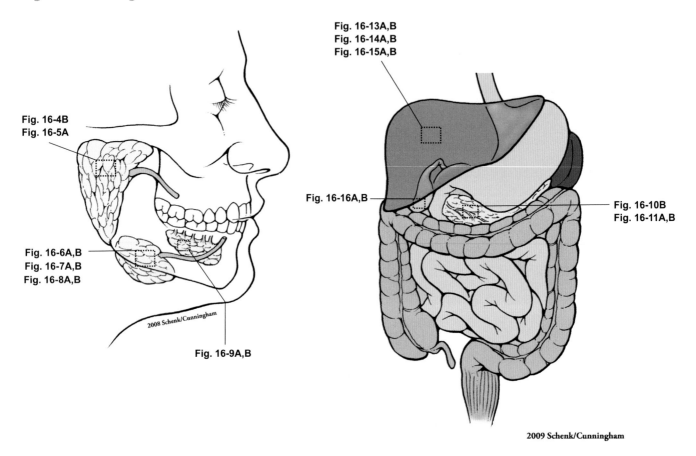

Figure 16-3. Orientation of detailed digestive glands and associated organs illustrations.

Digestive Glands and Associated Organs with Figure Numbers

Parotid Glands
Figure 16-4B
Figure 16-5A
Figure 16-5B
Figure 16-5C

Submandibular Glands
Figure 16-6A
Figure 16-6B
Figure 16-7A
Figure 16-7B
Figure 16-8A
Figure 16-8B

Sublingual Glands
Figure 16-9A
Figure 16-9B
Figure 16-9C

Pancreas
Figure 16-10A
Figure 16-10B
Figure 16-10C
Figure 16-11A
Figure 16-11B

Liver
Figure 16-12
Figure 16-13A
Figure 16-13B
Figure 16-13C
Figure 16-14A
Figure 16-14B
Figure 16-15A
Figure 16-15B
Figure 16-17A

Gallbladder
Figure 16-16A
Figure 16-16B
Figure 16-17B

Salivary Glands

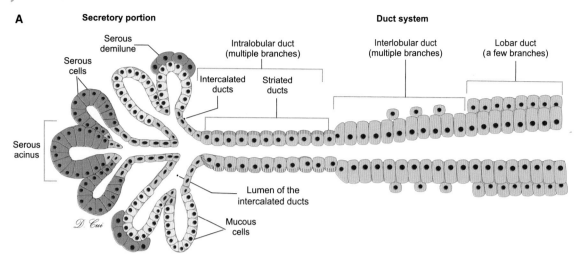

A

Secretory portion

Duct system

Serous demilune

Serous cells

Serous acinus

Intralobular duct (multiple branches)

Intercalated ducts

Striated ducts

Interlobular duct (multiple branches)

Lobar duct (a few branches)

Lumen of the intercalated ducts

Mucous cells

D. Cui

Figure 16-4A. General structure of the major salivary glands.

The **parotid, submandibular,** and **sublingual glands** are structurally very similar to one another, although they produce various secretions. Each unit of the salivary glands can be divided into a **secretory portion** and a **duct system**. The *secretory portion* contains **serous cells, mucous cells,** or a **mixture** of both. These secretory cells are arranged into acini resembling grapes on a stem (intercalated duct). Several serous cells form a cap, called a **serous demilune,** on the outer aspect of mucous cells; this arrangement can be found in the mixed glands. A capsule (dense connective tissue layer) surrounds an entire gland. Connective tissue septa penetrate the gland and subdivide it into **lobes** and **lobules.** The *duct system* includes **intralobular ducts** (located within the lobules), **interlobular ducts** (outside or between the lobules), **lobar ducts,** and a **main duct.** The *intralobular ducts* include **intercalated ducts** and **striated ducts.** The *main duct* empties the secretory products (saliva) into the oral cavity.

PAROTID GLANDS

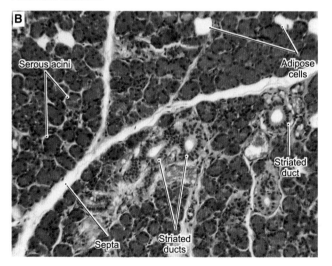

B

Serous acini

Adipose cells

Striated duct

Septa

Striated ducts

Figure 16-4B. Parotid gland. H&E, ×130.

The **parotid glands** are paired glands and are the largest of the major salivary glands. They are located anterior to and below the lower half of the ear, and superior, posterior, and deep to the ramus of the mandible. The **main duct** of each parotid gland passes through the cheek and opens into the oral cavity near the second upper molar tooth. The parotid glands are composed of **serous acini** and ducts. They are classified as **compound (branched) acinar glands** based on their duct shape and secretory units. This photomicrograph shows **striated ducts (intralobular ducts)** located in the lobules. The striated ducts are lined by taller cuboidal (or columnar) cells with centrally located nuclei. Connective tissue septa divide the gland into small lobules, and there are some adipose cells distributed in among the serous acini. Each acinus is formed by several serous cells with basally positioned dark nuclei.

CLINICAL CORRELATION

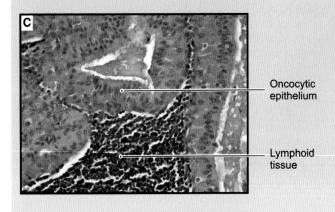

Oncocytic
epithelium

Lymphoid
tissue

Figure 16-4C. Warthin Tumor. H&E, ×400

Warthin tumor (papillary cystadenoma lymphomatosum) is a **benign neoplasm** of the parotid gland. Clinically, it presents as a painless swelling in the area of the parotid gland, and it has a strong association with cigarette smoking. The histologic appearance is striking and unique, with **multiple cystic spaces** and **papillary formations** set within a **lymphoid stroma**. The cysts and papillary areas consist of eosinophilic epithelial cells producing a two-layered epithelium. The basal layer is cuboidal, and the luminal layer is columnar. These epithelial cells are described as **oncocytic** and, upon ultrastructural examination, reveal abundant mitochondria. Surgical excision with an adequate margin is considered curative.

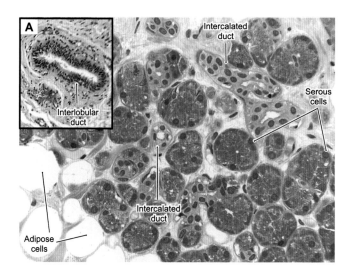

Figure 16-5A. Parotid glands. H&E, ×295; inset ×97

Parotid glands contain only serous secretory cells. There are some adipose cells scattered throughout the gland. All three types of salivary glands have similar duct systems. The intercalated ducts are shown here; they have a small lumen and are lined by lower cuboidal cells with basally located nuclei. The *inset* shows a large interlobular duct lined by **stratified columnar cells** and surrounded by a large amount of connective tissue. The diameter of the ducts gradually increases from the intercalated ducts to the large interlobular ducts, and their lining cells increase in height and in number of layers. The main duct (**duct of Stensen**) of the parotid gland traverses the buccinator muscles and opens opposite the secondary upper molars. All three types of salivary glands receive **parasympathetic** innervation. The parotid gland is innervated by the **glossopharyngeal nerve** (**cranial nerve [CN] IX**).

CLINICAL CORRELATIONS

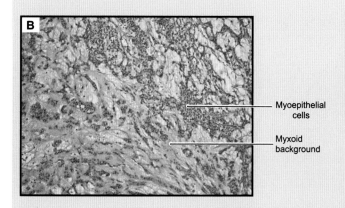

Figure 16-5B. Pleomorphic Adenoma. H&E, ×55

Pleomorphic adenoma, also called **benign mixed tumor**, is the most common benign salivary gland tumor. The majority, approximately 80%, occur in the parotid gland, most of which are in the superficial lobe, and are benign pleomorphic adenomas. The tumor may also involve submandibular, sublingual, and minor salivary glands. It is characterized by a slow-growing, mobile, and painless parotid mass. Most patients are not aware of the tumor for years. The mass itself is typically well demarcated but may be nodular in appearance. Histologically, the neoplasm is composed of epithelial and **myoepithelial cells** in a **chondromyxoid background**. Fine needle biopsy is useful in the diagnosis of pleomorphic adenoma. After surgery, pleomorphic adenomas may recur. Rapid growth of a mass in the same area after surgery may signify malignant transformation of the residual adenoma called **carcinoma expleomorphic adenoma**. This photomicrograph shows nests of **myoepithelial cells** in a **myxoid background**.

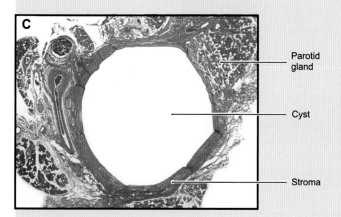

Figure 16-5C. Parotid Cyst. H&E, ×11

A **parotid cyst** is a fluid-filled closed cavity occurring within the parenchyma of the parotid gland and is usually caused by trauma, infections, salivary gland stones, or tumors. Physical exam usually reveals a painless lump or swelling. As the cyst enlarges, it may interfere with chewing, swallowing, and speaking. Additionally, parotid cysts may become infected. Histologically, the cyst is lined by an epithelium, and the cavity is filled with fluid or mucus. The surrounding **stroma** shows dense fibrosis and may be infiltrated by aggregates of lymphocytes, as shown in this slide. If necessary, surgical removal of the cyst is recommended.

SUBMANDIBULAR GLANDS

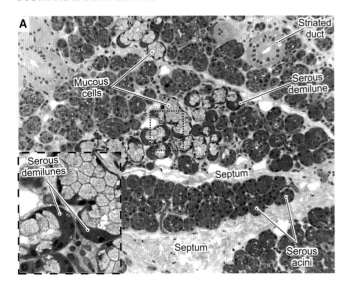

Figure 16-6A. **Submandibular glands.** H&E, ×136; inset ×408

Submandibular glands are also paired glands. They are smaller than the parotid glands, but larger than the sublingual glands. Each submandibular gland is divided into **superficial** (large) and **deep** (small) **lobes** and is located under the floor of the oral cavity adjacent to the mandible. The **main duct** of the submandibular gland drains **saliva** into the oral cavity at the **sublingual caruncles** on both sides of the frenulum linguae. The submandibular glands are mixed glands that contain predominantly **serous cells** but also some **mucous cells**. They are classified as **compound (branched) tubuloacinar glands**. Serous cells are arranged into many acini, and mucous cells are arranged as acini or tubular structures, which may have caps of serous cells (**serous demilunes**). Submandibular glands are innervated by **parasympathetic nerve fibers** from branches of the **facial nerve (CN VII)**.

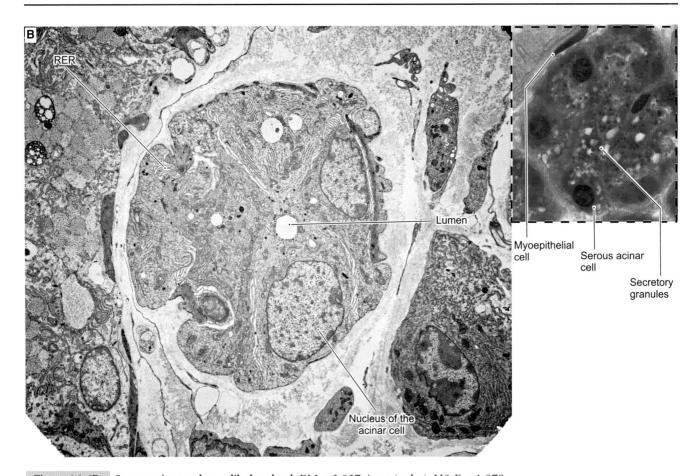

Figure 16-6B. **Serous acinus, submandibular gland.** EM, ×3,937; inset (*color*), H&E, ×1,079

Several **serous acinar cells** arranged in an **acinus** and sharing a common lumen are shown. The serous lumens are smaller than those of a mucous acinus. Each secretory cell has a relatively large nucleus and numerous **rough endoplasmic reticulum (RER)** cisterns in the basal portion of the cytoplasm. These features indicate their active protein synthesis. **Secretory granules** are usually located on the apical region of the cells (*color inset*). Secretory granules are not seen in this electron micrograph because they have already been discharged from these particular cells. The *inset* shows an acinus with secretory cells having round nuclei located basally and many secretory granules in the apical portions of the secretory cells. A **myoepithelial cell** with a flat nucleus is present here, located beneath the serous cell. It is a contractile cell and contains **smooth muscle myosin**. The myoepithelial cells contract and move the secretory products toward the intercalated duct.

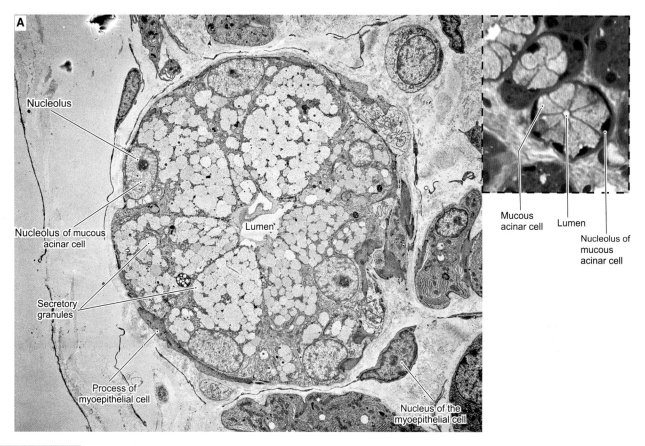

Figure 16-7A. **Mucous acinus, submandibular gland.** EM, ×6,818; inset (*color*) H&E, ×598

This is an example of a **mucous acinus,** showing numerous large **secretory granules** in the apical region of the cells. These granules contain **mucins,** which are synthesized within the cells. The nuclei of the mucous cells are flattened and lie against the basement membrane. Mucous cells have less RER than serous cells. **Myoepithelial cells** share the basement membrane with mucous cells. Myoepithelial cells have long **cellular processes** that can contract, promoting mucous cells to discharge their secretory products into the lumen of the intercalated ducts.

CLINICAL CORRELATION

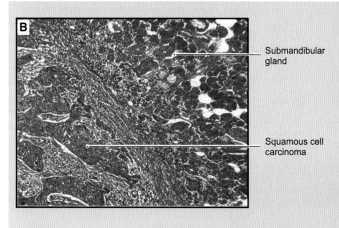

Figure 16-7B. **Squamous Cell Carcinoma of the Tongue.** H&E, ×83

Squamous cell carcinoma of the tongue is a **malignant oral neoplasm** representing the most common intraoral cancer. Squamous cell carcinoma is usually asymptomatic in the early stages, but local pain, difficulty swallowing, and **dysphagia** are common in the late stages. Clinically, the **neoplasm** may appear as a red or white nonhealing ulcer or exophytic mass, most commonly found on the lateral aspect of the tongue. This image shows a squamous cell carcinoma on the floor of the mouth invading the submandibular glands. The major risk factors for oral and tongue squamous cell carcinoma include **smoking** and **alcohol consumption, chronic irritation,** and **chewing tobacco.** Pathologically, the cancer cells show large, irregular and darkly stained nuclei. This cancer tends to metastasize through the lymphatic system. Surgical removal of the primary growth and related lymphatic nodes, chemotherapy, and radiation therapy are treatment options.

STRIATED DUCT

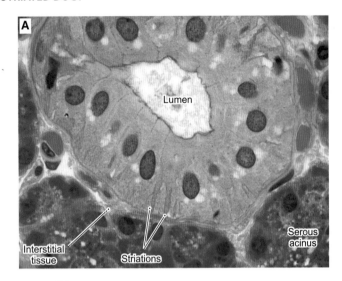

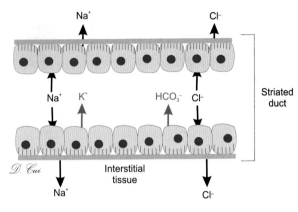

Figure 16-8A.   Striated duct, submandibular gland. H&E, ×845

Striated ducts are lined by **simple cuboidal** or **columnar cells** with **centrally positioned nuclei**. Their cytoplasm shows striations in the basolateral region, hence the name. The striations are due to deep indentations in the plasma membrane (**basolateral folds**), which increase the surface area occupied by pumps involved in **ion** and **fluid transport**. The folds contain many **mitochondria** that provide adenosine triphosphate for active transport. The **striated ducts** collect **primary saliva** (produced by acinar cells) from the **intercalated ducts**. The main function of the striated ducts is modulation of the **pH** and **ion composition** of the saliva. The striated ducts remove **Na⁺** and **Cl⁻ ions** in the primary saliva from the lumen and transport these ions to the interstitial tissues. Striated ducts also pump **K⁺** and **HCO₃⁻** into the saliva fluid. This results in a **hypotonic alkaline saliva** (secondary saliva), which moves from the striated ducts to the interlobular ducts, then to the main duct, and eventually enters the oral cavity. Saliva plays important roles in moistening and cleansing the oral cavity, helping to repair oral tissues, influencing the pH (**buffering**) in the oral cavity, stimulating the taste buds, helping to digest food, helping in the mineralization and hardening of the enamel of posterupted teeth, and destroying bacteria by antimicrobial action.

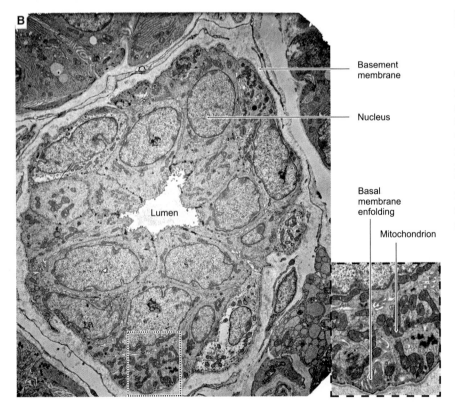

Figure 16-8B.   Intralobular duct, submandibular gland. EM, ×3,382; inset ×6,779

The duct shown here appears to be at the transition between a **striated intralobular duct** and an **interlobular duct**. Some of the lining cells, such as the one shown in the *inset*, have features of a striated duct in that there are extensive **basolateral folds** containing numerous mitochondria. These are the same features that account for the eosinophilic striations seen in these cells in H&E-stained sections for light microscopy.

SUBLINGUAL GLANDS

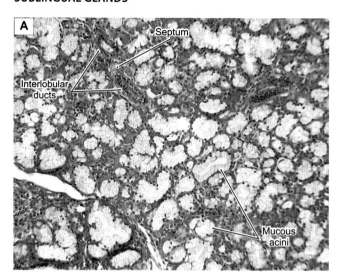

Figure 16-9A. Sublingual glands. H&E, ×123

Sublingual glands are the smallest of the three major salivary glands. They are paired glands and are located deep in the floor of the oral cavity, anterior to the submandibular glands. They are covered by the oral mucosa but have no capsule (dense connective tissue) enclosing them as the other two major salivary glands do. Sublingual glands have about 8 to 20 small ducts, which open into the crest of the sublingual fold on the floor of the oral cavity. They are **mixed glands** and contain **serous** and **mucous secretory cells**, but predominantly mucous cells. As in submandibular glands, **serous demilunes** are present; sublingual glands are also classified as **compound (branched) tubuloacinar glands.** Two intralobular ducts located inside connective tissue septa are labeled here. Sublingual glands are innervated by parasympathetic nerve fibers from branches of the **facial nerve (CN VII).**

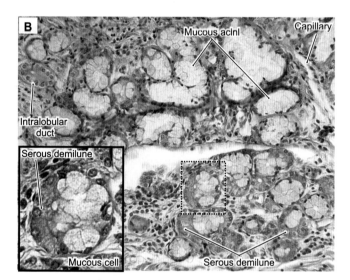

Figure 16-9B. Sublingual gland. H&E, ×179; inset ×408

Mucous cells make up the majority of the cells in the **sublingual glands** and are distributed throughout the gland. Some mucous cells may be capped with serous cells (**serous demilunes**); very occasionally, complete serous acini may be present. Mucous cells stain lighter than serous cells and they are often arranged in an elongated tubular structure (**mucous acinus**) with a flattened or round lumen. These mucous cells have dark nuclei located at the basal end of the cells. Nuclei of the mucous cells are smaller and flatter than in serous cells. The large intralobular ducts in the sublingual glands are short, and the striations of the ducts are not particularly obvious. The small intralobular ducts (**intercalated ducts**) are similar to those of the other two major salivary glands; they receive secretions directly from secretory cells.

CLINICAL CORRELATION

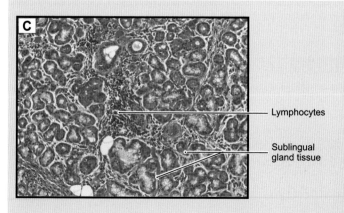

Figure 16-9C. Sialadenitis. H&E, ×109

Sialadenitis is the inflammation of salivary tissues or salivary glands caused by injuries, viral or bacterial infection, autoimmune disease, or stones within the salivary gland ducts. Ductal obstruction due to stones (**sialolithiasis**) may lead to painful gland enlargement and **abscess**, most often because of bacteria such as *Staphylococcus aureus*. Histologic findings in acute sialadenitis would show infiltration of glandular parenchyma by abundant neutrophils. The most common cause of viral sialadenitis is mumps, often affecting the parotid glands. **Sjögren syndrome** is an autoimmune disease characterized by periductal and periacinar **lymphocytic infiltrates**, formation of lymphatic nodules, periductal fibrosis, and destruction of the glands. This image shows chronic sialadenitis with a lymphocytic infiltrate within the glandular parenchyma.

Pancreas

A

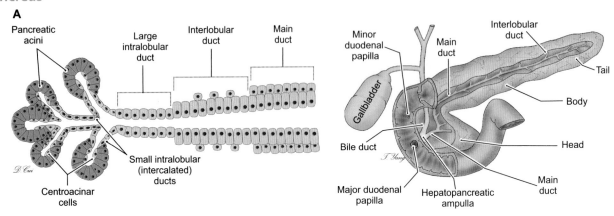

Figure 16-10A. A representation of the exocrine pancreatic duct system.

The **pancreas** is an elongated gland, which lies mostly posterior to the stomach. It can be divided into a **head, body,** and **tail**. The pancreatic duct begins in the tail of the pancreas, passes through the body, and enters the head of the pancreas. Most exocrine pancreatic secretions are carried by the **main duct,** which joins the bile duct of the gallbladder at the **hepatopancreatic ampulla** and empties the secretions into the duodenum through the **major duodenal papilla**. A small portion of the pancreatic secretion is released into the duodenum through the minor duodenal papilla. The exocrine portion of the gland has a duct system that is similar to that of the major salivary glands, except the pancreas does not have striated ducts and lobar ducts. Secretory products are released into the smallest portions of the intercalated ducts, formed by centroacinar cells, and then drained into the intralobular ducts, the interlobular ducts, and finally into the main duct.

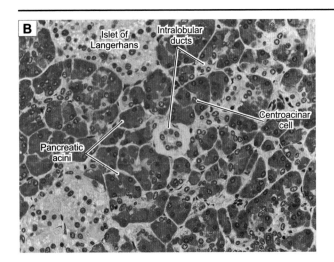

Figure 16-10B. Exocrine and endocrine pancreas. H&E, ×272

The **pancreas** consists of **exocrine** and **endocrine portions**. The *exocrine pancreas* has many serous secretory cells, which stain darkly, as in the major salivary glands. These secretory cells are often called **pancreatic acinar cells** and are arranged as acini. Each pancreatic acinar cell has a round nucleus and its cytoplasm contains many **zymogen granules**. These cells secrete enzymes that help in the digestion of proteins, lipids, and carbohydrates. The pancreas is innervated by parasympathetic nerve fibers from the right branch of the **vagus nerve (CN X)**. The *endocrine pancreas,* known as the **islets of Langerhans,** is found within the exocrine pancreas. The islets produce the hormones **insulin** and **glucagon,** which are released into the bloodstream to regulate blood glucose level. The endocrine portion of the gland does not have a duct system (see Chapter 17, "Endocrine System").

CLINICAL CORRELATION

C

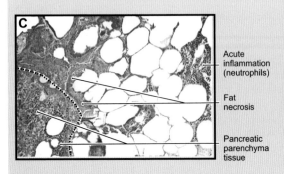

Figure 16-10C. Acute Pancreatitis. H&E, ×50

Acute pancreatitis is an acute inflammatory disease of the pancreas characterized by severe upper abdominal pain, nausea, and vomiting and elevated **serum pancreatic enzymes, amylase,** and **lipase**. Acute pancreatitis may be caused by **hypertriglyceridemia,** alcohol ingestion, infections, trauma, drugs, and **gallstones**. Gallstones may block the pancreatic duct, resulting in **autodigestion** of the pancreatic parenchyma by enzymes released because of disrupted cell membranes. Pathologic changes include interstitial and peripancreatic edema, fat necrosis with **saponification,** inflammatory infiltration of neutrophils, and **necrosis** of the **pancreatic parenchyma**. Based on the severity of the disease, treatment includes pain control, intravenous fluids, nasogastric suction, and reduction of food intake. In very severe cases, surgical removal of the damaged tissue may be necessary. This image shows acute pancreatitis with **fat necrosis,** an acute inflammatory infiltrate consisting of neutrophils, and inflamed pancreatic parenchyma.

EXOCRINE PANCREAS

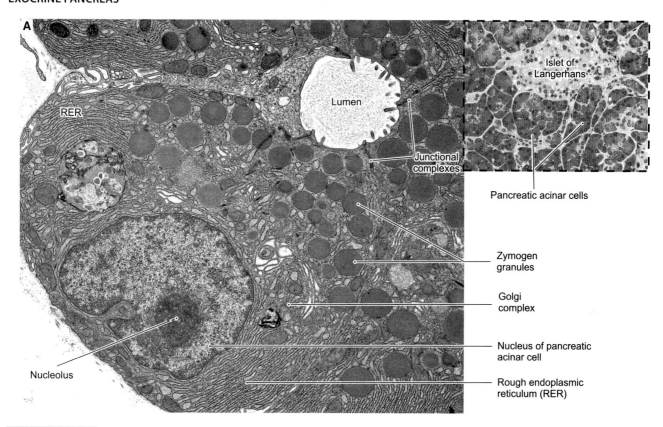

Figure 16-11A. **Pancreatic acinar cells.** EM, ×9,509; inset (*color*), H&E, ×157

Pancreatic acinar cells are protein-synthesizing cells and contain many **secretory (zymogen) granules** in the apical region of the cytoplasm and plentiful **RER** in the basal cytoplasm of the cells. A **Golgi complex** is seen close to the nucleus of the cell. A **lumen** is located at the apical region of the acinar cells, where zymogen granules are released. Several **junctional complexes** near the lumen indicate the fused borders between the neighboring acinar cells. The *inset color microphotograph* shows pancreatic cells arranged in **acini** as a secretory unit. These cells have basally positioned nuclei.

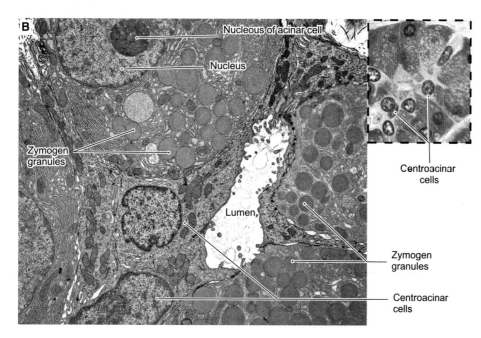

Figure 16-11B. **Centroacinar cells, pancreas.** EM, ×5,891; inset (*color*), H&E, ×628

Centroacinar cells are not protein-synthesizing cells and they do not have the features of active protein synthesis and secretion. They have many **mitochondria** but do not have much RER. These cells form the initial portions of the **intercalated ducts** and are located at the center of each **acinus**, hence their name. The centroacinar cells, along with intercalated ducts, play roles in transporting **primary pancreatic secretions**. They also secrete a large volume of fluid (rich in **sodium** and **bicarbonate**) into the pancreatic secretions to help neutralize acidic food contents entering the duodenum from the stomach.

Liver

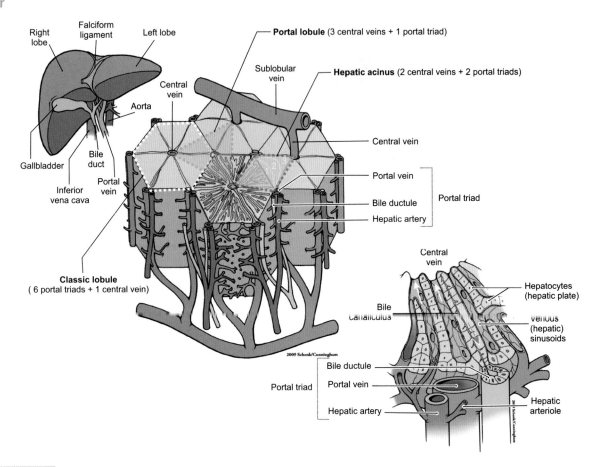

Figure 16-12.   General structure of the liver.

The **liver** is the largest gland and the largest visceral organ in the body. It has left and right lobes and is covered by a thin capsule called the **Glisson capsule**. The liver is located in the superior right and superior left quadrants of the abdominal cavity. The liver contains numerous **hepatocytes** arranged in plates; **venous sinusoids (hepatic sinusoids)** run between these hepatic plates. The liver has a rich vascular supply; it receives blood from both the **portal veins** and the **hepatic artery**. Secretory products and waste drain out of the liver by three routes: (1) the **hepatic venous system**, in which blood drains from the hepatic sinusoids (*white arrows in detail view above*) to the central vein, then to the sublobular vein, and finally to the large hepatic veins; (2) the **duct system for bile**, in which bile drains from bile canaliculi (*green arrow in the detail view above*) to the bile ductules, from the ductules into the hepatic ducts, which then join the **cystic duct** from the gallbladder; and (3) the **lymphatic vessel system**, in which lymph from the liver drains into the hepatic lymph vessels and passes through the lymph nodes near the liver to then drain into the thoracic duct. The liver has many lobules. These can be classified into three types based on their structure and function. (1) **Classic lobule** (*hexagon shape*) is the traditional way to describe liver lobules based on the direction of the blood flow. Each lobule contains six portal triads and one central vein; blood flows from portal triads into a central vein. (2) **Portal lobule** (*triangular shape*) emphasizes the exocrine functions of the liver (production of the bile). This classification is based on the direction of the bile flow. Each lobule contains three central veins and one portal triad in the center. The bile is produced by hepatocytes and enters the bile canaliculi to then drain into the bile ductule in the portal triad. (3) **Hepatic acinus** (*diamond shape*), which includes two central veins and two portal triads in each lobule. This classification is based on the blood oxygen level, nutrient supply, and metabolic activity. It is an important concept for liver pathology. The hepatic acinus can be subdivided into three zones: **zone 1, zone 2,** and **zone 3**.

SYNOPSIS 16-1 Functions of the Liver

- ■ *Exocrine function:* Secretion of bile into the duodenum to help digest fat and eliminate waste products, such as bilirubin and excess cholesterol. The main components of bile include water, bile salts, bilirubin, cholesterol, fatty acids, lecithin, and electrolytes.
- ■ *Endocrine function:* Synthesis of majority of plasma proteins such as fibrinogen, prothrombin, lipoproteins, and albumins, and their release into the bloodstream.
- ■ *Metabolism and detoxification:* Breakdown of proteins, toxic substances, and many drugs; oxidation and conjugation of toxins, estrogens, and other hormones; and elimination via bile or urine.
- ■ *Storage:* Storage of iron; blood; glycogen; triglycerides (lipid droplets); and vitamins A, D, and B12.

LIVER ACINUS AND PORTAL TRIAD

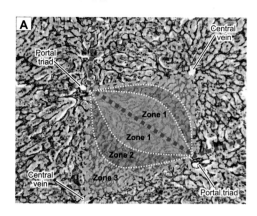 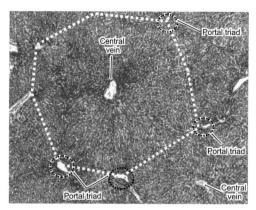

Figure 16-13A. **Liver acinus.** Silver stain, ×89 (*left*); H&E, ×42 (*right*)

Left: An example of the architecture and general pattern of the **liver** is shown. The hepatocytes are supported by a network of reticular fibers (*black*). The *red dotted line* indicates a portion of the classic lobule. The diamond-shaped **hepatic acinus** (*blue dotted line*) is located between two central veins and two portal triads. The hepatic acinus has three zones. **Zone 1** is closer to the portal triads and receives the most blood flow from the portal veins and hepatic arteries in the portal triads. Hepatocytes in this region are more likely to survive than cells in zone 3 in case of insufficient oxygen and nutrient supply in the liver, such as in heart failure. However, hepatocytes in zone 1 are also exposed to blood-borne toxins first and are more likely to be damaged than the cells in zone 3. **Zone 3** is far from the portal triads and close to the central veins; it has a poor oxygen and nutrient supply but is also less exposed to blood-borne toxins. In case of heart failure, hepatocytes in zone 3 lack oxygen and appear necrotic first. **Zone 2** has an intermediate response to oxygen and toxins.

Right: This image shows the general pattern of organization of the liver at a lower magnification. The classic lobule is indicated by the *white dotted line*.

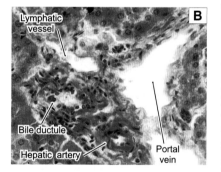

Figure 16-13B. **Portal triad, liver.** H&E, ×277

Six **portal triads** make up one hexagon-shaped, classic lobule. Each portal triad is composed of a **portal vein**, a **hepatic artery**, and a **bile ductule**. These structures are surrounded by connective tissues, which usually contains a **lymphatic vessel**. (1) The *portal vein* has a large lumen and thin vessel wall. The branches (portal venules) of the portal vein feed the hepatic sinusoids. (2) The *hepatic artery* has a small lumen and a wall of smooth muscle that is 2 to 3 cell layers thick. The hepatic artery also has branches (hepatic arterioles), which feed into the hepatic sinusoids. The hepatic sinusoids, therefore, receive glucose-rich blood from the portal vein and oxygen-rich blood from the hepatic artery. (3) The *bile ductule* is lined by cuboidal cells with dark, round nuclei. The bile ductule collects bile from the bile canaliculi and drains it into the hepatic duct.

CLINICAL CORRELATION

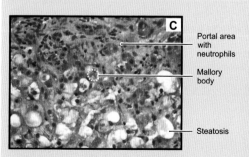

Figure 16-13C. **Alcoholic Fatty Liver (Steatosis).** H&E, ×186

Alcoholic fatty liver, or **steatosis**, is usually an asymptomatic and reversible liver condition associated with mild to moderate alcohol use in which lipid accumulates within hepatocytes. Severe steatosis may lead to **hepatomegaly** and mildly elevated serum bilirubin and alkaline phosphatase levels. Grossly, a fatty liver appears yellow and greasy compared to the normal red-brown appearance of liver tissues. Chronic alcohol abuse, particularly heavy binge drinking, may lead to **alcoholic hepatitis**, an inflammatory condition of the liver characterized by abdominal discomfort, malaise, hepatomegaly, and abnormal liver tests. Severe cases may result in fulminant hepatic failure. Histologic features of alcoholic hepatitis include a **neutrophilic infiltrate**, hepatocyte **edema** and **necrosis**, and the presence of **Mallory bodies**, which are cellular accumulations of cytokeratin intermediate filaments. Some patients will progress to **alcoholic cirrhosis** characterized by regenerating nodules of hepatocytes with intervening fibrous septae. This image shows **portal fibrosis**, infiltration by neutrophils, fatty change, and Mallory bodies.

HEPATOCYTES AND HEPATIC SINUSOIDS

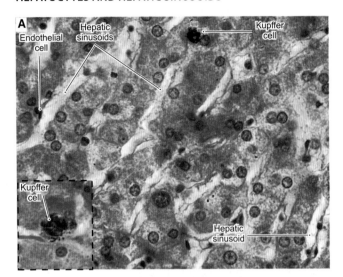

Figure 16-14A. Hepatocytes and hepatic sinusoids, liver. H&E, ×523; inset ×593

Hepatocytes are large polygonal cells with round nuclei positioned at the center of the cells. These cells have numerous functions that include modification and storage of ingested nutrients, production of many blood proteins, drug metabolism, and exocrine secretion of bile salts. This higher magnification view shows hepatocytes arranged in plates that are one or two cells thick. The **hepatic sinusoids** are located between the plates of hepatocytes. The endothelial cells that line the sinusoids are discontinuous, which allows proteins and other materials to pass through the walls of the sinusoids. **Kupffer cells** are specialized macrophages in the liver. They are irregular in shape with ovoid nuclei and often have ingested materials in their cytoplasm, making them distinguishable from hepatocytes and other cells. They move along the luminal surface of the hepatic sinusoids and clear (**phagocytose**) debris and damaged erythrocytes from the bloodstream.

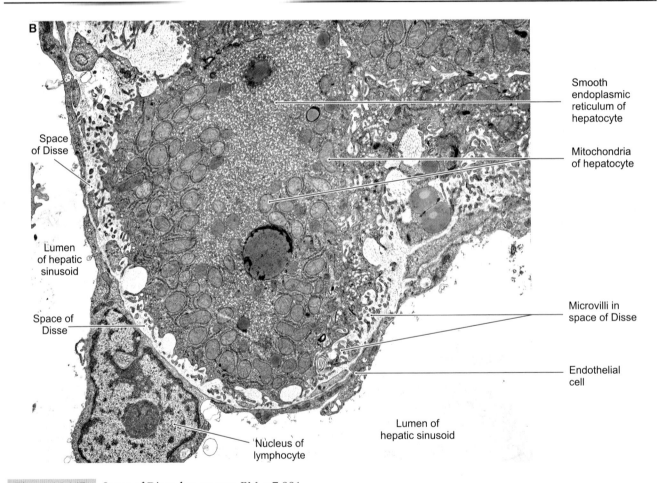

Figure 16-14B. Space of Disse, hepatocyte. EM, ×7,991

The **perisinusoidal space** known as the **space of Disse** is shown here. This space is formed by the surfaces of the hepatocytes and endothelial cells of the hepatic sinusoid. A nucleus of a lymphocyte is seen in the lumen of the hepatic sinusoid. The space of Disse contains many **microvilli**, which are extensions from the hepatocyte surface. Hepatocytes contain many **mitochondria** and much **smooth endoplasmic reticulum (SER)**. Hepatocytes are not directly in contact with the bloodstream; the space of Disse provides an environment for the exchange of proteins, plasma, and other material between the hepatocytes and blood in the hepatic sinusoid. The perisinusoidal space of Disse is also the main extracellular compartment from which liver lymph is derived.

HEPATOCYTES AND BILE CANALICULI

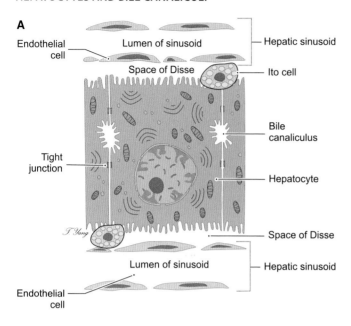

A

- Endothelial cell
- Lumen of sinusoid
- Space of Disse
- Tight junction
- T. Yang
- Lumen of sinusoid
- Endothelial cell

- Hepatic sinusoid
- Ito cell
- Bile canaliculus
- Hepatocyte
- Space of Disse
- Hepatic sinusoid

Figure 16-15A. A representation of bile canaliculi and hepatocytes.

The **bile canaliculi** are enlarged intercellular spaces, located between two adjacent **hepatocytes**. They receive bile after it is produced by hepatocytes and transport bile into the bile ductules. The **hepatic sinusoid** wall is lined by a thin, discontinuous endothelium. The hepatic sinusoids carry glucose-rich and oxygen-rich blood to supply the hepatocytes through the **space of Disse**. This is the space between the endothelial cells of the hepatic sinusoid and the hepatocytes. Short microvilli of the hepatocytes extend into the space of Disse; fat-storing cells called **Ito cells** or **hepatic stellate cells** are also located in the space. These cells contain many lipid droplets or vacuoles in their cytoplasm, which store vitamin A.

Jaundice is a condition in which the skin and sclera become markedly yellow. It results from a high level of bilirubin in the bloodstream. Bilirubin is normally removed from blood by hepatocytes and then modified and excreted into the bile. When excess bilirubin is released into the bloodstream (because of destruction of a large number of erythrocytes), or the elimination of bilirubin is interrupted (as in liver disease or gallstones), jaundice can develop.

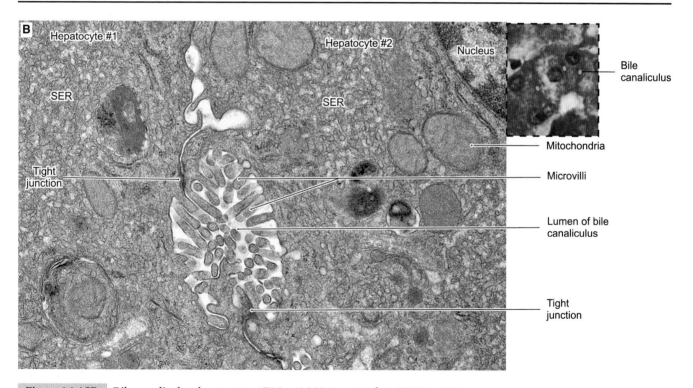

B

- Hepatocyte #1
- SER
- Tight junction

- Hepatocyte #2
- SER
- Nucleus

- Bile canaliculus
- Mitochondria
- Microvilli
- Lumen of bile canaliculus
- Tight junction

Figure 16-15B. Bile canaliculus, hepatocytes. EM, ×6,380; inset *(color)*, H&E, ×618

This image shows the lumen of a **bile canaliculus** between two neighboring **hepatocytes**. A small lumen of the canaliculus is filled with the **microvilli** of the two hepatocytes. A small portion of the nucleus, belonging to one of the hepatocytes, is visible in the upper right corner. The **SER** and mitochondria are shown in the cytoplasm of both hepatocytes. **Tight junctions (zonulae occludens)** seal each side of the bile canaliculus, preventing initial bile from leaking out of the canaliculus. The *inset color photomicrograph* shows the pink borders between neighboring hepatocytes. The positions of the **bile canaliculi** are indicated by *small circles* on the pink borders. The bile canaliculi are the smallest channels that collect bile in the hepatocyte plates.

Gallbladder

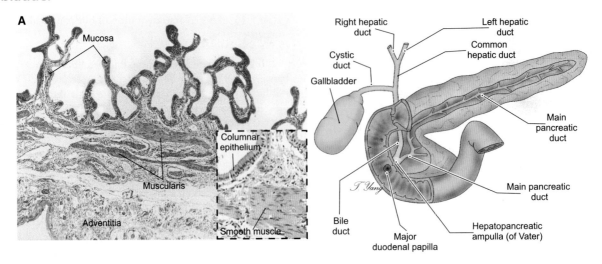

Figure 16-16A. **Gallbladder.** H&E, ×34; inset ×99

The gallbladder is a pear-shaped, saclike organ that stores, concentrates, and releases bile. It connects directly to the cystic duct, which is an extension of the gallbladder. Bile from the right and left hepatic ducts drains into the common hepatic duct, which connects to the cystic duct and enters the gallbladder. The gallbladder releases bile in response to **cholecystokinin**. The gallbladder has a thin wall, which is composed of three layers. (1) The **mucosa** is the innermost layer, lined by simple columnar epithelium, with many microvilli on the apical surfaces and a lamina propria (loose connective tissue) beneath the epithelium. The mucosa has many branching folds. (2) The **muscularis** consists of interlacing longitudinal and obliquely oriented bundles of smooth muscle fibers. The contraction of these muscle fibers helps empty bile through the cystic duct into the bile duct. The **spiral valve of Heister** (smooth muscle at neck of the gallbladder) controls the opening or closing of the gallbladder. The bile duct joins the pancreatic duct at the hepatopancreatic ampulla, and bile enters the duodenum through the major duodenal papilla. (3) The **serosa** is a connective tissue that covers most of the gallbladder. It contains mesothelium and is continuous with the covering of the liver. The **adventitia** attaches the gallbladder to the liver and lacks a mesothelium.

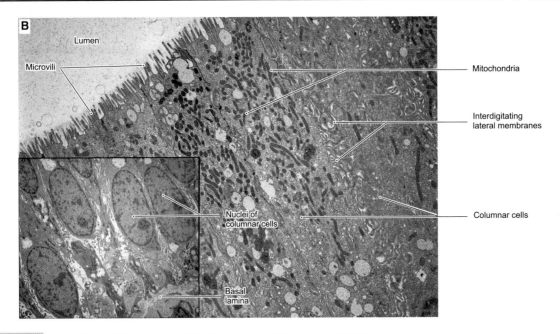

Figure 16-16B. **Epithelial cells lining the gallbladder.** EM, ×5,291; inset ×2,278

There are many short **microvilli** on the apical surfaces of the columnar cells that line the **gallbladder**. Numerous microvilli indicate the function of these cells, which is to absorb water from bile in the lumen and transport it into the interstitial tissue. Concentrating bile is one of the main functions of the gallbladder. The **interdigitating lateral membranes** at the lateral borders of the columnar cells are typical of water-transporting cells. Many **mitochondria** are in the cytoplasm of these cells and are more numerous in the superior region. The *inset* shows the basal region of the epithelium. Oval-shaped nuclei are located close to the basal lamina.

CLINICAL CORRELATIONS

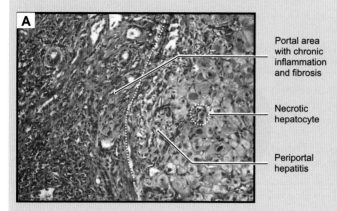

Portal area
with chronic
inflammation
and fibrosis

Necrotic
hepatocyte

Periportal
hepatitis

Figure 16-17A. Hepatitis C. H&E, ×53

Hepatitis C is an infectious liver disease caused by the **hepatitis C virus**, which may result in **chronic hepatitis** and **cirrhosis**. The hepatitis C virus is spread primarily by blood-to-blood contact. Common signs and symptoms may include fatigue, nausea, poor appetite, muscle and joint pains, jaundice, low fever, and tenderness in the liver. In some patients, the disease is self-limiting, but in others it becomes chronic with serious consequences. In the later stages of the disease, **cirrhosis** may ensue with resultant liver failure and ascites. Pathologic changes to the liver include **portal tract expansion** with **lymphocytes**, **portal fibrosis**, **periportal hepatitis**, **steatosis** (fatty change), and **lobular parenchymal inflammation**. In time, fibrosis becomes marked, surrounding nodules of regenerating hepatocytes to produce hepatic cirrhosis. Treatment options include injections of pegylated interferon-α, the antiviral drug ribavirin, and liver transplantation. This image shows a portal area and adjacent hepatocytes with **portal fibrosis** and a lymphocytic inflammatory infiltrate along with **periportal hepatitis** (or **"piecemeal" necrosis**) and scattered necrotic hepatocytes.

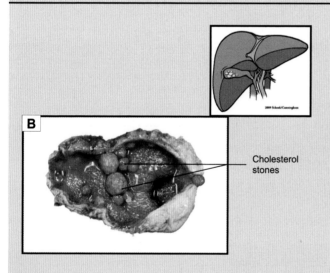

Cholesterol
stones

Figure 16-17B. Gallstones.

Gallstones are a condition in which stones are formed in the gallbladder or in the bile ducts. There are two major types of gallstones: **cholesterol stones** and **pigment stones**. *Cholesterol stones* are far more common than *pigment stones* in Western countries and the United States. Risk factors for gallstones include female gender, obesity, oral contraceptives, and being of Northern European, Mexican American, or Native American descent. Most patients are asymptomatic until stones obstruct the **cystic** or **common bile ducts**, causing severe pain, called **biliary colic**, because of smooth muscle contraction of the duct against the stone. The pain is colicky (wavelike) because of the intermittent nature of the contraction. Gallstones can cause acute or chronic **cholecystitis**, and blockage of the **hepatopancreatic ampulla (ampulla of Vater)** may lead to **acute pancreatitis**. The size of gallstones can range from that of a grain of sand to a golf ball. Cholesterol stones are pale yellow, radiolucent, and large (1–3 cm), whereas pigment stones are black, radiopaque, and smaller (<1 cm). Open surgical or laparoscopic removal of the gallbladder is the most common treatment for gallstones. This gross photograph shows a fresh cholecystectomy specimen containing multiple **cholesterol stones**.

SYNOPSIS 16-2 Pathologic and Clinical Terms for the Digestive Glands and Associated Organs

■ *Sialolithiasis:* The presence of sialoliths, or stones within the ducts of salivary glands; may cause obstruction resulting in inspissated secretions and swelling as well as infection.

■ *Autodigestion:* In reference to acute pancreatitis, the destruction of pancreatic tissues and surrounding adipose tissues by the release of pancreatic enzymes as a result of damage to exocrine pancreas cells.

■ *Saponification:* In reference to acute pancreatitis, the necrosis of adipose tissues by lipolytic pancreatic enzymes released as a result of damage to exocrine pancreas cells; free fatty acids react with calcium to form insoluble salts.

■ *Mallory body:* An intracellular accumulation of intermediate keratin filaments seen in hepatocytes in cases of alcoholic hepatitis.

■ *Periportal hepatitis:* Also called "piecemeal" necrosis in cases of hepatitis; inflammatory process in a portal area transgresses the limiting plate and involves the surrounding hepatocytes causing cell injury and death.

From Histology to Pathology

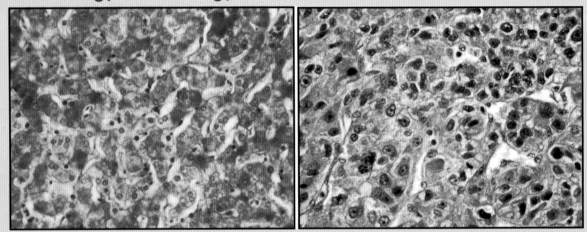

Figure 16-18. Normal liver and hepatocellular carcinoma. H&E, ×400

Normal liver on the *left*. Hepatocellular carcinoma (HCC) of liver on the *right*, also known as hepatoma, is the most common primary malignant neoplasm of the liver. There are many known causes of HCC, but the most common causes are chronic hepatitis B or C infections, alcoholic cirrhosis, toxins, and a form of hepatitis called nonalcoholic steatohepatitis (NASH). In patients with hepatitis, routine monitoring of blood alpha-fetoprotein can provide surveillance for the development of HCC in some patients. HCC may be solitary, multifocal, or diffuse, and invasion of intrahepatic vascular structures is commonplace.

Clinical Vignette Questions

1. A 67-year-old African American man discovered that the white part of his eyes (sclera) had been slowly turning yellow over the last 2 weeks. In addition, he had been experiencing malaise and upper central abdominal pain for about 2 months with an unintended 18-pound weight loss over the last 6 months. The patient's eyes were notably jaundiced, and laboratory evaluation showed elevated bilirubin. The patient was sent for a computed tomography scan, which showed a 3.8-cm mass in the head of the pancreas. A needle biopsy of the pancreas revealed infiltrating ductal adenocarcinoma of the pancreas. Which of the following tumor markers is characteristically elevated in patients with pancreatic adenocarcinoma?

A. Alpha-fetoprotein
B. CA19-9 antigen
C. CA125 antigen
D. Human chorionic gonadotropin
E. Placental alkaline phosphatase

2. A 54-year-old man with a long history of cigarette smoking notices a slowly enlarging, painless mass on the right side of his face anterior to his ear. Over a period of several months, the mass continues to enlarge, and he makes an appointment to see a clinician. Physical examination reveals a somewhat mobile mass in the region of the right parotid gland. Palpation of the mass does not elicit a pain response from the patient. The physician suggests excision of the mass, so the patient is referred to a surgeon. The tumor is removed and sent to pathology, where gross examination reveals a well-circumscribed mass within the parotid gland that appears cystic and exudes a fluid with the consistency and color of used motor oil. Histologically, the mass contains multiple cystic areas of varying sizes set within lymphoid tissue. The cystic areas are lined by an epithelium consisting of two layers of eosinophilic cells, a cuboidal basal layer, and a columnar luminal layer. Based on the clinical presentation and pathologic examination, which of the following is the most likely diagnosis of this lesion?

A. Acinic cell carcinoma
B. Mucoepidermoid carcinoma
C. Pleomorphic adenoma
D. Squamous cell carcinoma
E. Warthin tumor

17 Endocrine System

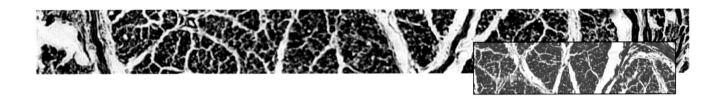

Introduction and Key Concepts for the Endocrine System
Pituitary Gland
Thyroid Gland
Parathyroid Glands
Adrenal Glands
Pineal Gland
Endocrine Pancreas (Islets of Langerhans)

Endocrine Organs and Figures/Images Orientation

Introduction and Key Concepts for the Endocrine System

The **endocrine system** is very closely associated with the nervous system and is much like the **nervous system** in some ways. The *nervous system* sends messages related to sensation, thought, and motor control using electrochemical signals (**action potentials**) that are carried by neurons and axons. The *endocrine system* sends messages to control and regulate the metabolic activity of the body using chemical signals (**hormones**) that are released by endocrine secretory cells and carried by the blood circulatory system. The endocrine system includes (1) **endocrine glands**, such as the pituitary gland, thyroid and parathyroid glands, adrenal glands, and the pineal gland; (2) **clusters of endocrine cells** located in the organs such as **islets of Langerhans** in the pancreas; and (3) **isolated endocrine cells** in certain tissues, such as the **enteroendocrine cells** in the epithelium of the respiratory and digestive tracts (see Chapters 11, "Respiratory System," and 15, "Digestive Tract"). The

endocrine organs that are discussed in this chapter include the pituitary gland, parathyroid glands, adrenal glands, and the endocrine pancreas (islets of Langerhans). Other endocrine organs, such as the testes and ovaries, are discussed in Chapters 18, "Male Reproductive System," and 19, "Female Reproductive System."

Endocrine secretions (hormones) are delivered through the capillary network of the vascular system to the target organs rather than through a series of ducts as in the exocrine system. The timing of hormone release is controlled by the **hypothalamus**. The hypothalamus acts as a command center, controlling the activity of the pituitary gland. The **pituitary gland** functions as a master gland, releasing hormones to control other endocrine glands and organs. The organs or tissues that are activated by released hormones are called **target organs** or **tissues**. The cells in the target organ/tissue have appropriate **receptors**, which are able to recognize and respond to specific hormones.

The hormones can be divided into three classes based on their structure:

1. **Steroid hormones** are lipid hormones that have the characteristic ring structure of steroids (terpenoid lipids) and are formed from cholesterol. Examples of these hormones include estrogen, testosterone, cortisone, and aldosterone.
2. **Peptide hormones** are composed of amino acids and are usually produced by the partial hydrolysis of proteins. The majority of hormones of this type are secreted by the pituitary gland (e.g., adrenocorticotropic hormone [ACTH], thyroid-stimulating hormone [TSH], follicle-stimulating hormone [FSH], prolactin, and growth hormones) and parathyroid glands (parathyroid hormone [PTH], or parathormone).
3. **Amine hormones** are derived from the amino acid **tyrosine**. Examples include triiodothyronine (T_3) and thyroxine (T_4) released by the thyroid and sympathomimetic hormones (adrenaline/epinephrine and noradrenaline/norepinephrine) secreted by the adrenal medulla.

Pituitary Gland

The **pituitary gland** is a neuroendocrine organ located inside the skull and considered a part of the brain. It consists of two divisions: the **adenohypophysis** (anterior lobe) and the **neurohypophysis** (posterior lobe). The pituitary gland produces various types of hormones that act on many target organs, many of which also secrete hormones. Secretion of the pituitary gland is controlled and regulated by **releasing hormone** and **inhibitory hormone** secreted by the hypothalamus or by nervous system signals from the hypothalamic nuclei, including the paraventricular nuclei, the supraoptic nuclei, and the arcuate nuclei. The hypothalamus itself receives signals from many areas of the brain, including the amygdala, hippocampus, brainstem tegmentum, and the infralimbic and cingulate cortices. The hypothalamus maintains body homoeostasis by regulating production of the hypothalamic hormones, which, in turn, control the secretion of the pituitary hormones from the pituitary gland.

ADENOHYPOPHYSIS, also called the **anterior pituitary**, is the anterior division of the gland and is derived from the ectoderm of the roof of the developing oral cavity (**Rathke pouch**). It is composed of glandular tissue. The adenohypophysis can be divided into three regions based on their anatomic positions: the **pars distalis**, **pars tuberalis**, and **pars intermedia**, three classes based on their structure.

1. The **pars distalis** is the main body of the adenohypophysis, containing blood vessels, a capillary network, and two main types of secretory cells supported by a network of reticular connective tissues. These secretory cells are classified as **chromophobes** and **chromophils**. The chromophobes do not effectively take a stain, so they appear clear in the Mallory trichrome stain. These cells are undifferentiated cells but are capable of differentiating into chromophils. The chromophils include **basophils** and **acidophils**.
2. **Basophils** appear blue in Mallory stain and include three subtypes of hormone secretory cells: **corticotrophs, thyrotrophs,** and **gonadotrophs.** Various hormones are produced by these cells, including ACTH, TSH, FSH, and **luteinizing hormone (LH)**. These hormones stimulate various target organs including the cortex of the adrenal glands, the thyroid, the testes, and the ovaries. The secretion of hormones by cells in the adenohypophysis is controlled by

hypothalamic releasing hormones and inhibitory hormones. *Corticotrophs* are stimulated by corticotropin-releasing hormone (CRH) from the hypothalamus. *Thyrotrophs* are stimulated by thyrotropin-releasing hormone. *Gonadotrophs* are stimulated by gonadotropin-releasing hormone.
3. **Acidophils** appear red in Mallory stain and contain two subtypes of hormone secretory cells: **somatotrophs** and **mammotrophs.** *Somatotrophs* secrete somatotropin (growth hormone), which stimulates the liver to produce the **insulin-like growth factor (IGF-1)** that promotes cartilage and bone growth, protein deposition, and cell reproduction. *Mammotrophs* secrete **prolactin,** which increases mammary gland size and promotes milk production.
4. The **pars tuberalis** is the neck of the adenohypophysis; it wraps around the infundibular stalk of the pituitary gland. It contains a rich capillary network and some low columnar basophilic cells that are commonly arranged in cords.
5. The **pars intermedia** is located between the pars distalis and pars nervosa. It contains cuboidal follicular cells and colloid cysts called **Rathke cysts,** which are lined by follicular cells. Rathke cysts are derived from the ectoderm of the dorsal portion of the **Rathke pouch;** these cysts are considered to be the remnants of the Rathke pouch that was present during development. The secretory cells may be involved in producing **melanocyte-stimulating hormone (MSH).** These cells are usually lightly stained by basophilic dye.

NEUROHYPOPHYSIS is derived from the inferior surface of the developing diencephalon. It is considered to be nervous tissue. It can be divided into the **infundibular stalk,** the **median eminence,** and the **pars nervosa.**

1. The **infundibular stalk** connects the median eminence to the pars nervosa.
2. The **median eminence** connects the inferior portion of the hypothalamus to the infundibular stalk of the neurohypophysis. It contains long axons that carry **antidiuretic hormone (ADH)** and **oxytocin hormone** produced by nuclei in the hypothalamus. These axons pass through the median eminence and terminate in the pars nervosa. The median eminence also contains short axons and axon terminal endings from the hypothalamus that release neurosecretory hormones (hypothalamic releasing and inhibiting hormones). These hormones are transported through the hypophyseal portal system from the primary capillary plexus to the secondary capillary plexus, thereby regulating the secretion of the secretory cells in the adenohypophysis.
3. The **pars nervosa** is the main body of the neurohypophysis. It contains a fenestrated capillary plexus, pituicytes (glial cells), and axons and axon terminal endings from neuron cell bodies in the hypothalamus. **Pituicytes** provide support and nutrition to the axons of the neurons. The enlarged axon terminal endings are filled with neurosecretory granules that are called **Herring bodies.** The neurosecretory hormones released in the pars nervosa include **ADH** or **vasopressin, oxytocin hormone,** and **neurophysins.**

Thyroid Gland

The **thyroid gland** has two lobes that are located inferior to the thyroid cartilage and anterior to the trachea. It contains thyroid follicles that produce T_3 and T_4, which regulate body metabolism. The **parafollicular cells** located between the follicles are known as **clear cells (C cells)** and produce **calcitonin** hormone. This hormone is released in response to high blood calcium and inhibits the activity of the osteoclasts. Calcitonin is involved in calcium and phosphorus metabolism. It decreases blood calcium levels and has opposing effects to the parathormone or PTH.

Parathyroid Glands

There are typically four small **parathyroid glands,** most commonly lying posterior to the thyroid gland. They consist of **chief cells** and **oxyphil cells.** Chief cells are hormone-producing cells that secrete **parathormone,** also called **PTH.** PTH is released in response to low blood calcium levels and indirectly promotes the proliferation and activity of osteoclasts, which remove bone. PTH also inhibits the activity of osteoblasts, which help to build up new bone.

PTH indirectly promotes osteoclasts by stimulating osteoblasts to produce **osteoclast differentiation factor,** also known as **RANKL,** which stimulates precursors (monocytes) to differentiate and fuse to become multinuclear osteoclasts. Increased numbers of osteoclasts cause active bone resorption, which results in more Ca++ being released into the blood. PTH also affects the distal tubules of the kidney to increase blood calcium levels by enhancing the reabsorption of calcium from distal tubules.

Adrenal Glands

The **adrenal glands** lie on the superior tips of the kidneys, in the posterior portion of the abdominal cavity. The adrenal glands can be divided into the **cortex** and the **medulla.** The *cortex* has three zones: (moving from external to internal) the **zona glomerulosa, zona fasciculata,** and **zona reticularis.** Cells in the cortex produce various corticosteroid hormones including **mineralocorticoids, glucocorticoids,** and **weak androgens** (see Table 17-1). The *medulla* contains **ganglion neurons** and **chromaffin cells.** The chromaffin cells produce **adrenaline (epinephrine)** and **noradrenaline (norepinephrine).** These hormones are known as **sympathomimetic hormones.**

Pineal Gland

The **pineal gland** is located inside the skull and lies above the superior colliculi of the midbrain. It is considered part of the epithalamus of the brain. It contains **pinealocytes, neuroglial cells,** and calcified structures called **brain sand (corpora arenacea).** The corpora arenacea are derived from the organic matter in the pineal gland and are rich in calcium and phosphate. The pineal gland has a rich blood supply. Pinealocytes, modified neurons that produce **melatonin,** are the predominant cells in the pineal gland. Melatonin is an important hormone in the regulation of the day and night cycle called the **circadian rhythm.**

Endocrine Pancreas (Islets of Langerhans)

There are many **islets of Langerhans** interspersed in the exocrine portion of the pancreas. The islets of Langerhans contain **alpha cells, beta cells, delta cells,** and **pancreatic polypeptide (PP) cells.** These hormone secretory cells produce **glucagon, insulin, somatostatin,** and PP, important hormones in regulating blood glucose levels.

Endocrine Organs and Figures/Images Orientation

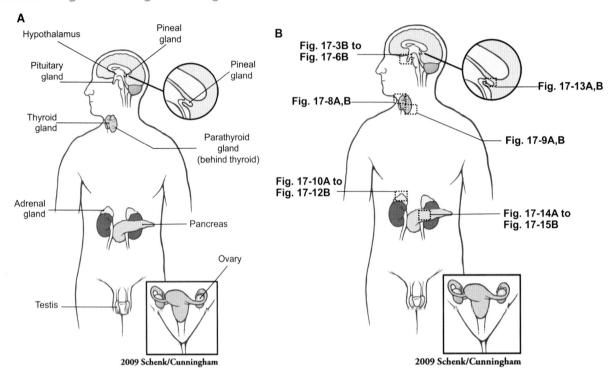

Figure 17-1. Overview and orientation of detailed endocrine organ illustrations.

The illustration on the *left* shows the location of the **endocrine organs**, which include the **pituitary gland, pineal gland, thyroid gland, parathyroid glands, adrenal glands, endocrine pancreas** (islet of Langerhans), **testes** (see Chapter 18, "Male Reproductive System"), and **ovaries** (see Chapter 19, "Female Reproductive System"). The *pituitary* and *pineal glands* are neuroendocrine organs; they are located inside the skull and are considered part of the brain. The *thyroid gland* has two lobes and is located inferior to the thyroid cartilage and anterior to the trachea. There are four *parathyroid glands* located behind (posterior to) the thyroid gland. The *adrenal glands* and *pancreas* are located in the abdominal cavity. The *islet of Langerhans* is the endocrine portion of the pancreas. The *ovaries* and *testes* produce sex-related hormones and also are part of the reproductive system; the details are discussed in Chapters 18 and 19. The illustration on the *right* shows the orientation of detailed endocrine organ illustrations presented in different figures.

Endocrine Organs with Figure Numbers

Pituitary glands
Figure 17-2
Figure 17-3A
Figure 17-3B
Figure 17-3C
Figure 17-4A
Figure 17-4B
Figure 17-5A
Figure 17-5B
Figure 17-6A
Figure 17-6B
Figure 17-7A,B,C

Thyroid glands
Figure 17-8A
Figure 17-8B
Figure 17-8C

Parathyroid glands
Figure 17-9A
Figure 17-9B

Figure 17-9C

Adrenal glands
Figure 17-10A
Figure 17-10B
Figure 17-11A
Figure 17-11B
Figure 17-12A
Figure 17-12B

Pineal glands
Figure 17-13A
Figure 17-13B
Figure 17-13C

Endocrine pancreas (islet of Langerhans)
Figure 17-14A
Figure 17-14B
Figure 17-15A
Figure 17-15B
Figure 17-16

Pituitary Gland

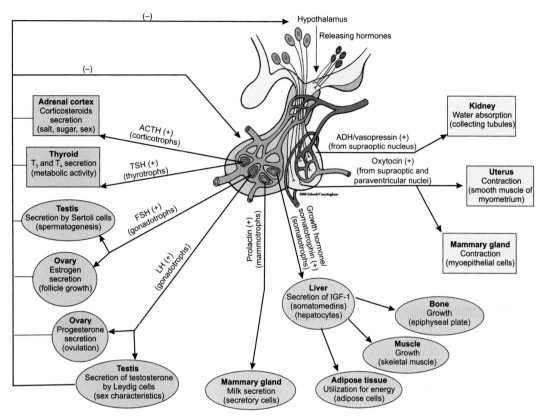

Figure 17-2.   Overview of hormone regulation by the pituitary gland.

The hormones released by the **basophils** in the **adenohypophysis** of the **pituitary gland** include **ACTH, TSH, FSH,** and **LH.** *ACTH* is synthesized by **corticotrophs,** which are stimulated by CRH from the hypothalamus. ACTH is synthesized by **thyrotrophs,** which stimulates the adrenal cortex to produce corticosteroids (glucocorticoids, androgens) and indirectly influences aldosterone. *TSH* is also synthesized by **thyrotrophs;** it stimulates production of T_3 and T_4 by the thyroid. *FSH* and *LH* are secreted by **gonadotrophs;** these hormones promote secondary sex characteristics and stimulate the development of ovarian follicles (ovary) and spermatogonia (testis). The hormones released by **acidophils** include prolactin and growth hormone. Prolactin is secreted by **mammotrophs (lactotrophs)** and stimulates the mammary glands to produce milk. The growth hormone (somatotropin) is secreted by **somatotrophs;** it stimulates the liver to produce **IGF-1,** also known as **somatomedins,** which promotes protein deposition, cell reproduction, and cartilage and bone growth and enhances fat utilization for energy by increasing fatty acids in the bloodstream. The hormones released by the neurohypophysis include **ADH** (or **vasopressin**) and **oxytocin,** which are produced by neurons whose cell bodies lie in the hypothalamus. *ADH* promotes water absorption by collecting tubules and ducts. *Oxytocin* stimulates contraction of smooth muscle fibers in the myometrium of the uterus.

Pituitary Gland

I. **Adenohypophysis (anterior pituitary gland)**
   A. Pars distalis
      1. Chromophobes
      2. Chromophils
         a. *Acidophils*: Somatotrophs (secrete growth hormone), mammotrophs/lactotrophs (secrete prolactin)
         b. *Basophils*: Corticotrophs (secrete ACTH), thyrotrophs (secrete TSH), gonadotrophs (secrete FSH and LH)
   B. Pars tuberalis: Gonadotrophs (secrete FSH and LH)
   C. Pars intermedia
      1. Rathke cysts (colloid-containing cysts)
      2. Basophilic cells/melanotrophs (secrete MSH)

II. **Neurohypophysis (posterior pituitary gland)**
   A. Neural (infundibular) stalk
   B. Median eminence
   C. Pars nervosa
      1. Herring bodies (contain neurosecretory granules)
      2. Neurohypophyseal hormones: ADH (secreted by neurons whose cell bodies are in the supraoptic nucleus), **oxytocin** (secreted by neurons whose cell bodies are in both supraoptic and paraventricular nuclei)

Abbreviations
ACTH: adrenocorticotropic hormone
TSH: thyroid-stimulating hormone
FSH: follicle-stimulating hormone
LH: luteinizing hormone
MSH: melanocyte-stimulating hormone

ANATOMY OF THE PITUITARY GLAND

A

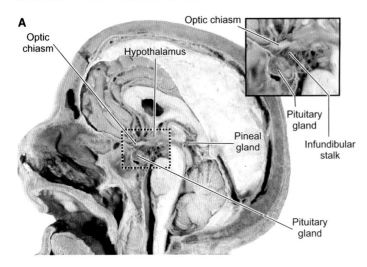

Figure 17-3A. Anatomy of the pituitary gland.

The **pituitary gland** is a small, bean-shaped gland, about 1 cm in diameter, located inferior to the **hypothalamus** and separated from it by the **diaphragma sellae** through which the **infundibular stalk (infundibulum)** passes. The pituitary gland lies within the sella turcica. Various important surrounding structures are visible in the photograph and *inset*. The pituitary gland is located inferior, and slightly caudal, to the **optic chiasm**; this is a particularly important anatomical relationship that is applicable to clinical medicine.

A **pituitary tumor**, as it enlarges, may impinge on the crossing fibers within the optic chiasm, causing visual field deficits. This most commonly results in **bitemporal hemianopia**, a loss of the temporal visual fields of both eyes. Other visual field deficits can also result from pituitary tumors.

B

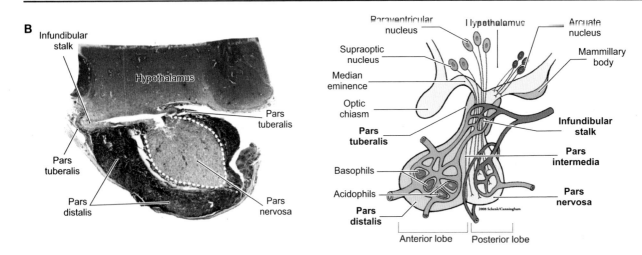

Figure 17-3B. **Pituitary gland.** Mallory trichrome and H&E, ×10

The **pituitary gland** is closely associated with the hypothalamus; it can be divided into two regions based on embryonic origins: the **adenohypophysis (anterior pituitary gland)** and the **neurohypophysis (posterior pituitary gland)**. The adenohypophysis arises from the **ectoderm** of the **Rathke pouch** (roof of the developing oral cavity). It includes the **pars distalis, pars tuberalis,** and **pars intermedia**. The neurohypophysis is differentiated from the neural ectoderm of the inferior surface of the developing diencephalon. It includes the **median eminence, infundibular stalk,** and **pars nervosa** and contains axons whose cell bodies are located in the hypothalamus.

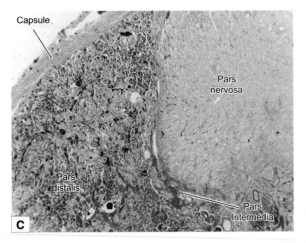

Figure 17-3C. **Pituitary gland.** Mallory trichrome and H&E, ×31

The **adenohypophysis (anterior pituitary gland)** with its connective tissue capsule is shown on the *left* of the microphotograph. It stains red-blue because it contains **chromophils** (acidophils and basophils) and **chromophobes**. The pars nervosa of the **neurohypophysis (posterior pituitary gland)** is nervous tissue; it is shown on the *right*. It contains **axons, pituicytes,** and **capillaries**. It stains much lighter than the adenohypophysis. The cell bodies of these axons are located in the **supraoptic** and **paraventricular nuclei** of the **hypothalamus**. These neurons have long axons that extend from the hypothalamus into the neurohypophysis of the pituitary gland. The axons contain neurosecretory granules consisting of two types of hormones: **oxytocin** (supraoptic and paraventricular nuclei) and **ADH** (supraoptic nucleus). Enlarged axon terminal endings are known as **Herring bodies**.

ADENOHYPOPHYSIS (ANTERIOR PITUITARY)

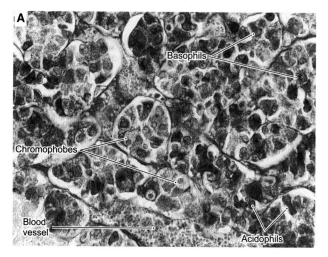

Figure 17-4A. Pars distalis, adenohypophysis (anterior pituitary gland). Mallory trichrome and H&E, ×281

The **pars distalis**, the largest part of the **adenohypophysis**, contains two major types of cells: **chromophobes** and **chromophils**. *Chromophobes* are so named because the cytoplasm does not absorb chromium salt stains, whereas the cytoplasm of *chromophils* does absorb chromium salts. In a Mallory trichrome–stained specimen, the chromophils can be divided into **acidophils** and **basophils** according to the staining (red or blue, respectively) of the granules in the cytoplasm. Overall cell composition is about 50% chromophobes, 15% basophils, and 35% acidophils. Acidophilic granules are characteristic of cells that secrete polypeptide hormones, such as growth hormone (**somatotrophs**) or prolactin (**mammotrophs**), and basophilic granules are characteristic of cells that secrete glycoprotein hormones such as TSH (**thyrotrophs**), LH, and FSH (**gonadotrophs**). **Corticotrophs,** which secrete molecules of the proopiomelanocortin family, also have basophilic granules. In this photomicrograph, chromophobes have pale cytoplasm, basophils have blue-staining granules in their cytoplasm, and acidophils have red-staining granules.

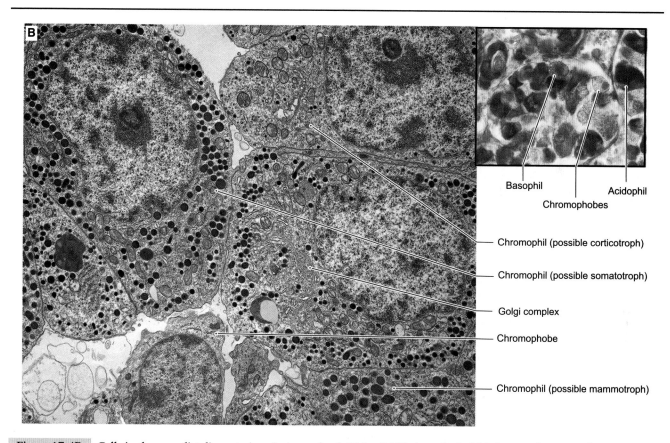

Figure 17-4B.   Cells in the pars distalis, anterior pituitary gland. EM, ×7,700; inset (*color*) Mallory trichrome and H&E, ×423

The five types of hormone-secreting (**chromophil**) cells in the anterior pituitary are most reliably identified by immunocytochemistry using antibodies against the specific hormone or hormones that each cell type secretes. However, an expert can also identify cell types on the basis of the size, density, and distribution of secretory granules in transmission electron micrographs. This image has an apparent **chromophobe** and at least three different types of **chromophils**. Note the differences in the features of the granules in the three chromophils that have been labeled. Note also that the nuclei of the chromophils have **nucleoli** and substantial **euchromatin**, features of cells that are actively synthesizing **polypeptides**. A moderate amount of **rough endoplasmic reticulum (RER)** and prominent **Golgi complexes** can also be seen in the chromophils. The rich capillary bed in the adenohypophysis consists of capillaries that are fenestrated, a feature that allows ready movement of both releasing factors and hormones between the blood plasma and the endocrine cells. The relative proportions of the specific cell types vary significantly according to specific location within the anterior lobe.

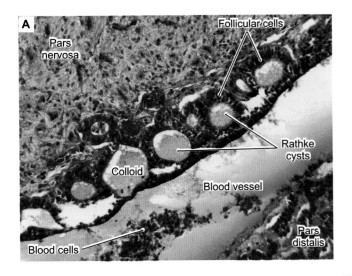

Figure 17-5A. Pars intermedia, anterior pituitary gland. Mallory trichrome and H&E, ×127

The **pars intermedia** originates from the ectoderm of the **Rathke pouch** and is part of the adenohypophysis. This bandlike structure lies between the **pars distalis** and **pars nervosa**. It is of the same embryonic origin as the pars distalis. The pars intermedia contains colloid cysts called **Rathke cysts**, which are lined by cuboidal to columnar follicular cells. These cells are associated with the formation of **MSH** in the fetus. This photomicrograph shows several colloid-filled cysts (Rathke cysts). Most cells in the pars intermedia resemble **basophilic cells** (**melanotrophs**). A blood vessel separates the pars intermedia and the pars distalis.

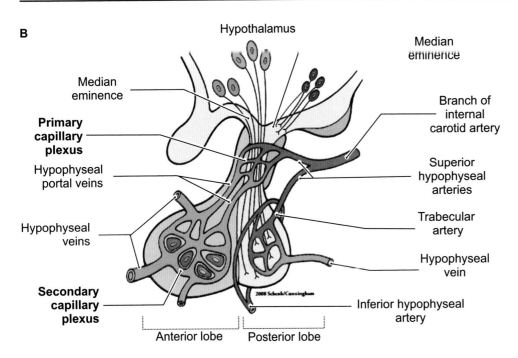

Figure 17-5B. Blood supply of the pituitary gland.

The **superior hypophyseal arteries**, which arise from the internal carotid artery and posterior communicating artery of the circle of Willis, supply the pars tuberalis, the infundibular (neural) stalk, and the median eminence. The *darker shaded area* indicates the **primary capillary plexus**, which receives blood from the superior hypophyseal arteries, drains blood into the hypophyseal portal veins supplying the **secondary capillary plexus** (*white shaded area*), and, finally, drains into the hypophyseal veins. Both primary and secondary capillary plexuses contain fenestrated capillaries. The portal blood circulation (from primary to secondary capillary plexuses) carries neurosecretory hormones from the median eminence into the pars distalis where they stimulate or inhibit basophils and acidophils to produce hormones. The pars nervosa receives blood mainly from the **inferior hypophyseal arteries**, which arise from the internal carotid artery. This artery also receives blood from the trabecular artery, which arises from the superior hypophyseal artery. The hormones released by **Herring bodies** enter the blood circulation through the capillary plexuses of the inferior hypophyseal and trabecular arteries.

NEUROHYPOPHYSIS (POSTERIOR PITUITARY GLAND)

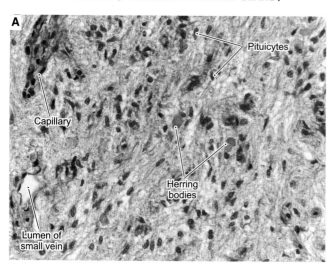

Figure 17-6A. **Pars nervosa, neurohypophysis (posterior pituitary gland).** Masson trichrome stain, ×281

The **neurohypophysis** is an outgrowth of the diencephalon and includes the **median eminence**, the **infundibular stalk**, and the **pars nervosa**. The median eminence is the termination site of short axons carrying factors from the arcuate nuclei that regulate activity of cells in the **adenohypophysis**. Long axons from the **supraoptic** and **paraventricular nuclei** of the hypothalamus pass through the **infundibular stalk** and terminate in the pars nervosa. The **pars nervosa** contains **unmyelinated axons, axon terminals, pituicytes,** and **capillaries.** Precursors of hormones (**ADH/vasopressin** and **oxytocin**) and carrier proteins (**neurophysins**) are synthesized in the cell bodies of neurons in the two hypothalamic nuclei and are transported through the axons in the infundibular stalk to the axon terminal endings in the pars nervosa, where processing is completed and secretion occurs adjacent to fenestrated capillaries. **Herring bodies** are large dilated axon terminal endings that are filled with accumulated neurosecretory granules. **Pituicytes** are glial cells that provide support and nutrition to the axons of the neurons.

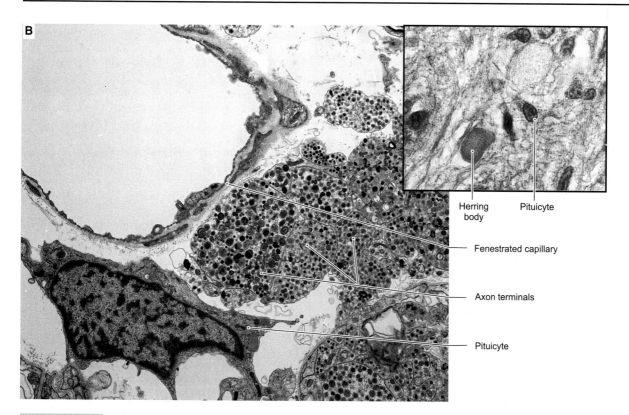

Figure 17-6B. **Pars nervosa, posterior pituitary gland.** EM, ×30,000; inset (*color*) Masson trichrome stain, ×791

Major components of the **posterior lobe** can be seen in this electron micrograph. **Terminals** of hormone secreting neurons are seen as vesicle-filled, membrane-bounded profiles of widely varying shapes and sizes. The largest, most distended profiles appear as **Herring bodies** in ordinary sections for light microscopy. The vesicles have been transported in **unmyelinated axons** to this site from the **supraoptic** and **paraventricular nuclei** of the **hypothalamus**, where they were constructed in the cell bodies of the neurons. **ADH** or **oxytocin** is released when action potentials are conducted from the hypothalamus in response to neural signals acting on the cell bodies and dendrites in the hypothalamus. The two secreted hormones have only a short distance to diffuse to reach the wall of a **fenestrated capillary**. There are no neuronal cell bodies in the posterior lobe, so any nuclei seen in the posterior lobe most likely will belong either to endothelial cells of capillaries or to **pituicytes**, as is the case with the nucleus in this view. Like astrocytes in other parts of the central nervous system, pituicytes have processes that contact nerve processes and the walls of capillaries.

CLINICAL CORRELATIONS

Prolactinoma—H&E

Normal

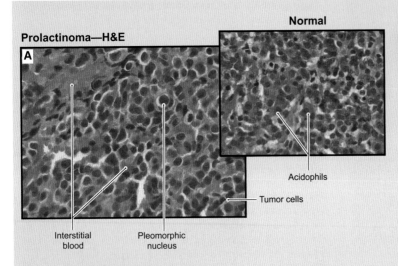

A

Interstitial blood

Pleomorphic nucleus

Acidophils

Tumor cells

Prolactinoma—immunocytochemistry

Normal

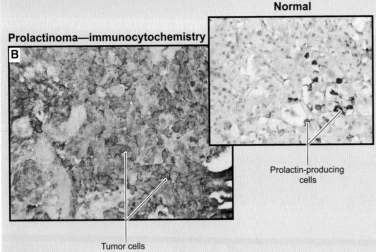

B

Tumor cells

Prolactin-producing cells

Figure 17-7A,B. Pituitary Adenoma. **A:** H&E, (*left*) ×213; (*right*) ×154. **B:** Immunocytochemistry, (*left*) ×213; (*right*) ×154

Pituitary adenomas are benign tumors of the anterior pituitary gland. Clinically, they can be divided into nonsecreting and secreting forms. Historically, adenomas were classified by their staining properties, the degree to which they took up the stains hematoxylin and eosin. They were classified as **basophilic, acidophilic,** or **chromophobic adenomas.** With modern immunocytochemical techniques, however, tumor cells can be classified by the type of hormone they produce. Some cells do not mark with any antibody, and their tumors are called **null-cell adenomas.** Pituitary tumors may compress the hypothalamus, cranial nerves, or the optic chiasm. A **bitemporal hemianopia** is commonly seen in patients suffering from compression of the optic nerve. Mutations are believed to play a role in the development of the tumors. Pathologically, the tumors are composed of uniform, polygonal cells arrayed in sheets or cords. They lack a reticular network of supporting connective tissue and show **monomorphism.** Treatment includes drug therapy and surgery, depending on the type and the size of the tumors. **A:** The **prolactinoma** lacks acidophils and has tumor cells with **pleomorphic nuclei** (variable size nuclei). The normal tissue of the pars distalis of the pituitary gland shows individual or clusters of acidophils interspersed among basophils and chromophobes (*right*). **B:** The cell membranes of **prolactin-producing tumor cells** have been stained brown using an immunocytochemical reaction. The majority of the cells in this sample are tumor cells. By contrast, in the normal tissue sample shown on the *right*, only a small number of prolactin-producing cells are stained.

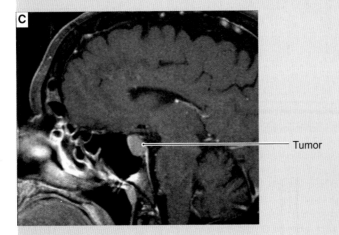

C

Tumor

Figure 17-7C. Pituitary Adenoma in Magnetic Resonance Imaging.

Pituitary tumors, called **adenomas,** can be classified according to their size, secretory status, histology, and general clinical picture of the patient. Regarding size, they can be **microadenomas,** which are less than 1 cm in size (about 50% of all tumors at diagnosis) and may be difficult to remove, and **macroadenomas,** which are greater than 1.0 cm in diameter, and may cause deficits related to hormone imbalance or compression of adjacent structures. Classification by secretory status may reflect, for example, excess **cortisol (Cushing disease)** or **prolactin (prolactinoma)** or the overproduction of **growth hormone (gigantism** or **acromegaly).** The MRI may reflect damage to the hypothalamus; the optic chiasm, nerve, or tracts; or increased intracranial pressure. Histologic classification relies on demonstrating particular abnormal cell types in biopsy samples.

Thyroid Gland

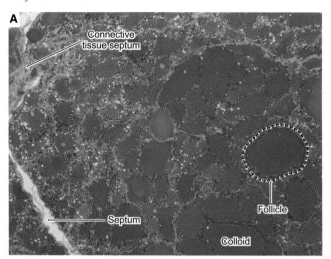

Figure 17-8A. Thyroid follicles, thyroid gland. H&E, ×70

The **thyroid gland** is derived from the developing endoderm of the foramen cecum of the tongue; it has two lobes and is one of the largest endocrine glands. Connective tissue **septa** divide the thyroid gland into lobules. Each lobule consists of numerous **thyroid follicles**. The thyroid follicles are the main functional components of the gland; they synthesize and release T_3 and T_4. Each follicle is filled with **colloid**, which is a gelatinous substance containing the stored form of T_3 and T_4. The follicular cells are usually simple cuboidal cells but may change to simple squamous (inactive) or columnar cells (active) depending on their states of secretion.

The thyroid hormones play an important role in regulating the basal metabolic activity of the body. **Iodine** is required for formation of thyroxine; **iodine deficiency** can lead to the development of **thyroid goiters (nodules)**.

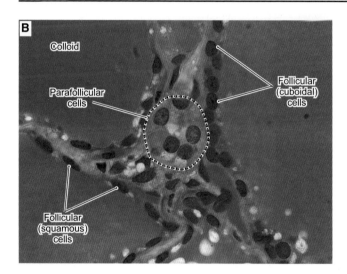

Figure 17-8B. Parafollicular cells, thyroid gland. H&E, ×702

Another type of endocrine cell located between the follicles of the thyroid gland is called a **parafollicular cell**. These cells are also called **clear cells** or **C cells** and are commonly located within the interstitial connective tissue septa. Parafollicular cells produce **calcitonin**, which inhibits osteoclasts from resorbing bone tissue, thereby decreasing blood calcium levels. High blood calcium levels stimulate parafollicular cells to secrete calcitonin. Parafollicular cells are relatively large cells with round nuclei and pale cytoplasm. They can be found scattered beneath the follicular cells or in small groups in the interstitial connective tissue between the follicles, as shown here.

Graves disease is an example of **hyperthyroidism** in which excessive amounts of thyroid hormones are secreted by follicular cells. In **hypothyroidism**, thyroid glands produce abnormally low levels of thyroid hormones, such as in **Hashimoto thyroiditis**.

CLINICAL CORRELATION

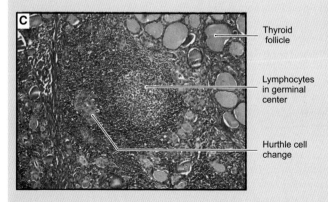

Figure 17-8C. Hashimoto Thyroiditis. H&E, ×55

Hashimoto thyroiditis is a chronic autoimmune disease, characterized by enlargement of the thyroid gland (**goiter**) and gradual failure of thyroid function. Hashimoto thyroiditis is the most common cause of hypothyroidism in the United States and primarily affects women. Autoantibodies against thyroid antigens, genetic susceptibility, and environmental factors are believed to play a role in the development of the disease. The signs and symptoms related to hypothyroidism include fatigue, increased sensitivity to cold, pale skin, constipation, muscle pain and weakness, and weight gain. Histologically, infiltrating lymphocytes form lymphoid follicles (lymphatic nodules) with germinal centers within the thyroid parenchyma. Some thyroid follicle cells show **Hurthle cell** change with abundant eosinophilic cytoplasm. Thyroid hormone replacement therapy is the treatment for the disease. Surgery may be indicated if enlargement of the thyroid gland causes compression of the airway.

Parathyroid Glands

A

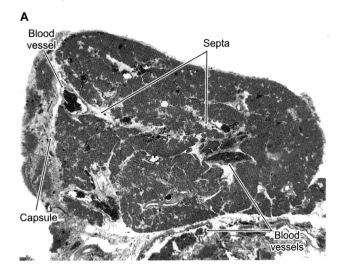

Blood vessel
Septa
Capsule
Blood vessels

Figure 17-9A. Overview of the parathyroid glands. H&E, ×37

The four small **parathyroid glands** typically lie on the posterior surface of the thyroid gland and are separated from the thyroid gland by a connective tissue capsule. Connective tissue septa with blood vessels divide each parathyroid gland into many incomplete lobules. The parathyroid glands are derived from the endoderm of pharyngeal pouch 3 (the inferior parathyroid glands) and pouch 4 (the superior parathyroid glands). There are two types of cells in the parathyroid glands: **chief cells** and **oxyphil cells**. Adipocytes are commonly found in the parathyroid glands in older individuals.

B

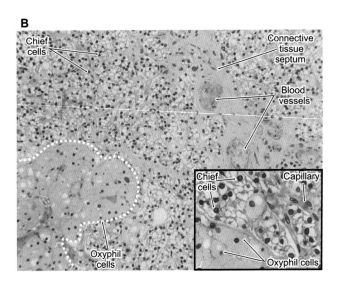

Chief cells
Connective tissue septum
Blood vessels
Chief cells
Capillary
Oxyphil cells
Oxyphil cells

Figure 17-9B. Chief cells and oxyphil cells of the parathyroid glands. H&E, ×139; inset ×296

The **chief cells** are smaller and more numerous than the **oxyphil cells**. They are distributed throughout the glands and are the principal cells in the parathyroid glands. Each *chief cell* has a large round nucleus with a small amount of clear cytoplasm. These chief cells produce **PTH**, also called **parathormone**, which is secreted in response to low blood calcium levels. PTH indirectly promotes osteoclast proliferation and increases their activity of absorption of bone tissue to increase blood calcium levels. The *oxyphil cells* are large cells with acidophilic (pink) cytoplasm as shown here. Each cell has a small nucleus and a large amount of cytoplasm containing numerous mitochondria. The oxyphil cells are often arranged in clusters; individual cells can also be found scattered among the chief cells. The oxyphil cells appear at puberty, and their numbers increase with age. Their functions are unclear.

CLINICAL CORRELATION

C

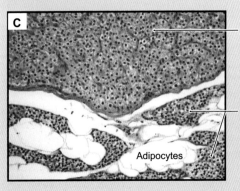

Adenoma composed of chief cells
Normal parathyroid gland with adipose tissue
Adipocytes

Figure 17-9C. Parathyroid Adenoma. H&E, ×96

Parathyroid adenomas are benign **neoplasms** of the parathyroid gland representing the most common cause of **primary hyperparathyroidism**, in which autonomous overproduction of parathyroid hormone occurs. The increased parathyroid hormone results in elevated blood calcium (**hypercalcemia**), which may cause constipation, kidney stones, neuropsychiatric issues, and bone diseases such as **osteitis fibrosa cystica**. The majority of cases are asymptomatic, discovered incidentally when hypercalcemia is detected on routine blood tests. Most cases are sporadic, but some cases may be related to inherited conditions like **multiple endocrine neoplasia** (MEN1 and MEN2). Parathyroid adenomas are usually solitary, whereas parathyroid hyperplasia tends to affect all four glands. Grossly, these adenomas are well circumscribed with a red-to-brown cut surface. Histologically, an adenoma is enveloped with a capsule, is usually composed of **monomorphic chief cells**, and tends to compress the surrounding normal parathyroid tissue. Definitive treatment is surgical removal of the parathyroid gland containing the adenoma.

Adrenal Glands (Suprarenal Glands)

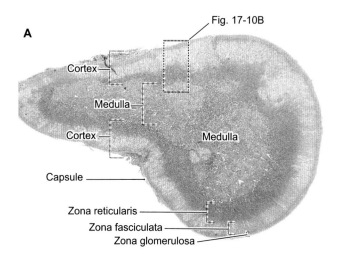

A

Fig. 17-10B

Cortex

Medulla

Cortex

Medulla

Capsule

Zona reticularis

Zona fasciculata

Zona glomerulosa

Figure 17-10A. Overview of the adrenal glands. H&E, ×7

An **adrenal gland** covers the apical region of each kidney. It is also called the **suprarenal gland**. Each adrenal gland is covered by a connective tissue **capsule** and has a **cortex** and a **medulla**. The *cortex* of the adrenal gland is derived from the **mesoderm** and can be divided into three zones: the **zona glomerulosa, zona fasciculata**, and **zona reticularis**. Hormone-producing cells in the cortex secrete several types of hormones: **mineralocorticoids, glucocorticoids**, and **weak androgens**. The *medulla* of the adrenal gland is derived from the **neural crest** and contains cell bodies of **sympathetic ganglion neurons** and their axons as well as **chromaffin cells**, which synthesize and release **adrenaline (epinephrine)** and **noradrenaline (norepinephrine)**.

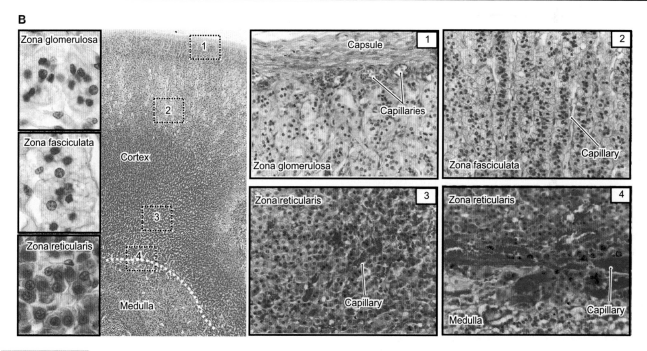

B

Figure 17-10B. Cortex of the adrenal gland. H&E, left ×41, left (*insets*) ×466; right (*4 panels*) ×163

The **cortex** of the adrenal gland contains many glandular cells. These cells are arranged in cords, which are formed by hormone secretory cells. The capillaries run parallel to these cords. (1) The **zona glomerulosa** lies beneath the connective capsule and consists of secretory cells that contain lipid droplets (**vacuoles**) and a pale-staining cytoplasm. These cells are arranged in round or ovoid clusters (like glomeruli); they secrete **mineralocorticoids**, mainly **aldosterone**, which control the electrolyte balance by acting on the distal tubules of the kidney to increase Na^+ and decrease K^+ absorption. (2) The **zona fasciculata** contains hormone-secreting cells that secrete **glucocorticoids** (mainly **cortisol** and **corticosterone**). The glucocorticoids stimulate glycogen synthesis in the liver; increase carbohydrate, fat, and protein metabolism; and suppress the immune response by slowing down immune cell (**lymphocyte**) circulation. ACTH stimulates the production of glucocorticoids. The cells in the zona fasciculata contain many lipid droplets, which make the cytoplasm appear light and vacuolated. These cells are arranged in long cords in which cell nuclei are packed close to one another with their pale-stained cytoplasm facing the capillaries. (3) The **zona reticularis** is adjacent to the medulla. Its secretory cells contain only a few lipid droplets, and their cytoplasm is stained dark and acidophilic in appearance. The cells are arranged in anastomosing cords, which are intermixed with by surrounding capillaries. These secretory cells secrete **androgens** (mainly dehydroepiandrosterone), which can be converted into testosterone or estrogen. ACTH also stimulates the secretion of the adrenal androgens. (4) The **junction** between the **zona reticularis** and the **medulla** is shown here. There are many blood vessels separating the zona reticularis of the cortex and the medulla. The cells in the medulla are stained lighter than the cells in the zona reticularis. The *left insets* show a high-power view of hormone secreting cells in the zona glomerulosa, zona fasciculata, and zona reticularis of the adrenal gland cortex. The *right panels* show regions of the adrenal gland that are indicated by the *dashed boxes*.

ADRENAL CORTEX

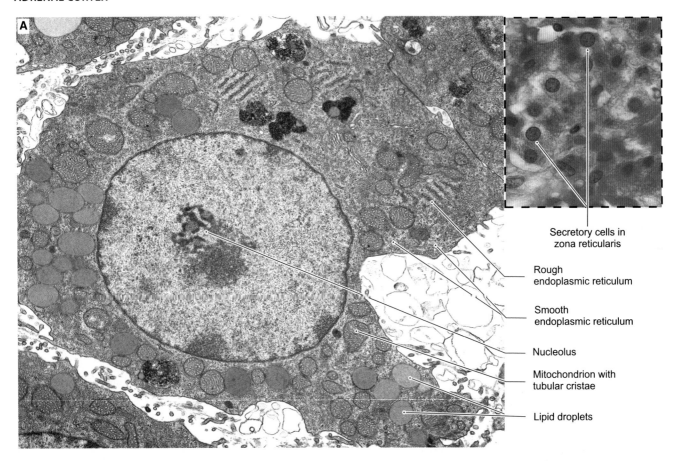

Secretory cells in
zona reticularis

Rough
endoplasmic reticulum

Smooth
endoplasmic reticulum

Nucleolus

Mitochondrion with
tubular cristae

Lipid droplets

Figure 17-11A. Adrenal cortical cells, adrenal cortex. EM, ×11,500; inset (*color*) H&E, ×680

Cells of the adrenal cortex have features common to all cells that synthesize and secrete steroid hormones. The three most prominent components of the cytoplasm are an abundance of **smooth endoplasmic reticulum (SER), mitochondria** that have peculiar **tubular cristae,** and **lipid droplets. Cholesterol,** the precursor of steroid hormones, is stored as esters in the lipid droplets. Enzymes necessary for synthesis of steroid hormones are located in the SER and in the inner mitochondrial membrane, so hormone production is a cooperative function of these two organelles. Although proteins are not secreted by these cells, protein synthesis is required to maintain structure and function. This is reflected by the prominent nucleolus and by the patches of RER.

CLINICAL CORRELATION

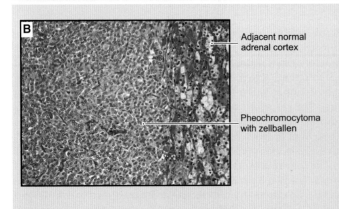

Adjacent normal
adrenal cortex

Pheochromocytoma
with zellballen

Figure 17-11B. Pheochromocytoma. H&E, ×96

Pheochromocytomas are **neoplasms** of the adrenal medulla characterized by the production of **catecholamines,** such as **epinephrine** and **norepinephrine,** which cause significant hypertension, often episodic, in affected patients. Most pheochromocytomas are sporadic, but about 10% are associated with familial syndromes such as **MEN (types 2A** and **2B),** and **von Hippel-Lindau.** Some pheochromocytomas are bilateral, and although most occur in adults, about 10% occur in children. Grossly, most of these tumors are well circumscribed and range in size from a few grams to kilograms. Microscopically, pheochromocytomas can have a diverse appearance, from spindle cells to large, bizarre cells. The cells are often arranged in nests, or cell packets called **zellballen.** Histologic features alone do not reliably separate benign tumors from malignant ones; therefore, the demonstration of metastases is necessary to ascertain malignancy. Definitive treatment is surgical removal of the tumor.

ADRENAL MEDULLA

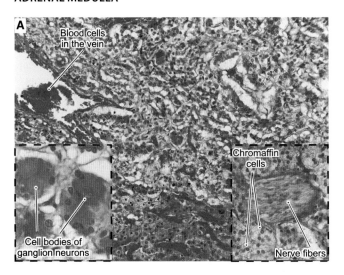

A
Blood cells in the vein

Cell bodies of ganglion neurons

Chromaffin cells

Nerve fibers

Figure 17-12A. Adrenal medulla. H&E, ×140; inset (*left*) ×340; inset (*right*) ×158

The **adrenal medulla** is derived from the neural crest; its embryonic origin is different from that of the adrenal cortex. The cells in the adrenal medulla include **chromaffin cells** and **ganglion neurons**. Large blood vessels (**veins**) are found in the medulla; these vessels drain blood out of the adrenal gland. Chromaffin cells are irregularly shaped neuroendocrine cells and are the predominant cells in the adrenal medulla. These cells have round nuclei with pale-staining cytoplasm as shown here. They have numerous plasma secretory granules that stain intensively with chromium salts; therefore, they are called **chromaffin cells**. These cells secrete the **sympathomimetic** hormones **adrenaline (epinephrine)** and **noradrenaline (norepinephrine)** in response to stress. The sympathetic ganglion neurons have large cell bodies that are surrounded by supporting cells as shown in the *left inset*. The adrenal medulla is innervated by sympathetic preganglionic nerves.

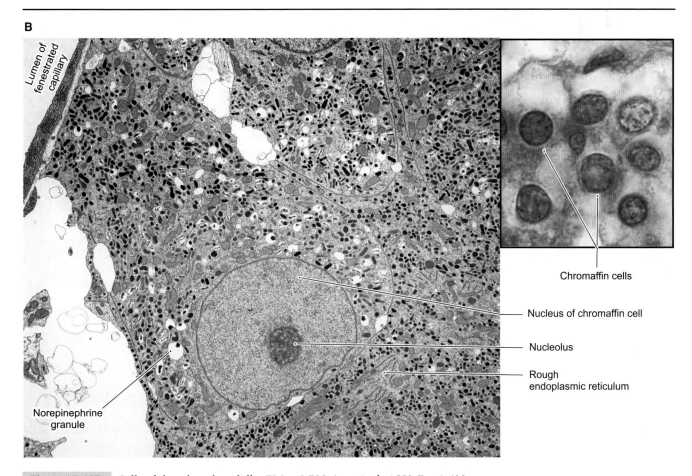

B
Lumen of fenestrated capillary

Chromaffin cells

Nucleus of chromaffin cell

Nucleolus

Rough endoplasmic reticulum

Norepinephrine granule

Figure 17-12B. Cells of the adrenal medulla. EM, ×5,700; inset (*color*) H&E, ×1,632

Cells of the adrenal medulla synthesize and secrete **adrenaline (epinephrine)** and **noradrenaline (norepinephrine)**, with adrenaline being the main product. These **catecholamines** are both synthesized from the amino acid **tyrosine** through a series of reactions that occur in the **cytosol** and within the granules in the cytoplasm. The generation of the granules, along with the enzymes, packaging proteins, and membrane proteins, involves the RER and **Golgi complex**, so these cells have equipment similar to a protein-synthesizing cell, although their product is not a protein. The granules vary greatly in size and appearance, a reflection partly of the current state of activity (synthesis, storage) and partly of the catecholamine (epinephrine, norepinephrine) stored in the granule. The granules that store norepinephrine (noradrenaline) are the large electron-lucent profiles containing a small electron-dense particle at the edge of the cavity. Like the cells of the cortex, the cells of the adrenal medulla are closely associated with the walls of fenestrated capillaries. However, the edge of the vessel in the *upper left corner* of this view does not show the fenestrations.

Pineal Gland

A

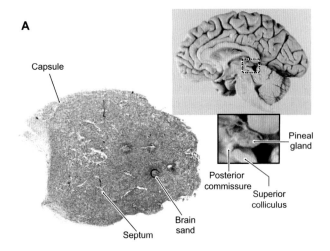

Capsule

Pineal gland

Posterior commissure

Superior colliculus

Brain sand

Septum

Figure 17-13A. Overview of the pineal gland. H&E, ×5

The **pineal gland** is a pinecone-shaped neuroendocrine gland about 8 mm in length that produces **melatonin** and is covered by a capsule of pia mater. The pineal gland is part of the epithalamus (a diencephalic structure) that extends caudally from its attachment immediately superior to the posterior commissure into the superior (quadrigeminal) cistern. It is superior to the colliculi of the midbrain. Secretion of melatonin is stimulated by darkness and inhibited by light. The level of this hormone increases during sleep. Connective septa divide the pineal into poorly defined lobules. This gland contains **pinealocytes, neuroglial cells,** and **blood vessels.** Calcified concretions called **brain sand** (also called **corpora arenacea**) may also be present in the pineal gland, especially in older patients.

The **calcifications (brain sand)** within the pineal gland increase with age. These calcifications appear white in computed tomography scan and magnetic resonance imaging and are commonly used as a natural landmark by radiologists and neurologists.

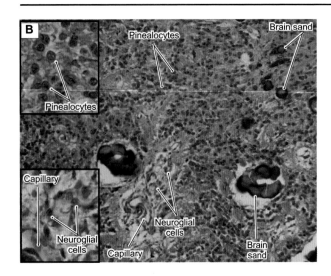

B

Brain sand

Pinealocytes

Pinealocytes

Capillary

Neuroglial cells

Neuroglial cells

Capillary

Brain sand

Figure 17-13B. Pinealocytes and brain sand of the pineal gland. H&E, ×140; insets ×363

The **pineal gland** is composed of two types of cells: **pinealocytes** and **neuroglial cells.** The *pinealocytes* are modified neurons, which have round or ovoid nuclei with pale-stained cytoplasm containing granules filled with **melatonin.** The pinealocytes synthesize **melatonin,** which is important in the regulation of the **circadian rhythms** (day and night cycles). The pinealocytes are larger than the neuroglial cells and have a long cytoplasmic process that extends to the capillaries; their secretory granules are released into the capillaries. The *neuroglial cells* are supportive cells with small, dark nuclei. They are also called **pineal astrocytes** and are commonly found near the capillaries. The particles of brain sand assume various sizes as shown here; their function is not known. Other functions of the pineal gland may relate to promoting sleep and sexual development; enhancing mood and slowing the aging process; and, possibly, inhibiting the growth of some tumors.

CLINICAL CORRELATION

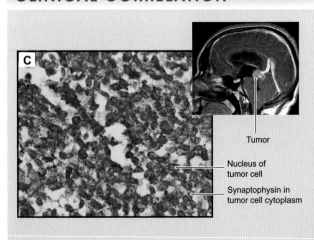

C

Tumor

Nucleus of tumor cell

Synaptophysin in tumor cell cytoplasm

Figure 17-13C. Pineoblastoma. Immunohistochemical preparation for synaptophysin, ×198

Pineoblastoma is an aggressive malignant tumor in children, which arises in the pineal gland. Because it commonly consists of cellular sheets that lack an architectural pattern, it is described as a **small blue cell tumor.** The term **embryonal** is also used to emphasize the rudimentary developmental stage of the tumor, although in some tumors the cells begin to show differentiation into neurons, or glial cells, or even rods and cones. The earliest stages of such specialization may be detectable before any architectural alteration. **Synaptophysin** is a protein associated with synapses. An antibody to this marker protein, conjugated to the enzyme peroxidase, creates a colored metabolite wherever synaptophysin appears in cell cytoplasm or membranes. In the image on the *left*, a brown compound marks the **tumor cells** that contain synaptophysin. Tumor treatments can be individually formulated based on the different cellular components.

Endocrine Pancreas

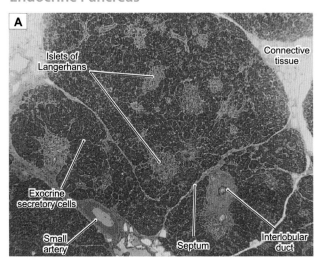

Figure 17-14A. Islets of Langerhans, endocrine pancreas. H&E, ×39

The pancreas has **endocrine** and **exocrine** components. The *endocrine* component consists of the **islets of Langerhans**, which are clusters of endocrine cells within a capillary network. There are numerous pale-staining islets of Langerhans scattered throughout the pancreas, and each of them is surrounded by an eosinophilic *exocrine* component of the pancreas as shown here. A connective tissue septum divides the pancreas into lobules. Two interlobular ducts, surrounded by the connective tissue, belong to the exocrine pancreas, from which they carry secretions. The endocrine pancreas does not have ducts; the hormones (**insulin** and **glucagon**) secreted by the islets of Langerhans are released into the capillaries and from there into the blood circulation. Insulin and glucagons play important roles in regulating blood glucose levels. Insulin stimulates glucose entry in many cells, thereby regulating carbohydrate metabolism and lowering blood glucose levels. Glucagon enhances the synthesis and release of glucose from the liver into the blood, thus increasing blood glucose levels.

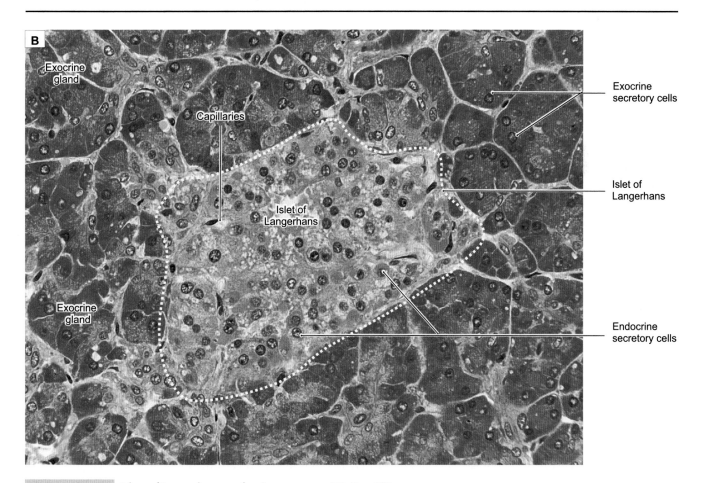

Figure 17-14B. Islets of Langerhans, endocrine pancreas. H&E, ×462

There are four types of endocrine cells in the **islets of Langerhans: alpha cells, beta cells, delta cells,** and **PP cells.** It is difficult to distinguish among them in H&E stain. However, the beta cells are usually distributed throughout the islets; the other three types of cells are commonly found at the periphery of the islets. *Alpha cells* secrete **glucagon**, *beta cells* secrete **insulin**, *delta cells* secrete **somatostatin** and **gastrin**, and *PP cells* secrete **pancreatic polypeptide**. Secretion of *insulin* occurs in response to high blood glucose levels; secretion of *glucagon* occurs in response to lower blood glucose levels.

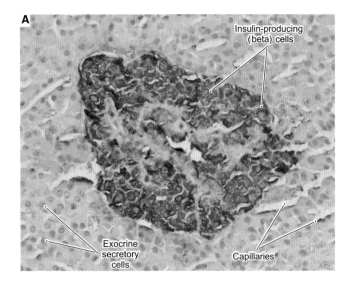

Figure 17-15A. Pancreatic islet cells, islets of Langerhans. Immunocytochemistry stain, ×189

This is an example of an **islet of Langerhans** prepared with a special immunocytochemistry stain for insulin. Cells with brown color are **insulin-producing cells** and are the predominant cells in the islets of Langerhans. Insulin-producing cells, also called **beta cells**, are distributed throughout the pancreatic islets. The background counterstain is hematoxylin, which makes the endocrine pancreatic cells appear light blue with darker blue–stained nuclei.

Type 1 diabetes mellitus is the most common type of diabetes in childhood and adolescence (65% of total cases). It is characterized by insulin deficiency and sudden onset of severe **hyperglycemia, diabetic ketoacidosis**, and death if patients are left without insulin treatment. Symptoms also include **polyuria, polydipsia, lethargy**, and **weight loss**. The major cause of the disease is autoimmune destruction of the insulin-secreting beta cells in the islets of Langerhans by T cells and humoral mediators (tumor necrosis factor, interleukin-1, nitric oxide). Treatment options depend largely on patient and physician preferences and include baseline doses of insulin plus adjustable premeal doses of short-acting insulin or rapid-acting insulin analogs.

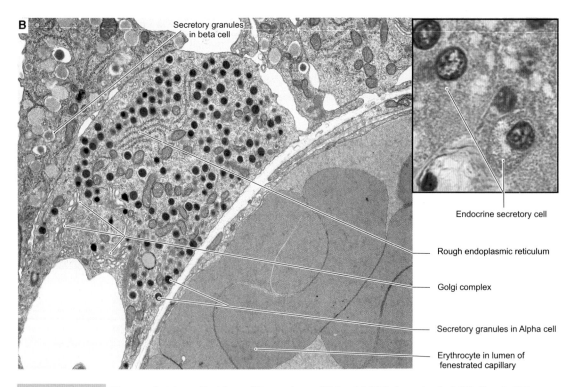

Figure 17-15B. Pancreatic islet cells, islets of Langerhans. EM, ×13,000; inset *(color)* H&E, ×1,632

Pancreatic islet cells, like other types of endocrine cells, are closely associated with **fenestrated** or **sinusoidal capillaries**. The granules of each of the four main types of cells have slightly different characteristic appearances in electron micrographs. Profiles of two different cells are visible in this view. The cell adjacent to the wall of the capillary appears to be an **alpha (glucagon-secreting) cell** with small-to-medium granules that have an electron-dense core with a very narrow electron-lucent surround. The profile in the *upper left* appears to belong to a **beta (insulin-secreting) cell** with larger granules, a less dense core, and a wide lucent area surrounding the core. The nuclei of the cells are not present in this view, but note that the cytoplasm of the alpha cell exhibits typical features of a polypeptide synthesizing and secreting cell. Both RER and a large **Golgi complex** are readily apparent.

CLINICAL CORRELATION

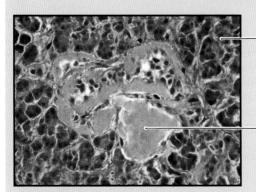

Exocrine pancreas

Amyloid replacing islet of Langerhans

Figure 17-16. **Type 2 Diabetes Mellitus.** H&E, ×195

Type 2 diabetes mellitus is characterized by **hyperglycemia** with normal or elevated **insulin** levels, in contrast to **type 1 diabetes** in which hyperglycemia is associated with little or no insulin production. In type 2 diabetes, insulin is present, but insulin-sensitive tissues, such as skeletal muscle and adipose tissues, manifest resistance to the action of insulin. Defects in **beta cell** function also contribute to the disease process. Type 2 diabetes generally has an insidious onset and typically affects adults. Risk factors include genetic factors and a strong association with obesity. Approximately 85% of type 2 diabetes is associated with obesity. Clinically, patients present primarily with **polyuria** and **polydipsia** due to the hyperglycemia. Chronic hyperglycemia leads to accelerated atherosclerosis and small vessel damage, which affects the eyes (**retinopathy**), kidneys (**nephropathy**), and nerves (**neuropathy**). Early in the disease, the islets of Langerhans become hyperplastic in order to produce more insulin. Later in the disease, the islets become atrophic with **amyloid** deposition. Treatment includes diet modification and exercise to induce weight loss and the use of oral hypoglycemic medications. Some patients may require insulin late in the disease process because of progressive loss of beta cells.

SYNOPSIS 17-1 Pathologic Terms for the Endocrine System

- *Bitemporal hemianopia*: A visual field deficit characterized by loss of both temporal visual fields, most often due to compression of the optic chiasm by a pituitary tumor or cyst.
- *Goiter*: A general term for enlargement of the thyroid gland; common causes include benign multinodular goiter, diffuse toxic goiter, and thyroiditis.
- *Osteitis fibrosa cystica*: A cystic bone lesion seen in patients with hyperparathyroidism due to increased osteoclast activity and bone resorption caused by elevated parathyroid hormone.
- *Polydipsia*: Term describing patients with excessive thirst, commonly seen in diabetes mellitus when hyperglycemia causes osmotic fluid diuresis with resultant dehydration and thirst.
- *Polyuria*: Term describing excessive urination, commonly seen in diabetes mellitus when hyperglycemia produces osmotic fluid diuresis with resultant dehydration and secondary polydipsia.
- *Amyloid*: Extracellular glycoproteins characterized physically by fibrillar ultrastructures and chemically by response to special staining reactions.

TABLE 17-1   Endocrine Organs

Gland Name	Hormone Producing Cells	Hormone Produced	Target Tissues and Organs	Main Functions
Pituitary Glands				
Adenohypophysis (anterior pituitary)	*Acidophils:* Somatotrophs	Growth hormone Somatotropin	Liver (primary); bone, muscle, and adipose tissue (secondary)	Stimulate body growth
	Mammotrophs	Prolactin	Mammary gland	Stimulate mammary glands to produce milk
	Basophils: Corticotrophs	ACTH and corticotropin	Adrenal cortex	Stimulate secretion of glucocorticoids and androgens
	Thyrotrophs	TSH	Thyroid gland	T_3 and T_4
	Gonadotrophs	FSH	Ovaries	Stimulate oocytes to develop and promote estrogen secretion
		LH	Testes	Stimulate testes to produce sperm
Neurohypophysis (posterior pituitary)	Neurosecretory cells from hypothalamus	Vasopressin/ADH	Collecting tubules of kidney; smooth muscle in arterioles	Promote collecting tubules' permeability to water
		Oxytocin	Uterus, mammary gland	Stimulate contraction of uterus and mammary gland
Thyroid Gland				
	Follicular cells	T_3 and T_4	Most tissues of body	Increase metabolic rate; influence body growth and development
	Parafollicular cells	Calcitonin	Bone	Inhibit osteoclasts' absorption activity and reduce blood calcium level
Parathyroid Gland				
	Chief cells	PTH	Bone; small intestine; kidney	Increase osteoclasts' absorption activity and increase blood calcium level
Adrenal Gland				
Adrenal cortex	Secretory cells in zona glomerulosa	Mineralocorticoids (aldosterone)	Renal tubules of the kidney	Influence salt and water balance by promoting renal tubule reabsorption of Na^+ and water and secretion of K^+
	Secretory cells in zona fasciculata	Glucocorticoids (cortisol or hydrocortisone; corticosterone)	Liver; immune cells (such as T and B lymphocytes and macrophages); muscle and adipose tissue	Involved in carbohydrate metabolism and stimulation of gluconeogenesis in the liver; immunosuppressive; reduces muscle and adipose tissue uptake of glucose
	Secretory cells in zona reticularis	Weak androgens (dehydroepiandrosterone, androstenedione)	Testes; uterine and mammary glands; other tissue, such as bone, hair, etc.	As weak androgens, can be converted to either testosterone or estrogen; contribute to sex characteristics and reproduction
Adrenal medulla	*Chromaffin cells:* Adrenaline secreting cells	Adrenaline (epinephrine)	Heart; blood vessel; liver and adipocytes	Increase heart rate and cardiac output; constrict blood vessels in organs and increase blood flow to heart and to skeletal muscle
	Noradrenaline secreting cells	Noradrenaline (norepinephrine)		Increase release of glucose and fatty acids into blood; dilate pupils, and prepare body for action
Pineal Gland				
	Pinealocytes	Melatonin Serotonin	Hypothalamus	Regulate circadian rhythms; promote sleep and control sexual activity; enhance mood and slow the aging process
Endocrine Pancreas				
	Alpha	Glucagon	Liver; gastric glands; exocrine pancreas	Regulate blood glucose levels; stimulate gastric gland secretion; inhibit exocrine pancreatic secretion
	Beta	Insulin		
	Delta	Somatostatin		
	PP cells	Pancreatic polypeptide		

ACTH, adenocorticotropic hormone; TSH, thyroid-stimulating hormone; FSH, follicle-stimulating hormone; LH, luteinizing hormone; ADH, antidiuretic hormone; T_3, triiodothyronine; T_4, thyroxine; PTH, parathyroid hormone; PP cells, pancreatic polypeptide cells.

From Histology to Pathology

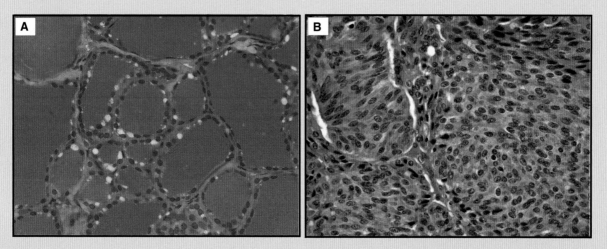

Figure 17-17. Normal thyroid glands and medullary carcinoma. H&E, ×400

Normal thyroid gland on the *left*. **Medullary carcinoma** on the *right*. Medullary carcinoma is a malignant neuroendocrine neoplasm of the thyroid gland arising from the parafollicular (C cells) that produce calcitonin. Most patients seek medical help due to an enlarging neck mass, but they may on occasion present with paraneoplastic symptoms due to the elaboration of **polypeptide hormones** like **vasoactive intestinal peptide (CIP)** and serotonin. Despite production of **calcitonin**, most patients do not experience **hypocalcemia**.

Grossly, medullary carcinoma appears gray to tan with infiltrative borders without a tumor capsule. The histologic appearance is quite variable, with **polygonal to spindle cells arranged in nests, cords**, and **follicles**. Some tumors may produce amyloid, appearing as an eosinophilic amorphous material that, when stained with congo red, appears apple-green under polarized light. The majority of sporadic and familial cases of medullary carcinoma involve point mutations in the rough endoplasmic reticula (RER) of its cells.

Clinical Vignette Questions

1. A healthy 56-year-old woman is attempting to obtain life insurance and must submit a blood specimen for analysis. The results of a basic metabolic profile were normal with the exception of calcium, which was 12.1 mg/dL (normal: 8.6–10.2 mg/dL). She makes an appointment with her internist, who verifies the hypercalcemia and who also finds her serum phosphorus concentration to be 2.1 mg/dL (normal: 2.7–4.5 mg/dL). In order to help elucidate the cause of the hypercalcemia, the physician orders a plasma parathyroid hormone (PTH) level, which is 210 pg/mL (normal: 11–72 pg/mL). A CT scan of the neck reveals a discrete, well-circumscribed mass in the region of the left inferior parathyroid gland. A radionuclide scan confirms the location of the mass and reveals no increased uptake in the other three glands. Based on this information, the most likely cause of the hypercalcemia is which of the following?

A. Excessive calcium supplementation
B. Excessive vitamin D supplementation
C. Parathyroid adenoma
D. Parathyroid carcinoma
E. Parathyroid hyperplasia

2. A 45-year-old woman noticed a lump on her anterior neck located to the left of midline. The lump grew progressively larger over the course of several months, but she did not seek medical attention until she began having difficulty swallowing (dysphagia). During the examination, the physician palpated a firm nodule in the left lobe of the thyroid gland. Ultrasound of the thyroid revealed a 3.7-cm solid mass involving the medial aspect of the left lobe of the thyroid gland. The patient was scheduled for surgery, at which time the left lobe of the thyroid gland and the isthmus were excised. Gross examination of the thyroid specimen revealed a tan mass with infiltrative borders. Histologic examination revealed polygonal to spindle-shaped cells with abundant cytoplasm arranged in nests. Which of the following is the most appropriate diagnosis in this case?

A. Adenoma
B. Anaplastic carcinoma
C. Follicular carcinoma
D. Medullary carcinoma
E. Papillary carcinoma

18 Male Reproductive System

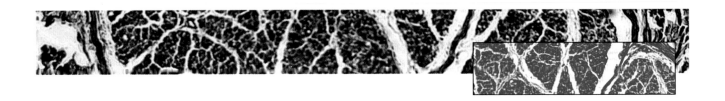

Introduction and Key Concepts for the Male Reproductive System
Testis
Intratesticular Genital Ducts
Extratesticular Genital Ducts
Accessory Genital Glands
Penis

Male Reproductive System

Structures of the Male Reproductive System

Figures and Images Orientation

Structures of the Urinary System with Figure Numbers
Testis

Hormone Regulation in the Male Reproductive System

Spermatogenesis

Intratesticular Genital Ducts

Extratesticular Genital Ducts

Pathway for Sperm Conduction through the Genital Ducts

Accessory Genital Glands

Penis

From Histology to Pathology

Clinical Vignette Questions

Introduction and Key Concepts for the Male Reproductive System

The **male reproductive system** is composed of (1) a pair of **testes** where spermatogenesis takes place; (2) a series of **genital ducts** that include **intratesticular genital ducts** and **extratesticular genital ducts** (which function to carry spermatozoa from the testes to their destination); (3) three major accessory genital glands: the **prostate gland, seminal vesicles,** and **bulbourethral glands;** and (4) the **penis,** which is the male copulatory organ. The main functions of the male reproductive system include production of spermatozoa, fertilization of the ovum in the female reproductive tract, production of sex hormones (testosterone) to develop and maintain secondary male sex characteristics, and performance of sexual activity (copulation).

Testis

The **testis** consists of numerous convoluted **seminiferous tubules** that are lined by **seminiferous epithelium** supported by a basement membrane. The seminiferous epithelium hosts various stages of **spermatogenic cells** (**spermatogonia, spermatocytes,** and **spermatids**), which are protected, nourished, and supported by **Sertoli cells**. The Sertoli cells also produce **testicular fluid**, anti-müllerian hormone, androgen-binding protein (ABP), etc. Between the seminiferous tubules, there is loose connective tissue that contains a special type of cells called the **interstitial cells of Leydig**. These cells mainly produce **testosterone** hormone that promotes **spermatogenesis** and the development of male sexual organs as well as maintains secondary male sexual characteristics. The testis is covered by the **tunica albuginea** (capsule), **tunica vaginalis** (mesothelial sac), and an outer layer of wrinkled thin skin, the **scrotum**. Spermatogenesis takes place in the seminiferous epithelium of the tubules.

Intratesticular Genital Ducts

The **intratesticular genital ducts** are located within the testis, including the **tubuli recti, rete testis, and ductuli efferentes.**

1. *Tubuli recti*: These are short, straight tubules lined by **simple cuboidal epithelium**. They carry the newly produced spermatozoa in testicular fluid from the seminiferous tubules to the rete testis in the mediastinum of the testis.
2. *Rete testis*: This is a maze of anastomosing tubules with an irregular lumen and is lined by **simple cuboidal epithelium** (Fig. 18-14C). This network of interconnecting tubules conducts the spermatozoa and testicular fluid into the ductuli efferentes.
3. *Ductuli efferentes*: These convoluted tubules are alternatively lined by two cell types: **nonciliated cuboidal cells** and **ciliated columnar cells**. The ductuli efferentes absorb some testicular fluid and move the spermatozoa to the head of the epididymis.

Extratesticular Genital Ducts

The **extratesticular genital ducts** located outside the testis include the **ductus epididymis, ductus deferens, ejaculatory ducts,** and **urethra**. These ducts are paired tubules except the urethra, which is a single tubule.

1. *Ductus epididymis*: Each **ductus epididymis** is a highly convoluted tube (about 6 m long) that has three regions: **head, body,** and **tail**. They are lined by **pseudostratified columnar epithelium** with **long stereocilia** that absorb large volumes of testicular fluid from the lumen and secrete a variety of substances, including **glycerophosphocholine**, which inhibits capacitation of spermatozoa from occurring in the male reproductive tract. The tail of the epididymis is the region where spermatozoa mature and are stored.
2. *Ductus deferens*: Each **ductus deferens** is a long tube that courses partly within a spermatic cord. Its proximal end connects with the tail of the epididymis. The distal portion becomes enlarged and is known as the **ampulla**. After its junction with the duct of the **seminal vesicle**, the **ductus deferens** continues its course to form the **ejaculatory duct**. The ductus deferens is lined by **pseudostratified columnar epithelium** and surrounded by a thick muscularis consisting of three layers of smooth muscle.
3. *Ejaculatory ducts*: The two **ejaculatory ducts** are surrounded by the prostate gland. They are straight tubes, lined by **pseudostratified columnar** and **simple columnar epithelium**. The ejaculatory ducts open into the **prostatic urethra** at the **colliculus seminalis**. The colliculus seminalis is a median elevation of the **verumontanum**, the portion of the male prostatic urethra where the ducts open.
4. *Urethra*: The **urethra** is a long tube (about 20 cm) lined by various types of **epithelium**. It is a common passage shared by the urinary system and reproductive system in the male. It can be divided into three regions: the **prostatic**, the **membranous**, and the **spongy** (**penile**) **urethra**. The *prostatic urethra*, lined by **transitional epithelium**, is connected with the bladder at its proximal end and passes through the prostate gland. The prostatic urethra is wider than other parts of the urethra and has two ejaculatory ducts opening into the urethra. The short *membranous urethra* is lined by pseudostratified columnar epithelium; it is the intermediate and narrowest part of the urethra. The membranous urethra connects the prostatic urethra to the spongy urethra. The *spongy urethra*, also called the **penile urethra**, is lined by stratified columnar epithelium. It passes through the penis and is the longest segment of the urethra.

Accessory Genital Glands

The **accessory genital glands** are exocrine glands that include the **prostate gland**, paired **seminal vesicles**, and **bulbourethral glands**. (1) The **prostate gland** is a collection of about 40 small tubuloalveolar glands lined by **simple columnar epithelium** and supported by a connective tissue stroma. **Prostatic secretions** contain **proteolytic enzymes, acid phosphatase, citric acid, fibrinolysin,** and **lipids**. (2) Each **seminal vesicle** has a single convoluted tube with a branched and folded mucosa lined by **pseudostratified columnar epithelium**. The epithelium is supported by a thin connective tissue layer that is surrounded by two layers of smooth muscle (**muscularis**). The seminal vesicle produces seminal fluid containing **fructose, prostaglandins, flavins, phosphorylcholine, vitamin C,** and **proteins**. **Semen** is a mixture of seminal fluid, prostatic secretion, spermatozoa, and testicular fluid. (3) The **bulbourethral glands** are a small pair of glands lined by **simple columnar epithelium**. They produce **preejaculate** (**preseminal**) fluid that lubricates the urethra before ejaculation.

Penis

The **penis** is an external genital organ that consists of three cylinders of **erectile tissue**, including the **corpora cavernosa** (two) and the **corpus spongiosum** (one). The corpus spongiosum contains the urethra in its center. The penis has a unique blood supply (dorsal arteries, deep arteries, and helicine arteries) and drainage (superficial veins, arteriovenous shunts) that are correlated with its erection.

Male Reproductive System

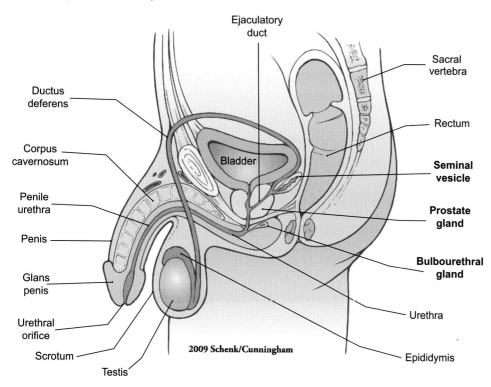

Ejaculatory
duct

Sacral
vertebra

Ductus
deferens

Rectum

Corpus
cavernosum

Bladder

**Seminal
vesicle**

Penile
urethra

**Prostate
gland**

Penis

**Bulbourethral
gland**

Glans
penis

Urethra

Urethral
orifice

2009 Schenk/Cunningham

Scrotum

Epididymis

Testis

Figure 18-1. Overview of the male reproductive system.

The **male reproductive system** includes the **testes, genital ducts, accessory genital glands,** and **penis.** There are two *testes* where spermatogenesis takes place and sex hormones (testosterone) are produced. The *genital ducts* include **intratesticular genital ducts** and **extratesticular genital ducts.** The *intratesticular genital ducts* comprise the **tubuli recti, rete testis,** and **ductuli efferentes,** which are located inside of the testis. The *extratesticular genital ducts* comprise the **ductus epididymis, ductus deferens, ejaculatory duct,** and **urethra.** The *accessory genital glands* include three major glands: the **seminal vesicles, prostate gland,** and **bulbourethral glands.** Two ejaculatory ducts meet with the **prostatic urethra** before it continues its course through the urogenital diaphragm as the **membranous urethra** and then through the penis as the **penile urethra.** The *penis* is composed of three cylinders of spongy erectile tissue including the two corpora cavernosa and the corpus spongiosum (containing the urethra).

Structures of the Male Reproductive System

I. **Testes**
    A. Testicular tunicate
        1. Tunica vaginalis
        2. Tunica albuginea
        3. Tunica vasculosa
        4. Mediastinum testis
        5. Special cells (interstitial cells of Leydig)
    B. Seminiferous tubules
        1. Spermatogenic cells
        2. Sertoli cells
II. **Genital ducts**
    A. Intratesticular genital ducts
        1. Tubuli recti
        2. Rete testis
        3. Ductuli efferentes

    B. Extratesticular genital ducts
        1. Ductus epididymis
        2. Ductus (vas) deferens with spermatic cord
        3. Ejaculatory ducts
        4. Urethra (prostatic, membranous, and spongy/penile
           urethra)
III. **Accessory genital glands**
    A. Prostate gland
    B. Seminal vesicles
    C. Bulbourethral glands
IV. **Penis**
    A. Tunica albuginea
    B. Corpus cavernosum
    C. Corpus spongiosum and spongy/penile urethra

Figures and Images Orientation

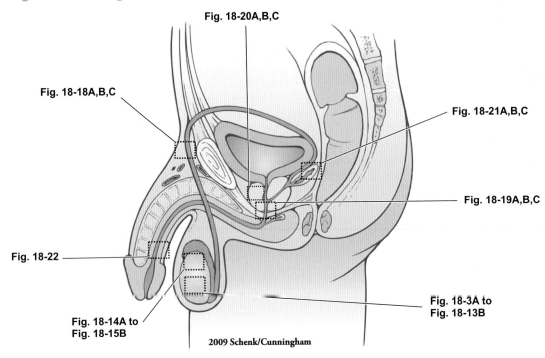

Fig. 18-20A,B,C

Fig. 18-18A,B,C

Fig. 18-21A,B,C

Fig. 18-19A,B,C

Fig. 18-22

Fig. 18-3A to
Fig. 18-13B

Fig. 18-14A to
Fig. 18-15B

2009 Schenk/Cunningham

Figure 18-2. Orientation of detailed male reproductive system illustrations.

Structures of the Urinary System with Figure Numbers

Testis:
Seminiferous tubules
Figure 18-3A
Figure 18-3B
Figure 18-3C
Figure 18-4A
Figure 18-4B
Figure 18-5
Figure 18-6A
Figure 18-6B
Figure 18-7
Figure 18-8

Spermatogenesis
Figure 18-9
Figure 18-10
Figure 18-11A,B
Figure 18-12A,B
Figure 18-13A,B

Intratesticular genital ducts:
Tubuli recti
Figure 18-14A
Figure 18-14B

Rete testis
Figure 18-14C

Ductuli efferentes
Figure 18-15A
Figure 18-15B
Figure 18-15C

Extratesticular genital ducts:
Ductus epididymis
Figure 18-16
Figure 18-17A
Figure 18-17B

Ductus deferens and spermatic cord
Figure 18-18A
Figure 18-18B
Figure 18-18C

Ejaculatory ducts
Figure 18-19A
Figure 18-19B

Prostatic urethra
Figure 18-19C

Accessory genital glands:
Prostate gland
Figure 18-20A
Figure 18-20B
Figure 18-20C

Seminal vesicles
Figure 18-21A
Figure 18-21B
Figure 18-21C

Penis:
Figure 18-22

Testis

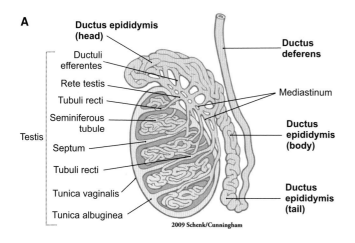

Figure 18-3A. Overview of the testis.

Each **testis** is composed of many convoluted **seminiferous tubules**. The anterior portion of the testis is covered by a closed sac of peritoneum called the **tunica vaginalis** (mesothelial sac). The **tunica albuginea** is a thick layer of capsule (dense connective tissue) that surrounds and divides the testis into small lobules; the connective tissue continues at the posterior part and becomes thicker and forms the vertically oriented connective tissue mass called the **mediastinum**. The mediastinum contains the **rete testis**, which consists of a labyrinth of small channels that collect sperm from the **tubuli recti**. The **ductus epididymis** is a single long, highly convoluted duct that receives sperm from the **ductuli efferentes**. The epididymis is divided into three parts: the head, body, and tail. The tail of the epididymis connects with the **ductus deferens**. The testes play important roles in the production of sperm and secretion of testosterone (sex hormone).

SEMINIFEROUS TUBULES

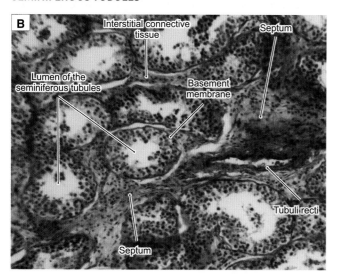

Figure 18-3B. Seminiferous tubules of the testis. H&E, ×122

Seminiferous tubules are the main functional components of the testis. Each of the several hundred seminiferous tubules in each testis is a highly coiled tubule lined by a stratified **germinal (seminiferous) epithelium** containing various stages of **spermatogenic cells**. The seminiferous epithelium is supported by the basement membrane. Cross sections of some seminiferous tubules and a connective tissue septum are shown here. The **tubuli recti** (straight tubules) are located in the connective tissue septa. The connective tissue between neighboring tubules, which contains small vessels and endocrine cells, is called **interstitial connective tissue**.

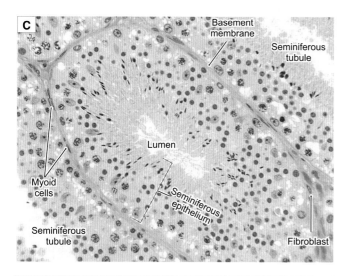

Figure 18-3C. Seminiferous tubule. H&E, ×281

This is an example of a single **seminiferous tubule**, consisting of germinal epithelium and its basement membrane. The seminiferous tubule is surrounded by a very thin connective tissue containing a few fibroblasts. Another type of cell, the **myoid cell**, has the appearance of smooth muscle cells, with flat and elongated nuclei. These cells surround the seminiferous tubules and contract to help the movement of the testicular fluid in which the spermatozoa are suspended. Neighboring seminiferous tubules are in close contact with one another. The various stages of the spermatogenic cells include **spermatogonia**, **spermatocytes** (primary and secondary), and **spermatids** (early, intermediate, and late). They are present in six different specific combinations of cell types that define the stages of the cycle of the seminiferous epithelium.

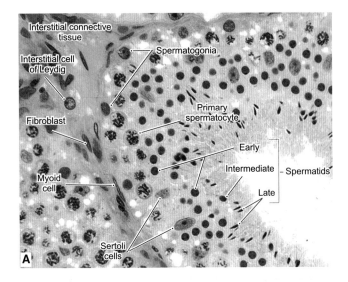

Figure 18-4A. Cells in the seminiferous tubules. H&E, ×458

There are two types of **cells in the seminiferous tubules**: spermatogenic (germ) cells and **supporting (Sertoli) cells**. The *spermatogenic cells* consist of

1. *Spermatogonia*: These cells have round or oval nuclei and are located near the basement membrane. They can be subdivided into **type A** and **type B** cells. *Type A cells* are stem cells that divide slowly and give rise to *type B cells*.
2. *Spermatocytes*: These derivatives of spermatogonia B cells undergo meiosis. They move toward the lumen and can be divided into **primary (first meiotic division)** and **secondary (second meiotic division) spermatocytes**. *Primary spermatocytes* in prophase are most commonly seen in sections. Their large nuclei contain strands of condensed chromosomes. *Secondary spermatocytes* complete the second meiotic division very quickly, so they are rarely seen.
3. *Spermatids*: These cells have small interphase nuclei that range from spherical to thin and elongated. They can be classified as **early, intermediate, or late spermatids**, based mainly on the appearance of the nucleus.

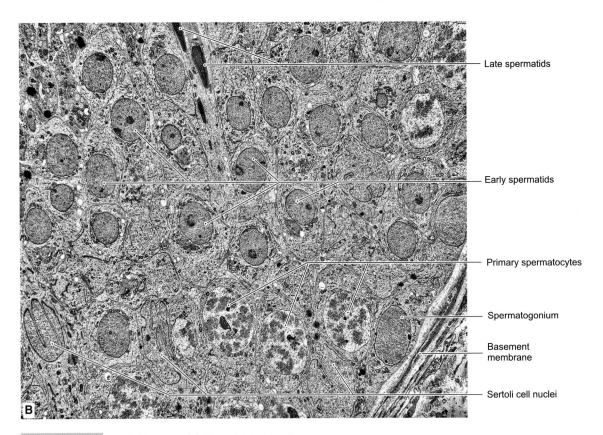

Figure 18-4B. Seminiferous epithelium. EM, ×4,600

This low-magnification view shows almost the full thickness of the **seminiferous epithelium**. **Sertoli cells** are the nongerm cells that organize the epithelium and divide it into two compartments, **basal** and **adluminal**. The only cell type in the *basal compartment* is the **spermatogonium**, which, like the Sertoli cells, contacts the basement membrane. This patch of epithelium appears to be in stage one of the six stages (cell associations) of seminiferous epithelium. The *adluminal compartment* contains three cohorts of cells, each at a different stage of **spermatogenesis**. The least advanced cells are **primary spermatocytes** in prophase of meiosis I. The chromosomes of these diploid cells have begun condensing, and homologous pairs have aligned into synaptonemal complexes. **Early spermatids,** which appear as small, undifferentiated cells, predominate in the middle and superficial regions of the epithelium. The third and most advanced cell type here is the **late spermatid**. The heads of a few can be seen surrounded by the cytoplasm of a Sertoli cell.

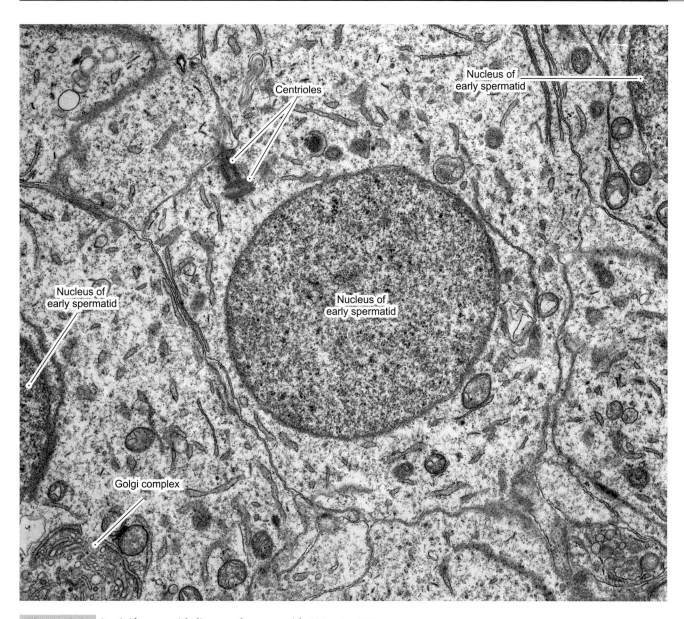

Centrioles

Nucleus of
early spermatid

Nucleus of
early spermatid

Nucleus of
early spermatid

Golgi complex

Figure 18-5. Seminiferous epithelium, early spermatid. EM, ×17,000

Completion of **meiosis II** by **secondary spermatocytes** produces **spermatids**. These are haploid cells that do not divide but undergo **spermiogenesis**, that is, morphological differentiation into **spermatozoa**. The cells in this image are **early spermatids** that have not yet acquired many of the specializations of spermatozoa. The interphase nucleus in the center is still spherical, and the chromatin is not yet highly condensed. The **Golgi complex**, visible in the cell on the *left*, will be the site of development of the acrosomal vesicle and, ultimately the acrosome, which will form a cap on one side of the nucleus. Note that the plane of section happens to pass through the central cell's centrosome with its pair of **centrioles**. One member of the pair will organize the development of the flagellum with its axoneme of microtubules. The other centriole will participate in the first cleavage division if the spermatozoan fertilizes a **secondary oocyte**. This **spermatid** is linked to its cohort spermatids by cytoplasmic bridges, although this is not evident in this image. Like all cells engaged in spermatogenesis, spermatids are embedded in cytoplasmic processes of Sertoli cells.

SERTOLI CELLS

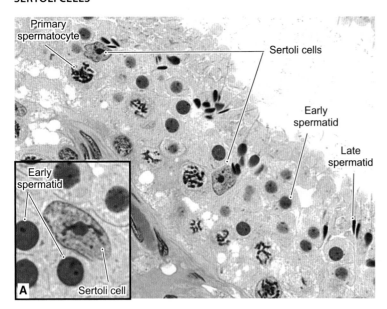

Figure 18-6A. Sertoli cells, seminiferous tubules. H&E, ×732; inset ×1,603

Sertoli cells have pale oval or irregularly shaped nuclei, and nucleoli are often present. They are irregular columnar cells with many folded cytoplasmic processes forming compartments for the spermatogenic cells. They form **tight junctions (zonulae occludentes)** with the neighboring Sertoli cells, thereby providing a blood-testis barrier to protect spermatogenic cells from being harmed by autoimmune reactions. Sertoli cells control hormones, nutrients, and other substances passing through the compartments and maintain the ideal environment for **spermatogenesis**. They play important roles in supporting, protecting, and nourishing spermatogenic cells as well as in secreting testicular fluid (rich in fructose) to help in transporting spermatozoa out of the seminiferous tubules. They also secrete **ABP, anti-müllerian hormone,** and **inhibin** and **activin hormones.**

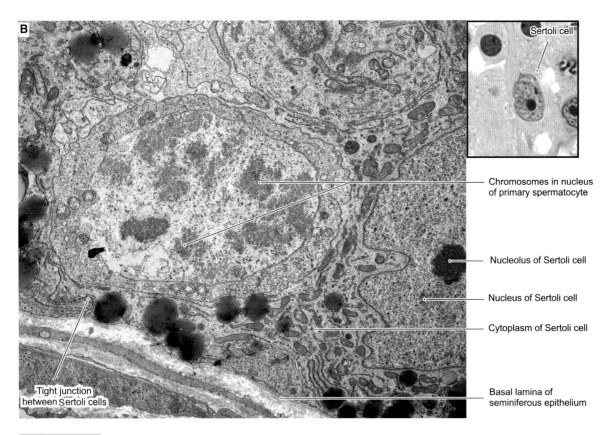

Figure 18-6B. Sertoli cell and primary spermatocyte, seminiferous epithelium. EM, ×7,900; inset (*color*) H&E, ×1,005

Sertoli cells, the only somatic cells of the seminiferous epithelium, are dynamic cells with a long list of functions in support of **spermatogenesis.** Their processes envelope and support the germ cells throughout the many stages of meiosis and spermiogenesis. In this view, cytoplasmic extensions of the Sertoli cell (with its nucleus at the left edge) enshroud the **primary spermatocyte** that has entered **prophase of meiosis I** and isolate it from the **basal compartment** so that it is no longer accessible to the immune system. Note also the example of the **junctional complexes** (including **tight junctions**) that couple adjacent Sertoli cells and, thereby, establish a controlled and specialized environment in support of the cells that are undergoing spermatogenesis. Other functions of Sertoli cells are secretion of testicular fluid, concentration of androgens, and phagocytosis of the residual bodies jettisoned by late spermatids as they complete spermiogenesis.

INTERSTITIAL CELLS OF LEYDIG

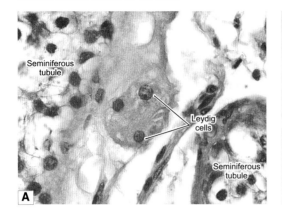

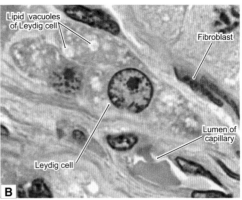

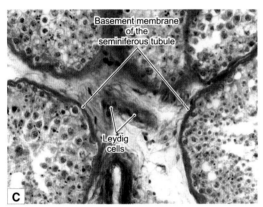

Figure 18-7. Interstitial cells of Leydig. H&E, *left* ×263; *right* ×2,016; iron hematoxylin stain, ×237

The **interstitial cells of Leydig** are located in the interstitial (connective) tissue near the blood capillaries and between the seminiferous tubules. These cells have round nuclei and pale-stained cytoplasm with lipid drops (lipid vacuoles) in the peripheral region of the cytoplasm, which give them a bubbly appearance (like many steroid-producing cells). These cells contain abundant smooth endoplasmic reticulum, which contributes to steroid hormone production. The interstitial cells of Leydig derive from the mesoderm and are usually large in size (about 20 μm in diameter) compared with other cells in the connective tissue. They are the endocrine cells that produce the important male sex hormone, **testosterone**. Testosterone plays important roles in developing and maintaining male sex characteristics, stimulating muscle and bone growth, and increasing bone density. A small amount of testosterone is also produced by the adrenal glands and ovaries in the female.

SYNOPSIS 18-1 Functions of Sertoli Cells

- *Support:* Provide physical support and nutrition for the different stages of spermatogenic cells.
- *Protection:* Form **blood-testis barrier** by tight junctions between adjacent Sertoli cells that protect spermatogenic cells from autoimmune destruction; also control hormones, nutrients, and other substances being transported in and out of the seminiferous tubules.
- *Phagocytosis:* Remove **residual bodies** after excess cytoplasm is shed from the spermatids during maturation of the spermatozoa.
- *Secretion:* (1) Secrete and release fructose-rich fluids (testicular fluid) to help nourish and move sperm from the seminiferous tubules to the epididymis; (2) secrete **anti-müllerian hormone** to prevent oviducts from developing from the müllerian duct in the early stages of the male embryo; (3) secrete **androgen-binding protein** (ABP) to maintain the concentration of testosterone in the seminiferous tubules, thereby promoting spermatogenesis; (4) secrete **glial cell–derived neurotrophic factor** (GDNF) to promote survival and differentiation of the spermatids (GDNF is better known for promoting development of neurons); and (5) produce **inhibin** and **activin** hormones to provide negative and positive feedback to the hypothalamus, thereby regulating follicle-stimulating hormone (FSH) secretion by the pituitary gland.

SYNOPSIS 18-2 Functions of Testosterone

The **interstitial cells of Leydig** secrete **testosterone**, which is the major male sex hormone. Its functions include the following:
- Promoting development of male sex organs in early fetal development.
- Promoting male sexual characteristics, such as growth of beard and axillary hair, enlargement of the larynx, and deepening the voice.
- Increasing muscle growth, thickness of the skin, and sebaceous gland secretion.
- Promoting bone growth and increasing bone density.
- Increasing basal metabolism and physical energy.
- Promoting spermatogenesis.

Hormone Regulation in the Male Reproductive System

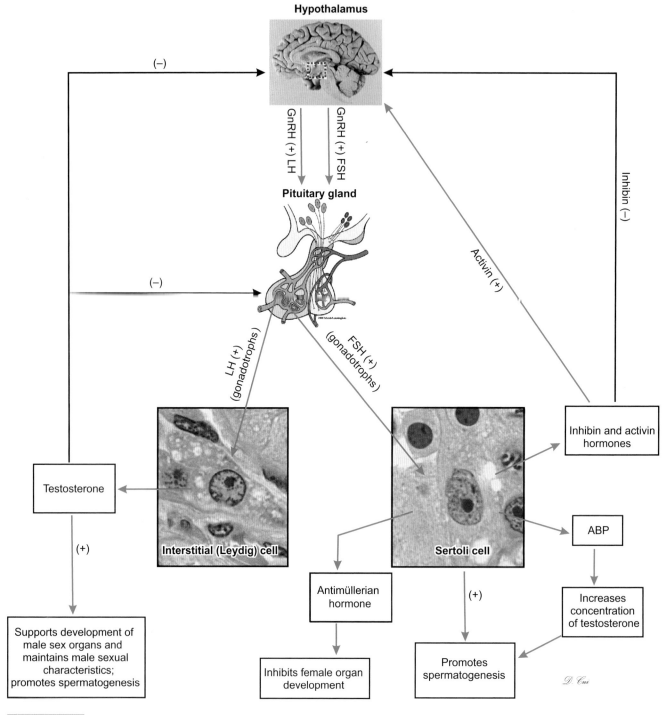

Figure 18-8. Hormone regulation involving the testicular cells (interstitial cells of Leydig and Sertoli cells). H&E, ×1,005

The preoptic nucleus in the hypothalamus secretes **gonadotropin-releasing hormone (GnRH)**, which stimulates the pituitary gland to produce and release **luteinizing hormone (LH)** and **FSH**. Secretion of **testosterone** by the **interstitial cells of Leydig** is stimulated by the **LH** produced by the **gonadotrophs** in the **adenohypophysis** of the pituitary gland. An excessive level of **testosterone** sends negative feedback to the hypothalamus to inhibit production of **GnRH**, resulting in decreased secretion of LH in the pituitary gland. **Sertoli cells** that release **ABP** are stimulated by **FSH**, which stimulates production of the **ABP**. Sertoli cells also secrete **anti-müllerian hormone** as well as **inhibin** and **activin hormones**. The **inhibin hormone** suppresses and **activin hormone** stimulates the production of GnRH, which influences FSH production by the gonadotrophs in the adenohypophysis of the pituitary gland.

Spermatogenesis

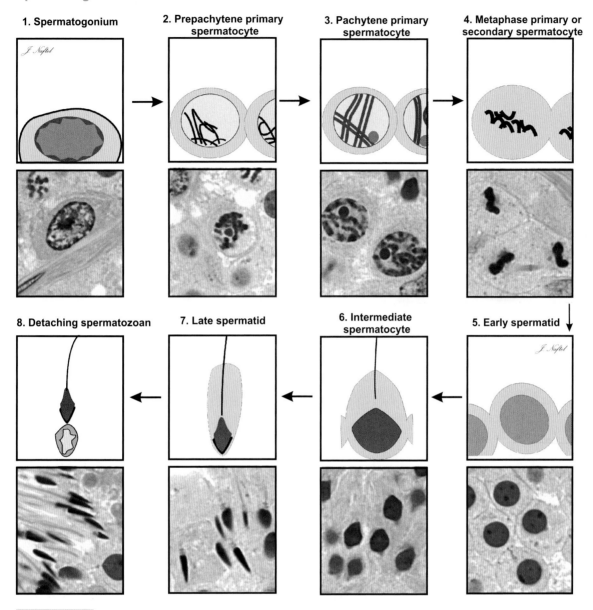

Figure 18-9. Overview of readily identifiable spermatogenic cells in the seminiferous epithelium. H&E, ×1,496

Spermatogenesis involves an orderly sequence of changes as cells proceed through **mitosis (spermatogonia)**, **meiosis (spermatocytes)**, and **spermiogenesis (spermatids)**. Only the eight most readily identifiable stages are illustrated here owing to their distinctiveness and adequate abundance in ordinary sections. *Spermatogonia* can be identified by their position (in contact with the basement membrane) and their oval interphase nuclei with the long axis parallel to the basement membrane. *Primary spermatocytes* undergo several substages of prophase I, but, here, the earlier substages are denoted as **prepachytene**. The condensing chromosomes in **prepachytene primary spermatocytes** tend to be clumped at one edge of the nuclear envelope. By contrast, the paired chromosomes of **pachytene primary spermatocytes** form broad bands that fill the nucleus. *Pachytene primary spermatocytes* are abundant in sections, because this is the phase of meiosis with the longest duration. After a primary spermatocyte completes pachytene, the remaining steps of meiosis I and meiosis II (by the daughter secondary spermatocytes) are completed very rapidly, so examples of cells in these stages of meiosis are more difficult to find in sections. Cells in either metaphase I or metaphase II are most conspicuous and easiest to locate. The products of meiosis II are *spermatids*. These haploid cells begin as **early spermatids**, recognizable by their small spherical interphase nuclei. The first clear evidence that spermiogenesis is underway is a change in shape of the nucleus from spherical to a broad diamond shape; a cell with such a nucleus can be designated an **intermediate spermatid**. When the nucleus has assumed the sharply pointed shape and dense appearance of a spermatozoan but remains inserted deeply into the epithelium, the cell can be denoted a **late spermatid**. Finally, nuclei of **detaching spermatozoa** can readily be recognized, because they form a row at the surface of the epithelium and overlie a layer of residual bodies.

SPERMATOGENESIS AND STAGES OF THE SEMINIFEROUS EPITHELIUM

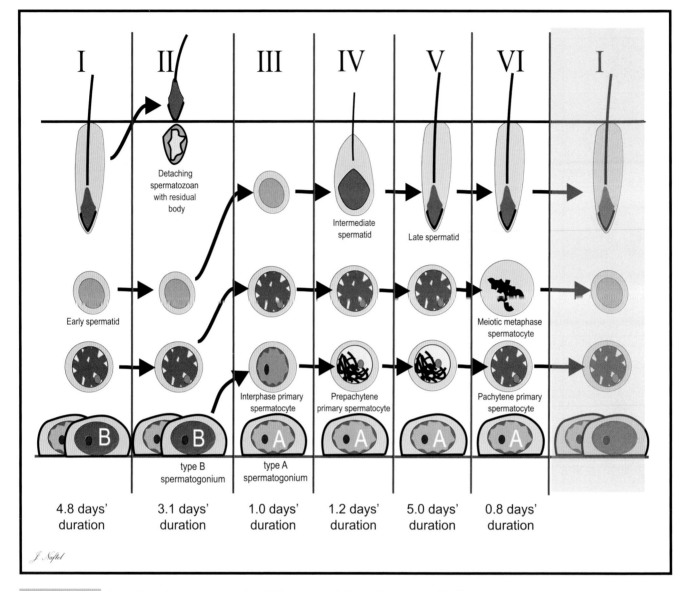

Figure 18-10. Overview of spermatogenesis and the stages of the seminiferous epithelium.

If small patches of **seminiferous epithelium** are examined, it can be seen that there are six recurring groupings of stages of developing gametes that populate the epithelium. These groupings (associations) represent recurring stages that a patch of epithelium cycles through over time, and their existence indicates that the many steps in **spermatogenesis** proceed with a very rigid timetable. If the composition of a bit of epithelium could be monitored over time, it would be seen that, as cohorts of germ cells begin and complete spermatogenesis within the epithelium, the epithelium itself will change in appearance and contain the six different groupings of developing germ cells. The ability to recognize the stages in the cycle of the epithelium has made it possible to undertake simple experiments that have revealed some important dynamics of spermatogenesis. Therefore, the time required for a patch of epithelium to complete the six stages of one cycle is 16 days, and it can be inferred that with each 16-day cycle a single patch of epithelium will release a group of new **spermatozoa** for only a brief period when it reaches the end of **stage II**. Likewise, the end of stage II is the only time during the 16-day cycle that a new cohort or generation of primary spermatocytes will enter the **adluminal compartment** to begin **meiosis I**. The time required for a new **type B spermatogonium** to generate completed spermatozoa is 56 days.

STAGES OF THE SEMINIFEROUS EPITHELIUM

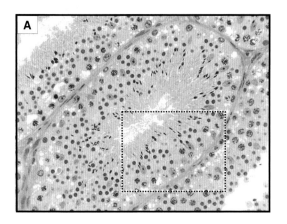

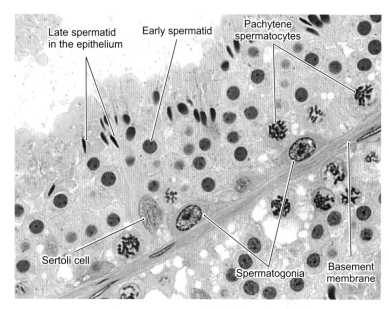

Figure 18-11A. Stage I seminiferous epithelium. H&E, *left* ×207; *right* ×747

Stage I seminiferous epithelium is shown at low magnification (*left*), and a detailed representation of the region is indicated by the box (*right*). Stage I seminiferous epithelium is characterized by the following: (1) **Spermatogonia** are located at the basement membrane; both **type A** and **B spermatogonia** are present, although the two types are not easily distinguished in H&E-stained sections. (2) A layer of **pachytene primary spermatocytes** is present. Although some of these cells are near the basement membrane, they are not in direct contact with it. (3) A prominent layer of round, undifferentiated **early spermatids** has moved toward the surface of the epithelium. (4) The **late spermatids** have their heads inserted deep into the epithelium.

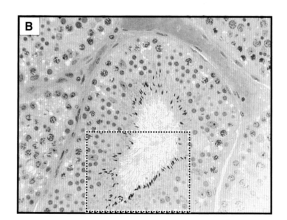

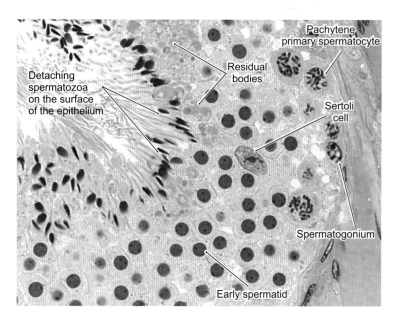

Figure 18-11B. Stage II seminiferous epithelium. H&E, *left* ×207; *right* ×747

Stage II seminiferous epithelium is shown at low magnification (*left*), and a detailed representation of the region is indicated by the box (*right*). The composition of the spermatogenic cell in stage II seminiferous epithelium is similar to that of stage I. The most characteristic features of this stage are the following: (1) **Detaching spermatozoa** (very late spermatids) have completed differentiation and are in the process of shedding their excess cytoplasm. (2) The small leftover cytoplasmic masses that have been shed are called **residual bodies** and are present in the luminal border of the epithelium, beneath the heads of the detaching spermatozoa. (3) These detaching spermatozoa are positioned in a row on the surface of the epithelium ready to be released from the epithelium into the lumen. (4) **Early spermatids** with round nuclei and pachytene primary spermatocytes are present. (5) Both **type A** and **B spermatogonia** are present.

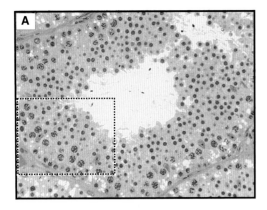

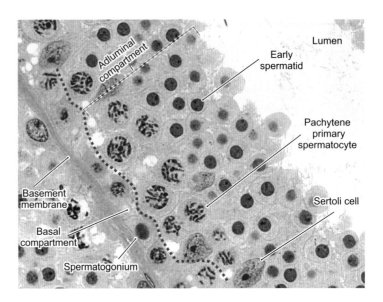

Figure 18-12A.   Stage III seminiferous epithelium. H&E, *left* ×207; *right* ×747

Stage III seminiferous epithelium is shown at low magnification (*left*), and a detailed representation of the region is indicated by the box (*right*). Stage III has a similar composition of spermatogenic cells as that of stage II, except for the absence of the detaching spermatozoa at the surface and the added presence of a new generation of primary spermatocytes near the basement membrane (not readily apparent). This stage is characterized by the following: (1) There is an absence of **detaching spermatozoa,** which have been released into the lumen to be suspended in testicular fluid and transported along the genital ducts. (2) **Early spermatids** with round nuclei have moved to the surface of the epithelium. (3) There is the continued presence of a generation (cohort) of **primary spermatocytes** in the pachytene stage of prophase I. (4) A new generation of primary spermatocytes has moved from the **basal compartment** into the **adluminal compartment,** although they are difficult to distinguish. Compartments are created by **tight junctions** of neighboring **Sertoli cells.** The *basal compartment* is situated on the basement membrane side of the tight junctions between **Sertoli cells,** and it contains spermatogonia. The *adluminal compartment* is situated above the junctions and toward the lumen and contains spermatocytes and spermatids. The tight junctions establish a **blood-testis barrier** that prevents immunoglobulins from entering the adluminal compartment. Newly formed primary spermatocytes are lefted from the basal compartment and into the adluminal compartment by outgrowth of processes extended from the local Sertoli cells.

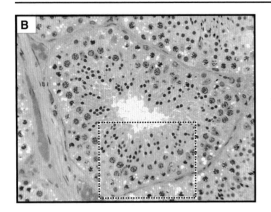

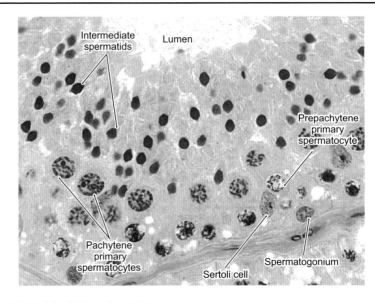

Figure 18-12B.   Stage IV seminiferous epithelium. H&E, *left* ×207; *right* ×747

Stage IV seminiferous epithelium is shown at low magnification (*left*), and a detailed representation of the region is indicated by the box (*right*). Stage IV differs from stage III mainly in the progression of the generation of early spermatids (in stage III) to intermediate spermatids (in stage IV). Stage IV has the following composition: (1) **intermediate spermatids** with diamond-shaped or irregular nuclei; (2) one generation of primary spermatocytes in **pachytene** of prophase I; (3) a separate generation of primary spermatocytes at an early (**prepachytene**) stage of prophase I; and (4) **type A spermatogonia** in the basal compartment.

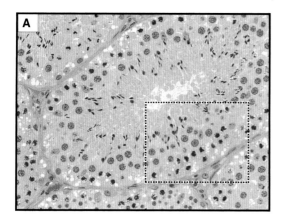

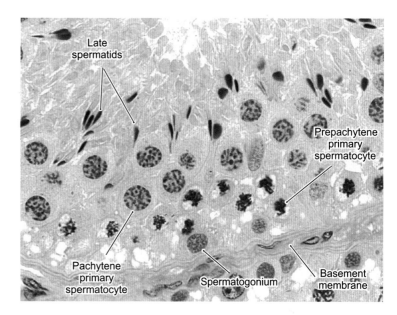

Figure 18-13A.   **Stage V seminiferous epithelium.** H&E, *left* ×207; *right* ×747

Stage V seminiferous epithelium is shown at low magnification (*left*), and a detailed representation of the region is indicated by the box (*right*). In this example, stage V has newly developed late spermatids and two generations of primary spermatocytes. Stage V is characterized by the following: (1) There are no early or intermediate spermatids; only **late spermatids** are present. The cytoplasm of each late spermatid extends from the sharply pointed nucleus toward the lumen. (2) Two generations (both **pachytene** and **prepachytene**) of **primary spermatocytes** are present. (3) **Type A spermatogonia** are present, as always, in the basal compartment.

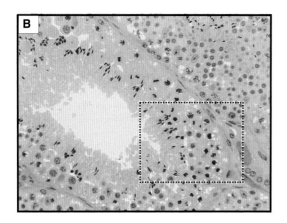

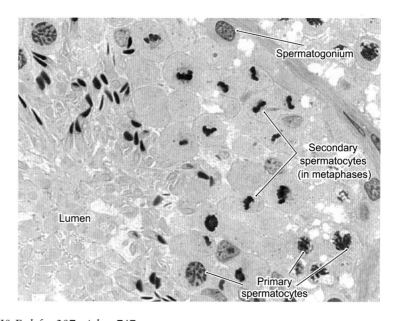

Figure 18-13B.   **Stage VI seminiferous epithelium.** H&E, *left* ×207; *right* ×747

Stage VI seminiferous epithelium is shown at low magnification (*left*), and a detailed representation of the region is indicated by the box (*right*). The most characteristic feature of stage VI is the presence of **metaphases** of either **primary** or **secondary spermatocytes**, which are present only in this stage. Interphase secondary spermatocytes also occur in stage VI, but these are rarely apparent. The characteristics at this stage are as follows: (1) **Late spermatids** are present at the epithelium near the lumen. (2) Dividing **spermatocytes** with their chromosomes clumped in the center of the cytoplasm. (3) A separate generation of primary spermatocytes in **prophase** is present, although they are not easily distinguished. (4) **Type A spermatogonia** are present. This is a very active stage during which each member of the older cohort of primary spermatocytes completes the first meiotic division to produce two secondary spermatocytes, and, in a very short time, each secondary spermatocyte completes the second meiotic division to produce two spermatids.

Intratesticular Genital Ducts

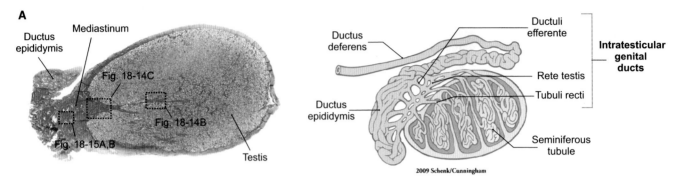

Figure 18-14A. Intratesticular genital ducts. H&E, ×6

The series of ducts that transport spermatozoa from the seminiferous tubules to the outside of the male body are called **genital ducts**. They include **intratesticular genital ducts** and **extratesticular genital ducts**. The *intratesticular genital ducts* refer to ducts within the testis. They are composed of the **tubuli recti, rete testis,** and **ductuli efferentes**. The *extratesticular genital ducts* include the **ductus epididymis, ductus deferens, ejaculatory ducts,** and **urethra**.

TUBULI RECTI AND RETE TESTIS

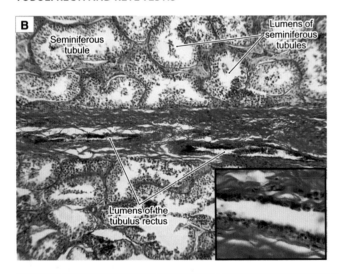

Figure 18-14B. Tubuli recti. H&E, ×71; inset ×210

The **tubuli recti** are short (about 1 mm), straight tubules that carry the spermatozoa from the seminiferous tubules into the rete testis. *Rectus* means "straight." Each tubulus rectus is lined by a single layer of cuboidal epithelial cells and is supported by a layer of dense connective tissue. It is located in the septum (connective tissue) and opens into the rete testis in the mediastinum. The terminal portion of the seminiferous tubules is lined by Sertoli cells. The germinal cells in the seminiferous tubules are gradually reduced in number near the tubuli recti and disappear at the terminal portion. The **spermatozoa** are pushed forward by the flow of the testicular fluid through the tubuli recti and into the **rete testis**. An example here shows two segments of a tubulus rectus.

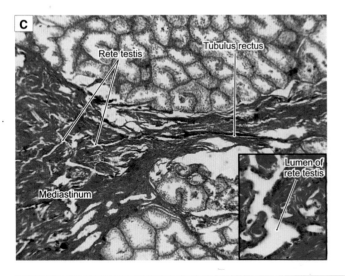

Figure 18-14C. Rete testis. H&E, ×35; inset ×163

The **rete testis** is an interconnecting network of tubules located in the mediastinum. These tubules have an irregular lumen and are lined by simple cuboidal epithelium and supported by a dense connective tissue. This example shows the terminal portion of the tubulus rectus opening into the tubule of the rete testis.

DUCTULI EFFERENTES

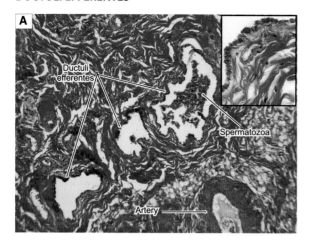

Figure 18-15A. Ductuli efferentes. H&E, ×68; inset ×234

There are 15 to 20 tubules of **ductuli efferentes** leading from the rete testis in the mediastinum to the head of the epididymis. They are also called **efferent ducts**. The ductuli efferentes are lined by two types of epithelial cells: **nonciliated cuboidal cells** with **microvilli (absorptive cells)** and **ciliated columnar cells**. They are alternately distributed on the luminal surface of the ductuli efferentes. The epithelium of the ductuli efferentes is supported by a thin layer of connective tissue; beneath it is a thin layer of circular smooth muscle that contracts to move testicular fluid and spermatozoa toward the ductus epididymis (*inset*). Smooth muscle cells are interspersed with some elastic fibers. The muscle layer becomes thicker as it nears the ductus epididymis.

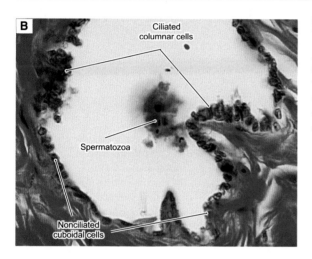

Figure 18-15B. Ductuli efferentes. H&E, ×463

An example of **ductuli efferentes** at high magnification is shown. The **nonciliated cuboidal cells** have an absorptive function, absorbing excess testicular fluid secreted by seminiferous tubules and increasing the concentration of spermatozoa in the lumen of the ductuli efferentes. The **ciliated columnar cells** of the ductuli efferentes have a motile function, sweeping spermatozoa and testicular fluid toward the epididymis.

CLINICAL CORRELATION

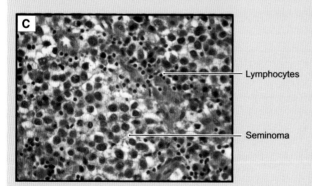

Figure 18-15C. Testis Seminoma. H&E, ×192

Most tumors of the testes arise from the germinal epithelium of the seminiferous tubules; therefore, this group is termed **germ cell tumors**. These germ cell tumors can be divided into **seminomas**, and all other germ cell tumors are called **nonseminomatous**, examples of which include **choriocarcinoma, embryonal carcinoma, yolk sac tumor,** and **teratoma**. Seminomas are the most common germ cell tumor of the testis and are most likely to occur in the pure form, because germ cell tumors commonly contain multiple tumor types (**mixed germ cell tumors**). Germ cell tumors tend to arise from *in situ* lesions of the germinal epithelium called **intratubular germ cell neoplasia (IGCN)**. The incidence of seminoma peaks in the fourth and fifth decades of life. **Cryptorchidism** and **gonadal dysgenesis** are risk factors for germ cell tumors. Patients present with painless enlargement of the testis. Grossly, classic seminomas are circumscribed and fleshy. Histologically, classic seminoma consists of sheets of large cells with distinct cell borders and nucleoli, infiltrated with **lymphocytes**. These cells are typically positive for **placental alkaline phosphatase** on immunohistochemical preparations. Because of the potential for seeding across fascial planes, biopsy is not recommended. Seminomas are very sensitive to radiation and chemotherapy.

Extratesticular Genital Ducts

DUCTUS EPIDIDYMIS

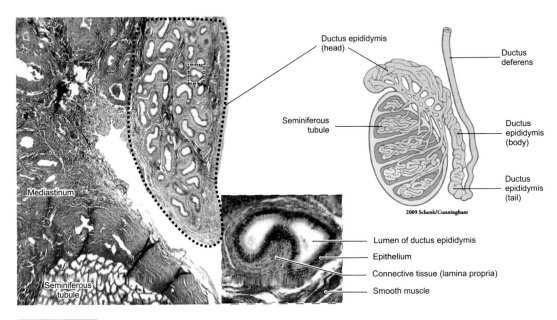

Figure 18-16.   Ductus epididymis. H&E, ×11; inset ×75

This is an example of the **ductus epididymis** in the head region. The ductus epididymis is a single highly convoluted tube about 4 to 5 m in length. It connects the **ductuli efferentes** to the **ductus deferens**. The ductus epididymis is lined by pseudostratified columnar epithelium with long stereocilia and is supported by connective tissue (lamina propria) and a circular smooth muscle layer in its wall. The ductus epididymis can be divided into three regions: **head, body,** and **tail.** The *head* of the ductus epididymis, also called the **initial region,** receives spermatozoa from the ductuli efferentes. The spermatozoa in the head of ductus epididymis are weak and unable to function effectively in fertilization. They pass through the *body* region with the help of contraction of the smooth muscle in the wall of the ductus epididymis and are stored in the *tail* region, where the spermatozoa undergo maturation. The maturation of the spermatozoa is influenced by androgenic hormones. The final step of maturation is called **capacitation** and occurs only after the spermatozoa enter the female reproductive tract. Capacitation enables sperm to penetrate and fertilize an egg.

Epididymitis is an inflammation of the epididymis. Common causes include *Chlamydia trachomatis, Escherichia coli,* and *Neisseria gonorrhoeae* infections. In the male, **urethritis** (an inflammation of the urethra) is often associated with epididymitis. Chronic epididymitis may result in infertility, because spermatozoa are stored and mature in the tail of the ductus epididymis.

Pathway for Sperm Conduction through the Genital Ducts

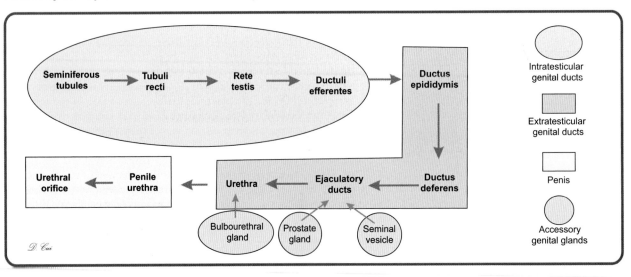

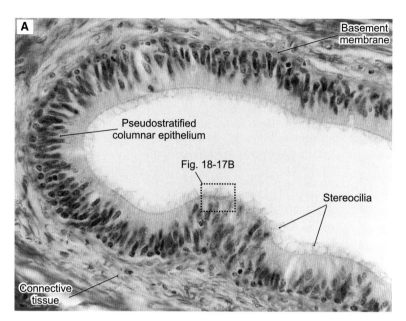

Basement membrane

Pseudostratified columnar epithelium

Fig. 18-17B

Stereocilia

Connective tissue

Figure 18-17A. Epithelium of the ductus epididymis. H&E, ×305

The **epithelium of the ductus epididymis** is a **pseudostratified columnar epithelium** composed of **basal cells** and **principal cells**. The *basal cells* are short with round nuclei; they are stem cells and are capable of differentiating into principal cells. The *principal cells* are columnar cells with elongated nuclei and apical stereocilia (long microvilli, 10 μm or more in length, which function in absorption but have no motile function). They absorb large volumes of testicular fluid. The principal cells also play an important role in the secretion of glycerophosphocholine, which inhibits **capacitation** of the premature sperm in the male reproductive tract. Normally, capacitation happens only after the sperm enters the female reproductive tract.

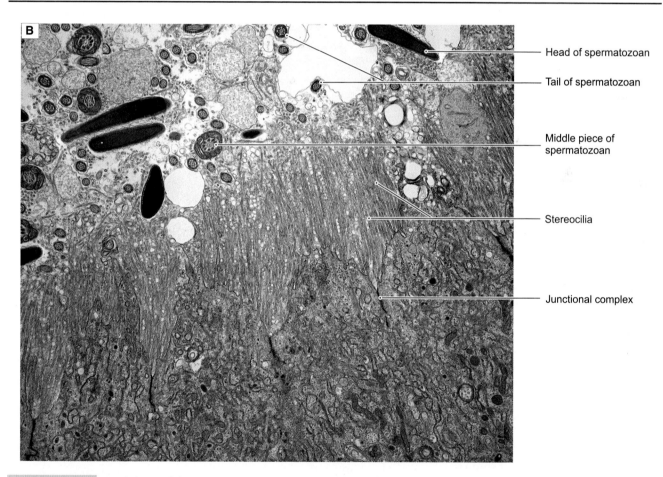

Head of spermatozoan

Tail of spermatozoan

Middle piece of spermatozoan

Stereocilia

Junctional complex

Figure 18-17B. Epithelium of the ductus epididymis. EM, ×5,900

The view here is limited to part of the lumen and the apical ends of the columnar epithelial cells forming the wall of the **ductus epididymis. Junctional complexes** between neighboring epithelial cells seal the contents of the lumen from the interstitial compartment underlying the epithelium. The extremely long microvilli (**stereocilia**) are a reflection of the large amount of testicular fluid that is resorbed by the ductus epididymis. The lumen is the site of storage and final maturation of the spermatozoa that have been delivered to the epididymis by the flow of the testicular fluid. Note the randomly oriented sections through the **heads, middle pieces,** and **tails** of **spermatozoa** in the lumen.

DUCTUS DEFERENS AND SPERMATIC CORD

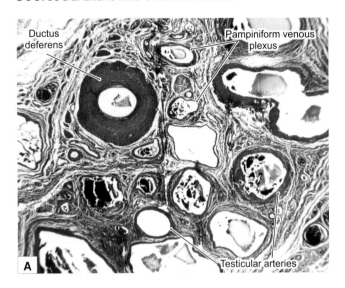

A

Labels: Ductus deferens; Pampiniform venous plexus; Testicular arteries

Figure 18-18A. Ductus deferens, spermatic cord. H&E, ×11

The **ductus deferens (vas deferens)** consists of bilateral tubes that continue from the tails of the left and right **ductus epididymis**. Each tube is about 30 to 40 cm long and is surrounded by a thick wall of smooth muscle. Each ductus deferens resides within a **spermatic cord** in its course from the testis through the abdominal wall to the penis. The distal portion of the ductus deferens becomes enlarged and is called the **ampulla**. The spermatic cord contains the **ductus deferens, testicular artery, pampiniform venous plexus, nerves**, and **lymphatic vessels** within the connective tissue.

The spermatic cord is a very long vascular strand containing the testicular vessels that provide the blood supply to the testis. If **testicular torsion** (twisted spermatic cord) occurs, acute testicular pain and necrosis of testis tissue may result because of interrupted blood supply from arteries or, more commonly, because of venous infarction.

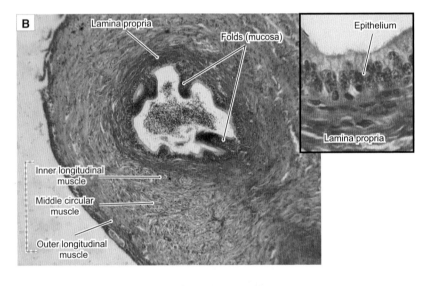

B

Labels: Lamina propria; Folds (mucosa); Epithelium; Lamina propria; Inner longitudinal muscle; Middle circular muscle; Outer longitudinal muscle

Figure 18-18B. Ductus deferens. H&E, ×69; inset ×476

The lining of the **ductus deferens**, like that of the epididymis, is pseudostratified columnar epithelium. The ductus deferens is characterized by fingerlike mucosal folds extending into the lumen. The thick muscularis contains inner longitudinal muscle, middle circular muscle, and outer longitudinal muscle, although these muscle layers are not easy to distinguish from one another. The outer longitudinal muscle is covered by an adventitia (connective tissue layer). The smooth muscle of the ductus deferens is richly innervated by postganglionic sympathetic nerve fibers, which initiate ejaculation when activated. The *inset* shows pseudostratified columnar epithelium with stereocilia of the ductus deferens.

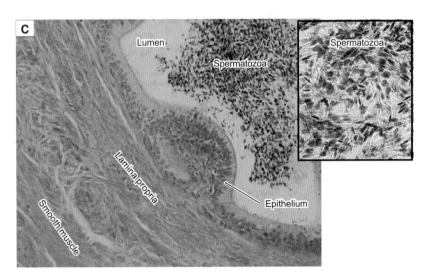

C

Labels: Lumen; Spermatozoa; Spermatozoa; Lamina propria; Smooth muscle; Epithelium

Figure 18-18C. Ductus deferens. van Gieson stain, ×139; inset ×476

An example of the **ductus deferens** with van Gieson stain is shown. The nuclei of the spermatozoa are brownish to black and are located in the lumen of the ductus deferens. Smooth muscle lies beneath the lamina propria.

A **vasectomy (deferentectomy)** is a surgical procedure for sterilization of the male. In this minor surgical procedure, both sides of the proximal portion of the ductus deferens are typically severed and sealed. The procedure prevents sperm from entering the urethra of the penis.

EJACULATORY DUCT AND PROSTATIC URETHRA

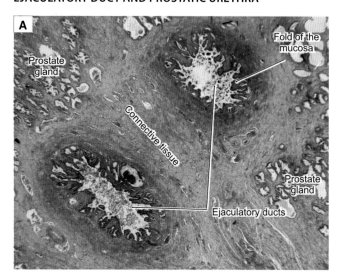

Figure 18-19A. Ejaculatory duct, prostate gland. H&E, ×11

The ampulla of the ductus deferens continues after it joins with the duct of the seminal vesicle to form the **ejaculatory duct**. The two ejaculatory ducts pass through the prostate gland to join with the urethra. Each ejaculatory duct is a short, straight tube (1–2 cm in length) and has a thin wall lined by **pseudostratified** (or **simple**) **columnar epithelium** and supported by connective tissue. Smooth muscle is present in the initial segment but disappears in most of the ejaculatory ducts. Here is an example of the two ejaculatory ducts within the prostate gland, surrounded by large amounts of connective tissue. The mucosa forms many folds extending into the lumen. The lumen may contain **prostatic concretions** (secretory material of the prostatic gland and often seen in older male patients).

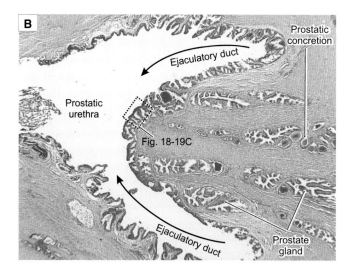

Figure 18-19B. Ejaculatory duct, prostate gland. H&E, ×34

The **ejaculatory ducts** penetrate the prostate gland and open into the **prostatic urethra**, at the **seminal colliculus** (also called the **verumontanum**), on the posterior wall of the prostatic urethra. This portion of the urethra has thick mucosa and shallow folds as shown here. The function of the ejaculatory ducts is to transport spermatozoa and seminal fluid into the prostatic urethra. The urethra includes three parts: the **prostatic urethra** (proximal part, near the bladder), the **membranous urethra** (intermediate part), and the **penile** (spongy) **urethra** (distal part). Prostatic concretions, also called **corpora amylacea**, are present in the lumen of the prostate gland shown here.

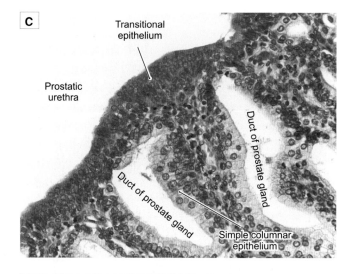

Figure 18-19C. Epithelium of the prostatic urethra. H&E, ×272

Where the two ejaculatory ducts merge with the prostatic urethra, the epithelium changes from simple or pseudostratified columnar to the transitional epithelium that is characteristic of the urinary system. Here is an example of **prostatic urethral epithelium** at higher magnification; it is taken from the *dashed box* indicated in Figure 18-19B. The epithelium of the duct of the prostate gland is simple columnar epithelium with round nuclei. The prostatic secretions are delivered into the prostatic urethra through numerous small ducts of the prostate gland.

Accessory Genital Glands

PROSTATE GLAND

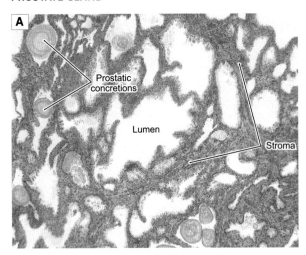

A Prostatic concretions
Lumen
Stroma

Figure 18-20A. Prostate gland. H&E, ×34

The **prostate gland** is similar to a chestnut in size and shape. It surrounds the initial portion of the urinary urethra (**prostatic urethra**) where the urethra exits the bladder. The prostate gland is penetrated by two **ejaculatory ducts** and the **urethra**. It contains many (about 30–50) highly **branched tubuloalveolar glands (compound tubuloalveolar glands)**. Each gland has a duct that empties its products into the **prostatic urethra**. The mucosa of the prostate gland is highly folded and is lined by simple columnar epithelium, which is supported by a stroma (thin layer of connective tissue strands with many smooth muscle cells). Here is an example of the prostate gland with its characteristically irregular lumen that may contain **prostatic concretions**. These concretions are also known as **corpora amylacea** and are more prominent in older men; they are composed of material secreted by the prostate gland.

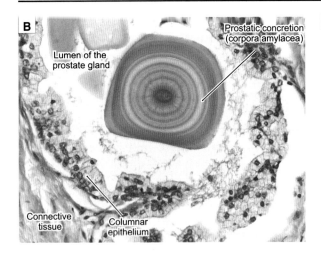

B Lumen of the prostate gland
Prostatic concretion (corpora amylacea)
Connective tissue
Columnar epithelium

Figure 18-20B. Prostate gland. H&E, ×272

A lumen in the **prostate gland** is shown housing a **prostatic concretion (corpora amylacea)**. This is composed of calcified prostatic secretions that typically display concentric rings. These structures increase in number with age. The secretion of the prostate gland contains **proteolytic enzymes, acid phosphatase, citric acid, fibrinolysin,** and **lipids**. The epithelial cells are columnar in shape with basally located round nuclei. The prostate gland produces secretions that empty into the urethra to mix with **spermatozoa** and **seminal vesicle fluid** to form semen. The prostatic secretion plays important roles in liquefying the coagulated semen, helping to expel the spermatozoa, and increasing their motility and survival rate after the semen has been transported into the female reproductive tract.

CLINICAL CORRELATION

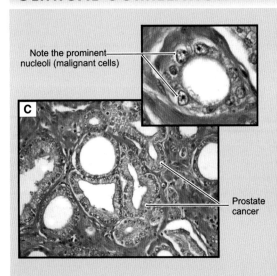

Note the prominent nucleoli (malignant cells)
C
Prostate cancer

Figure 18-20C. Prostate Cancer. H&E, ×96; inset ×164

Prostate cancer is the most common cancer in men and typically affects men over the age of 50 years. It can be seen in younger men but is unusual before the age of 40. The etiology of prostate cancer is elusive, but known risk factors include a positive family history, African American race, androgenic hormonal influences, and environmental factors. The majority of prostate cancers are adenocarcinomas arising from the glandular component of the prostate. Patients may present with urinary symptoms, such as difficulty initiating or stopping the urine stream, or **dysuria** (pain on urination). Other patients may first present with bone pain due to advanced metastatic disease. Many patients are diagnosed with prostate cancer through screening programs utilizing the digital rectal exam and the serum **prostate-specific antigen (PSA) test**, and a needle biopsy if indicated. Histologically, the appearance of prostate cancer is highly varied, from **well-formed tubular structures** to individual infiltrating **malignant cells**. Prostate cancers are graded histologically on the **Gleason system**, from 1 (well differentiated) to 5 (poorly differentiated). Treatment of prostate cancer may involve chemotherapy, hormonal manipulation, radiation therapy (external beam and radioactive implants), or radical prostatectomy. For some patients, particularly the elderly, watchful waiting may be a reasonable alternative.

SEMINAL VESICLES

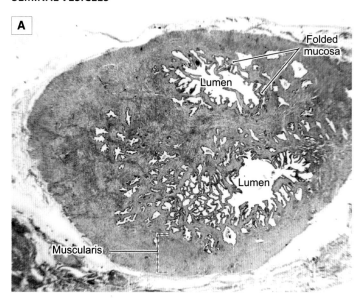

Figure 18-21A. Seminal vesicles. H&E, ×11

The **seminal vesicles** are paired glands that develop from the ductus deferens. Each seminal vesicle consists of a single highly convoluted tube with a duct that connects to the terminal portion (**ampulla**) of the **ductus deferens**. The ampulla of the ductus deferens is continuous with the ejaculatory duct. The mucosa of the seminal vesicles is extensively branched and folded and lined mostly by pseudostratified columnar epithelium. The epithelium is supported by a thin layer of connective tissue (**lamina propria**), and beneath it is the **muscularis** composed of **inner circular** and **outer longitudinal smooth muscle**. Contraction of the muscularis pushes the seminal secretion into the ejaculatory duct during ejaculation.

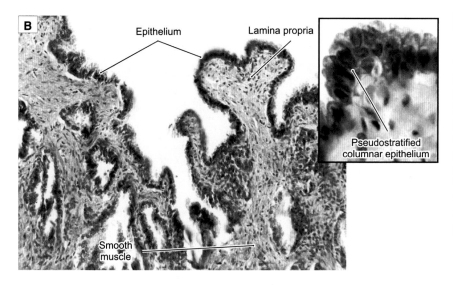

Figure 18-21B. Seminal vesicle. H&E, ×278; inset ×635

This is an example of the mucosa of the **seminal vesicle**. The **nonciliated, pseudostratified columnar epithelium** (*inset*), underlying **lamina propria**, and some **smooth muscle fibers** are shown here. The epithelium of the seminal vesicle varies from simple to pseudostratified columnar epithelium. The mucosa appears branched and folded. The epithelium contains basal cells and secretory cells with abundant rough endoplasmic reticulum and well-developed Golgi complexes.

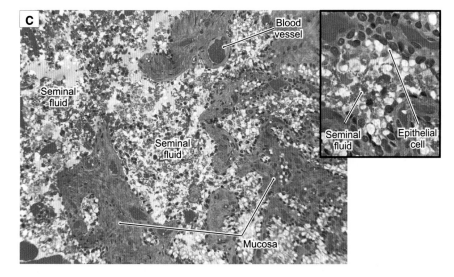

Figure 18-21C. Seminal vesicle with seminal fluid. H&E, ×139; inset ×328

The **seminal vesicles** produce large volumes of **seminal fluid**, which contributes about 70% of the volume of semen. Seminal fluid contains **fructose** and other **sugars, prostaglandins, flavins, phosphorylcholine, mucus, vitamin C,** and **proteins.** The *fructose* provides an energy source for sperm motility; the *flavins*, also known as **lipochrome pigment,** add a yellowish color to the seminal fluid and have a strong fluorescent quality under the ultraviolet light. The *inset* shows seminal epithelium and seminal fluid (viscous material) filling the lumen of a seminal vesicle.

Penis

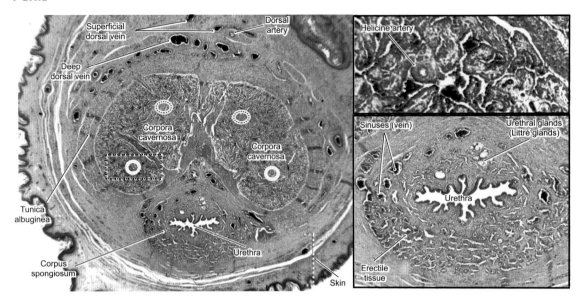

Figure 18-22.   Overview of the penis. H&E, ×13; inset (*upper*) ×67; inset (*lower*) ×26

The **penis** is composed of three cylinders of erectile tissue: the two **corpora cavernosa** and the **corpus spongiosum** as shown on the *left*. Each *cavernosa* is surrounded by a **tunica albuginea** (thick and dense connective tissue); the *corpus spongiosum* is surrounded by a thin layer of connective tissue with some smooth muscle fibers. The **penile (spongy) urethra** is enclosed in the center of the corpus spongiosum and extends into the terminal end (**glans**) of the penis. Each cylinder contains erectile tissue composed of a trabecular network of veins (**sinuses**) surrounded by collagen, elastic fibers, and smooth muscle cells. The three cylinders, with their tunica albuginea, are surrounded by hairless **thin skin** containing arteries, veins, nerves, and connective tissue and covered by stratified squamous epithelium. The two *red circles* indicate the position of the **deep arteries**; the *yellow circles* indicate the position of the **helicine arteries** in the corpora cavernosa.

The penis is supplied by the **dorsal arteries**, and blood drains into the **dorsal veins**. A special blood vessel arrangement called an **arteriovenous (A-V) shunt** allows blood to flow directly from arteries to veins. In the erect state, the arteriovenous shunt closes, which results in blood being forced from the **helicine arteries** into the sinuses (cavernous spaces) in the erectile tissue (*right upper inset*). Dilation of the sinuses produces **penile erection**. Erection is activated by parasympathetic stimulation through the spinal nerves and the sacral parasympathetic preganglionic motor neurons in the spinal cord (S2–S4). The *right lower* photomicrograph shows the penile urethra surrounded by **erectile tissue** and **sinuses** (veins) filled with blood. The **urethral glands** (**Littré glands**) are mucous glands in the submucosa of the penile urethra, also called **paraurethral (periurethral) glands**. The secretion of the urethral glands lubricates the urethra and contributes to the semen during ejaculation.

A clinical condition called **erectile dysfunction** is characterized by the inability to produce or maintain an erection of the penis. This happens due to insufficiency of dilation of the sinuses in the erectile tissue. The causes are varied, including hormonal disorders, neurological problems, hypertension, psychological factors, smoking, and alcohol use.

SYNOPSIS 18-3 Clinical and Pathologic Terms for the Male Reproductive System

- **IGCN:** Noninvasive intratubular or *in situ* lesions within the seminiferous tubules that give rise to the majority of adult germ cell tumors of the testis; IGCN is often found adjacent to testicular germ cell tumors on histologic examination.
- **Cryptorchidism:** Lack of, or incomplete, descent of a testis, from the abdominal cavity into the scrotum; the testis may remain intra-abdominal or be found in the inguinal canal; an undescended testis is a risk factor for the development of testicular tumors.
- **Gonadal dysgenesis:** Abnormal development of the gonads with resultant alterations in sexual development; gonadal dysgenesis is a risk factor for the development of testicular tumors; the underdeveloped gonad is often referred to as a "streak gonad."
- **PSA:** A protein synthesized by prostatic epithelial cells; elevated serum PSA levels are associated with benign processes such as benign prostatic hypertrophy as well as adenocarcinoma of the prostate; the PSA test is used as a screening test for prostate cancer as well as a tumor marker in patients with a history of prostate cancer who have received treatment.

From Histology to Pathology

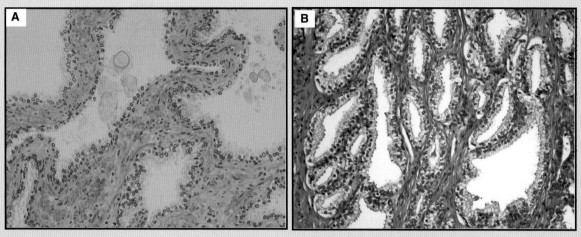

Figure 18-23.   Normal prostate glands and benign prostatic hyperplasia. H&E, ×100

Normal prostatic glands on the *left*. **Benign prostatic hyperplasia (BPH)** on the *right*. BPH is a common disorder that is usually seen in men older than age 50 years. Signs and symptoms of BPH are usually limited to the lower urinary tract, which include frequency of urination, nocturia, hesitancy, urgency, and weak urinary stream. Histologic examination of BPH specimens reveals hyperplasia with crowded and hyperplastic prostatic glands.

Clinical Vignette Questions

1. A 32-year-old man presented with an enlarging testicular mass that had been present for 8 months. He also complained of abdominal pain of slow onset, weakness, and numbness in the right lower extremity for 3 months. The patient was in good health until this episode had occurred, and he had never had any surgery. Physical examination revealed a 6-cm nontender mass in the right testis and tenderness over the right lower quadrant. Inguinal lymphadenopathy was palpable. Human α-fetoprotein level was within normal range. Ultrasonographic imaging showed a mass 6 cm in diameter. CT body scans showed a 12-cm retroperitoneal lesion encompassing the aorta and renal vasculature and pushing the right kidney laterally. No metastatic lesions were found above the diaphragm. A right orchiectomy was performed, followed by chemotherapy. What is the most likely diagnosis for this patient?

A. Testicular abscess
B. Testicular choriocarcinoma
C. Testicular hydrocele
D. Testicular seminoma
E. Testicular tuberculosis

2. A 62-year-old man was referred for further evaluation of urinary retention. The patient had a history of hypertension and obesity, and he smoked 15 cigarettes a day. He had been taking captopril, an angiotensin-converting enzyme inhibitor (ACEI) for his blood pressure. Findings at physical examination showed a blood pressure of 148/94 and an extremely enlarged prostate gland on digital rectal examination. Lab tests revealed slight proteinuria (30 mg/dL) without hematuria. Prostate-specific antigen (PSA) and α-fetoprotein were slightly elevated (5.60 and 52.5 ng/mL, respectively). CT scan showed an ~10-cm mass in the pelvis, which seemed to be arising from the prostate. No signs of metastasis in other parts of the urinary system were identified. Radical prostatectomy was performed 3 days later, and the prostatectomy specimen was fixed for 24 hours prior to sectioning and processing. Pathological examination revealed well-formed tubular structures with moderately differentiated cells showing prominent nucleoli. What is the most likely diagnosis for this patient?

A. Benign prostatic hyperplasia
B. Prostate adenocarcinoma
C. Prostatic sarcoidosis
D. Prostatitis
E. Urothelial carcinoma

19 Female Reproductive System

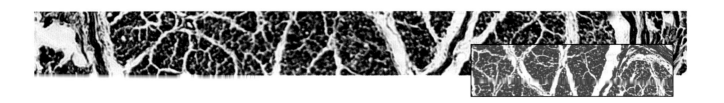

Introduction and Key Concepts for the Female Reproductive System

The **female reproductive system** comprises the **ovaries, uterine (fallopian) tubes, uterus, vagina, external genitalia,** and **mammary glands.** The *external genitalia* (vulva) includes the **labia minora, labia majora, mons pubis, clitoris,** and **vestibule.** Female secondary sex characteristics appear at puberty, along with the monthly menstrual cycle. This cycle of changes in the reproductive system is influenced by interactions among the hypothalamus, pituitary gland, ovaries, and uterus; related events occur periodically during each menstrual cycle. The menstrual cycle is influenced by hormones including **follicle-stimulating hormone (FSH), luteinizing hormone (LH), estrogen,** and **progesterone.** These hormones cause changes in the female reproductive organs and their functions, promote development of follicles and oocytes, and produce an ideal environment for fertilization, implantation, and fetal growth. The female reproductive system plays an important role in the **production** and **regulation** of female hormones (estrogen and progesterone) and in the development and maintenance of female sex characteristics.

Ovaries

The **ovaries** are paired, almond-shaped structures located in the upper part of the pelvic cavity. Their size and position vary depending on the age and reproductive state of the individual. The ovaries are suspended by the **mesovarium** of the broad ligament and are attached to the uterus by the ligament of the ovary. Each ovary has a **cortex** and **medulla**. The *cortex* contains numerous **developing follicles** in various stages as well as **postovulatory structures**, a **corpus luteum**, and several **corpora albicans**. Each developing follicle contains an **oocyte**. The *medulla* is composed of loose connective tissue and blood vessels, nerve fibers, and lymphatic vessels.

1. *Primordial follicles:* In the earliest stage of follicular development, **primordial follicles** rest at the periphery of the cortex. Each primordial follicle consists of a **primary oocyte** surrounded by a single layer of squamous supporting cells called **follicular cells**. The **oocyte** is small (about 20–30 μm) and is in prophase (**dictyotene**) of meiosis I. The nucleus of the oocyte has a pale appearance and contains decondensed chromatin.
2. *Primary follicles:* At puberty, the primordial follicles begin to grow, the oocyte increases its size, and the supporting follicle cells also increase in size and become cuboidal cells. These follicle cells are now called **granulosa cells**. When the oocyte of the **primary follicle** is surrounded by a single layer of granulosa cells, the follicle is called a **unilaminar primary follicle**. As the oocyte increases in size, the granulosa cells build up more layers, and the follicle is called a **multilaminar primary follicle**. The **zona pellucida**, a gel-like layer between the oocyte and the granulosa cells, first appears in the multilaminar primary follicle.
3. *Secondary follicles:* As granulosa cells continue to proliferate, the follicle size increases, and spaces filled with follicular fluid (**liquor folliculi**) develop among the cells. These spaces merge to become a single large space called the **antrum**. The stromal cells that cover the follicle develop into a layer called the **theca folliculi**. The theca folliculi is well developed in the **secondary follicle**, and it includes the **theca interna** and **theca externa**.
4. *Graafian (preovulatory) follicle:* In its final stage, the follicle reaches a maximum size of up to 25 mm (2.5 cm). This follicle has a large antrum filled with liquor folliculi. It has reached its mature stage and is ready to release the oocyte (**ovulation**). The oocyte has reached its maximum size and is embedded in a mound of granulosa cells that protrude into the antrum. The granulosa cells that are in immediate

contact with the oocyte are called the **corona radiata** and remain with the oocyte at ovulation. The **graafian follicle** bulges from the surface of the ovary. In response to a sharp increase in the level of LH (**LH surge**), the oocyte resumes meiotic division, becomes arrested as a **secondary oocyte**, and ovulation then occurs.
5. *Postovulatory structures:* After ovulation, the remainder of the graafian follicle develops into the **corpus luteum** and continues to produce steroid hormones. If fertilization and implantation occur, the corpus luteum will remain active and continue to produce progesterone during the first 6 months of pregnancy. If fertilization does not occur, the corpus luteum degenerates after 10 to 14 days and becomes the **corpus albicans**.

Uterine (Fallopian) Tubes (Oviducts)

The uterine (fallopian) tubes, also called oviducts, are paired, muscular, open-ended tubes that receive the ovum and provide an ideal environment for fertilization. Each **uterine (fallopian) tube** has four regions: the **infundibulum, ampulla, isthmus,** and **intramural portion**. Fertilization usually occurs in the ampulla of the uterine (fallopian) tube. The uterine (fallopian) tube wall has a **mucosa** containing ciliated cells and secretory (peg) cells in its epithelium, a **muscularis layer**, and a **serosa** outer covering.

Uterus

The **uterus** is a pear-shaped muscular organ that connects to the two uterine (fallopian) tubes and to the vagina via the cervix. It is the site for **implantation** and **placentation**. *Implantation* is the attachment of the **blastocyst** to the uterine wall; *placentation* is the establishment of a **placenta** that nourishes the developing embryo and fetus via the **umbilical cord**. The uterus has a thick wall, which consists of **endometrium** (mucosa), **myometrium** (muscularis), and **serosa**. The uterus can be divided into three regions: the **fundus, body,** and **cervix**. The endometrium undergoes the following morphological and functional changes during the menstrual cycle.

1. *Menstrual phase:* This is the initial stage (from days 1 to 4 of the cycle). The functional layer (**functionalis**) of the endometrium sloughs off and bleeds about 2 weeks after ovulation if fertilization does not occur.
2. *Proliferative phase:* Following the menstrual phase (days 5–14 of the cycle), the functionalis of the endometrium recovers and rebuilds itself. Its glands appear straight, and its surface is smooth.
3. *Secretory phase:* At this phase (days 15–28 of the cycle), the endometrium becomes ready for implantation. The endometrium thickens, and the glands appear coiled with large lumens and a sawtooth appearance. These changes are mainly influenced by **progesterone**. If a **blastocyst**

becomes embedded in the endometrium (**implantation**), the development of the placenta takes place within a short time.

Vagina

The **vagina** is a muscular tube that connects the cervix to the external genitalia. It consists of **mucosa, muscularis,** and **adventitia** and functions as a copulatory organ and birth passage.

Mammary Glands

The **mammary glands** are paired exocrine glands located beneath the skin on the chest. These glands can be classified as **compound tubuloalveolar glands**. In the female, the mammary glands undergo morphological and functional changes in response to female hormones (**estrogen, progesterone**). In later pregnancy, the mammary glands prepare to produce milk (**lactation**) for the newborn infant.

SYNOPSIS 19-1 Clinical and Pathologic Terms for the Female Reproductive System

- *Endophytic:* Term to describe an inward-growing process such as a neoplasm that grows on the interior of an organ.
- *Exophytic:* Term to describe an outward-growing process such as a neoplasm that grows externally on an organ or within the lumen of an organ.
- *Hemoperitoneum:* Blood within the peritoneal cavity because of a variety of causes including trauma, rupture of a tumor, or rupture of an ectopic pregnancy.
- *Menorrhagia:* Refers to excessive or prolonged uterine bleeding at regular intervals during menstruation; some causes include uterine leiomyomas, anovulation and ovarian dysfunction, hormonal imbalance, bleeding tendency, and malignancy.
- *Metrorrhagia:* Refers to uterine bleeding at irregular intervals often at times between the expected menstrual periods; causes may be similar to menorrhagia and include hormonal imbalance, malignancy, uterine polyps, and bleeding tendency.
- *Nulliparity:* Term used to describe never having given birth to a child; by contrast, a woman who has given birth to two or more children is termed *multiparous.*

Anatomy of the Female Organs

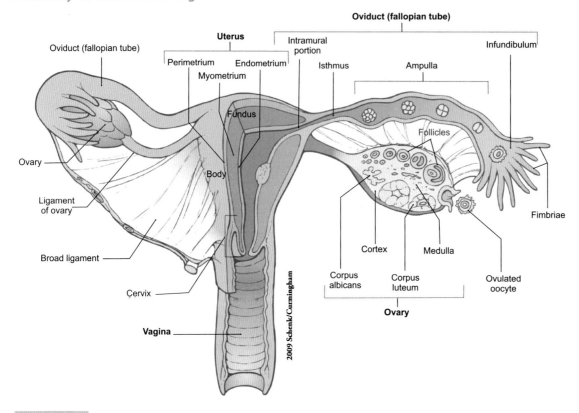

Figure 19-1. Overview of the female organs.

The **female reproductive system** functions in reproduction and the secretion of female hormones that maintain female sex characteristics. It consists of two **ovaries**, two **uterine (fallopian) tubes**, the **uterus**, the **vagina, external genitalia**, and two **mammary glands**. Each *ovary* has a **medulla** and **cortex** that contain different stages of the **developing follicles, corpus luteum**, and **corpus albicans**. The uterine (fallopian) tube is a muscular tube, which captures and transports the ovulated oocyte and functions as the normal site of fertilization. It can be divided into the **infundibulum, ampulla, isthmus**, and **intramural portions**. The *uterus* is a thick-walled chamber that can be divided into three regions: the **fundus, body**, and **cervix**. The *fundus* and *body* of the uterus are composed of **endometrium, myometrium**, and **serosa**; the endometrium undergoes extensive changes during the menstrual cycle. The mucosa of the *cervix* does not undergo structural changes during the menstrual cycle; however, secretions of the mucosa change based on hormone levels during the menstrual cycle. Most of the female organs undergo some degree of change during the menstrual cycle in response to changes in levels of various hormones.

Structures of the Female Reproductive System

I. **Ovaries**
   A. Cortex (contains ovarian follicles and connective tissue)
      1. Primordial (resting) follicles
      2. Primary (growing) follicles
      3. Secondary (antral) follicles
      4. Graafian follicle
      5. Corpus luteum (postovulatory structure)
      6. Corpus albicans (postovulatory structure)
   B. Medulla (contains loose connective tissue, blood vessels, lymphatic vessels, and nerve fibers)

II. **Uterine/fallopian tubes** (contain mucosa, muscularis, and serosa)
   A. Infundibulum
   B. Ampulla
   C. Isthmus
   D. Intramural portion

III. **Uterus** (contains endometrium, myometrium, and serosa)
   A. Menstrual cycle
      1. Proliferative phase
      2. Secretory phase
      3. Menstrual phase

IV. **Cervix** (contains mucosa, branched cervical glands, dense connective tissue, and a few smooth muscle cells)
   A. Internal os (opening of cervix)
   B. Endocervical canal (portion between uterus and external os)
   C. External os (opening of ectocervix)
   D. Ectocervix (portion that projects into the vagina)

V. **Vagina** (contains mucosa, muscularis, and adventitia)

VI. **Mammary gland**
   A. Compound tubuloalveolar glands
   B. Lactiferous sinuses
   C. Lactiferous ducts
   D. Nipple

Figures and Images Orientation

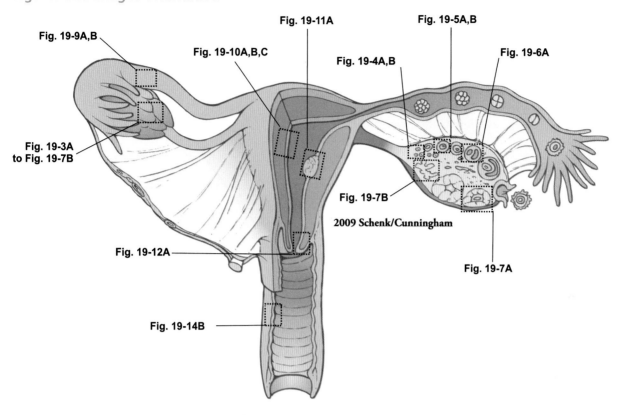

Fig. 19-11A

Fig. 19-5A,B

Fig. 19-9A,B

Fig. 19-10A,B,C

Fig. 19-6A

Fig. 19-4A,B

Fig. 19-3A to Fig. 19-7B

Fig. 19-7B

2009 Schenk/Cunningham

Fig. 19-12A

Fig. 19-7A

Fig. 19-14B

Figure 19-2. Orientation of detailed female reproductive system illustrations.

Structures of the Female Reproductive System with Figure Numbers

Ovaries
Figure 19-3A
Figure 19-3B
Figure 19-4A
Figure 19-4B
Figure 19-5A
Figure 19-5B
Figure 19-6A
Figure 19-6B
Figure 19-7A
Figure 19-7B
Figure 19-7C

Uterine (Fallopian) Tube (Oviduct)
Figure 19-9A
Figure 19-9B

Uterus
Figure 19-10A
Figure 19-10B
Figure 19-10C
Figure 19-11A
Figure 19-11B

Figure 19-12A
Figure 19-12B
Figure 19-12C

Cervix
Figure 19-13A
Figure 19-13B

Placenta
Figure 19-14A
Figure 19-14B

Umbilical cord
Figure 19-15A

Vagina
Figure 19-15B

Mammary glands
Figure 19-16A
Figure 19-16B
Figure 19-16C
Figure 19-16A
Figure 19-16B

Ovaries

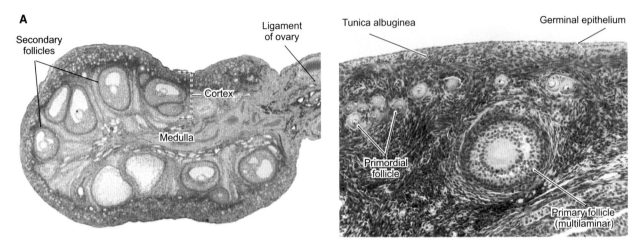

Figure 19-3A.   Overview of the ovary. H&E, left ×17; right ×129

The **ovaries** are paired organs covered by a simple, usually cuboidal, mesothelium (sometimes called **germinal epithelium**) and a tunica albuginea (connective tissue). Each ovary is divided into a **cortex** and a **medulla**. The *cortex* contains various stages of follicles including **primordial follicles, primary follicles, secondary follicles**, and, occasionally, **graafian follicles**. It may also contain the **corpus luteum**, a temporary endocrine gland formed by components of an ovulated follicle. A degenerated corpus luteum persists in the ovary as the **corpus albicans**. Most follicles degenerate (undergo **atresia**) before ovulation and are then called **atretic follicles**. The *medulla* contains connective tissue with blood vessels, nerve fibers, and lymphatic vessels.

STAGES OF OVARIAN FOLLICLES

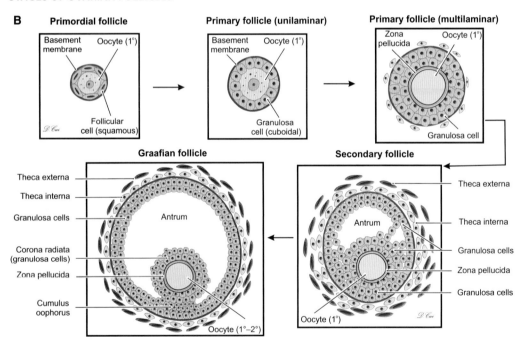

Figure 19-3B.   Development of the ovarian follicles.

This illustration shows **ovarian follicles** from early to late stages: the **primordial (resting) follicle**, the unilaminar **primary follicle**, the multilaminar **primary (growing) follicle**, the **secondary (antral or vesicular) follicle**, and the graafian (preovulatory) follicle. Each of these follicles contains a **primary (1 degree) oocyte**, which is an immature ovum. A **secondary oocyte** is formed shortly before ovulation, when the oocyte completes the first meiotic division. The secondary oocyte does not undergo the second meiotic division unless fertilization occurs. Note that the follicles are not drawn to scale; a graafian (preovulatory) follicle is ~1,000 times the diameter of a primordial follicle.

PRIMORDIAL FOLLICLES

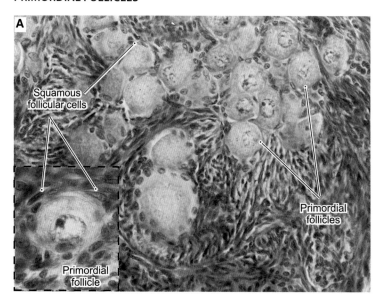

Figure 19-4A. Primordial follicles, ovary. H&E, ×290; inset ×110

Primordial follicles are the smallest and most numerous types of follicles in the cortex of the ovary. Each primordial follicle contains a **germ cell** (**primary oocyte**) in a resting state that may persist for as long as 50 years. The primary oocyte is surrounded by a layer of **squamous cells** called **follicular cells**. These follicular cells are somatic cells that support the oocyte. The oocyte has a pale appearance and a large nucleus with a prominent nucleolus. About 1 million follicles are present in the ovaries at the time of birth; however, only a few hundred of these follicles become mature. The follicles begin to grow at puberty, and there is a constant loss of follicles throughout the reproductive years. At menopause, only a few follicles remain.

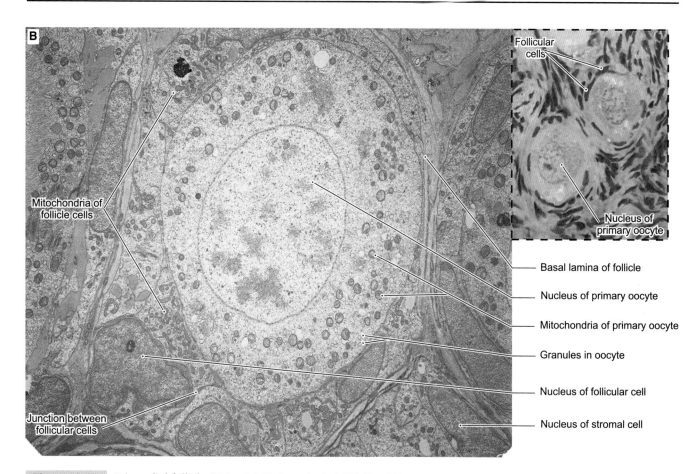

Figure 19-4B. Primordial follicle. EM, ×3,900; inset (*color*) H&E, ×500

The **primary oocyte** at the center of this **primordial follicle** may appear to be in interphase of the cell cycle, but it is arrested in **dictyotene** of prophase I of meiosis. What appear to be patches of heterochromatin in the nucleus are partially decondensed tetrads composed of paired homologous chromosomes. The oocyte has been in prophase of meiosis I before birth of the individual. Follicular cells form a simple squamous epithelium that surrounds the oocyte. Note that these cells adhere tightly to the surface of the oocyte. Indeed, there are junctions between the oocyte and the follicle cells, although they are not readily identifiable here. Neighboring follicular cells are also connected by junctional complexes, and there is a basal lamina between the follicular cells and the surrounding interstitial tissue of the ovarian cortex.

PRIMARY FOLLICLES

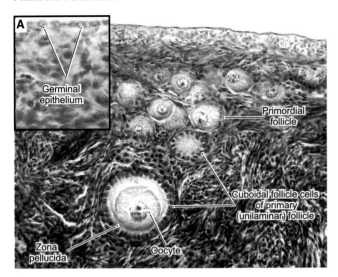

Figure 19-5A. Primary follicles, ovary. H&E, ×202; inset ×438

Primary follicles develop from primordial follicles. Each primary follicle consists of a **primary oocyte** and **cuboidal follicle cells**. These follicle cells increase in height (from squamous cells to cuboidal cells), and their cellular layers gradually increase as the follicle continues to grow. At this stage, follicle cells are called **granulosa cells**, because their cytoplasm begins to have a granular appearance. The primary follicles can be classified into **unilaminar primary follicles** and **multilaminar primary follicles**. The *unilaminar primary follicle* has a single layer of cuboidal granulosa cells with a smaller oocyte. The *multilaminar primary follicle* has several layers of cuboidal granulosa cells surrounding a relatively large oocyte. As the oocyte increases its size, the **zona pellucida** emerges as an amorphous layer between the surface of the oocytes and the surrounding granulosa cells. Situated outside of the basement membrane of the granulosa cells are stromal cells that flatten and develop into a sheath that surrounds the follicle; this layer is called the **theca folliculi.**

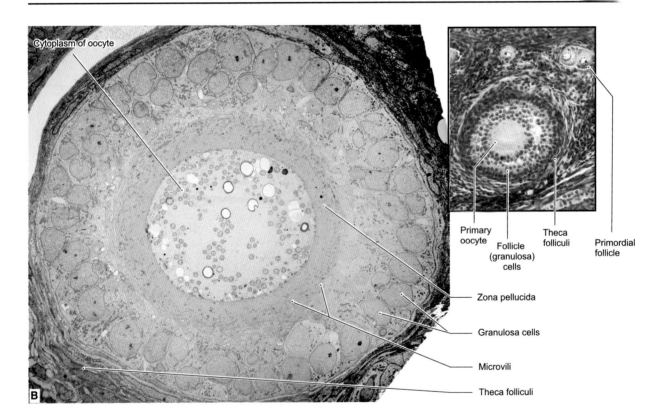

Figure 19-5B. Growing (primary) follicle. EM, ×3,200; inset (*color*); H&E, ×152

The **oocyte** in the center of this **growing follicle** has been sectioned off center so that the nucleus is not shown. Although the oocyte has begun to grow, it is still arrested in prophase of meiosis I. Note the membrane-bound vesicles in the cytoplasm of the oocyte; these will participate in the cortical granule reaction if the oocyte becomes fertilized. The follicle cells that surrounded the oocyte have proliferated and transformed into **granulosa cells**. At this stage, the granulosa comprises about two layers of cuboidal cells. The inner granulosa cells no longer have smooth close contact with the surface of the oocyte because a layer of amorphous extracellular material, the **zona pellucida**, has developed. As the granulosa cells continue to proliferate, several layers of cells will accumulate, and ultimately, a fluid-filled space, the **antrum**, will develop. Changes are also underway in the stroma adjacent to the growing follicle. The stromal cells (**fibroblasts**) have become concentrated and flattened against the basal lamina of the granulosa. These **theca folliculi cells** will develop properties of steroid hormone–synthesizing cells if development of the follicle continues.

SECONDARY AND GRAAFIAN FOLLICLES

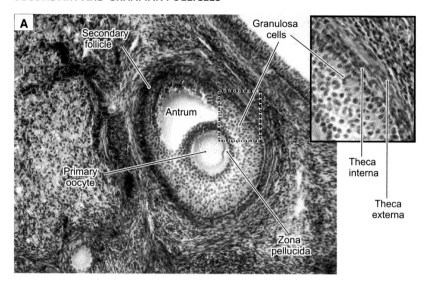

Figure 19-6A. Secondary follicles, ovary. H&E, ×108; inset ×211

The **secondary follicle** develops from the continued growth of the **multilaminar primary follicle**. Spaces filled with **follicular fluid (liquor folliculi)** appear among the granulosa cells within the secondary follicle. These spaces gradually merge to form a single large space called the **antrum**. The **zona pellucida** is distinct, and the theca folliculi (surrounding the follicle) develops into the **theca interna** and **theca externa**. The *theca interna* is the inner vascular layer containing cuboidal (steroid-producing) secretory cells. These cells secrete **androgens**, which diffuse into the granulosa cells where they are converted into **estrogens** in response to FSH. The *theca externa* is an outer connective tissue layer containing mainly collagen and some small squamous cells mixed with a few smooth muscle cells.

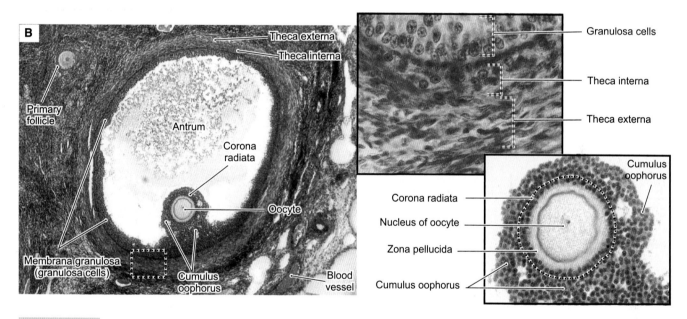

Figure 19-6B. Graafian follicles, ovary. H&E, ×54; inset (*upper*) ×429; inset (*lower*) ×178

The **graafian follicle** is a mature follicle; it is also called a **preovulatory follicle**. At this stage, the follicle has grown to a large size (about 25 mm) and bulges from the surface of the ovary. The decreased number of granulosa cells and increased volume of fluid in the **antrum** result in the oocyte being located at the periphery of the follicle. The **membrana granulosa** is formed by multiple cellular layers of granulosa cells lining the inner wall of the antrum. Some granulosa cells form a hillock called the **cumulus oophorus**, which supports and houses the oocyte. The inner granulosa cells of the **cumulus oophorus** form a single layer called the **corona radiata**, which immediately surrounds the oocyte. As the follicle grows, most of the granulosa cells gradually loosen from the cumulus oophorus, but the corona radiata remains in contact with the oocyte. Eventually, the oocyte, with the corona radiata, floats freely in the antrum before ovulation. The oocyte remains as a primary oocyte in the graafian follicle until pituitary secretion of LH increases sharply (**LH surge**); this stimulates the primary oocyte to complete the **first meiotic division** and become a **secondary oocyte**. The secondary oocyte with the corona radiata and **polar body** (from the first oocyte division) are released from the graafian follicle of the ovary. After the secondary oocyte reaches the **ampulla** of the uterine **(fallopian) tube**, the **second meiotic division** occurs, if fertilization takes place. A spermatozoan must penetrate the corona radiata and zona pellucida to complete the fertilization process. The *upper inset* shows the **theca folliculi** (**theca interna** and **theca externa**). The *lower inset* shows the oocyte surrounded by granulosa cells.

The **ovarian cycle** is under the control of the hormones **FSH** and **LH** produced by the **gonadotrophs** of the **anterior pituitary gland**. *FSH* stimulates **estrogen** production and follicular growth; *LH* stimulates meiotic division of the **primary oocyte**, ovulation, and development of the **corpus luteum**. The **estrogens** play an important role in the stimulation of follicle growth by promoting proliferation of the **granulosa cells**, and they also stimulate the mammary glands to prepare for **lactation**.

POSTOVULATION STRUCTURES: CORPUS LUTEUM AND CORPUS ALBICANS

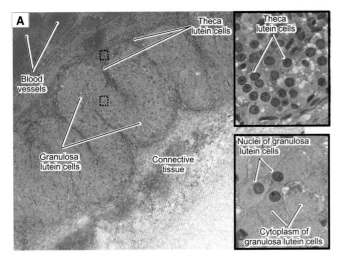

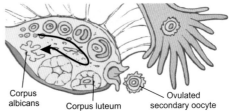

Figure 19-7A. Corpus luteum, ovary. H&E, ×36; insets ×363

After ovulation, the remaining portion (wall) of the graafian follicle transforms into the **corpus luteum** (yellow body). The wall of the corpus luteum is folded and contains **granulosa lutein cells** (derived from granulosa cells) and **theca lutein cells** (from the theca interna). The *granulosa lutein cells* are large and have pale cytoplasm; these cells have features of steroid hormone–producing cells, and they produce primarily **progesterone**. The *theca lutein cells* are smaller but also have features of steroid hormone–secreting cells; these cells secrete primarily progesterone and androgens.

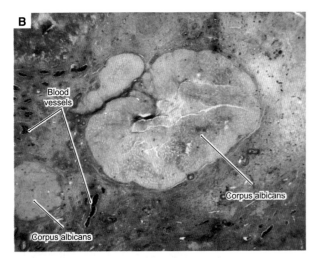

Figure 19-7B. Corpus albicans, ovary. H&E, ×34

In the absence of fertilization, the **corpus luteum** is active only for a short period of time (10–14 days). The corpus luteum degenerates, decreases in size, and forms a structure called the **corpus albicans**. The corpus albicans consists of dense connective tissue that appears as a white scar; it gradually decreases in size and remains in the ovary for months to years. However, if fertilization and implantation occur, the corpus luteum is rescued from degeneration by **human chorionic gonadotropin (hCG) hormone** from the **placenta**. During pregnancy, the corpus luteum will remain active until the placenta takes over progesterone secretion. The corpus luteum degenerates around the 12th week of pregnancy. Formation of the corpus luteum is stimulated by the **LH surge**.

CLINICAL CORRELATION

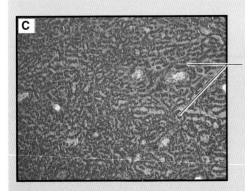

Granulosa cell tumor with neoplastic cells arranged in cords

Figure 19-7C. Granulosa Cell Tumor. H&E, ×52

Granulosa cell tumor of the ovary is a **neoplasm** composed of ovarian granulosa and, occasionally, theca cells. Granulosa cell tumors may arise at any age and are divided into **juvenile** and **adult** types. These tumors may produce excess **estrogen**, the result of which may cause **precocious puberty, endometrial hyperplasia,** and **endometrial cancer**. Symptoms may include abdominal pain, **hemoperitoneum** with hypotension, and mimicking an ectopic pregnancy in younger patients because of rupture of the tumor. Histologically, the tumor cells are small and cuboidal and may be arranged in a variety of patterns including solid, trabecular, and cordlike. The tumor cells often contain a groove resembling a coffee bean. Small follicle-like structures named **Call-Exner bodies** may be visible in well-differentiated tumors. The behavior of granulosa cell tumors is variable and may take an aggressive course in some patients. A total **abdominal hysterectomy** and **bilateral salpingo-oophorectomy** are the treatments of choice in the early stage.

Hormonal Regulation and the Female Reproductive Cycle

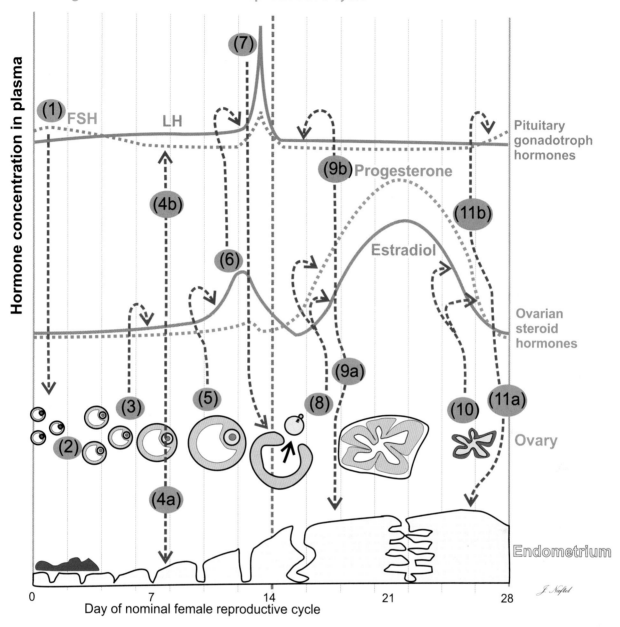

Figure 19-8. Events of the female reproductive cycle.

The following sequence of events refers to the numbered events labeled in *red* in the diagram above. (1) At the beginning of the **female reproductive cycle**, there are rising levels of **gonadotropic hormones** from the anterior pituitary, most importantly **FSH**. (2) This rise promotes ovarian recruitment of a cohort of antral follicles to proceed into advanced development and then selection of typically a single dominant follicle at about day 6. (3) These follicles secrete steroid hormones, most prominently estrogens, that (4a) promote rebuilding of the endometrium (**proliferative phase**) and (4b) exert a negative feedback on FSH secretion by pituitary gonadotropes. (5) In the latter part of the **follicular phase**, the dominant follicle secretes increasing amounts of estrogens (and, to a lesser extent, progesterone). (6) When circulating estrogen reaches a threshold level (about 200 pg/mL) for a duration of about 36 hours, pituitary gonadotropes are stimulated to sharply increase secretion of gonadotropic hormones—most importantly, LH. (7) This **LH surge** from the pituitary brings about final maturation of the dominant follicle culminating in ovulation (about 40 hours after initiation of the LH surge) and formation of the **corpus luteum** from the remaining components of the follicle. (8) The corpus luteum secretes progesterone as well as estrogens. (9a) This induces a change in the endometrium from the proliferative phase to the **secretory phase**. (9b) Meanwhile, gonadotropin secretion is greatly reduced, probably because of negative feedback effects of the high progesterone and estrogen levels coming from the corpus luteum. (10) Without LH support, the corpus luteum fails after about 10 days, and steroid hormone levels fall. (11a) This loss of steroid hormone support results in degenerative changes in the endometrium culminating in **menstruation**. (11b) The fall in progesterone also releases the pituitary gonadotropes from negative feedback with the result that FSH secretion starts to rise toward the end of the cycle, and this starts another round of follicle recruitment.

Uterine (Fallopian) Tube

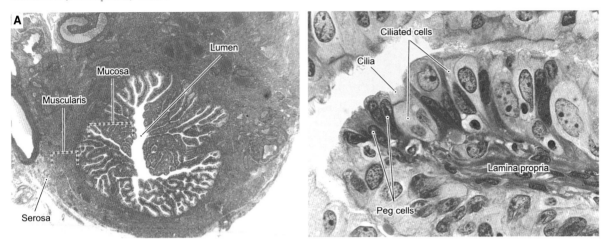

Figure 19-9A. Uterine (fallopian) tube (oviduct). H&E, left ×17; right ×680

The uterine (fallopian) tube is also called the **oviduct**. It can be divided into four regions: the **infundibulum, ampulla, isthmus**, and **intramural portion**. The *infundibulum* is a funnel-shaped opening that has a fringe of tentacle-like extensions called **fimbriae**. The *ampulla* has a relatively large, labyrinthine lumen where fertilization usually takes place. The *isthmus* is a narrow portion of the uterine (fallopian) tube, close to the uterus. The *intramural portion* is the terminal segment and is located within the uterine wall. The wall of the uterine (fallopian) tube consists of a **mucosa** (simple columnar epithelium and lamina propria), **muscularis** (inner circular and outer longitudinal smooth muscle), and **serosa**. The epithelium of the uterine (fallopian) tube contains **ciliated cells** and **peg cells**. The cells vary in height according to hormonal stimulation. The uterine (fallopian) tube provides an ideal environment for the fertilization of the oocyte and initial development of the embryo as well as transportation of the **zygote** (fertilized oocyte) to the uterus. On the *left* is a low-magnification view of the ampulla; on the *right* is a higher magnification view of the mucosa. *Ciliated cells* help sweep the oocyte toward the uterus. Each ciliated cell has a pale appearance with many cilia on its apical surface. These cells have a large nucleus and a fair amount of cytoplasm. *Peg cells* are secretory cells that produce nutrient-rich secretions to nourish and protect the oocyte and promote fertilization. They are small in size and interspersed among the ciliated cells.

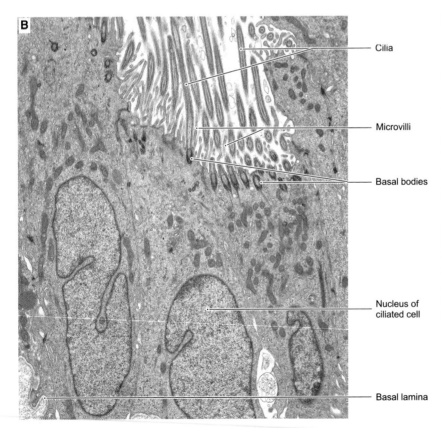

Figure 19-9B. Epithelial cells lining the uterine (fallopian) tube (oviduct). EM, ×8,900

The **simple columnar epithelium** that lines the uterine/fallopian tube (oviduct) is composed of two cell types (**ciliated cells** and **peg cells**); only *ciliated cells* are shown here. These ciliated cells function, along with smooth muscle of the muscularis, in mixing the contents (**gametes**) of the lumen and in transporting the oocyte and zygote at a precisely controlled rate along the length of the lumen of the uterine (fallopian) tube. The number and activity of cilia change in response to changes in the levels of steroid hormones throughout the reproductive cycle, reaching a peak at the time of ovulation when estrogens dominate. Note that these cells also bear numerous **microvilli**, suggesting an additional absorptive function.

Uterus

PHASE OF THE ENDOMETRIUM

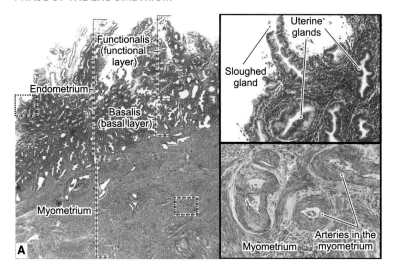

A

Figure 19-10A. Menstrual phase of the endometrium, uterus (days 1–4 of the cycle). H&E, ×13; insets ×93

The wall of the **uterus** includes the **endometrium**, the **myometrium**, and serosa. The endometrium, the mucosa of the uterus, is composed of a surface epithelium and simple tubular **uterine glands** within a stroma of connective tissue. The endometrium consists of the **basalis (basal layer)** and the **functionalis (functional layer)**. The functionalis is near the lumen and undergoes changes during the menstrual cycle. During the **menstrual phase**, the functionalis sloughs off as a result of **ischemia** and **necrosis** caused by contraction of the coiled arteries. This occurs when fertilization does not take place and the corpus luteum atrophies, causing the levels of **estrogen** and **progesterone** to fall. The menstrual phase is the initial stage of the menstrual cycle; the endometrium will begin to recover at the end of the menstrual phase.

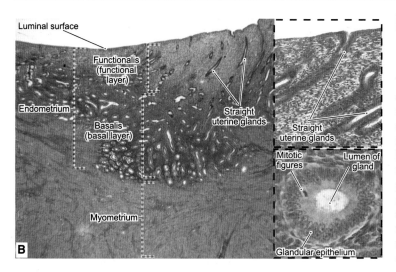

B

Figure 19-10B. Proliferative phase of the endometrium, uterus (days 5–14 of the cycle). H&E, ×18; inset (*upper*) ×68; inset (*lower*) ×293

The **proliferative phase** follows the menstrual phase. The epithelium, uterine glands, and connective tissue of the functionalis are rebuilt by proliferation and differentiation of cells that remained in the basalis. At this stage, the uterine glands are straight and have narrow lumens as shown here; the surface of the endometrium is smooth. The epithelial lining of the uterine glands commonly appears as **pseudostratified columnar epithelium** because of proliferation of the lining cells. **Mitotic figures** are occasionally seen (*inset*). The glands open onto the luminal surface of the uterus. During the proliferative phase, the changes in the endometrium are driven by **estrogens** that are produced by the granulosa cells of the developing follicles.

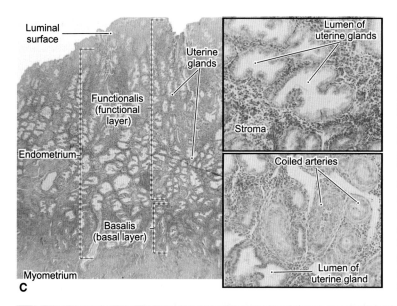

C

Figure 19-10C. Secretory phase of the endometrium, uterus (days 15–28 of the cycle). H&E, ×14; insets ×89

The **secretory phase** begins shortly after ovulation occurs. It is influenced by **progesterone** produced by the corpus luteum. At this stage, the endometrium becomes thickest (6–7 mm), and the uterine glands are coiled and have large sacculated lumens. The *upper inset* shows tortuous glands with large, irregular, sawtooth-shaped lumens. The *lower inset* shows coiled arteries found in the endometrial stroma. These coiled arteries are also called **spiral arteries** and extend transiently from the basalis into the functionalis of the endometrium. The coiled arteries arise from arcuate arteries of the myometrium. During the secretory phase, these spiral arteries become elongated and highly coiled and extend into the functionalis of the endometrium. The arcuate arteries also give rise to straight arteries that permanently supply the basalis.

BLOOD SUPPLY TO THE UTERUS

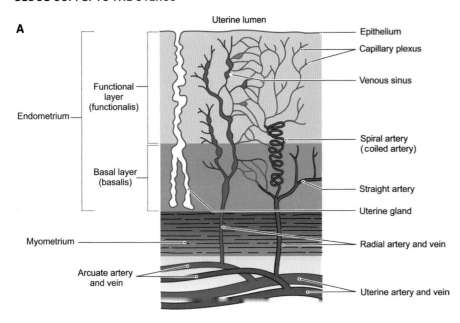

Figure 19-11A. Blood supply to the endometrium and uterus.

The **uterine artery** branches from the anterior trunk of the **internal iliac artery**. The **uterine artery** gives rise to the **arcuate artery**, and the arcuate artery further gives rises to the **radial artery** that supplies blood to the **myometrium** of the uterus. **Straight arteries** and **spiral arteries** branch from the radial artery and supply blood to the **endometrium**. **Spiral arteries**, also called **coiled arteries**, respond to progesterone hormone and grow quickly into the functional layer of the endometrium during the **secretory phase** when progesterone level is high. In the **menstrual phase**, when progesterone level drops, **spiral arteries** contract and cause ischemia and necrosis, and the **functional layer** of the **endometrium** sloughs off. The **straight artery** supplying the endometrium remains unchanged during the menstrual cycle. Oxygen and nutrient exchange occur via the **capillary plexus**, and blood drains into the **venous sinus**, then into the **radial veins**, and then the **uterine veins**.

Ectopic pregnancy is an **extrauterine pregnancy**. The majority of ectopic pregnancies occur in the **fallopian tube**, but other possible types of ectopic pregnancies include **cervical, interstitial, intramural, ovarian,** and **abdominal. Intrauterine and extrauterine pregnancies** can occur at the same time, although it is rare. Rupture of an **ectopic pregnancy** can cause life-threatening hemorrhage. A typical ectopic pregnancy appears 6 to 8 weeks after the last normal menstrual period. Sudden abdominal pain and/or vaginal bleeding are typical presenting signs and symptoms. Symptoms early in an ectopic pregnancy may be less common because **progesterone, estradiol,** and **human chorionic gonadotropin (hCG)** levels tend to be lower than in normal pregnancy. Ultrasound helps to diagnose an ectopic pregnancy, but for severe bleeding, time may not allow physicians to perform further tests, and emergency surgery must be performed.

CLINICAL CORRELATION

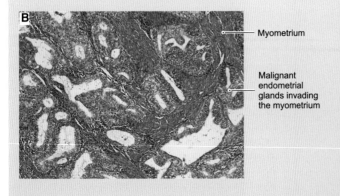

Myometrium

Malignant endometrial glands invading the myometrium

Figure 19-11B. Endometrial Adenocarcinoma. H&E, ×100

Endometrial adenocarcinoma is a malignancy arising from the **endometrial glandular epithelium**, and it is usually seen in postmenopausal women. Endometrial adenocarcinomas are broadly divided into **types I and II.** Most **type I** adenocarcinomas are the endometrioid histologic type due to their resemblance to proliferative endometrial glands, especially well-differentiated examples. These **adenocarcinomas** typically arise in the background of endometrial hyperplasia as proliferation of the **endometrial glands.** Some risk factors for type I adenocarcinoma include unopposed estrogen, obesity, diabetes, cigarette smoking, and infertility. **Type II** endometrial adenocarcinomas tend to occur in the setting of **endometrial atrophy.** They are often poorly differentiated, and they consist of the aggressive serous type. Treatment involves radical hysterectomy, lymph node dissection, and, in some cases, chemotherapy.

IMPLANTATION

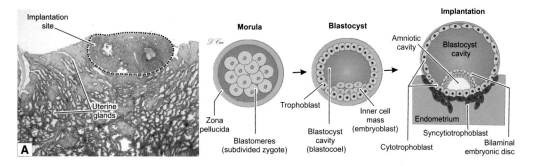

Figure 19-12A. Implantation, endometrium of the uterus. H&E, ×8

After an ovum has been successfully fertilized by a spermatozoan in the ampulla of the uterine (fallopian) tube, the **zygote** (fertilized oocyte) undergoes mitotic cell division (**cleavage**) and becomes a multicellular structure called the **morula**. The morula develops into the **blastocyst**, which is transported into the uterus. The process of the **blastocyst** attaching to the endometrium of the uterus is called **implantation**. Implantation occurs at the end of the secretory phase; the endometrium during this period of time is also called the **premenstrual endometrium** (days 25–28). Implantation usually occurs on the posterior wall of the body of the uterus. If implantation succeeds, the trophoblast differentiates into two cell layers: an inner **cytotrophoblast layer** and an outer **syncytiotrophoblast layer**. The **syncytiotrophoblast** attaches to and invades the endometrium of the uterus, and the process of placentation begins. hCG secreted by the placenta stimulates the **corpus luteum** to remain active and continue to secrete **estrogen** and **progesterone** during the pregnancy. The photomicrograph on the *left* shows an implantation site enclosed within the connective tissue of the endometrium.

CLINICAL CORRELATIONS

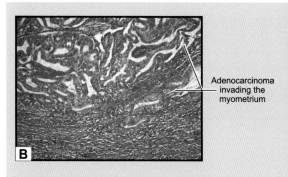

Figure 19-12B. Endometrial Adenocarcinoma. H&E, ×48

Endometrial adenocarcinoma is the most common form of endometrial cancer, accounting for ~80% of cases. The majority of cases of endometrial adenocarcinoma arise in the setting of elevated levels of **estrogen** unopposed by the action of **progesterone**, causing **endometrial hyperplasia**. Some cases, however, arise in postmenopausal women with atrophy of the endometrium. Excess or unopposed estrogen may be due to chronic anovulation, obesity, ovarian granulosa cell tumors, or exogenous hormone intake. In the early stage, the cancer is usually asymptomatic. Common symptoms include vaginal bleeding, **menorrhagia, metrorrhagia,** and lower abdominal pain. Histologically, the cancer is characterized by the presence of cells resembling the glandular cells of the endometrium and range from well differentiated with gland formation to poorly differentiated with solid sheets of **neoplastic cells.** Endometrial biopsy is widely used in the diagnosis of the cancer. Treatment options include surgical removal of the uterus, radiation therapy, and chemotherapy.

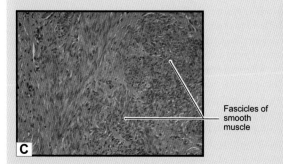

Figure 19-12C. Uterine Leiomyoma. H&E, ×95

Uterine leiomyoma, or **fibroid,** is a benign neoplasm, derived from smooth muscle cells of the uterine myometrium. Leiomyomas represent the most common benign neoplasm in women and occur more frequently in African Americans. Leiomyomas occur in the reproductive years when estrogen levels are high and tend to regress during menopause. Most patients with fibroids are asymptomatic, but, as the tumor enlarges, symptoms may include abnormal bleeding, menorrhagia, lower abdominal pain, and increased urinary frequency. Grossly, leiomyomas are well circumscribed and may be in subserosal, intramural, or submucosal locations. Leiomyomas can be single but are often multiple and may become quite large. The cut surface is typically white to tan, with a whorled, bulging appearance. Histologically, the tumor cells appear as well-differentiated, spindle-shaped smooth muscle cells, often with increased extracellular matrix, such as **collagen, proteoglycan,** and **fibronectin.** Leiomyomas rarely become their malignant counterpart, **leiomyosarcomas,** which usually develop *de novo*. Treatment options include **hysterectomy, myomectomy** (removal of the fibroid), and hormone therapy.

CERVIX

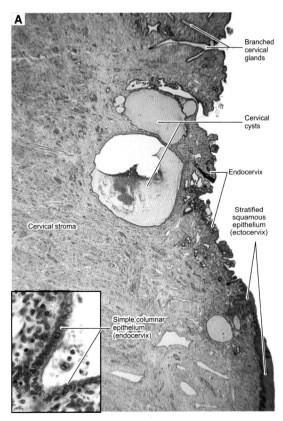

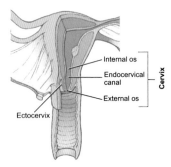

Figure 19-13A. Cervix. H&E, ×17; inset ×350

The inferior part of the uterus forms the **cervical canal**, which bulges into the vagina. The **internal os** is the opening from the endocervical canal to the uterus; the **external os** is the opening to the vaginal canal. The surface of the **endocervix** is lined by simple columnar epithelium, which consists of mucus-secreting cells (*inset*); the **ectocervix** is lined by stratified squamous epithelium. The cervix contains long branched mucous glands known as **cervical glands**; when these glands become obstructed, they form cervical cysts (**nabothian cysts**). The secretion of the cervix changes depending on the stage of the menstrual cycle; however, the mucosa of the cervix does not slough off as does the endometrium of the uterus. The **cervical stroma** is composed of dense connective tissue mixed with a small amount (about 15%) of smooth muscle. Usually, the cervix has a narrow canal; however, during delivery, dilation of the cervix allows the baby to pass through the canal.

The **cervical transformation (transition) zone** is the area of the cervical mucosa between the original **squamocolumnar junction** and the restored or new squamocolumnar junction that is formed through the processes of squamous metaplasia and squamous epithelialization. The majority of **cervical carcinomas** arise in this zone, and it is important that this area be sampled during screening with a **Papanicolaou smear**.

CLINICAL CORRELATION

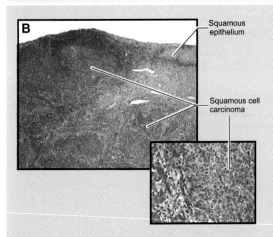

Figure 19-13B. Cervical Cancer. H&E (*upper left*), ×20; (*lower right*), ×115

Cervical cancer is a malignant neoplasm of the uterine cervix, the majority of which are **squamous cell carcinomas**. Risk factors include the early onset of sexual activity, multiple sexual partners, and exposure to **human papillomavirus (HPV)**. **Invasive squamous cell carcinoma** is preceded by precursor lesions called **cervical intraepithelial neoplasia**, in which dysplastic epithelial changes are present. The majority of intraepithelial lesions are related to infection by HPV. The introduction of screening using the **Papanicolaou smear**, or "Pap" smear, has dramatically reduced the incidence of invasive cervical lesions. Symptoms of cervical cancer include abnormal vaginal bleeding, postcoital bleeding, and vaginal discharge. Histologically, the cancer typically arises in the **cervical transformation zone** and may show superficial ulceration with **endophytic** or **exophytic** growth patterns. The cancer can spread by direct invasion to nearby tissues and organs or metastasize through hematogenous or lymphatic routes. Gardasil, a vaccine against certain HPV types, is used in young women to prevent infection by the virus. Treatment options include surgical removal of the uterus (hysterectomy), radiation therapy, and chemotherapy.

Placenta

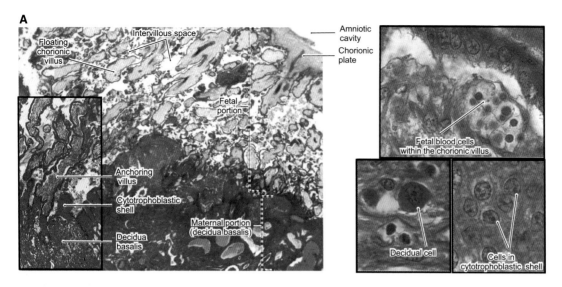

Figure 19-14A. **Overview of the placenta.** H&E, left ×13; left inset ×55; right *(upper)* ×704; right *(lower)* ×748

The **placenta** consists of the **maternal portion** and the **fetal portion**. It is a temporary organ that provides a bridge for exchanging gases, nutrients, hormones, and other materials between the maternal and fetal blood circulations. The *maternal portion* is the **decidua basalis.** The *fetal portion* consists of the **chorionic plate, chorionic villi,** and **cytotrophoblastic shell.** Fetal blood flows within the blood vessels of the chorionic villi; maternal blood is contained within the intervillous space. The placental barrier prevents the fetal blood from mixing with the maternal blood. The decidua basalis forms when stromal fibroblasts of the endometrium are transformed into decidual cells at the site of implantation. The syncytiotrophoblast invades the maternal blood vessels replacing smooth muscle in the vessel walls. Syncytiotrophoblasts also line the surface of the intervillous space. The cytotrophoblast forms an interface (**cytotrophoblastic shell**) between the maternal and fetal tissues.

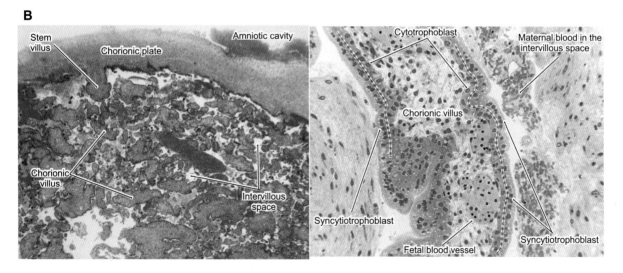

Figure 19-14B. **Fetal portion of the placenta.** H&E, left ×18; right ×136

The chorionic plate consists of connective tissue and forms the wall of the amniotic cavity; it contains chorionic arteries and veins. The chorionic villi can be classified on the basis of their developmental stages: (1) **Primary chorionic villi** are newly formed villi at an early stage (about the 2nd week of implantation) and consist of only a trophoblast layer. (2) **Secondary chorionic villi** develop at the end of the 2nd week when mesenchymal tissue grows into the villi and forms a mesenchymal core within the trophoblastic shell. (3) **Tertiary chorionic villi** develop at the 3rd week, at which time the fetal blood and blood vessels are formed within the chorionic villi. By the end of the 3rd week, the fetal blood begins to flow, and gas and nutrient exchange takes place between the fetal and maternal blood by diffusion through the placental barrier. The **placental barrier** is composed of the **syncytiotrophoblast, cytotrophoblast, connective tissue** of the **villus, endothelium** of the **fetal capillary,** and the **basement membranes** of the trophoblast and endothelium. The syncytiotrophoblast produces **hCG** hormone, which plays an important role in maintaining pregnancy via stimulation of the **corpus luteum** to secrete **progesterone.**

Umbilical Cord

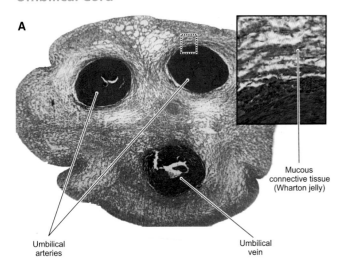

A

Mucous connective tissue (Wharton jelly)

Umbilical arteries

Umbilical vein

Figure 19-15A. Umbilical cord. H&E, ×12; inset ×79

The **umbilical cord** is a ropelike structure that connects the developing fetus to the placenta. It contains two **umbilical arteries** and one **umbilical vein**. These vessels carry oxygen and nutrients from the mother to the fetus and waste products away from the fetus. The blood vessels are surrounded by a **mucous connective tissue** (**Wharton jelly**). The umbilical arteries carry **deoxygenated fetal blood** to the placenta by way of the chorionic arteries and the chorionic villi. After gas and nutrient exchange with the maternal blood, the **oxygenated blood** is transported from chorionic veins to the umbilical vein, which returns blood to the fetus.

Funisitis is inflammation of the umbilical cord that often accompanies **chorioamnionitis** (inflammation of the fetal membranes). Funisitis typically occurs after 20 weeks of gestation, often because of a bacterial infection. Neutrophils migrate through the umbilical vessels and may enter the Wharton jelly. Another possible complication in pregnancy is an **umbilical knot**. In severe cases, obstruction of blood supply can result in the fetal death.

Vagina

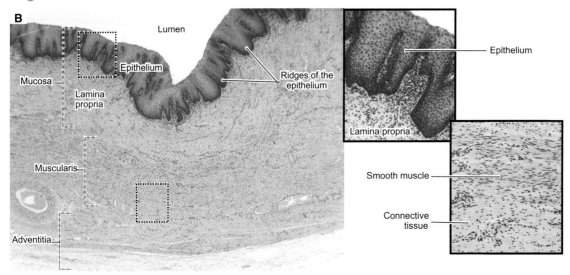

B

Lumen

Epithelium

Mucosa

Lamina propria

Ridges of the epithelium

Epithelium

Lamina propria

Muscularis

Smooth muscle

Connective tissue

Adventitia

Figure 19-15B. Vagina. H&E, ×41; inset (*upper*) ×63; inset (*lower*) ×74

The **vagina** is a tubular organ that connects the cervix of the uterus to the external genitalia. The wall of the vagina consists of the **mucosa, muscularis,** and **adventitia**. The *mucosa* comprises a **nonkeratinized stratified squamous epithelium** and an underlying **lamina propria** (dense irregular connective tissue with many **elastic fibers**). The *muscularis* contains mainly longitudinal smooth muscle and some oblique smooth muscle bundles. The *adventitia layer* is composed of both dense connective tissue (near the muscularis) and loose connective tissue (outer layer). The vagina is moistened by cervical secretions, and it has many sensory nerve endings in the inferior part near the entrance. The epithelium of the vagina undergoes minimal change during the menstrual cycle. There are numerous elastic fibers in the connective tissue, and **ridges** (folds) in the mucosa, enabling the vaginal canal to expand during sexual intercourse and during the delivery of a baby.

The **Papanicolaou (Pap) smear** is a very important diagnostic method used for screening early signs of **cervical cancer**. Cells from the epithelial surface of the vagina and cervix are collected by using a brush and spatula while the vagina is opened by a speculum. Examination of these sample cells provides valuable information for detecting precancerous changes that may require treatment.

Mammary Glands

A

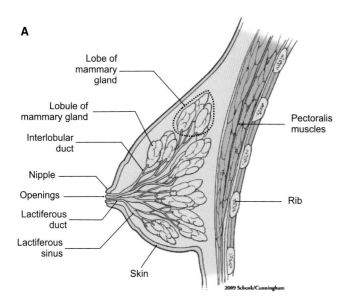

Lobe of mammary gland

Lobule of mammary gland

Interlobular duct

Nipple

Openings

Lactiferous duct

Lactiferous sinus

Skin

Pectoralis muscles

Rib

2009 Schenk/Cunningham

Figure 19-16A. Overview of the mammary gland.

In humans, there are two multilobed **mammary glands**, one located within the connective tissue of each breast. These exocrine glands produce milk after a pregnancy. Each gland is composed of 15 to 25 lobes of **compound tubuloalveolar glands**. Each lobe is separated from others by dense connective tissue and adipose tissue and opens into a **lactiferous duct**. The secretory alveoli produce milk and drain it into the **intralobular ducts** and then to the **interlobular ducts**. The interlobular ducts merge into **lactiferous sinuses** from which the milk empties into the **lactiferous ducts** (15–25). The female mammary glands begin to enlarge during puberty and undergo changes at different times based on hormone (**estrogen, progesterone, prolactin**, and **human placental lactogen**) levels.

B

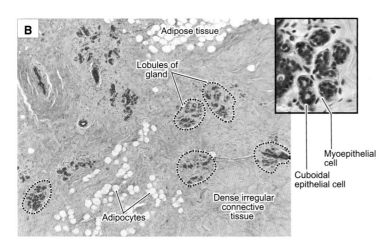

Adipose tissue

Lobules of gland

Myoepithelial cell

Cuboidal epithelial cell

Dense irregular connective tissue

Adipocytes

Figure 19-16B. Inactive (resting) mammary gland. H&E, ×41; inset ×359

An example of a **resting mammary gland** shows a large amount of dense irregular connective tissue and adipose tissue with small mammary gland lobules. The glandular tissue contains mainly **intralobular ducts**, which are lined by **cuboidal epithelial cells** and underlying **myoepithelial cells** (*inset*). The resting mammary gland has only a few secretory alveoli, some undeveloped intralobular ducts, interlobular ducts, lactiferous sinuses, and lactiferous ducts.

C

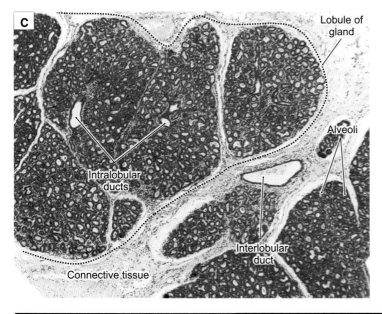

Lobule of gland

Alveoli

Intralobular ducts

Interlobular duct

Connective tissue

Figure 19-16C. Active (during pregnancy) mammary gland. H&E, ×41

An example of a **mammary gland during pregnancy** shows large lobules and a relatively small amount of interlobular connective tissue. The glandular tissue contains many proliferated **alveoli** and **intralobular ducts**. A large interlobular duct is located within the connective tissue shown here. When the mammary glands begin to secrete milk (**lactation**), the lumina of the alveoli and the ducts are dilated and filled with milk. The milk contains many lipid droplets and proteins (caseins, lactalbumin, and immunoglobulin A) as well as lactose, ions, vitamins, and water. Secretion of milk is initiated by hormonal changes: decrease of **estrogen** and **progesterone** and increase of **prolactin** after delivery and the loss of the placenta. The milk is released by the **milk ejection reflex** when stimulated by suckling.

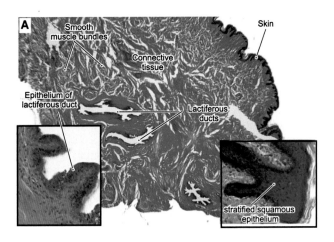

Figure 19-17A. Nipple, mammary gland. H&E, ×11; left inset ×146; right inset ×136

The **nipple** is a small projection at the center of the breast. It contains 15 to 25 openings of **lactiferous ducts** within its connective tissue and smooth muscle bundles. It is covered by thin skin and surrounded by the **areola** (pigmented skin). The nipple has many sensory nerve endings that receive stimulation during **suckling**. This stimulation results in release of **oxytocin** from the pars nervosa of the pituitary; the oxytocin stimulates contraction of the myoepithelial cells in the mammary gland. The contraction of the myoepithelial cells pushes milk out of the alveoli and ducts and through the lactiferous ducts to the surface of the nipple. This process is called the **milk ejection reflex**. The lactiferous ducts shown here are from the proximal portion of the ducts near the lactiferous sinuses.

CLINICAL CORRELATIONS

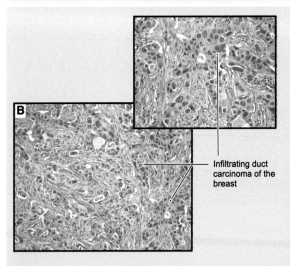

Figure 19-17B. Adenocarcinoma of the Breast (Breast Cancer). H&E, left (*lower*) ×44; right (*upper*) ×71

Infiltrating duct carcinoma, or **invasive ductal carcinoma**, is the most common **adenocarcinoma of the breast (breast cancer)**; it contains no features to further classify it into special types of breast carcinoma, such as **lobular, tubular,** and **mucinous carcinomas**. Risk factors for the development of breast cancer include female gender, increasing age, family history, long reproductive life, **nulliparity**, and the presence of proliferative breast lesions or ductal hyperplasia. Approximately 5% of breast cancers are related to specific gene mutations, including *BRCA1* and *BRCA2*. Common signs and symptoms include a palpable breast mass, bloody discharge from the nipple, change in size or shape of a breast, skin dimpling, inverted nipple, peeling of the nipple skin, and redness or pitting of the skin over the breast. Mammograms and breast exams are used to screen for breast cancer. Biopsy is performed on suspicious lesions to determine a tissue diagnosis. Histologically, breast cancer varies from well-formed glandular structures to sheets of poorly differentiated cells. Histologic grading of breast cancer is based on tubule formation, nuclear **pleomorphism**, and the mitotic rate. Treatment includes surgical removal of a tumor (**lumpectomy**), removal of the entire breast (**mastectomy**) and lymph nodes, radiation therapy, chemotherapy, and hormone therapy.

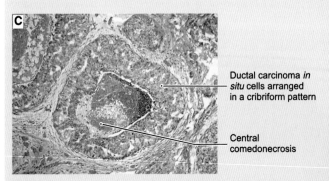

Figure 19-17C. Ductal Carcinoma *in Situ*. H&E, ×100

Ductal carcinoma *in situ* (DCIS) represents ductal adenocarcinoma of the breast confined to the ductal system with no transgression of the basement membrane and invasion of the adjacent fibrous stroma. Most DCIS results from changes in the ducts beginning as a proliferation of ductal cells. In time, these proliferating ductal cells may show signs of **cellular atypia** and eventually become DCIS, the precursor to invasive ductal carcinoma. DCIS may be subdivided into low, moderate, and high grade based on the cellular arrangements and the degree of atypia. High-grade DCIS often shows necrosis in the center of the duct lumen called **comedonecrosis**. **Microcalcifications** often form in this necrotic material. Cellular patterns include solid, cribriform, papillary, **micropapillary,** and **comedocarcinoma**. Treatment for DCIS may be conservative (**lumpectomy** with radiation) if the disease is localized, but mastectomy may be required for extensive disease.

From Histology to Pathology

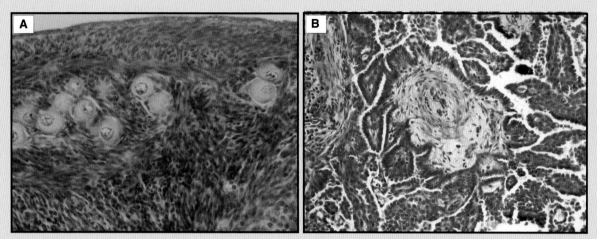

Figure 19-18. Normal Ovary on the left (A). Serous Carcinoma on the right (B). H&E, ×100

Normal ovary on the *left*. **Serous carcinoma** on the *right*. Serous carcinoma is the most common malignant neoplasm of the ovary and arises from the ovarian surface epithelium. Clinically, ovarian tumors often do not become apparent until they have reached considerable size. Symptoms include abdominal pain, gastrointestinal and urologic problems, and abdominal distension. Often, malignant ovarian tumors have already metastasized by the time of diagnosis. Histologically, **serous carcinoma** shows a papillary architecture and varying degrees of differentiation. Psammoma bodies, calcified concentric laminations, are often present but are not specific to this neoplasm. Treatment consists of surgery, chemotherapy, and radiation. Epithelial tumors of the ovary often express the tumor marker CA125, which is useful in following patients after treatment for evidence of recurrence.

Clinical Vignette Questions

1. A 45-year-old woman presents to her gynecologist for her annual gynecologic and breast exam. The patient has a history of proliferative fibrocystic changes including ductal cysts, stromal fibrosis, and duct epithelial hyperplasia. During the breast exam, the physician notes generally nodular breasts, but no discrete masses suspicious for malignancy are palpated. The patient is sent for mammography, and the radiologist notes numerous microcalcifications, the nature of which are concerning for malignancy. The patient is scheduled for a stereotactic breast biopsy to assess the nature of the tissue associated with the microcalcifications. Which of the following is the most appropriate diagnosis in this case?

A. Ductal carcinoma *in situ*
B. Fibrocystic changes
C. Infiltrating duct carcinoma
D. Invasive lobular carcinoma
E. Lobular carcinoma *in situ*

2. A 68-year-old woman with a history of progressive abdominal pain and increasing abdominal girth presents to her family physician. Physical exam reveals a protuberant abdomen, which is more prominent on the left side. Palpation of the abdomen does elicit pain. The physician orders a CT of the abdomen and pelvis, which reveals a 32-cm cystic and solid mass in the left pelvis which extends superiorly into the abdomen. The patient is referred to a gynecologic surgeon who schedules the patient for an exploratory laparot-omy. At surgery, the surgeon encounters a cystic mass in the region of the left adnexa (ovary and tube). The mass is excised and sent immediately to pathology for an intraoperative consultation. Further examination of the abdominal cavity reveals nodules on multiple serosal surfaces. Gross examination of the mass reveals multiple cysts containing watery fluid and intervening solid areas. Papillary excrescences (projections or outgrowths) cover the surface of the mass and the adjacent fallopian tube. Which of the following is the most appropriate diagnosis?

A. Endodermal sinus tumor
B. Granulosa cell tumor
C. Mature cystic teratoma
D. Mucinous cystadenoma
E. Papillary serous cystadenocarcinoma

3. A 75-year-old woman begins to experience episodes of vaginal bleeding. She makes an appointment with her gynecologist, where an ultrasound shows a thickened endometrium. The gynecologist performs an endometrial biopsy, and ample tissue is retrieved for pathologic examination. Results of microscopic pathologic examination reveal a high-grade serous carcinoma of the endometrium. Which of the following is a major risk factor for serous carcinoma of the endometrium?

A. Endometrial atrophy
B. Endometrial hyperplasia
C. Obesity
D. Unopposed estrogen

20 Eye

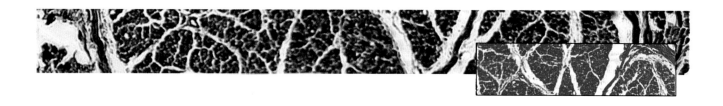

Introduction and Key Concepts for the Eye
Eyelids
Tunica Fibrosa (Tunica Externa)
Refractive Media of the Eye
Tunica Vasculosa (Tunica Media)
Retina (Tunica Interna)
Optic Nerve

Anatomy of the Eye

Structures of the Eye

Figures and Images Orientation

Structures of the Eye with Figure Numbers

Eyelid

Tunica Fibrosa (Tunica Externa)

Clinical Vignette Questions

Introduction and Key Concepts for the Eye

The **eye** is the organ of vision, perhaps the most important of the sensory modalities. The eye converts light into nerve impulses in a way that allows the brain to be aware of the individual's visual surroundings. In our study, we divide the structure of the eye into three general categories: those structures that **protect** the eye (eyelids); those structures that help **form a visual image** of what the individual is looking at (**cornea, lens, sclera,** and associated structures); and those structures that **convert the visual image into nerve impulses** and conduct the impulses to the brain (**retina** and **optic nerve**), where they are analyzed to produce the sensation of vision.

The basic structure of the eye is that of a hollow sphere with optical elements on the anterior surface that focus an inverted image of the surroundings onto the inside of the posterior wall. The primary structural element of the sphere is the **tunica fibrosa**, or **tunica externa**, which consists of the **sclera** and the **cornea**. Lining the inside of the tunica externa is the **tunica vasculosa**, consisting of the **choroid**, the **ciliary body**, and the **iris**. The eye is filled with a transparent liquid (**aqueous humor**) and a transparent gel (**vitreous body**). In the anterior portion of the eye is the **lens**, which is flexible and can adjust the focus of the image depending on the distance from the eye to the object being viewed. The image is focused on the **retina**, a layer of neurons and neural receptors that line the internal surface of the posterior two thirds of the eye. The axons of the **ganglion cell neurons** in the retina leave the eye and form the **optic nerve**.

Eyelids

The **eyelids** protect the eyes from injury by foreign objects and also maintain a thin film of **moisture** on the surface of the cornea that prevents the cornea from drying out and becoming opaque. Each eyelid consists of an outer layer of **skin**; a middle layer of **muscle, glands,** and **connective tissues** (**tarsal plate**); and an inner layer of **conjunctival tissue** (**palpebral conjunctiva**). There are several types of glands in the eyelid that aid in keeping the cornea moist, including **meibomian glands, glands of Zeis, glands of Moll,** and **accessory lacrimal glands**.

Several muscles are associated with the eyelids. These include (1) the **orbicularis oculi muscle**, a circular sheet of striated muscle that is innervated by the facial nerve (cranial nerve [CN] VII) and functions to close the eyelids; (2) the **levator palpebrae superioris muscle**, a thin flat striated muscle that originates in the orbit, passes forward, and inserts into the upper eyelid. It is innervated by the oculomotor nerve (CN III) and is responsible for opening the eyelid and holding it open; and (3) the **superior tarsal muscle** (**Müller muscle**), a bundle of smooth muscle that arises from the interstitia of the levator muscle and inserts on the upper end of the tarsal plate and superior conjunctiva of the eyelid. The superior tarsal muscle is innervated by sympathetic nerve fibers from the superior cervical ganglion and helps to raise the upper eyelid.

Tunica Fibrosa (Tunica Externa)

The outermost structures of the eye are the **cornea** and **sclera**.

CORNEA is a transparent tissue that covers the anterior sixth of the eye. The cornea contains no blood vessels and aids in focusing the visual image onto the retina. It consists of five layers. The thickest layer, the **stroma**, comprises 90% of the thickness of the cornea and consists of collagen fibers and fibroblasts embedded in an extracellular matrix. The anterior surface of the cornea is covered by a thin layer of **pavement epithelium** (stratified squamous epithelium) resting on the **Bowman membrane**. The posterior surface of the cornea is covered by a layer of corneal **endothelium** (simple squamous epithelium) that is only one cell thick and rests on the **Descemet membrane**.

SCLERA is a tough, thin structure consisting of dense, irregular, opaque connective tissue that comprises the posterior five sixths of the outer surface of the eyeball. The cornea and sclera are continuous with each other at the **limbus**. The extraocular muscles, which move the eyes in their orbits, insert in the sclera. The conjunctival tissue, which covers the inner surfaces of the eyelids, also attaches to the sclera.

Refractive Media of the Eye

LENS is a transparent, flexible, biconvex structure that is suspended from the ciliary processes by **zonular fibers**. The curvature of the lens can be changed by contraction or relaxation of the **ciliary muscles** (under control of **parasympathetic** nerve fibers of the oculomotor nerve) so that the image of nearby or distant objects can be focused on the retina. The lens has three components: the **lens capsule**, the **subcapsular epithelium**, and the **lens fibers**. The *lens capsule* is a transparent basement membrane that surrounds the entire lens. Immediately beneath it, on only the anterior surface of the lens, is a single layer of squamous cells, the *subcapsular epithelium*. In the region of the equator of the lens, proliferating epithelial cells become elongated, are displaced toward the center of the lens, and lose their nuclei. They are then called *lens fibers* and comprise the major bulk of the lens.

AQUEOUS HUMOR is a thin, watery, transparent fluid that is produced continuously by the **ciliary body** and fills the **anterior chamber**. It exits the anterior chamber in the region of the **angle of the anterior chamber**. It is produced by the **ciliary processes**, which are rich in capillaries.

VITREOUS BODY is a transparent gelatinous substance that fills the eye between the **posterior surface of the lens** and the **retina**. Its composition is predominantly **water** with small amounts of **collagen** and **hyaluronic acid**. The surface of the vitreous body is covered by a layer of condensed vitreous fibers called **hyaloid membrane**. It is in contact with the posterior lens capsule, the zonular fibers, the posterior portion of the ciliary epithelium (pars plana), the retina, and the optic nerve head. The vitreous body is important in maintaining the transparency and shape of the eye.

Tunica Vasculosa (Tunica Media)

The **tunica vasculosa** (sometimes called the **uveal tract**) lies just internal to the tunica externa and consists of the **iris** (anteriorly), the **ciliary body**, and the **choroid** (posteriorly).

IRIS is a thin diaphragm of tissue in the anterior chamber, composed of a highly vascularized, loose connective tissue **stroma**, two groups of **contractile elements**, the **anterior iridal border**, and the **posterior iridal border**. The *posterior iridal border* contains two layers of **pigmented epithelium**, the anterior iridal epithelium (anterior pigmented epithelium) and the **posterior iridial epithelium** (posterior pigmented epithelium). Two groups of muscle fibers regulate the diameter of the **pupil**, the circular hole in the center of the iris, and adjust the amount of light entering the eye. The circular **constrictor pupillae muscle** (smooth muscle fibers) reduces the size of the pupil under the influence of parasympathetic nerve fibers; the radial fibers of the **dilator pupillae muscle** (myoepithelial cells) act to increase the size of the pupil under the influence of **sympathetic nerve fibers**.

CILIARY BODY lies interior to the anterior margin of the sclera, between the choroid and the iris. It is composed of two concentric rings of tissue, the **pars plicata** and the **pars plana**, and includes epithelial tissue, a stroma of connective tissue, and smooth muscle fibers. The muscles of the ciliary body control the curvature of the lens and, therefore, function to focus the visual image on the retina. The epithelium of the ciliary body has two layers, a **pigmented layer** and a **nonpigmented layer**. The latter secretes the **aqueous humor**, which fills the anterior chamber of the eye and leaves the anterior chamber in the region of the **anterior chamber angle**.

CHOROID is a highly vascularized tissue containing some collagen fibers that is loosely attached to the overlying sclera. The inner surface of the choroid adheres tightly to the pigment epithelium layer of the retina. The innermost layer of the choroid is the **choriocapillaris**, which supplies oxygen and nutrients to the outer layers of the retina. The **Bruch membrane** delineates the junction between the choriocapillaris and the **retinal pigment epithelium**.

Retina (Tunica Interna)

The **retina** consists of a thin sheet of neurons that covers the inner surface of the posterior two thirds of the eye and a layer of cuboidal epithelial cells that sit on the choroid and contain melanin (**retinal pigment epithelium**). In general, the **retina** can be divided into an **optic (neural) retina** and a **nonoptic (nonneural)** retina. The *neural retina*, often referred to as simply "retina," contains neural elements and has the visual functions described below. The *nonneural retina* has no neural elements and no visual function. It is the anterior continuation of the pigmented layer, which covers the surface of the ciliary body and the posterior surface of the iris.

Unlike the rest of the eye, the retina develops as a part of the central nervous system (CNS). It contains five types of neural elements: **photoreceptor cells** (**rods** and **cones**), **bipolar cells**, **horizontal cells**, **amacrine cells**, and **ganglion cells**. The retina can be divided into 10 layers, some of which contain the nuclei of cells and others of which contain cell processes and synapses.

The retina is not homogeneous throughout its extent. Over most of the retina, the focused light of the visual image must pass through all of the neural layers, as well as small blood vessels, before reaching the **photoreceptors**. This degrades the image to a certain extent. However, in the **fovea centralis**, a small region near the posterior pole of the eye, the superficial layers are displaced to the side, and light strikes the photoreceptors directly. The visual image in this region is perceived with the greatest detail. The area immediately surrounding the fovea centralis is the **macula lutea**. This is the thickest region of the retina and contains a high concentration of both **cones** (for **color vision**) and **rods** (for **low-light vision**). More peripherally, the retina becomes thinner. There are fewer ganglion cells, fewer cones, and a relatively higher proportion of rods. These changes cause visual acuity to be reduced but sensitivity to low light levels to increase.

Optic Nerve

The **ganglion cells** are the output cells of the retina. The axons of ganglion cells travel in the nerve fiber layer to the **optic disk**, where the nerve fibers exit the eye and form the **optic nerve**. There are no photoreceptors in the optic disk; this absence produces a small **blind spot** in the visual field. The appearance of the optic disk when viewed through an ophthalmoscope is an important diagnostic aid.

Anatomy of the Eye

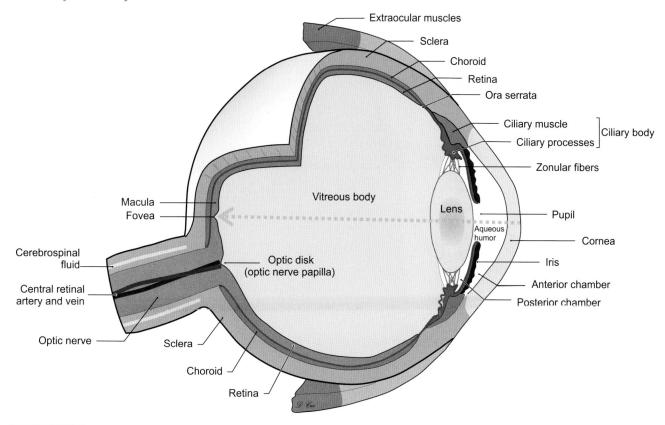

Figure 20-1. Overview of the eye.

The *yellow dashed line* indicates light coming in and projecting on the **fovea**.

Structures of the Eye

I. **Tunica fibrosa (tunica externa)**
  A. Cornea
    1. Pavement epithelium (anterior corneal epithelium)
    2. Bowman membrane
    3. Corneal stroma (corneal substantia propria)
    4. Descemet membrane
    5. Endothelium (posterior corneal epithelium)
  B. Sclera
    1. Episclera (blood vessels and adipose tissue)
    2. Sclera proper
II. **Tunica vasculosa (tunica media)**
  A. Choroid
    1. Bruch membrane
    2. Choriocapillaris
    3. Choroid propria
  B. Iris
    1. Pigment epithelium
    2. Stroma
    3. Constrictor pupillae muscle
    4. Dilator pupillae muscle
  C. Ciliary body
    1. Ciliary processes
    2. Ciliary epithelium
    3. Ciliary muscle

III. **Refractive media of the eye**
  A. Lens (biconvex, flexible, transparent structure)
    1. Lens capsule
    2. Subcapsular epithelium
    3. Lens fibers
    4. Zonular fibers
  B. Aqueous humor (transparent fluid occupying the space between the lens and cornea)
  C. Vitreous body (refractive gel filling the interior of the globe posterior to the lens)
IV. **Retina (tunica interna)**
  A. Fovea
  B. Macula
  C. Peripheral retina
V. **Optic nerve**

Figures and Images Orientation

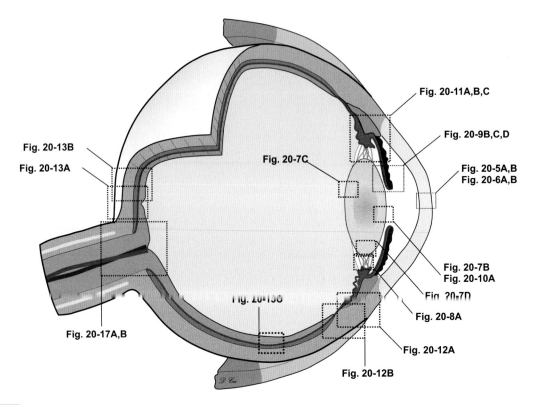

Fig. 20-11A,B,C

Fig. 20-9B,C,D

Fig. 20-13B

Fig. 20-13A

Fig. 20-7C

Fig. 20-5A,B
Fig. 20-6A,B

Fig. 20-7B
Fig. 20-10A

Fig. 20-7D

Fig. 20-8A

Fig. 20-17A,B

Fig. 20-13B

Fig. 20-12A

Fig. 20-12B

Figure 20-2. Orientation of detailed eye illustrations.

Structures of the Eye with Figure Numbers

Eyelid

Figure 20-3A
Figure 20-3B
Figure 20-3C
Figure 20-4A
Figure 20-4B
Figure 20-4C

Cornea

Figure 20-5A
Figure 20-5B
Figure 20-5C
Figure 20-6A
Figure 20-6B

Lens

Figure 20-7A
Figure 20-7B
Figure 20-7C
Figure 20-7D
Figure 20-8A
Figure 20-8B
Figure 20-8C
Figure 20-10A

Iris

Figure 20-9A
Figure 20-9B

Figure 20-9C
Figure 20-9D
Figure 20-10B

Ciliary Body

Figure 20-11A
Figure 20-11B
Figure 20-11C
Figure 20-12A
Figure 20-12B
Figure 20-12C

Retina

Figure 20-13A
Figure 20-13B
Figure 20-13C
Figure 20-14A
Figure 20-14B
Figure 20-15A
Figure 20-15B
Figure 20-15C
Figure 20-16A
Figure 20-16B

Optic Nerve

Figure 20-17A
Figure 20-17B

Eyelid

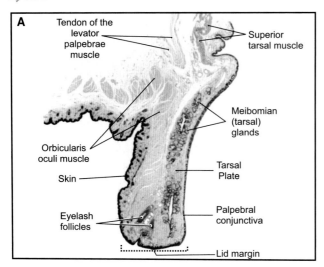

Figure 20-3A. Overview of the upper eyelid. H&E, ×7.6

A low-power photomicrograph of the **upper eyelid** is shown. The eyelids contain an outer layer of **skin**; a middle layer of **muscles, glands,** and **tarsal plate**; and an inner layer of **conjunctival tissue (palpebral conjunctiva)**. Eyelids cover and protect the eye from the environment, injury, and intense light. They also maintain a smooth corneal surface by spreading a film of lacrimal fluid (**tears**) evenly over the cornea to moisten the eye. The skin of the eyelids is thin, loose, and delicate and, therefore, may permit extreme swelling. The internal lid is covered by a **palpebral conjunctiva**, a layer of stratified low columnar epithelium. It is continuous with the **bulbar conjunctiva** where it covers the sclera of the eyeball. The **tarsal plate** is a dense fibroelastic tissue, which provides flexible support. The **tarsal glands (meibomian glands)** are embedded in it. The **eyelashes** are located in the anterior margins of the eyelids.

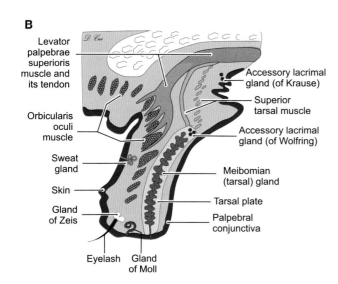

Figure 20-3B. Representation of the upper eyelid, glands, and muscles that control eyelid movements.

Several types of **glands** in the eyelids include (1) **meibomian (tarsal) glands,** sebaceous glands that produce a lipid-rich substance; (2) **glands of Zeis,** modified sebaceous glands associated with the follicles of the eyelashes; (3) **glands of Moll,** modified sweat glands, associated with eyelash follicles; and (4) **accessory lacrimal glands,** serous glands that contribute to tears. The **muscles** associated with upper eyelids are the (1) **orbicularis oculi muscle,** a circular sheet of striated muscle which functions to close the eyelids; (2) **levator palpebrae superioris muscle,** a thin, flat, striated muscle that arises from the apex of the orbit and inserts into the posterior surface of the orbicularis oculi muscle and the skin of the upper eyelid, and which opens the eyelid; and (3) **superior tarsal muscle (Müller muscle),** smooth muscle that arises from the interstitia of the levator muscle and inserts on the upper end of the tarsal plate and superior conjunctiva of the lid. It joins the levator palpebrae superioris muscle in raising the upper eyelid.

CLINICAL CORRELATION

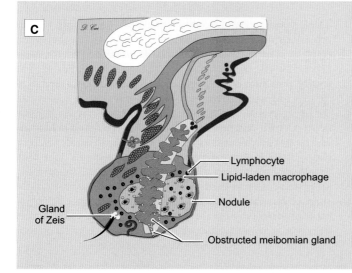

Figure 20-3C. Chalazion.

Chalazion is a chronic eyelid inflammatory lesion that results from the obstruction of the ducts of either the **Zeis** or **meibomian glands,** or both. Trapped sebaceous secretions leak into the surrounding tissue and cause a **granulomatous inflammation.** This is frequently associated with **blepharitis** and occasionally becomes secondarily infected. Early symptoms and signs include **eyelid swelling** and **erythema.** In time, it changes into a firm nodule within the eyelid or the tarsal plate. Histologic examination reveals granulation tissue characterized by focal aggregation of epithelium-like (**epithelioid**) cells, **lymphocytes, giant cells of Langerhans,** and yellow **lipid-laden macrophages.** Treatment options include warm compresses applied to the outer lid until acute symptoms disappear, topical antibiotics, and surgical incision if the lesion is large and disturbs vision.

GLANDS OF THE EYELID

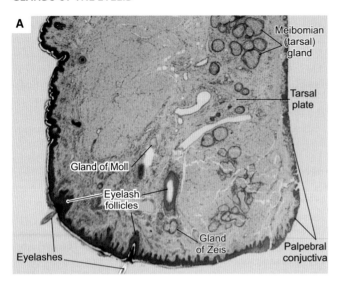

Figure 20-4A.   Upper eyelid (lower part), glands of the eyelid. H&E, ×68

Eyelids (palpebrae) consist of upper and lower eyelids. The structural components of the **upper eyelid** are similar to those of the **lower eyelid**, although the upper eyelid is more mobile. **Eyelashes** and their follicles are visible at the margin of the eyelid. The **tarsal glands**, also called **meibomian glands**, are large sebaceous glands embedded in the tarsal plate. The glands associated with eyelashes are (1) **glands of Moll** and (2) **glands of Zeis**. The glands of Moll are modified sweat glands near the base of the eyelash. They have unbranched tubules, which begin in a simple spiral rather than coiling in a glomerular shape, as do ordinary sweat glands. The glands of Zeis are small, modified sebaceous glands that are sometimes called **ciliary glands**. They are close to the eyelash follicles and empty their secretions into the follicles.

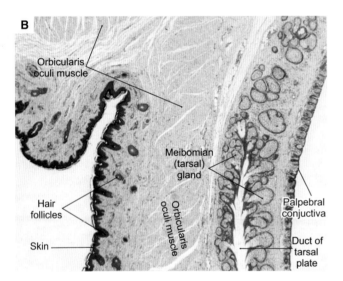

Figure 20-4B.   Upper eyelid (middle part). H&E, ×68

The **outer layer of the eyelid** is covered by **thin skin** (see Chapter 13, "Integumentary System"), a keratinized stratified squamous epithelium, over a loose elastic connective tissue layer. The skin contains **hair follicles**, which are much smaller than eyelash follicles (found only in the lid margin). **Orbicularis oculi muscle fibers** are located beneath the skin. The inner surface of the lid is a layer of **palpebral conjunctiva**, covered by stratified low columnar epithelium, which is in contact with the eyeball. The **tarsal (meibomian) glands**, embedded in the tarsal plate, lie between the orbicularis muscles and palpebral conjunctiva. Each gland has a single duct that opens at the lid margin. Their lipid secretion creates a surface on the tear film that prevents lacrimal fluids (**tears**) from evaporating from the surface of the eyeball. This secretion also lubricates the cornea and edges of the eyelids.

MUSCULAR CONTROL OF UPPER EYELID MOVEMENT

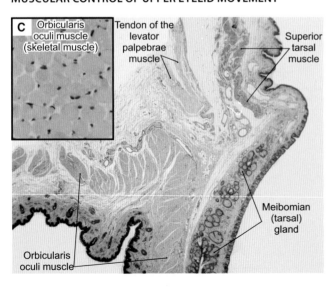

Figure 20-4C.   Upper eyelid (upper part), muscular control of upper eyelid movement. H&E, ×68; inset ×272

Three types of **muscles** control **upper eyelid movement**. (1) The **orbicularis oculi muscle** is a sheet of striated muscle that is oriented in a circle around the eye. It is innervated by the facial nerve (CN VII) and is responsible for closing the eyelids. (2) The **levator palpebrae superioris muscle** is a band of striated muscle that originates in the orbit, passes forward, and inserts into the upper eyelid. This muscle is innervated by the oculomotor nerve (CN III) and functions to open the eyelid and hold it up. The levator palpebrae muscle is not visible here, but its tendon is clearly seen. (3) The **superior tarsal muscle**, also called the **Müller muscle**, is a smooth muscle that inserts on the superior tarsal plate. It is innervated by sympathetic nerve fibers from the superior cervical ganglion and works with the levator palpebrae superior muscle to raise the upper eyelid. Damage to the levator palpebrae superior muscle, the superior tarsal muscle, or their innervation can cause **ptosis** (drooping of the eyelid).

Tunica Fibrosa (Tunica Externa)

CORNEA

A

Anterior

Pavement epithelium
(anterior corneal epithelium)

Bowman membrane

Stroma

Descemet membrane

Corneal endothelium

Posterior

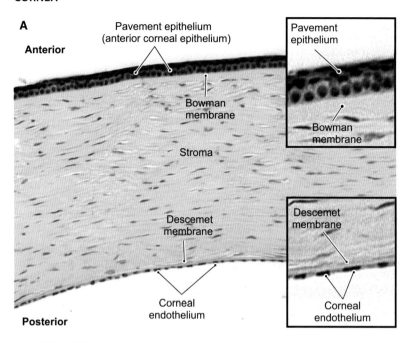

Pavement epithelium

Bowman membrane

Descemet membrane

Corneal endothelium

Figure 20-5A. Cornea. H&E, ×77.5; insets ×173

The **cornea** is a transparent and avascular tissue, which is composed of five layers: three cellular layers (epithelial layers and stroma) and two noncellular layers (Bowman membrane and Descemet membrane). These include (1) **pavement epithelium (anterior corneal epithelium)**; (2) the **Bowman membrane** (basement membrane of the pavement epithelium); (3) **stroma**, consisting of fibroblasts (also called **keratocytes** in the cornea) and alternating lamellae of collagen fibers; (4) the **Descemet membrane** (basement membrane of the **posterior corneal epithelium (endothelium)**; and (5) the **corneal endothelium** (posterior corneal epithelium). The cornea has a rich nerve supply from CN V. The superficial corneal layer contains numerous sensory nerve fibers, and irritation can cause severe eye pain. CN V also carries the afferent limb of the corneal reflex.

B

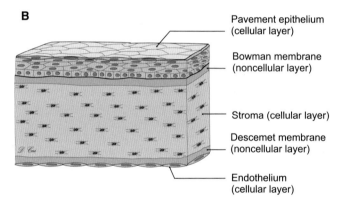

Pavement epithelium
(cellular layer)

Bowman membrane
(noncellular layer)

Stroma (cellular layer)

Descemet membrane
(noncellular layer)

Endothelium
(cellular layer)

Figure 20-5B. A representation of the cornea.

Pavement epithelium is formed by stratified squamous epithelium consisting of four to six layers and is about 50 mm in thickness; it has a high capacity for regeneration. The transparency of the cornea is due to its avascularity and due to its state of relative dehydration. **Corneal endothelium** is a single layer of squamous cells. This layer functions in the regulation of water in the stroma. The primary task of corneal endothelium is to pump the excess fluid out of the stroma and, therefore, is critical for keeping the cornea clear. If this endothelium is damaged, the result may be corneal swelling due to fluid retention within the stroma and loss of its transparency.

CLINICAL CORRELATION

C

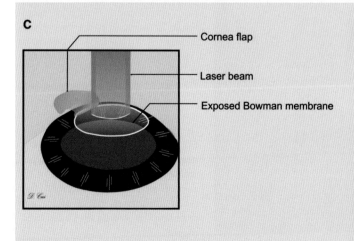

Cornea flap

Laser beam

Exposed Bowman membrane

Figure 20-5C. LASEK.

Laser refractive surgery reshapes the cornea in order to focus images more accurately onto the retina. The most common procedures include **laser *in situ* keratomileusis (LASIK)** and **laser-assisted epithelial keratomileusis (LASEK)**. Laser techniques have been continuously modified to reduce complications and enhance surgical outcomes. Unlike with LASIK, the most recent LASEK surgery saves the epithelium by using an alcohol solution to weaken epithelial cell adhesion so the epithelial layer can be lifted as a flap. After the **epithelial flap** is moved out of the way, excimer laser energy is applied through the **Bowman membrane layer** and into the upper stroma to reshape the cornea. The epithelial flap is then returned to its original position. The advantages of LASEK are a reduction of postoperative discomfort, a decreased risk of infection, and an increase in the overall thickness of the untouched area of the cornea.

ANTERIOR AND POSTERIOR CORNEAL EPITHELIUM

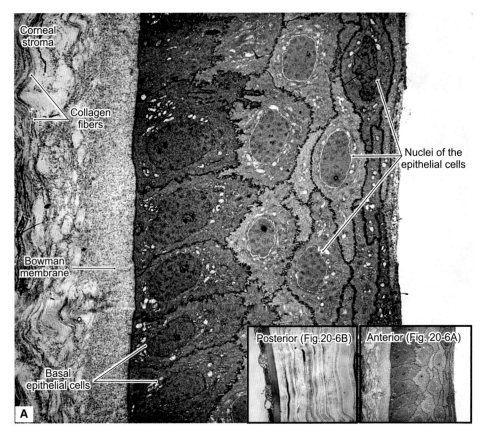

A

Figure 20-6A. Pavement epithelium (anterior epithelium). EM, ×6,000

The **anterior corneal epithelium** is a **stratified squamous epithelium** that covers the external surface of the cornea. The lack of keratinization and the uniform thickness of the epithelium contribute to the essential transparency of the cornea. The epithelial cells have a fairly fast turnover rate of about 1 week. The surface cells are not perfectly smooth, but rather have small **microvilli** (only a few are preserved here) that serve to anchor the vitally important tear film. Not shown in this field are free nociceptive nerve endings that penetrate the epithelium and provide the afferent limb of the corneal blink reflex. **Bowman membrane** is the commonly used term for the thick **basement membrane** at the interface between the anterior corneal epithelium and the **corneal stroma.**

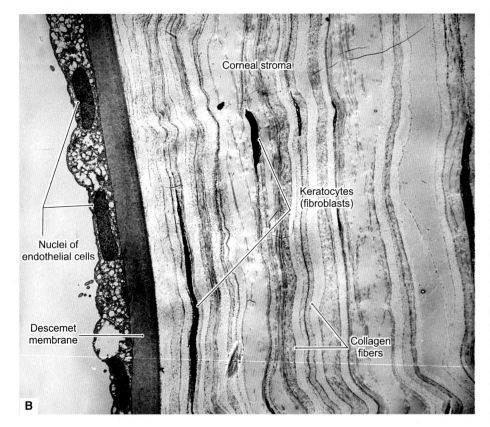

B

Figure 20-6B. Corneal endothelium (posterior corneal epithelium). EM, ×4,500

The **posterior corneal epithelium** is sometimes called the **corneal endothelium.** It is a simple squamous epithelium that faces the aqueous humor of the anterior chamber. **Descemet membrane** is the commonly used term for the sharply defined **basement membrane** of the posterior epithelium. Descemet membrane is unusual in that it consists largely of an orderly network of **type VIII collagen,** a relatively rare collagen type. The epithelial cells are joined by **tight junctions,** and they control the movement of water, ions, and metabolites between the stroma and the aqueous humor, the source of nutrition for the **corneal stroma.** Orderly layers of **type I collagen** fibrils form the bulk of the corneal stroma. The extremely flattened **fibroblasts** that produce and maintain the stroma are called **keratocytes.**

Refractive Media of the Eye

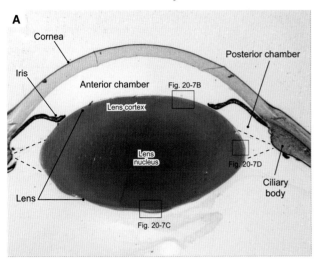

A

Cornea

Iris

Anterior chamber

Posterior chamber

Fig. 20-7B

Lens cortex

Lens nucleus

Fig. 20-7D

Ciliary body

Lens

Fig. 20-7C

ANTERIOR REGION OF THE LENS

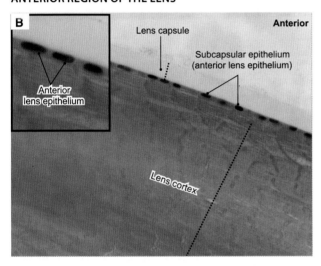

B

Anterior

Lens capsule

Subcapsular epithelium (anterior lens epithelium)

Anterior lens epithelium

Lens cortex

POSTERIOR REGION OF THE LENS

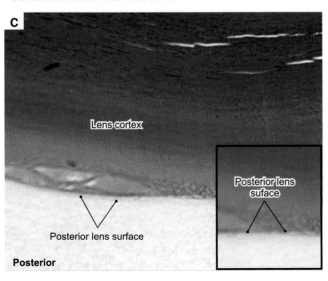

C

Lens cortex

Posterior lens suface

Posterior lens surface

Posterior

Figure 20-7A. Overview of the lens. H&E, ×11

The **lens** is a biconvex, avascular, flexible, and colorless transparent structure. Anterior to the lens is aqueous humor and posterior to it is the vitreous body. The lens is composed of the **lens capsule, subcapsular epithelium,** and **lens fibers.** The peripheral region of each lens fiber contains a nucleus and organelles, which form the bulk of the lens called the **lens cortex.** In the central part of the lens, the fibers lose their nuclei and organelles; this region is filled with crystalline proteins and is called the **lens nucleus.** The lens is held in place by zonular fibers (position indicated by *dashed lines*). The **anterior chamber** is the space between the cornea and the iris. The **posterior chamber** is a narrow space between the iris and the posterior zonular fibers of the lens. These chambers are filled with aqueous humor and communicate through the pupil.

Figure 20-7B. Anterior region of the lens. H&E, ×272; inset ×680

The **anterior lens** is covered by a **thickened lens capsule,** a transparent basement membrane that envelops the entire lens. Beneath it is a single layer of flat, squamous cells (**subcapsular epithelium**).

Figure 20-7C. Posterior region of the lens. H&E, ×272; inset ×680

The **posterior lens** is covered by a **thin lens capsule** (see Fig. 20-8B). No subcapsular epithelium lies beneath the capsule in this region. The **posterior lens surface** is in contact with the **vitreous body,** a transparent gel, which contains water, collagen, and hyaluronic acid and fills the interior of the globe posterior to the lens.

Figure 20-7D. Equatorial region of the lens. H&E, ×272; inset ×544

The cells of the **subcapsular epithelium** in the **equatorial region of the lens** are increased in height, and most cells are cuboidal in shape. The sizes of the **lens fibers** and their **nuclei** are increased in this region. The equatorial surface of the capsule is connected to the zonular fibers, which hold the lens in place.

EQUATORIAL REGION OF THE LENS

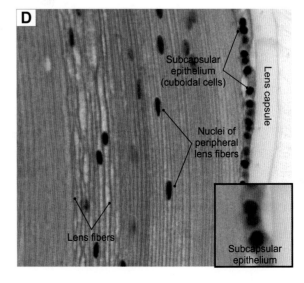

D

Subcapsular epithelium (cuboidal cells)

Lens capsule

Nuclei of peripheral lens fibers

Lens fibers

Subcapsular epithelium

REFRACTIVE FUNCTION OF THE LENS

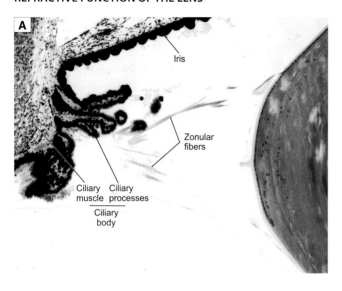

A

Iris

Zonular
fibers

Ciliary   Ciliary
muscle   processes
Ciliary
body

Figure 20-8A. Lens and zonular fibers. H&E, ×34

The **zonular fibers** are also called the **zonules of Zinn**. The combination of all the zonular fibers is referred to as the **suspensory ligament** of the eye. These fibers form a connection between the ciliary body and the equatorial (lateral) region of the lens. One end of each zonular fiber is attached to a **ciliary process**, and the other end of the fiber is embedded in the **capsule of the lens**. The capsule is thicker on the anterior and lateral surfaces than on the posterior surface. The zonular fibers have an important function during **accommodation**, which is to adjust the tension of the lens (thereby changing the curvature of the lens) to enable an object to be focused on the retina. Some ciliary muscle fibers are arranged in a circle at the base of the iris. Contraction of these fibers decreases the diameter of the circle and, therefore, decreases the tension on the zonular fibers so the lens becomes more round (the curvature *increases*). Relaxation of the ciliary muscle increases tension on the zonular fibers and the lens becomes flattened (curvature *decreases*).

B

Anterior

Zonular
fibers (relaxed)

Lens curvature
increases

Lens
cortex   Lens nucleus

Lens curvature
decreases

Zonular
fibers (stretched)

Anterior lens capsule

Subcapsular
epithelium

Nucleus of
lens fibers

Lens
fibers

Posterior
lens capsule

Posterior

Figure 20-8B. Representation of the lens and its function.

The **lens** is transparent and is composed of a **lens capsule, subcapsular epithelium**, and **lens fibers**. The function of the lens is to focus light on the retina. When *focusing on a distant object*, the ciliary muscle is relaxed, tension on the zonular fibers increases, and the anteroposterior thickness of the lens decreases. To *focus on a near object*, the ciliary muscle contracts to release the tension on the zonular fibers and the thickness of the lens increases. Ciliary muscle contraction also pulls the choroid forward to aid in focusing objects on the retina. The ability of the lens to accommodate decreases with age (**presbyopia**). The most common disorder associated with the lens is the **cataract**.

CLINICAL CORRELATION

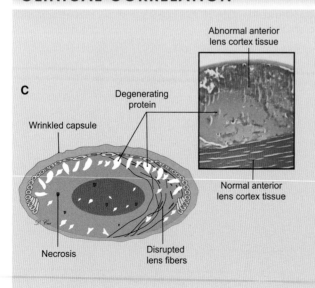

C

Wrinkled capsule

Degenerating
protein

Necrosis

Disrupted
lens fibers

Abnormal anterior
lens cortex tissue

Normal anterior
lens cortex tissue

Figure 20-8C. Cataract. H&E, ×51

Cataract is a condition of opacity in the lens of the eye. **Crystallin protein** in the lens degenerates, becoming insoluble and opaque. In cataractous lenses, lens fibers are edematous and sometimes necrotic. These changes alter the normal continuity of the lens fibers. The capsule may become wrinkled. The *inset* photomicrograph shows a cluster of altered protein in the anterior lens cortex. Cataract is usually an age-related disorder that causes partial or total blindness if left untreated. Risk factors include age, smoking, alcohol use, sunlight exposure, diabetes mellitus, and systemic corticosteroid use. Cataracts are usually bilateral and progress slowly. The visual acuity decrease is directly related to the density of the cataract. Types of cataracts include **senile cataract, congenital cataract, traumatic cataract, toxic cataract**, and **cataract associated with systemic disease**. The *senile cataract* is the most common form. Medical intervention consists of removing the opacified lens from the eye and implanting an artificial intraocular lens.

Tunica Vasculosa (Tunica Media)

IRIS

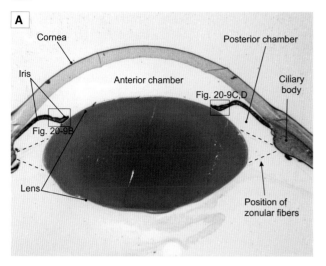

Figure 20-9A.   Overview of the iris and nearby structures. H&E, ×11

A low-magnification photomicrograph of the anterior part of the eye is shown. The **cornea, iris, lens, ciliary body,** and their anatomical relationships are reviewed here. The iris arises from the anterior part of the ciliary body and separates the **anterior** and **posterior chambers.** The iris covers part of the anterior surface of the lens and forms the pupil, which regulates the amount of light that enters the eye.

Figure 20-9B.   Iris. H&E, ×136

The **anterior iridial border** (**anterior surface of the iris**) consists of a discontinuous layer of fibroblasts and melanocytes. Beneath it is a thick layer of loose connective tissue, called the **iris stroma** (**stroma iridis**), which contains some fibers, cells (fibroblasts and melanocytes), and blood vessels. The **posterior surface of the iris** is covered by two layers of heavily **pigmented epithelial cells,** which completely block light coming into the eye (except the light through the pupil). These are the **anterior iridial epithelium** (**anterior pigment epithelium**) and the **posterior iridial epithelium** (**posterior pigment epithelium**).

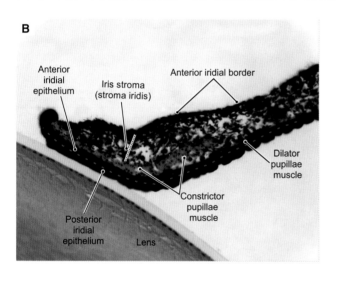

Figure 20-9C.   Constrictor pupillae muscle and its function. H&E, ×272; inset ×628

The pigment epithelium of the iris is partially in contact with the **lens capsule.** There is a thick layer of concentrically oriented smooth muscle in the stroma of the iris, which is called the **constrictor pupillae muscle** (**sphincter muscle**). It is innervated by **postganglionic parasympathetic fibers** from the **ciliary ganglion** and serves to decrease the pupillary size when the eye is exposed to strong light.

Figure 20-9D.   Dilator pupillae muscle and its function. H&E, ×473; inset ×680

The **dilator pupillae muscle** of the iris is composed of radially arranged myoid processes of myoepithelial cells of the anterior pigmented epithelium, located more peripherally in the iris than the constrictor pupillae muscle. It is innervated by **postganglionic sympathetic fibers** from the **superior cervical ganglion** and serves to increase pupillary size when the light is dim.

CONSTRICTOR PUPILLAE MUSCLE

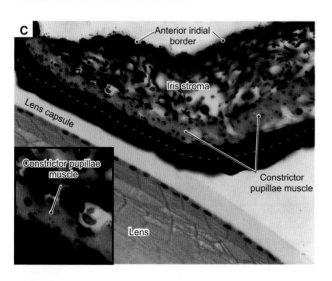

DILATOR PUPILLAE MUSCLE

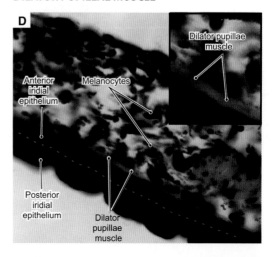

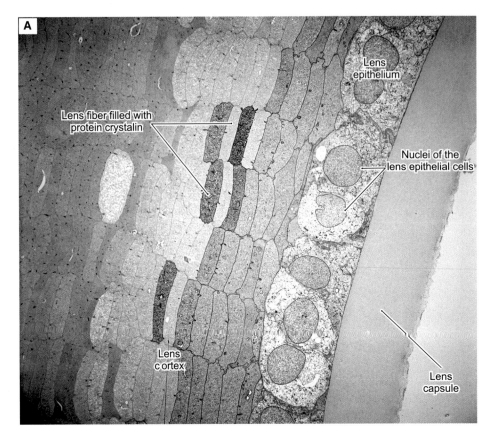

Figure 20-10A. Anterior surface of the lens. EM, ×3,600

A simple epithelium, the **lens epithelium**, covers the **anterior surface of the lens**. The heights of the cells vary, ranging from squamous near the center of the anterior surface to columnar at the edge (**equator**) of the lens. Because the lens develops from a ball of **epithelial cells** (**lens vesicle**) that invaginate from the surface ectoderm (**lens placode**), the basement membrane of the epithelium covers the surface of the lens as the **lens capsule**. The part of the lens capsule at the equator of the lens serves as the insertion for **zonule fibers** of the lens suspensory ligament. Behind the lens epithelium is an orderly array of lens fibers. Each lens fiber is a highly elongated, **crystallin-filled** remnant of an epithelial cell that extends the full thickness of the lens. The lens fibers in this view are seen in cross section.

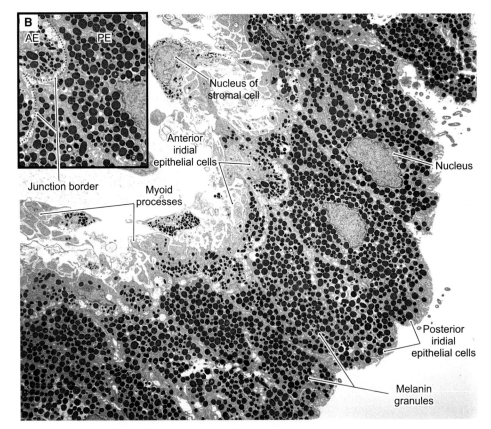

Figure 20-10B. Posterior surface of the iris. EM, ×4,600

The **posterior surface of the iris** is covered by double epithelium derived from the inner and outer layers of the lip of the original optic cup. The cells of the **posterior iridial epithelium** are tall and densely packed with melanin granules. The cells of the **anterior iridial epithelium** are more complicated in shape. Part of the cytoplasm of these cells contains **melanin granules**, similarly to the posterior epithelial cells; however, these cells also extend contractile processes into the adjacent iridial stroma. These **myoid processes** are filled with **actin filaments**, and, because of their radial orientation, the diameter of the pupil is increased when they contract. Therefore, the **myoepithelial cells** of the anterior iridial epithelium collectively constitute the pupillary dilator. At the border between the posterior and anterior iridial epithelia ([PE and AE, respectively] *inset*), the apices of the epithelial cells contact each other.

CILIARY BODY

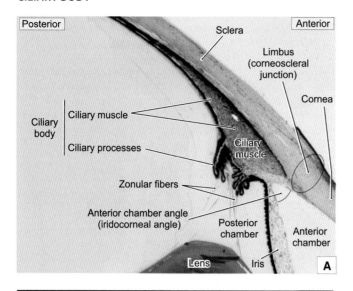

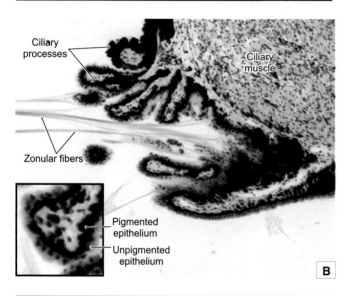

Figure 20-11A. Overview of the ciliary body and nearby structures. H&E, ×19

The **ciliary body** is located internally to the anterior margin of the sclera. The transition between the cornea and sclera is the **limbus (corneoscleral junction).** This is an important landmark for eye surgery procedures. The surface of the anterior portion of the ciliary body (**ciliary process**) has zonular fibers attached to it and is in contact with the aqueous humor. The surface of the posterior portion of the ciliary body is in contact with the vitreous body.

Figure 20-11B. Ciliary processes and the ciliary muscle. H&E, ×87; inset ×348

Ciliary processes have loose connective tissue cores and are covered by two layers of epithelium: (1) a **nonpigmented layer** and (2) a **pigmented layer.** The apical surfaces of the two epithelial layers face each other. Their basal surfaces each rest on a basement membrane, one bordering the ciliary stroma and the other bordering the aqueous humor. The cells are firmly connected by junctional complexes. The **ciliary muscle** contains three smooth muscle fiber groups: (1) **longitudinal muscle fibers,** which stretch the choroid to alter the opening of the anterior chamber angle for drainage of aqueous humor; (2) **radial muscle fibers,** which increase tension on the zonular fibers and cause the lens to flatten, allowing the eyes to focus for distant vision; and (3) **circular muscle fibers,** which relax the tension on the zonular fibers and cause the lens to become more convex to accommodate for near vision. Ciliary muscles are innervated by **parasympathetic nerve fibers** of the oculomotor nerve.

Figure 20-11C. Ciliary body, transverse and posterior views. H&E, ×34; inset ×62

The **ciliary body** consists of (1) the **ciliary ring (pars plana),** the region that contains a ring of smooth muscle (**ciliary muscle**) surrounded by loose connective tissue and covered by the ciliary epithelium and (2) the **ciliary processes (pars plicata),** fingerlike structures, which contain many fenestrated capillaries that produce aqueous humor. Aqueous humor flows from the posterior chamber through the pupil to the anterior chamber, then passes into the **trabecular meshwork** and finally into the **canal of Schlemm.**

CILIARY RING (PARS PLANA) AND CILIARY PROCESS (PARS PLICATA)

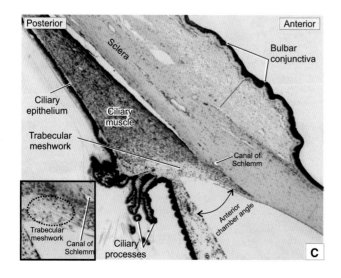

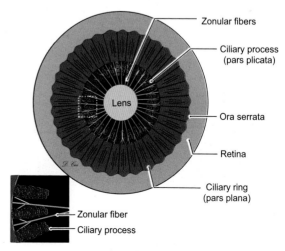

CILIARY BODY AND OUTFLOW OF AQUEOUS HUMOR

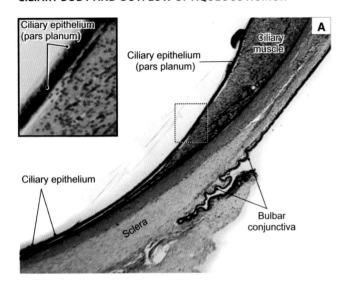

Figure 20-12A. Posterior portion of the ciliary body. H&E, ×34; inset ×102

The **ciliary body** lies posterior to the root of the **iris**, anterior to the **ora serrata**, and interior to the **sclera**. The ciliary body is triangular in shape. The anterior portion is thick, and the **posterior portion** gradually becomes thinner and ends at the ora serrata. The two cell layers of the **ciliary epithelium** cover the entire surface of the ciliary body.

Figure 20-12B. Ora serrata. H&E, ×34; inset ×102

The **ora serrata** is a **denticulate border (junction)** between the ciliary body and the retina; this is an important anatomic landmark for the ophthalmologist. The extended **ciliary epithelium** from the ciliary body is shown on the *right side* of the picture. The anterior portion of the **retina** is shown on the *left side* of the picture. The **pigmented ciliary epithelium** and its **basement membrane** are continuous with the **retinal pigmented epithelium** and the **Bruch membrane**.

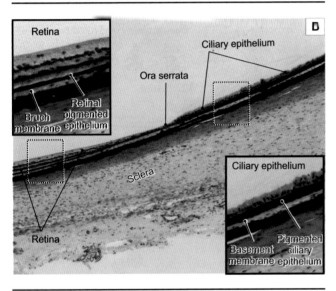

Aqueous humor is produced in the **posterior chamber** by the epithelium that lines the **ciliary processes** of the ciliary body. It flows through the pupil from the posterior chamber to the anterior chamber (*yellow arrow*), where it is absorbed into the **trabecular meshwork**. The aqueous humor then diffuses through connective tissue and epithelial tissue into the **canal of Schlemm**. **Aqueous veins** connect the canal of Schlemm to episcleral veins, where the aqueous humor is absorbed into the body's venous circulation.

Interference with the normal flow of aqueous humor leads to **increased intraocular pressure,** and a serious medical condition, **glaucoma,** may result. The most likely sites of blockage of the flow of aqueous humor are at the trabecular meshwork and the endothelial lining of the canal of Schlemm rather than the venous collector system.

CLINICAL CORRELATION

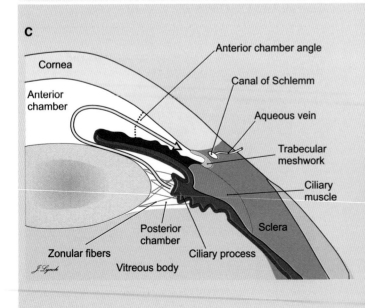

Figure 20-12C. Glaucoma.

Glaucoma is a group of eye diseases that produce elevated **intraocular pressure,** usually because of obstruction of the aqueous humor outflow. Glaucoma results in damage to the optic nerve and is a major cause of blindness. (1) **Open-angle glaucoma** is the most common type. Fragments from normal cell degeneration become deposited within the trabecular meshwork and endothelial lining of the canal of Schlemm and reduce the absorption of aqueous fluid. Intraocular pressure rises slowly over a long period of time. **Peripheral vision** may be reduced before the patient is aware of the loss. As the pressure rises, the optic disk becomes cupped. (2) **Acute angle-closure glaucoma** is also common. Occlusion of the anterior chamber angle occurs when the peripheral iris obstructs aqueous outflow. Intraocular pressure can rise quickly and reach very high levels. Patients may present with **severe headache and eye pain,** malaise, nausea, and vomiting. Immediate medical intervention is necessary to prevent vision loss.

Retina (Tunica Interna)

FOVEA

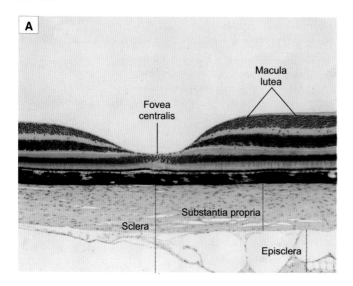

Figure 20-13A. Overview of the retina; fovea. H&E, ×17

The **retina** is a multilayered sheet of neural tissue covering the inner aspect of the posterior two thirds of the eyeball. There are regional variations in its structure: the **macular** (**central**) **region** is generally thicker than the **peripheral region**, and cone receptors predominate in the central retina, whereas rods are more numerous in the periphery. The **fovea centralis** is a small depression in the central retina caused by the displacement of the superficial layers, thereby allowing incoming light more direct access to the photoreceptors in this area. The photoreceptors here consist entirely of miniature cones, and there are no blood vessels in this region. These characteristics permit maximum visual acuity to be achieved in the fovea. The **macula lutea** is the region immediately surrounding the fovea centralis. *Macula lutea* means "yellow spot"; this region appears yellow in the living retina when viewed with an ophthalmoscope.

MACULAR RETINA

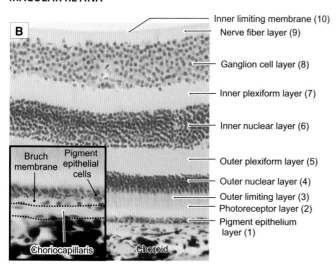

Inner limiting membrane (10)
Nerve fiber layer (9)

Ganglion cell layer (8)

Inner plexiform layer (7)

Inner nuclear layer (6)

Outer plexiform layer (5)
Outer nuclear layer (4)
Outer limiting layer (3)
Photoreceptor layer (2)
Pigment epithelium layer (1)

Bruch membrane Pigment epithelial cells
Choriocapillaris Choroid

Figure 20-13B. Macular region of the retina and the retinal layers. H&E, ×184; inset ×368

The **macular region of the retina** is relatively thick, and its ganglion cell layer contains many layers of nuclei. However, both the macular and peripheral regions of the retina have the same histologic layers: (1) the **pigment epithelium layer**, a layer of cuboidal cells that contain melanin granules; (2) the **photoreceptor layer**, external segments of rods and cones; (3) the **outer limiting layer**, a junction complex between the Müller cells and photoreceptor cells; (4) the **outer nuclear layer**, containing nuclei of the photoreceptor cells; (5) the **outer plexiform layer**, containing processes of photoreceptor cells, bipolar cells, and horizontal cells; (6) the **inner nuclear layer**, containing nuclei of bipolar cells, horizontal cells, amacrine cells, and Müller cells; (7) the **inner plexiform layer**, containing processes of the cells in the adjacent layers; (8) the **ganglion cell layer**, containing nuclei of the ganglion cells; (9) the **nerve fiber layer**, containing axons of the ganglion cells; and (10) the **inner limiting membrane**, which is the basement membrane of the Müller cells.

PERIPHERAL RETINA

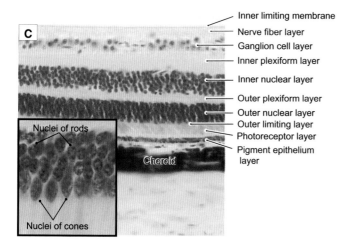

Inner limiting membrane
Nerve fiber layer
Ganglion cell layer
Inner plexiform layer
Inner nuclear layer
Outer plexiform layer
Outer nuclear layer
Outer limiting layer
Photoreceptor layer
Pigment epithelium layer

Nuclei of rods
Choroid
Nuclei of cones

Figure 20-13C. Peripheral region of the retina and distribution of the rods and cones. H&E, ×184; inset ×694

The **peripheral part of the retina** is thinner than the macular region and its **ganglion cell layer** becomes a single layer of nuclei. The **rod photoreceptors** are more numerous in the peripheral retina. The **nuclei of rod cells** are small and round and spread throughout the depth of the outer nuclear layer. The **cone photoreceptors** are present in both the center and periphery of the retina but are most highly concentrated in the **fovea** and **macula**. The **nuclei of cone cells** are large and ovoid in shape and often located at the base of the **outer nuclear layer**. **Rod and cone cells** are both **photoreceptor neurons**. *Rods* are specialized for motion detection and vision in dim light. *Cones* are specialized for fine visual acuity and color vision. Note the difference in thickness between the macular and peripheral regions of the retina and the relatively low number of ganglion cells in the peripheral retina.

A **Rod cell**

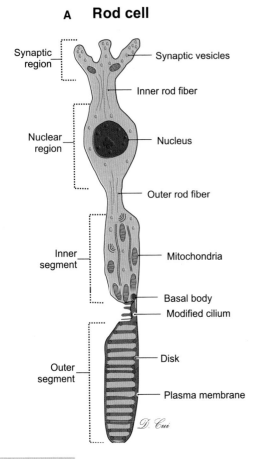

B **Cone cell**

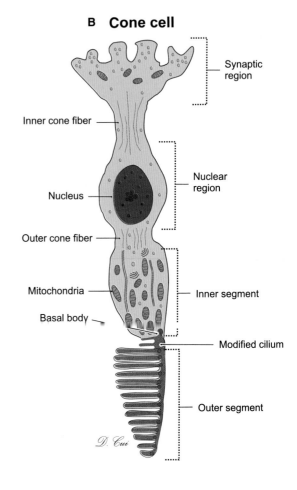

Figure 20-14A,B. Representation of rods and cones.

Rods and cones are photoreceptor cells in the retina. They are similar in structure, and both have (1) a **synaptic region**, (2) a **nuclear region**, (3) **inner segments**, and (4) **outer segments**. There are numerous **synaptic vesicles** in the synaptic regions, where the photoreceptors synapse with the dendrites of bipolar cells. The nuclear regions of rods and cones lie in the outer nuclear layer. The **inner** and **outer segments** form the photoreceptor layer of the retina. The *inner segments* contain **mitochondria, rough endoplasmic reticulum, Golgi apparatuses**, and other organelles that support the synthesis of proteins. The *outer segments* are in contact with the apical region of the pigmented epithelium cells. **Outer segments of rods** are composed of a series of superimposed **disks**, which have individual membranes, are stacked on each other, and are enclosed within the **plasma membrane**. **Outer segments of cones** have **disks** that are formed by invaginations of the **plasma membrane**. The membranes of the disks are continuous with the plasma membrane of the cell. The inner region is much wider than the outer region, which gives a cone appearance. Other differences between rods and cones are listed in Table 20-1.

TABLE 20-1 Comparison of Rods and Cones

Types of Photoreceptor Cells	Synaptic Region	Nuclear Region	Inner Segment	Outer Segment	Distribution in the Retina	Main Function
Rods	Spherule synapses with dendrites of one bipolar neuron	Small, round nucleus	Fewer mitochondria than cones; synthesized proteins passed only to newly forming disks	Cylindrical in shape; disk membranes are separate and are not connected to the outside plasma membrane; disks contain rhodopsin protein	Numerous in the peripheral retina; none in fovea	Vision in dim light; motion detection
Cones	Pedicle synapses with dendrites of several bipolar neurons	Large, ovoid nucleus	More mitochondria than rods; synthesized proteins passed to entire outer segment	Cone shaped; disk membranes are connected to the plasma membrane and form invaginated membranes; disks contain iodopsin protein	Highly concentrated in the fovea and macula lutea; less numerous in periphery	Color vision; perception of fine detail

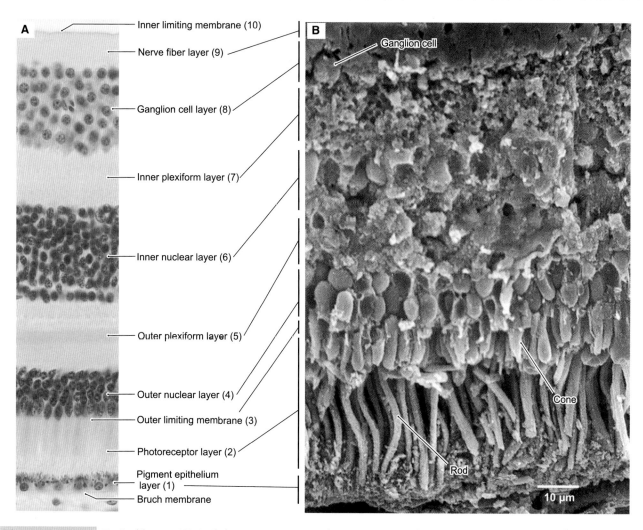

A

- Inner limiting membrane (10)
- Nerve fiber layer (9)
- Ganglion cell layer (8)
- Inner plexiform layer (7)
- Inner nuclear layer (6)
- Outer plexiform layer (5)
- Outer nuclear layer (4)
- Outer limiting membrane (3)
- Photoreceptor layer (2)
- Pigment epithelium layer (1)
- Bruch membrane

B — Ganglion cell, Cone, Rod, 10 µm

Figure 20-15A,B. **Retinal layers.** H&E (*left*), ×463; Scanning electron micrograph (SEM), freeze-fracture preparation (*right*) ×1,200

There are 10 histologic layers in the retina: (1) **pigment epithelium layer** (cells contain melanin granules); (2) **photoreceptor layer** (contains the external segments and part of the internal segments of the photoreceptor cells: rods and cones); (3) **outer limiting membrane** (border formed by the Müller cell processes); (4) **outer nuclear layer** (contains the somata and nuclei of the photoreceptor cells); (5) **outer plexiform layer** (contains the processes of photoreceptor, bipolar, horizontal, and interplexiform cells); (6) **inner nuclear layer** (contains the nuclei of bipolar, horizontal, amacrine, interplexiform, and Müller cells); (7) **inner plexiform layer** (contains the processes of bipolar, amacrine, interplexiform, and ganglion cells); (8) **ganglion cell layer** (contains the somata and nuclei of the retinal ganglion cells); (9) **nerve fiber layer** (contains the axons of the retinal ganglion cells, Müller cell processes, and astrocytes); and (10) **inner limiting membrane** (basement membrane of the Müller cells). Within the outer plexiform layer, the photoreceptor cell processes synapse on the bipolar and horizontal cell processes, and the horizontal and interplexiform cell processes synapse on the bipolar cell processes. Within the inner plexiform layer, the bipolar cell processes synapse on the amacrine, interplexiform, and retinal ganglion cell processes, and the amacrine cell processes synapse on the retinal ganglion cell processes. The freeze-fracture preparation of the peripheral retina in image B shows the 3D shapes of the various cells in the retina. This section from the peripheral retina has fewer ganglion cells than the macular retina illustrated in image A.

FUNCTIONAL RETINAL LAYERS

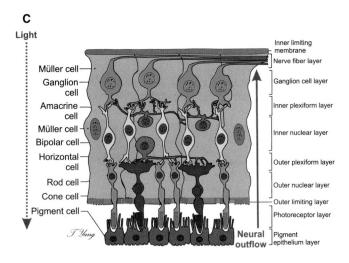

Figure 20-15C. Representation of the functional retinal layers.

Light passes through all **retinal layers** to activate the **photoreceptor cells** (rods and cones), and excess light is absorbed by pigmented epithelial cells. The photoreceptors transduce the light into electrochemical signals, which pass to the **conducting neurons** (bipolar cells, then **ganglion cells**). Horizontal and amacrine cells are **association neurons** that have long dendrites. The dendrites of the **horizontal cells** synapse with photoreceptors and contribute to the elaborate neuronal connections in the **outer plexiform layer**. The dendrites of **amacrine cells** are in contact with bipolar and ganglion cells and modulate signals in the **inner plexiform layer**. The ganglion cells collect all visual information and send it along their axons in the optic nerve. **Müller cells** are large supporting neuroglial cells and extend from the **inner limiting membrane** to the **outer limiting membrane**. Their processes surround all the neuronal elements of the retina.

SYNOPSIS 20-1 Retinal Layers

- *Pigment epithelium layer*, a layer of cuboidal cells, which are rich in melanin granules. This layer is important in absorbing excess light and in esterifying vitamin A.
- *Photoreceptor (rods and cones) layer*, consists of inner and outer segments of the photoreceptor cells.
- *Outer limiting layer*, a plexus of junction complexes that joins the membranes of the photoreceptor cells and Müller cells (retinal glial cells).
- *Outer nuclear layer*, contains nuclei of the photoreceptor cells (rods and cones).
- *Outer plexiform layer*, consists of axodendritic synapses between the axons of the photoreceptor cells and dendrites of the bipolar and horizontal cells.
- *Inner nuclear layer*, contains nuclei of bipolar cells, horizontal cells, amacrine cells, and Müller cells.
- *Inner plexiform layer*, composed of axodendritic synapses between the bipolar cell axons, ganglion cell dendrites, and processes of the amacrine cells.
- *Ganglion cell layer*, contains nuclei of the ganglion cells.
- *Nerve fiber layer*, contains axons of the ganglion cells.
- *Inner limiting membrane*, the basement membrane of the Müller cells.

The ganglion cells and their axons are part of the central nervous system. They cannot regenerate following severe damage. Embryologically, the pigmented epithelium layer and the neural layers of the retina originate from different layers of the optic vesicle. Therefore, **retinal detachment** may occur between the pigmented epithelium layer and the rest of the neural retina.

CLINICAL CORRELATIONS

A

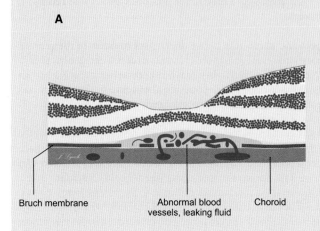

Bruch membrane   Abnormal blood   Choroid
                        vessels, leaking fluid

Figure 20-16A. Age-Related Macular Degeneration.

Age-related macular degeneration (ARMD) is a degenerative eye disease affecting the central portion of the retina. Symptoms include blurred vision, distortion of straight lines, and worsening of color vision. There are two forms: **exudative (wet)** and **nonexudative (dry)**. *Wet ARMD* is characterized by the growth of new vessels from the choroidal circulation and **serous fluid leakage** from the new vessels. This causes detachment of the retina and macula, producing a rapid and irreversible loss of central vision. Treatment options include laser photocoagulation, surgery, and drugs. *Dry ARMD* is characterized by subretinal drusen deposits (focal eosinophilic material arising from the **Bruch membrane** and lying between the pigment epithelium and the Bruch membrane), atrophy and degeneration of the outer retina, including the retinal pigment epithelium, Bruch membrane, and choriocapillaris. The causes of ARMD are not well understood, but risk factors include age, smoking, family history, hypertension, and ethnicity (higher in non-Hispanic Caucasians).

B

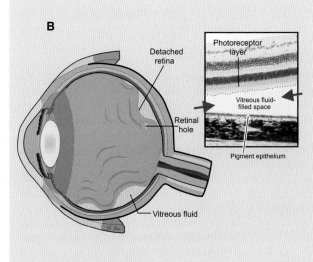

Detached
retina

Photoreceptor
layer

Retinal
hole

Vitreous fluid-
filled space

Pigment epithelium

Vitreous fluid

Figure 20-16B. Retinal Detachment. H&E, ×62

Retinal detachment is an eye condition in which the sensory retina separates from the underlying retinal pigment epithelium and choroid (see *red arrows*). It is categorized into three major types: (1) **rhegmatogenous retinal detachment ([RRD]** illustrated) is the most common; it occurs when **vitreous fluid** leaks into the subretinal space through a break in the retina; (2) **exudative** or **serous detachment** occurs in association with inflammation or a tumor; and (3) **traction detachment** occurs when scar tissue on the retina's surface contracts and causes the retina to separate from the retinal **pigment epithelium**. Retinal detachment is a medical emergency that can lead to permanent vision loss. Time is critical for surgical reattachment of the retina, which will usually preserve vision. Symptoms include flashes, floaters, and visual field distortion or loss. Treatment options include laser photocoagulation, cryoretinopexy, vitrectomy, and silicone oil repair.

Optic Nerve and Optic Disk

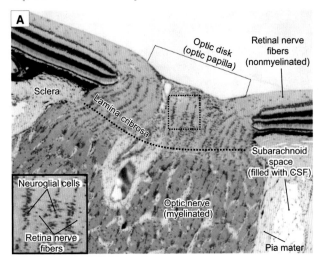

Figure 20-17A. Optic nerve and optic disk. H&E, ×22; inset ×83

The **optic nerve** is a nerve fiber trunk formed by the convergence of retinal ganglion cell axons at the posterior pole of the eye. From there, they leave the globe on their way to the brain. Each optic nerve contains about one million **myelinated axons** and even more **neuroglial cells**. The surface of the optic nerve is covered by pia mater, which is continuous with that on the surface of the brain. The **optic disk** (**optic nerve papilla**) is the small circular site in the retina where the retinal nerve fiber layer (**nonmyelinated nerve fibers**) continues into the optic nerve. The nonmyelinated nerve fibers begin to acquire myelin at the level of the **lamina cribrosa** (*thin dotted line*), a perforated, sievelike region of the sclera through which optic nerve fibers and blood vessels pass. The myelinated segments of ganglion cell axons, therefore, form the optic nerve. The **neuroglial cells** include **oligodendrocytes**, which produce myelin for axons in the CNS, and **astrocytes**, which perform several nutritive and supportive functions.

CLINICAL CORRELATION

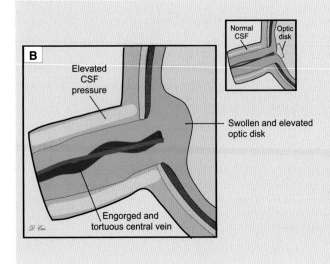

Figure 20-17B. Papilledema.

Papilledema is a noninflammatory swelling of the optic disk. It is produced by **increased intracranial pressure** that is transmitted along the optic nerve sheath as elevated **cerebrospinal fluid** pressure, and it is, therefore, a sign of a potentially life-threatening condition. The increased pressure disrupts blood circulation within the optic nerve, causing leakage of water, protein, and other contents into the extracellular spaces of the optic disk. The most noticeable symptoms of increased intracranial pressure are headache and vomiting. Clinical findings include a **swollen and elevated optic disk** (papilledema), **engorged and tortuous retinal veins**, and focal hemorrhages. **Cerebral tumors, subdural hematoma, malignant hypertension**, and **hydrocephalus** are the most common causes of increased intracranial pressure and papilledema. Because papilledema is a sign of many systemic intracranial and spinal diseases, the correct diagnosis of the underlying disease is essential for proper treatment.

SYNOPSIS 20-2 Clinical Terms for the Eye

- *Blepharitis:* Inflammation of the eyelids and especially of their margins.
- *Ptosis:* Drooping or falling down, usually of the upper eyelid, because of muscle weakness or paralysis.
- *Open angle (glaucoma):* Raised intraocular pressure in which obstruction to aqueous flow occurs at the ultrastructural level, within the walls of the tiniest interstices of the trabecular meshwork.
- *Closed angle (glaucoma):* The flow of aqueous fluid is blocked by the root of the iris. This can be a generalized closure (hyperopic eyes) or in multiple focal adhesions caused by inflammation (peripheral anterior synechiae).
- *Cupping of the optic disk:* Glaucoma destroys retinal axons as they traverse the optic disk in the walls of a central, cup-shaped conduit. As the walls disappear, the cup enlarges.
- *Dry macular degeneration:* Scattered drusen damage the pigment epithelium of the macula, gradually decreasing visual acuity.
- *Wet macular degeneration:* Abnormal capillaries break through the retinal pigment epithelium and leak underneath the retina. When close to the fovea, they can decrease visual acuity.
- *Limbus:* An anatomic transition zone between cornea and sclera (corneoscleral junction), which is an important landmark for eye surgery procedures.
- *Ora serrata:* A denticulate border (junction) between the ciliary body and the retina; this is an important anatomic landmark for the ophthalmologist.

From Histology to Pathology

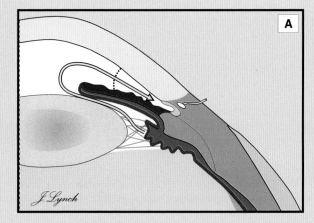 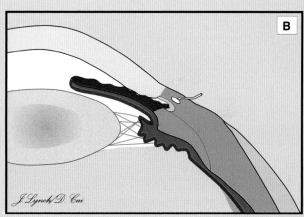

Figure 20-18.   Normal outflow of aqueous humor and acute angle-closure glaucoma. H&E, ×100

Normal outflow of aqueous humor on the *left*. **Acute angle-closure glaucoma** on the *right*. Acute angle-closure glaucoma is a form of glaucoma characterized by a sudden increase in intraocular pressure because the angle of the anterior chamber is blocked, and the aqueous humor cannot drain from the anterior chamber. It is usually unilateral and excruciating pain may radiate to areas of trigeminal distribution.

Atrophy of the optic nerve head ("cupping") along with peripheral vision defects is the common finding with acute angle-closure glaucoma. Treatment may involve surgery and medications to lower the intraocular pressure and reverse angle closure. The normal flow of aqueous humor is indicated by the curved **yellow arrow** in image A. In image B, drainage of aqueous humor into the canal of Schlemm is blocked.

Clinical Vignette Questions

1. A 54-year-old Asian woman was brought to your clinic with a sudden onset of excruciating pain and vision loss in the right eye. She was complaining of nausea, and she had vomited several times in the past 2 hours. The patient had no history of eye injury. An eye exam showed conjunctival redness, a swollen right upper eyelid, and tearing. Under the slit lamp, you see the swollen and cloudy cornea, a shallow anterior chamber, and a dilated and fixed pupil that reacts poorly to light. The intraocular pressure is 28 mm Hg (normal = 10–21 mm Hg) on the left side of the eye and 45 mm Hg on the right side. What is the most likely diagnosis?

A. Acute angle-closure glaucoma
B. Bacterial keratitis
C. Blepharitis
D. Iritis
E. Viral conjunctivitis

2. A 40-year-old woman with myopia (nearsightedness) was involved in a mild motor accident 5 hours ago. She was wearing a seatbelt, but the impact of the airbag deployment caused discomfort in her left eye with tearing, flashes of light, and blurred vision. Her husband brought her to the emergency department for a check-up. The patient told you she was wearing contact lenses when the accident happened. Eye examination showed a minor corneal abrasion, edema, and visual field loss. Binocular indirect ophthalmoscopy examination revealed elevation of the translucent detached retina with a large horseshoe tear. Prior to this accident, the patient was healthy except for myopia, and she never had an injury to her eye. Your diagnosis is rhegmatogenous retinal detachment and corneal abrasion, and emergency eye surgery is scheduled. Histologically, where does this retinal detachment most likely occur in the retina for this patient?

A. Ganglion cell layer and inner plexiform layer
B. Inner nuclear layer and outer plexiform layer
C. Nerve fiber layer and inner limiting membrane
D. Outer nuclear layer and outer limiting layer
E. Photoreceptor layer and pigment epithelium layer

21 Ear

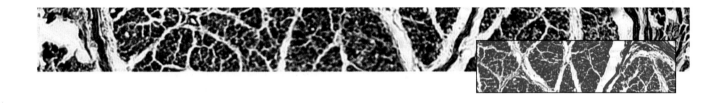

Introduction and Key Concepts for the Ear
Auditory System
Vestibular System

Clinical Vignette Questions

Introduction and Key Concepts for the Ear

The **ear** is a complex structure that serves two important sensory functions, **hearing** (through the **auditory system**) and **balance** (through the **vestibular system**). Sensory receptor organs that serve the two functions are supplied by two distinct branches of cranial nerve (CN) VIII, the **acoustic branch** and the **vestibular branch**. The ear can be divided into three general regions, the **outer ear**, **middle ear**, and **inner ear**. (1) The *outer ear* consists of a **pinna** (**auricle**), an irregularly shaped structure with a core of cartilage covered on both sides by thin skin, and an **external auditory meatus** that conducts sound to the middle ear. (2) The *middle ear* includes the **tympanic membrane**, the **tympanic cavity** containing the **ossicles**, and the **auditory tube**. The *tympanic membrane*, the landmark between the outer ear and middle ear, covers the medial end of the external auditory meatus and converts sound waves in the air to mechanical vibrations. The *tympanic cavity* is an air-filled space that contains the *ossicles*, three tiny bones that conduct the mechanical vibrations of the tympanic membrane to the **oval window** of the cochlea. The tympanic cavity is connected to the nasopharynx by the *auditory tube* (eustachian tube), thereby allowing the air pressure on each side of the tympanic membrane to be equalized when the ambient air pressure changes (e.g., by changes in altitude). (3) The *inner ear* consists of structures contained within the **bony labyrinth**, a system of tunnels and cavities in the petrous portion of the **temporal bone,** the hardest bone in the body. The structures include the **cochlear labyrinth** or **cochlea** (Latin for "snail shell"), which subserves hearing. It contains a spiral, fluid-filled tunnel within which a membranous tube, the **cochlear duct**, is suspended. The sensory receptors that detect sound are located in a strip of specialized epithelium, the **organ of Corti** (**spiral organ**), in the cochlear duct. The **vestibular labyrinth** consists of a complex group of fluid-filled tunnels and cavities in the temporal bone that contain a group of interconnected membranous structures, the **semicircular ducts, utricle,** and **saccule.** The sensory receptors that are involved in balance are located in specialized regions of the semicircular ducts (**rotation**) and in the utricle and saccule (**static head position** and **acceleration**).

Auditory System

Sound is normally produced by compression and rarefaction waves in air, of various frequencies, that impinge upon the tympanic membrane where they are converted into mechanical vibrations in the ossicles. The mechanical vibrations, in turn, are transferred to the fluid of the **vestibule** at the **oval window.** This fluid is **perilymph**, a sodium-rich fluid that is similar in composition to cerebrospinal fluid and extracellular fluid. The resulting vibrations, or pressure waves, in the perilymph spread into the **scala vestibuli** of the cochlear labyrinth and act upon mechanoreceptors in the **cochlear duct** to produce the sensation of **hearing.** The cochlear duct is a membranous tube, triangular in cross section, that coils inside the spiral tunnel in the cochlea. It is suspended within the cochlear labyrinth so that it divides the labyrinth into two tunnels, the **scala vestibuli** (above) and the **scala tympani** (below), which are connected with each other by a small opening, the **helicotrema.** The cochlear duct encloses the **scala media**, a space containing **endolymph**, a potassium-rich fluid similar in composition to intracellular fluid. The scala media is bounded above by the **vestibular membrane**, below by the **basilar membrane**, and externally by the **spiral ligament** and **stria vascularis**. The sensory receptors for hearing are specialized epithelial cells (**hair cells**) in the **organ of Corti**. The hair cells get their name from clumps of **stereocilia** that project from their apical surfaces and contact an overlying gelatinous structure, the **tectorial membrane**. The organ of Corti sits on the basilar membrane and extends its entire length, from the base of the cochlea to the apex. It contains a single row of **inner hair cells** and three or four rows of **outer hair cells**. In humans, there are about 3,500 inner hair cells and 12,000 outer hair cells, yet 95% of the afferent axons in the auditory nerve contact only inner hair cells. The primary function of the inner hair cells appears to be basic frequency and loudness discrimination, whereas the outer hair cells appear to be primarily concerned with the fine-tuning of frequency discrimination in the cochlea. When sound waves cause pressure waves to occur in the scala vestibuli and scala media, the basilar membrane vibrates up and down, and a shearing force is generated between the surface of the organ of Corti and the tectorial membrane. The shearing force bends the stereocilia of the hair cells, leading to the release of neurotransmitters by the hair cells and the initiation of action potentials in auditory nerve axons.

Vestibular System

The sense of **balance** is critical to our ability to walk, run, jump, or even just stand still with eyes closed. One important source of neural signals that aid in controlling such behaviors is the **peripheral vestibular apparatus**. This includes the **vestibular labyrinth**, consisting of the **vestibule**, a cavity within the temporal bone, and three **semicircular canals**, curved tunnels that connect with the vestibule. One canal is in approximately the horizontal plane; the other two are in approximately the vertical plane and at right angles to each other. These cavities in the bone are filled with **perilymph**. Floating within the vestibule are two membranous saclike structures, the **utricle** and **saccule**. Within each of the semicircular canals is a membranous tube called a **semicircular duct**, which joins the utricle at each of its ends. The utricle, saccule, and semicircular ducts contain **endolymph**. The **semicircular ducts** detect rotational movements of the head. Each duct has an enlargement at one end where it joins the utricle. This swelling is called the **ampulla** and contains the sensory receptors that are stimulated by rotational movements. A short wall of connective tissue, the **crista ampullaris**, extends across part of each ampulla. Hair cells, similar to those of the organ of Corti, cover the upper surface of the crista. Their **stereocilia** and **kinocilia** are embedded in a gel-like structure, the **cupula**, which blocks the ampulla. When the head turns, the inertia of the endolymph in the semicircular ducts causes the fluid to push against the cupula and deflect the cilia of the hair cells, thereby initiating action potentials in axons in the vestibular nerve. **Vestibular hair cells** are also clustered in a small region of the **utricle**, the **macula utriculi**. The stereocilia and kinocilia of these hair cells are embedded in a gelatinous structure, the **otolithic membrane**. Thousands of tiny calcium carbonate crystals, **otoconia**, are clustered on the surface of the otolithic membrane. These crystals are heavier than the surrounding endolymph. **Gravity** or **linear acceleration**, therefore, exerts a force on the otoconia, causing the underlying cilia to be deflected and consequently sending a neural signal to the central nervous system (CNS) related to head position or acceleration. The **saccule** contains a similar region, the **macula sacculi**.

Anatomy of the Ear

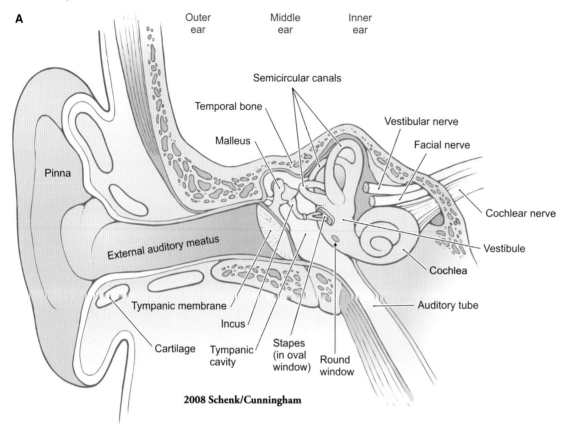

Figure 21-1A. Overview of the ear: outer (external), middle, and inner ear.

The **ear** is divided into three regions: the **outer ear, middle ear,** and **inner ear.** The *outer ear* includes the **pinna** and the **external auditory meatus.** The *pinna* (or **auricle**) is an irregularly shaped structure of elastic cartilage covered by a layer of **perichondrium** (connective tissue) and thin skin. One important function of the pinna is to selectively filter higher frequency sound waves and, therefore, aid in spatial localization of sounds in the environment. The *external auditory meatus* is a tunnel that carries sound waves to the **tympanic membrane,** where the compressions and rarefactions of air are converted into mechanical vibrations. The outer third of the meatus is lined with a continuation of the cartilage of the pinna and a continuation of the perichondrium and thin skin that covers the pinna. In the inner two thirds of the meatus, the skin adheres directly to the periosteum of the temporal bone. The *middle ear* is an air-filled cavity (**tympanic cavity**) that is separated from the outer ear by the **tympanic membrane.** It contains three tiny bones, the **ossicles,** which are the smallest bones in the body. These ossicles transfer sound-induced movement of the tympanic membrane to the fluid contained in the **cochlea,** where the vibrations are transduced into nerve impulses. The middle ear is connected to the posterior region of the nasopharynx by the **auditory tube** (**eustachian tube**), which allows the equalization of air pressure on each side of the tympanic membrane. The *inner ear* contains the **cochlea** and the **vestibular apparatus.** The cochlea, the snail shell–shaped organ of hearing, includes a membranous tube lying within a fluid-filled tunnel in the temporal bone. **Auditory hair cells** in the cochlea are excited by vibratory movements of the fluid and generate action potentials in auditory nerve fibers. The **vestibular apparatus** is the body's sensory organ for balance and consists of membranous structures contained within the three **semicircular canals** and the **vestibule** as well as some accessory structures. **Vestibular hair cells** within the **semicircular ducts** (inside the semicircular canals) detect rotational movement of the head in three dimensions. Vestibular hair cells within the **utricle** and **saccule** (inside the vestibule) detect static head position and linear acceleration in the horizontal and vertical planes, respectively. The auditory and vestibular branches of CN VIII innervate these structures.

Outer (External) Ear

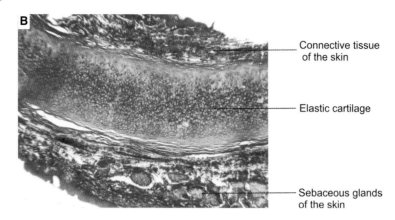

Connective tissue
of the skin

Elastic cartilage

Sebaceous glands
of the skin

Figure 21-1B.   Pinna (auricle). H&E, ×40

The **pinna**, also called the **auricle**, is the flexible, visible part of the external ear, which consists of an irregularly shaped plate of **elastic cartilage** covered by thin skin on both sides. It is attached to the skull by muscle and ligament, and **sebaceous glands, sweat glands,** and **hair follicles** can be found in the skin of the pinna. The shape of the pinna facilitates collecting, locating, and amplifying sound waves. The pinna is largely innervated by the **auriculotemporal (CN V$_3$), lesser occipital (C2),** and **auricular (CN X) nerves.** The **superficial temporal artery** and **posterior auricular artery** supply blood to the pinna.

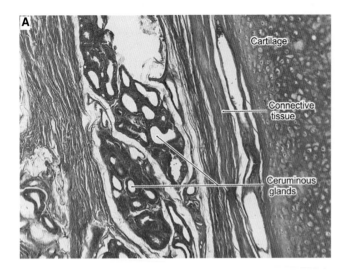

Figure 21-2A.   External auditory meatus. H&E, ×40

The **external auditory (acoustic) meatus**, also called the **external auditory (acoustic) canal**, is a tubular structure lined by skin. The outer one third of the canal is comprised of cartilage as supporting tissue, and the inner two thirds, located within the **temporal bone**, extends continuously to the **tympanic membrane**. Hair follicles, sebaceous glands, and **ceruminous glands (apocrine glands)** can be found in the skin of the external auditory meatus. The **ceruminous gland** produces **cerumen (ear wax)** to moisturize, clean, and protect the canal and keep foreign materials away from the tympanic membrane. The external auditory meatus is innervated by the **intermedius nerve** of **CN VII** as well as the mandibular division of the trigeminal nerve (CN V$_3$) and the auricular branch of the vagus nerve (CN X).

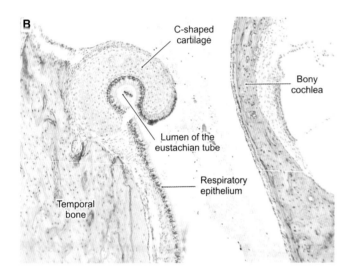

Figure 21-2B.   Pharyngotympanic (eustachian/auditory tube), H&E, ×100

The **pharyngotympanic (eustachian) tube**, also called the **auditory tube**, is located within the **tympanic cavity**. It is covered by **ciliated pseudostratified columnar epithelium (respiratory epithelium)**, and it connects the middle ear to the nasopharynx. Its external opening can be found in the back of the **nasal cavity**, within the **nasopharynx**, inferior to the gross anatomical feature called the **torus tubarius**. The **pharyngotympanic tube** plays an important role in regulating the air pressure within the middle ear and balancing the air pressure between the middle ear and outside air pressure.

The **pharyngotympanic tube** can become swollen and blocked when a patient has an allergy or catches a bad cold. The patient can experience **ear pain, fullness, tinnitus** (ringing tone in the ear), and conductive hearing loss, especially during air travel when a plane is taking off and landing.

CLINICAL CORRELATION

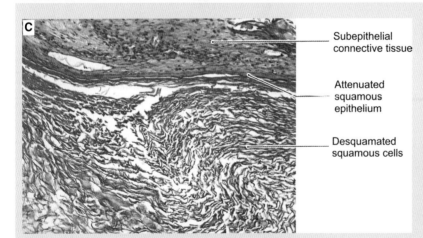

Figure 21-2C.   Cholesteatoma. H&E, ×200

Cholesteatoma is a mass of keratin-producing squamous epithelium that often grows from the **tympanic membrane** in the middle ear. As cholesteatoma progresses, it can cause damage to the **ossicles, inner ear, mastoid air cells,** and the **external auditory canal** leading to **sepsis, meningitis, brain abscess, sensorineural hearing loss, vertigo, facial paralysis,** and even death. Trauma and chronic inflammation of the tympanic membrane may increase the incidence of **cholesteatoma**. Surgery involving a **tympanomastoidectomy** remains the primary treatment for this condition.

Middle Ear

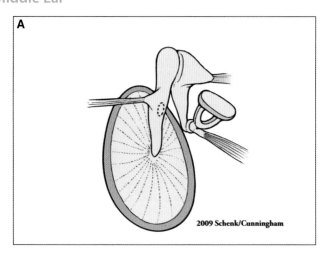

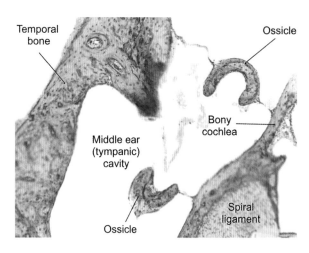

Figure 21-3A. Middle ear structures. H&E, ×100

The **tympanic membrane** (viewed here from its medial side within the middle ear) is a thin, semitransparent cone-shaped sheet of collagenous fibers and fibroblasts, covered on the lateral (outer) surface by a very thin layer of skin and on the medial (inner) surface by the mucosa that lines the rest of the tympanic cavity. The most lateral ossicle, the **malleus** (hammer), is attached to the upper half of the tympanic membrane. The **incus** (anvil) is attached to the malleus by a saddle-shaped synovial joint, and the **stapes** (stirrups) is attached to the incus by a ball-and-socket synovial joint. The footplate of the stapes is attached to the oval window of the **vestibule**. When sound waves cause the tympanic membrane to vibrate, the chain of ossicles rotates about the **anterior malleal** and **posterior incudal ligaments**, causing the footplate of the stapes to rock on the **oval window** producing waves of compression in the fluid that fills the **bony labyrinth**. This lever arrangement increases the pressure on the oval window ~20-fold compared to the air pressure on the tympanic membrane in a phenomenon known as impedance matching. The **tensor tympani muscle** and the **stapedius muscle** contract during very loud sounds, reducing the movement of the ossicles and the oval window.

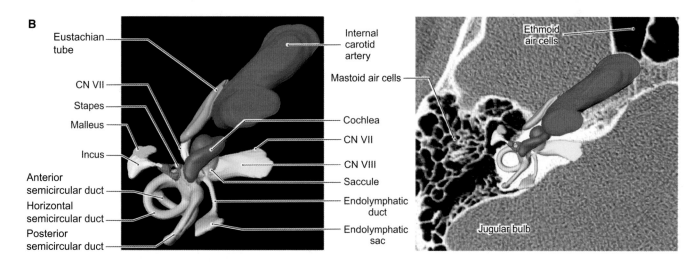

Figure 21-3B. Middle ear 3D structures. Stereoscopic model (*left*); stereoscopic model with computed tomography (CT) image.

The 3D structures of the middle and inner ear are labeled in the image on the *left*. The image on the *right* depicts an axial CT slice through the temporal region of the skull overlain on 3D structures of the middle and inner ear. Inner ear structures such as the bony **cochlea** and several of the structures comprising the vestibular apparatus are visible, such as the **superior (anterior)**, **horizontal (lateral)**, and **posterior semicircular ducts**, which are the membranous structures found within the bony superior (anterior), horizontal (lateral), and posterior semicircular canals, respectively. The membranous **endolymphatic duct**, which courses through the bony vestibular aqueduct and its associated membranous **endolymphatic sac** are also visible. The **utricle** can be partially seen where the horizontal and posterior semicircular ducts converge. The **superior semicircular duct** (*left*) also has a connection to utricle. The **saccule** can also be seen in *image A* near the cochlea. Additional associated structures depicted include the **pharyngotympanic (eustachian) tube** (*orange*) and several structures of extreme surgical importance, including the jugular bulb (*right image*), internal carotid artery (*red*), facial nerve (CN VII; *light yellow*), and vestibulocochlear nerve (CN VIII; *yellow*).

Inner Ear

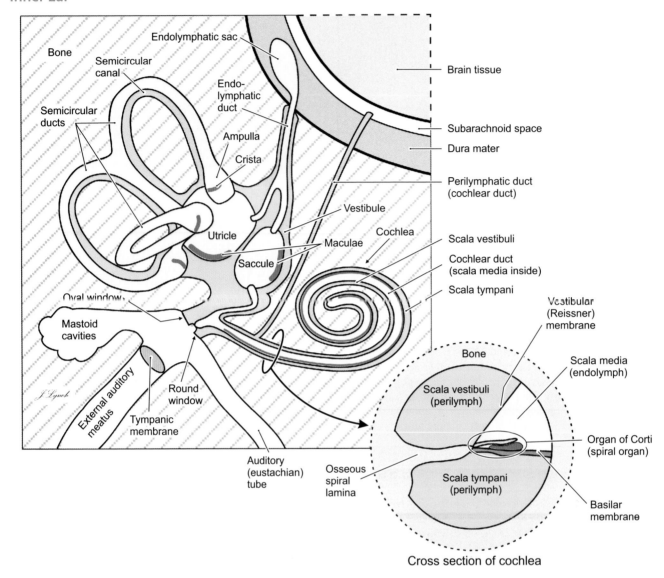

Cross section of cochlea

Figure 21-4. **Major structures of the inner ear.**

The **bony labyrinth** is a complex cavity in the petrous portion of the **temporal bone**, the hardest bone in the body. The cavity is lined with endosteum and contains **perilymph** (*blue shading*), a clear fluid with a composition very similar to that of cerebrospinal fluid. The bony labyrinth is divided into three portions, the **vestibule**, the **cochlea** (anteriorly), and the **semicircular canals** (posteriorly). The **membranous labyrinth**, consisting of the three **semicircular ducts**, the **utricle**, and the **saccule**, lies within the bony labyrinth. The walls of the membranous labyrinth are, in general, composed of a thin layer of fibrous connective tissue; a thin layer of more delicate, more vascularized connective tissue; and an internal lining of simple epithelium. Two saclike structures, the **utricle** and **saccule**, are found in the vestibule. A **semicircular duct** lies within each of the semicircular canals. A similar but more complicated structure, the **cochlear duct**, lies within the bony cochlea. These membranous structures are continuous with each other and contain **endolymph** (*yellow shading*), a fluid with a high concentration of K+ (potassium) ions that is unique in the body. Specialized regions within the membranous labyrinth (indicated by *thick orange lines*) contain receptor cells innervated by branches of the vestibulocochlear nerve (CN VIII). These include the **cristae** (singular, *crista*, from Latin for "crest") in each of the **ampullae** (singular, *ampulla*, from Latin for "flask" or "bottle") of the semicircular ducts, the **maculae** (singular, *macula*, from Latin for "spot") of the utricle and saccule, and the **organ of Corti** (**spiral organ**) in the cochlear duct. The receptor cells in all these regions are specialized epithelial cells (**hair cells**) that transduce movements of the basilar membrane into nerve impulses.

MEMBRANOUS LABYRINTH

A

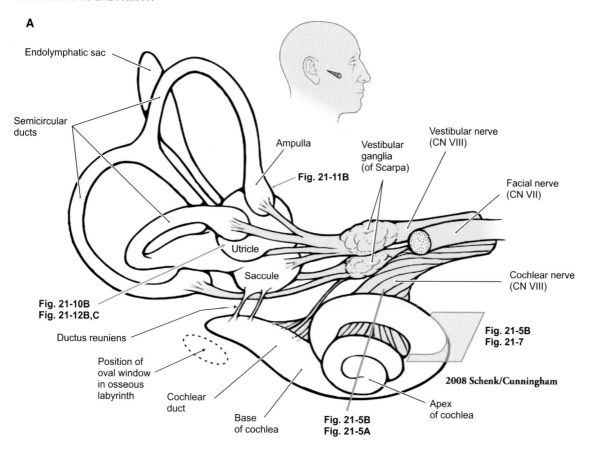

Figure 21-5A. Membranous labyrinth: utricle, saccule, cochlear duct, and semicircular ducts.

The endolymph-filled **membranous labyrinth** floats within the perilymph-filled **osseous (bony) labyrinth**. This anatomically correct drawing shows the position of the cochlea and semicircular canals within the head. The labyrinth is viewed from the direction indicated by the *pointer* in the *small inset* of the head. The position of the nerves that innervate the **cochlea, cristae of the ampullae**, and **maculae of the utricle and saccule** are illustrated. The positions and planes of section of the photomicrographs that follow in this chapter are indicated by *blue lines, arrows,* or *boxes*. The *dashed oval* indicates the position of the oval window in the osseous labyrinth.

B

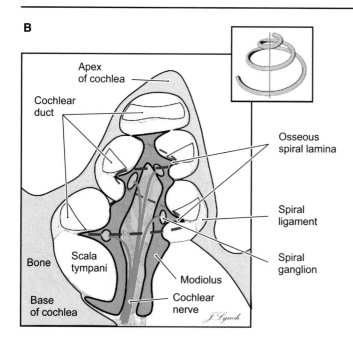

Figure 21-5B. Cochlear duct and modiolus.

The membranous **cochlear duct** lies within a spiral-shaped tunnel in the temporal bone. In this illustration, the cochlea has been cut in half along the plane indicated by the *single blue line* in Figure 21-5A and in the *inset*. The spiral of the cochlear duct makes about two and one-half turns from the base of the cochlea to its apex. The outer bony surface of the cochlea is indicated in *light gray*. A spiral, screw-shaped bony structure, the **modiolus**, forms the central core of the cochlea and is indicated in *darker gray*. A spiral cavity within the modiolus contains the cell bodies of the **spiral ganglion** (*green*) and the proximal axons of the **cochlear nerve (CN VIII)**. The **osseous (bony) spiral lamina** curves around the modiolus like the threads of a screw (*red dashed line* and *inset*). The central edge of the cochlear duct is attached to the spiral lamina; the outer wall of the cochlear duct is attached to the spiral ligament. Histologic sections of these structures are shown in Figures 21-6A,B.

AUDITORY SYSTEM
COCHLEA

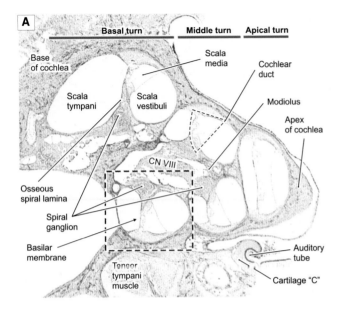

Figure 21-6A. Cross section of cochlea. H&E, ×22

The **cochlea** consists of a spiral tunnel in the temporal bone and associated membranous structures within that tunnel. The tunnel makes two and three-quarter turns as it proceeds from the wide **base** of the cochlea to its **apex**. The cross section shows the cochlea in its approximate anatomical orientation (plane of section is indicated by the *blue line* through the cochlea in Fig. 21-5A). The tunnel is lined with endosteum and is larger at the base, becoming progressively narrower toward the apex. It is divided into two sections, the **scala** ("staircase") **vestibuli** and the **scala tympani**. These two sections are separated by the membranous **cochlear duct** (Figs. 21-4 and 21-5A,B), which encloses the **scala media**. The cochlear duct contains the sensory receptors of the cochlea. The vestibule opens into the scala vestibuli, and sound waves are transmitted from the oval window to the sensory receptors by this route. The *scala vestibuli* is continuous with the scala tympani at the cochlear apex via a small opening, the **helicotrema** (see Fig. 21-8A). The *scala tympani* extends from the helicotrema to the round window of the tympanic cavity. The **auditory tube** connects the middle ear cavity with the nasopharynx to allow air pressure in the middle ear to equilibrate with that of the surrounding environment. The auditory tube runs in a groove in a C-shaped band of cartilage. The structures associated with the scalae vestibuli, tympani, and media (*dashed rectangle*) are shown at higher magnification in Figure 21-6B.

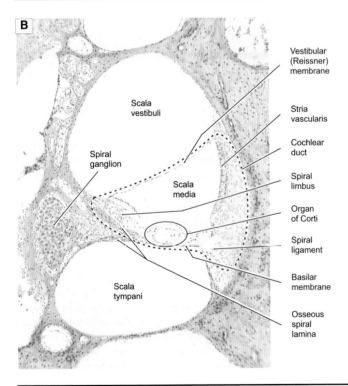

Figure 21-6B. Scala media and organ of Corti. H&E, ×84

It is traditional to represent the internal structures of the cochlea as if the basilar membrane is horizontal. This photomicrograph has, therefore, been rotated 90 degrees counterclockwise from its position in Figure 21-6A. The **cochlear duct** (*dotted line*) is a roughly triangular structure that lies between the **scala vestibuli** and the **scala tympani**. The fluid-filled space within the cochlear duct is the **scala media** (*yellow shading*). In this photomicrograph, the cochlear duct is bounded by the **bony labyrinth** and **basilar membrane** below, the **stria vascularis** on the right, and the **vestibular membrane (Reissner membrane)** above. The basilar membrane supports the **organ of Corti**. The **stria vascularis** is a specialized, thickened region of stratified epithelium. In contrast to most types of epithelium, it is highly vascularized by a dense meshwork of capillaries. The stria vascularis is instrumental in maintaining the high K$^+$ concentration of the endolymph in the scala media. Lateral to the stria vascularis, the endosteum is much thickened and forms the **spiral ligament**, to which the outer edge of the basilar membrane connects. The **vestibular membrane** consists of two layers of squamous epithelial cells on either side of a basal lamina. The **tectorial membrane** (*not labeled*) normally rests on the hair cells of the organ of Corti. However, it is often distorted or damaged during tissue processing.

ORGAN OF CORTI

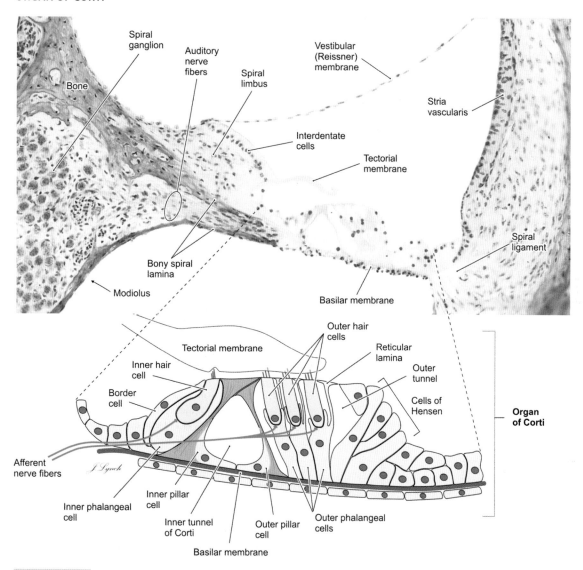

Figure 21-7. Organ of Corti and associated structures. H&E, ×189

The **organ of Corti** is a band of specialized epithelial cells that rest on the **basilar membrane**, a thin sheet of fibrous connective tissue that extends from the **osseous (bony) spiral lamina** to the **spiral ligament**. The surface of the basilar membrane in the scala tympani is covered by a thin layer of vascularized connective tissue and elongated mesothelial cells. The organ of Corti contains the **auditory hair cells,** the receptor cells for hearing, as well as several types of supporting cells. The hair cells have bundles of 50 to 100 stereocilia (hairs) protruding from their upper surfaces. The **transduction of sound waves** to nerve impulses is based upon changes in the polarization of the hair cell membrane that occur when their apical stereocilia are bent during the vibration of the basilar membrane by sound waves. The hair cells are in synaptic contact with **afferent** and **efferent nerve fibers** of the auditory branch of CN VIII (*efferent fibers not illustrated*). Auditory hair cells are divided into two groups: **inner hair cells** and **outer hair cells.** In humans, there are about 3,500 inner hair cells arranged in a single row and about 12,000 outer hair cells arranged in three or sometimes four rows. The hair cells are surrounded by a variety of **supporting cells,** including **pillar cells, phalangeal cells, border cells,** and **cells of Hensen.** The inner and outer hair cells are separated by **inner** and **outer pillar cells.** These cells have long, thin processes that include dense bundles of microtubules and extend from the basilar membrane to the upper surfaces of the hair cells. Pillar cells surround a triangular, fluid-filled space, the **inner tunnel of Corti.** The basal and lateral aspects of inner hair cells are surrounded by **inner phalangeal cells.** By contrast, **outer phalangeal cells** cup only the lower third of each outer hair cell, whereas the upper two thirds of each outer hair cell is surrounded by a fluid-filled space. The spaces between the upper surfaces of the outer hair cells are filled by processes of phalangeal cells. These processes form the **reticular lamina. Tight junctions** connect the phalangeal cell processes and the apical surfaces of the hair cells to form a barrier that separates the endolymph of the scala media from the cells of the organ of Corti. Columnar epithelial cells called **border cells** mark the medial extent of the organ of Corti; columnar epithelial cells called **cells of Hensen** mark its lateral extent. The **tectorial membrane** hangs over the organ of Corti and deflects the stereocilia of the hair cells when sound waves move the basilar membrane. The tectorial membrane is a gelatinous structure, containing fine filaments, which is secreted by columnar epithelial cells (**interdentate cells**) on the surface of the **spiral limbus.** It is commonly distorted during tissue processing; its normal position is illustrated.

SOUND TRANSDUCTION

A

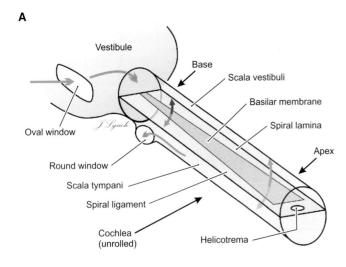

Figure 21-8A. Sound transduction.

As shown in this diagram of a straightened cochlea, **sound waves** are transmitted into the **perilymph** (*blue*) of the **scala vestibuli** by movements of the footplate of the **stapes** on the **oval window**. The membranous **round window** provides pressure relief for the sound waves within the closed chamber of the **bony labyrinth**. The **basilar membrane** (*gray*) is a thin sheet of fibrous connective tissue that supports the **organ of Corti**. The basilar membrane is narrower at the **base** of the cochlea (about 0.21 mm) than at the **apex** of the cochlea (about 0.36 mm). It is also stiffer at the base of the cochlea than at the apex. These properties cause the basilar membrane to vibrate preferentially (**resonate**) near the base when stimulated at high frequencies (*red arrows*) and near the apex (*blue arrows*) when stimulated at low frequencies. This arrangement creates a **tonotopic map** along the organ of Corti and is one of the ways in which the cochlea encodes sound waves of different frequencies into trains of nerve impulses that can be processed by the nervous system to produce the sensation of **pitch**.

B

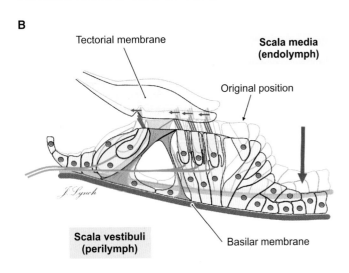

Figure 21-8B. Stereocilia displacement.

When a **sound wave** increases the pressure in the perilymph of the scala vestibuli, the pressure in the **endolymph** of the **scala media** increases simultaneously, because the vestibular membrane is very thin and delicate. This increased pressure moves the tectorial membrane and basilar membrane downward (*large red arrow*) and away from their original positions (indicated by the *ghost outline*). Because the centers of rotation of the **tectorial membrane** and **basilar membrane** are different, the downward movement of the two membranes induces a transverse displacement of the tips of the hair cells (*small red arrows*). This bending of the **stereocilia** opens K⁺ channels and causes a change in the **membrane potential** of the hair cells. The potential change (**depolarization**) induces the release of transmitter molecules and produces **action potentials** in the afferent nerve fibers of the **cochlear nerve**.

AUDITORY HAIR CELLS

C

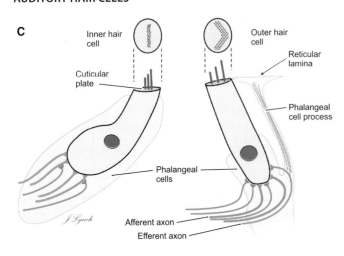

Figure 21-8C. Auditory hair cells.

There are several differences between the **inner** and **outer hair cells**. The stereocilia of inner hair cells are arranged in a straight line, whereas the stereocilia of the outer hair cells are arranged in a "V" or "W" pattern. Inner hair cells are completely surrounded by inner phalangeal cells; only the lower third of outer hair cells is cupped by the cell bodies of outer phalangeal cells. About 95% of the sensory nerve fibers in the auditory nerve contact inner hair cells. A single afferent axon typically contacts only one inner hair cell, and each inner hair cell has synaptic contact with at least 10 afferent axons (*green*). By contrast, a single afferent axon may branch and contact as many as 10 outer hair cells. In addition, there are efferent nerve fibers (*orange*) that originate in auditory centers in the brainstem and make synaptic contacts on hair cells or on afferent nerve endings. These efferent fibers play a role in tuning the excitability of the hair cells. The majority of the efferent endings are on outer hair cells.

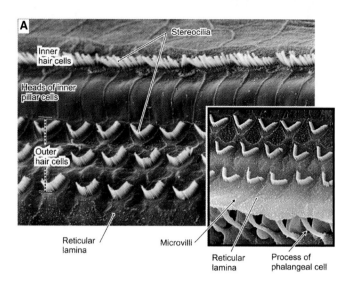

Figure 21-9A. Inner and outer hair cells. SEM, ×1,300

The arrangement of **inner** and **outer hair cells** is illustrated in these scanning electron micrographs. The row of **stereocilia** of the inner hair cells is separated from the outer hair cells by the heads of the inner pillar cells. The "V" or "W" pattern of the stereocilia of the outer hair cells is clearly seen. Outer hair cells are particularly important for **frequency discrimination**. They possess the unique property of being able to actively change their physical length in response to changing electrical fields. This property contributes to the frequency selectivity of hair cell responses. The *inset* shows the thin processes of the outer **phalangeal cells** that flatten out to form the **reticular lamina**. This lamina serves to isolate the endolymph in the scala media from the perilymph in the scala tympani. The upper surfaces of the hair cells are smooth, whereas the surrounding processes of phalangeal cells are covered with **microvilli**.

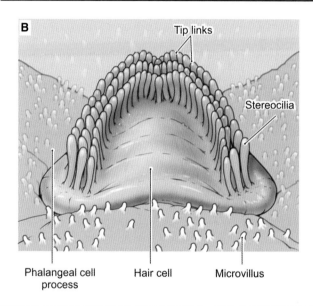

Figure 21-9B. Stereocilia of an outer hair cell. SEM, ×5,000

The **stereocilia of outer hair cells** are typically arranged in three rows, with the tallest row on the outside of the "V." Each stereocilium is narrower at its base than in its body. The stereocilia are connected at their tips by fine filaments (**tip links**), which play a critical role in changing the ionic permeability of the cell membrane when the stereocilia are bent. The permeability change initiates a sequence of events that result in the release of neurotransmitter molecules, leading to action potentials in the afferent nerve fibers. Outer hair cells vary in length along the basilar membrane, with the shortest at the basal end of the cochlea and the longest at the apical end.

CLINICAL CORRELATION

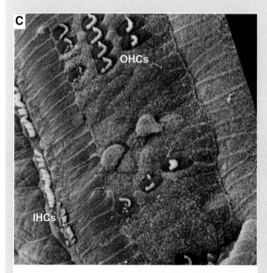

Inner and outer hair cells damaged by loud, prolonged noise

Figure 21-9C. Sensorineural Hearing Loss. SEM, ×376

Extended exposure to loud sounds can impair hearing. This scanning electron micrograph shows hair cells damaged by high-intensity sound for several days (*right*). **Outer hair cells** are more subject to damage than inner hair cells. Durations of loud noise as short as a few minutes can produce detectable damage to **stereocilia**; longer duration exposure (as illustrated here) causes death of hair cells. Damaged hair cells are not replaced in mammals, although they are replaced in some birds and reptiles. In mammals, the holes left by dying hair cells are filled by the processes of phalangeal cells in order to maintain the barrier between the endolymph and perilymph. Hair cells are normally lost with advancing age (**presbycusis**). Hair cell damage can also be produced by prolonged exposure to high dosages of aminoglycoside antibiotics (e.g., gentamicin, streptomycin, neomycin), some diuretics (e.g., furosemide), and some chemotherapy agents. When only outer hair cells are damaged, there is an overall loss of sensitivity and a profound loss of frequency discrimination (e.g., ability to understand speech). A loss of both inner and outer hair cells leads to complete deafness, which cannot be ameliorated by hearing aids.

Vestibular System

SENSORY RECEPTORS

A

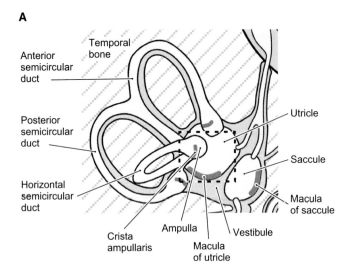

Figure 21-10A. Sensory receptors: crista ampullaris, maculae of the utricle and saccule.

The vestibular apparatus of the inner ear contains **sensory receptors** that detect rotation of the head in space, linear acceleration, and the static position of the head. The sensory receptors are **hair cells** that are similar in many, but not all, respects to the hair cells of the auditory system. **Rotational movements** of the head are detected by hair cells located in the **crista ampullaris** of the anterior, posterior, and horizontal **semicircular ducts** (located within their respective semicircular canals). **Horizontal acceleration** is detected by hair cells in the macula of the utricle; **vertical acceleration** is detected by hair cells in the macula of the saccule. **Static head position** is detected by combining signals from the maculae of the utricle and saccule. The *dashed rectangle* indicates the approximate position of the photomicrograph in Figure 21-10B.

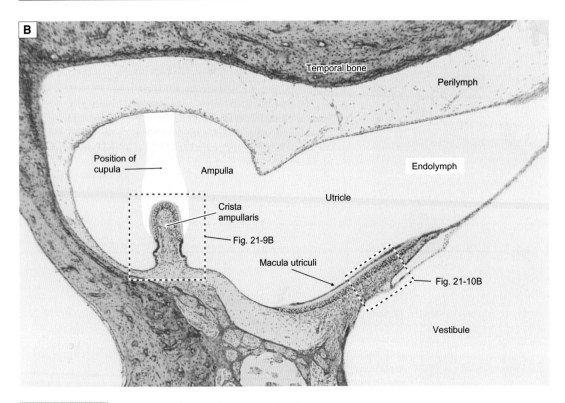

Figure 21-10B. Crista ampullaris and macula utriculi. H&E, ×60

A low-power photomicrograph that includes the **ampulla** of a semicircular canal, the **utricle**, and a portion of the **vestibule** is shown. The semicircular canal within the temporal bone is filled with **perilymph**. The membranous labyrinth, filled with endolymph, floats within this bony canal. The sensory receptors of both the vestibular system and the auditory system are in contact with the endolymph. The **crista ampullaris** contains vestibular hair cells and the sensory receptors of the vestibular system and is described in detail in Figure 21-11A,B. A gelatinous structure, the **cupula**, surrounds the crista ampullaris and forms a wall across the ampulla. The cupula is normally lost during tissue processing. Movement of the endolymph during head rotation deflects the cupula and, thereby, bends the cilia of the hair cells. The large fluid-filled utricle contains the **macula utriculi**, a sense organ that measures linear acceleration and static position of the head. The macula utriculi contains vestibular hair cells with cilia that are embedded in a gelatinous structure, the **otolithic membrane**. This membrane is covered by tiny crystals (**otoconia**), which have a higher specific gravity than the surrounding endolymph and, consequently, are influenced by gravity and acceleration.

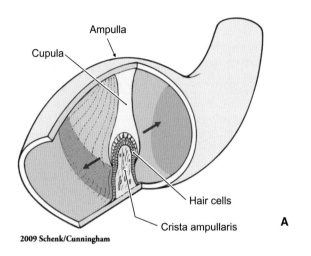

Ampulla
Cupula
Hair cells
Crista ampullaris
A
2009 Schenk/Cunningham

Figure 21-11A. **Ampulla of the semicircular canal.**

Each of the three semicircular ducts has an enlargement called the **ampulla** near one of the points at which the duct joins the utricle. There is a ridge, the **crista ampullaris**, on the floor of each ampulla. Partially surrounding the ridge and extending to the ceiling of the ampulla is a wall, the **cupula**, which completely blocks the duct. The cupula consists of a firm gel of proteins and polysaccharides. This structure is normally dissolved during the tissue preparation process and only remnants are typically seen in histological sections. When the head rotates, the **endolymph** within the semicircular ducts moves (*red arrows*) and exerts pressure on the cristae and their respective cupulae, causing them to deflect slightly. This deflection bends the hair cells in the cristae and modulates the frequency of action potentials that are going to the brainstem vestibular centers, thereby producing the sensation of motion.

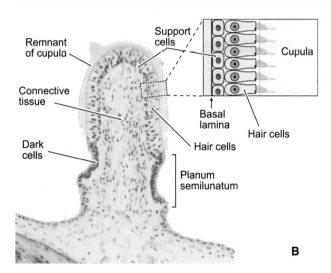

Remnant of cupula
Connective tissue
Dark cells
Support cells
Cupula
Basal lamina
Hair cells
Hair cells
Planum semilunatum
B

Figure 21-11B. **Crista ampullaris.** H&E, ×166

The **crista ampullaris** (also known as the **ampullary crest**) is a projection of connective tissue covered with epithelium within the ampulla. The epithelium consists of **hair cells, support cells,** and **dark cells.** The cilia of the *hair cells* are embedded in the gelatinous material of the **cupula.** The hair cells are cradled by *supporting cells* that rest on the **basal lamina** of the epithelium. There are two distinct types of hair cells in the cristae, termed **type I** and **type II hair cells.** The **planum semilunatum** is a region of endothelium composed of a single layer of cells called "dark cells," because they stain more intensely than other epithelial cells in the internal ear. *Dark cells* display cytological characteristics of cells with high metabolic activity and are believed to be important in controlling the ionic composition of the endolymph. They are found in several other locations within the labyrinthine ducts, including the stria vascularis.

CLINICAL CORRELATION

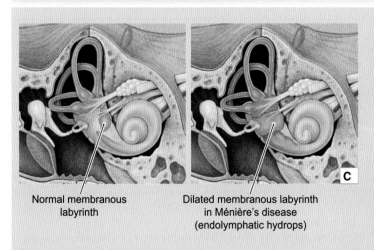

Normal membranous labyrinth
Dilated membranous labyrinth in Ménière's disease (endolymphatic hydrops)
C

Figure 21-11C. **Ménière Disease.**

Ménière disease is a disorder of the labyrinth of the inner ear, characterized by intermittent episodes of **hearing loss, tinnitus, aural pressure,** and **vertigo.** Its causes are uncertain but may include autoimmune disorders, viral infections, genetic predisposition, allergies, and head trauma. Disorders of secretory cells in the membranous labyrinth and endolymphatic sac may produce ionic imbalance between endolymph and perilymph, resulting in **endolymphatic hydrops** (swelling of the membranous labyrinth) and producing many of the above symptoms. Diagnosis is based on history, clinical symptoms, audiometry, and vestibular testing. Postmortem histopathologic findings may include perisaccular fibrosis, atrophy of the endolymphatic sac, and other membranous changes. Treatments include reduction of caffeine and salt intake, diuretics, antinausea medications, glucocorticoid therapy, intratympanic gentamicin injection, surgical labyrinthectomy, and vestibular nerve section.

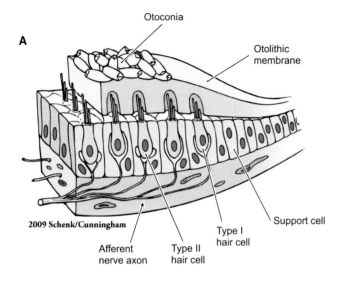

A

Otoconia

Otolithic membrane

Support cell

Type I hair cell

Type II hair cell

Afferent nerve axon

2009 Schenk/Cunningham

Figure 21-12A. Macula of the utricle.

The **utricle** and **saccule** are similar in structure. The walls consist of an outer fibrous layer, an intermediate layer of vascularized connective tissue, and an inner epithelial lining. In both the utricle and the saccule, there is a region of specialized epithelium termed the **macula**, which is 2 to 3 mm in diameter. The macula contains two types of **sensory hair cells**, classified as **type I** and **type II**. The sensory epithelium of the macula is overlaid by a gelatinous structure, called the **otolithic membrane**, which is similar in makeup to the cupula of the ampulla. The stereocilia and kinocilia of the hair cells are embedded in the membrane. Hundreds of tiny crystals, **otoconia**, are attached to the surface of the otolithic membranes. These crystals have a higher specific gravity than the surrounding **endolymph** and are consequently affected by gravity or linear acceleration. Changes in head position or acceleration, therefore, cause the otoconia-weighted otolithic membrane to deflect the cilia of the hair cells and, thus, trigger changes in the frequency of nerve impulses generated by the hair cells.

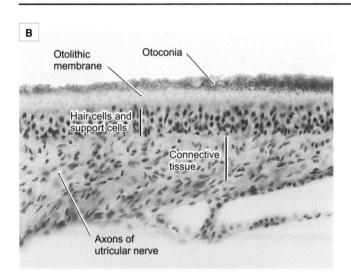

B

Otolithic membrane

Otoconia

Hair cells and support cells

Connective tissue

Axons of utricular nerve

Figure 21-12B. Macula of the utricle with otoconia. H&E, ×260

This photomicrograph shows a cross section of the **macular region of the wall of the utricle** (an enlargement of the area indicated by the *dashed rectangle* in Fig. 21-10B). The **otoconia**, which stain darkly in this H&E stain, lie on the surface of the **otolithic membrane**; the otolithic membrane itself is almost transparent. The support cells provide mechanical support to the hair cells and also secrete the substance of the otolithic membrane.

Dizziness is one of the most common reasons adults seek medical care. The term has two general meanings: (1) a feeling of **light-headedness** or "about to faint" or (2) a feeling that the individual is spinning or that the room is spinning. This latter feeling is properly called **vertigo**. Twenty percent of all complaints of dizziness involve problems related to the otoconia of the utricle and saccule.

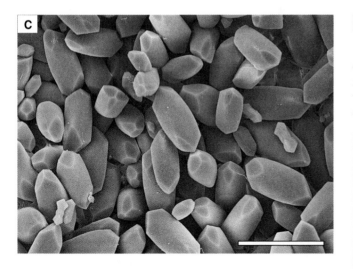

C

Figure 21-12C. Otoconia from the macula of the utricle. SEM, scale bar = 10 μm

Otoconia are crystals of almost pure calcium carbonate that form in the region of the macular hair cells. The otoconia lie on the surface of the otolithic membrane, attached by a proteinaceous substance that is not well understood.

The number of **otoconia** present decreases with age, contributing to the balance difficulties often experienced by older individuals. In addition, crystals or small groups of crystals sometimes become detached from the otolithic membrane and drift into a semicircular canal or even become attached to the hair cells in a canal. This dislocation can disrupt the normal neural signals from the labyrinth and produce a type of severe **vertigo** termed **benign paroxysmal positional vertigo**. Treatment that involves sequences of different head positions and movements can usually improve or eliminate the symptoms. The exact maneuver depends upon which semicircular canal is involved.

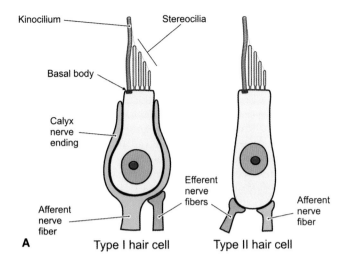

Figure 21-13A. Vestibular hair cells.

Type I hair cells are **pyriform** (pear shaped) and have basally located nuclei. They are almost completely surrounded by a single, chalice-shaped synaptic terminal (**calyx**) of a large afferent nerve fiber. Each type I hair cell is innervated by a single nerve axon, and each axon branches to innervate only a few hair cells. Type I hair cells receive few efferent endings, which contact the afferent nerve endings rather than the hair cell itself. **Type II cells** are more cylindrical in shape, with more centrally located nuclei. These cells are contacted by multiple small bouton-like synaptic endings associated with both afferent and efferent nerve fibers. Type II cells receive axon terminals from multiple nerve fibers, each of which branches to contact many type II hair cells. Both types of vestibular hair cells have a single **kinocilium** (with a typical **basal body** and a ring of nine double microtubules) on one side of the apical surface. A group of 40 to 100 **stereocilia** of various lengths are arranged in a hexagonal array next to the kinocilium.

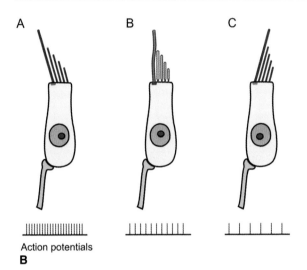

Figure 21-13B. Excitation and inhibition in hair cells.

Vestibular hair cells continuously release a small amount of neurotransmitter at the afferent terminal synapses, producing a moderate frequency of action potentials in afferent nerve fibers in the resting state (**B**). When movement of endolymph causes the cupula or otolithic membrane to deflect the hair cell stereocilia *toward* the kinocilium, the amount of neurotransmitter released goes up and the frequency of action potential discharge *increases* (**A**). When the stereocilia are deflected *away from* the kinocilium, less neurotransmitter is released, and the frequency of the action potentials *decreases* (**C**). Hair cells in different regions of the peripheral vestibular apparatus have their kinocilia and stereocilia oriented in different directions. The CNS integrates information from the various hair cells to form a central representation of the position of the head in space, the direction of any movement of the head, and the rate of change (acceleration) of any movement.

CLINICAL CORRELATION

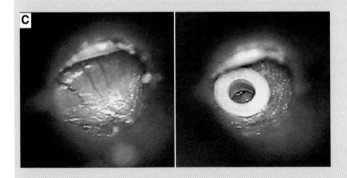

Figure 21-13C. Ventilation Tubes for Otitis Media.

Otitis media refers to an accumulation of fluid in the middle ear. This buildup may be caused by bacterial or viral infection (acute otitis media) or by noninfectious conditions, including allergies and developmental issues (otitis media with effusion). In either case, the mucosal lining of the middle ear produces serous exudate and pus. The consequent buildup of fluid in the middle ear produces pressure on the tympanic membrane, which may cause severe pain (**otalgia**) and temporary conductive hearing loss. Most cases resolve spontaneously, although antibiotics are often prescribed to speed recovery. Occasionally, the hearing loss may persist and may affect speech development. In cases of severe and repeated episodes, a ventilation tube (ear tube, tympanostomy tube) may be inserted into an incision made in the tympanic membrane to reduce the pressure in the middle ear (*right*). This procedure, called a myringotomy, relieves the pain and reduces other adverse effects of fluid buildup. These tubes usually stay in place for 6 to 9 months before they spontaneously fall out. The hole in the tympanic membrane typically heals shut on its own.

CLINICAL CORRELATIONS

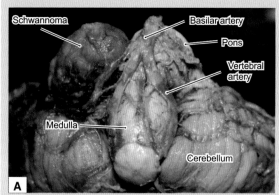

A

Ventral (anterior) surface of the brain

Figure 21-14A. Vestibular Schwannoma.

Vestibular schwannoma (sometimes called **acoustic schwannoma** or, incorrectly, **acoustic neuroma**) is a Schwann cell–derived **benign tumor**, usually arising from the vestibular branch of CN VIII during the fifth or sixth decade of life. Risk factors include prolonged exposure to loud noise, childhood exposure to low-dose radiation, and possible links to parathyroid adenoma. Symptoms include **hearing loss, headache, vertigo, tinnitus,** and **facial pain.** The tumor is usually unilateral. It appears as a well-circumscribed, encapsulated mass. The tumor attaches to the nerve but can usually be separated from the nerve. Histologically, schwannomas arise from perineural elements of Schwann cells. Areas of alternately dense and sparse cellularity, called **Antoni A** and **Antoni B regions,** are characteristic of the tumor. Treatment options include surgical removal of the tumor, stereotactic radiosurgery, stereotactic radiotherapy, and proton beam therapy.

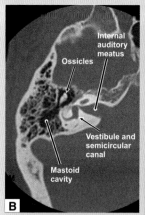

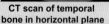

B

CT scan of temporal bone in horizontal plane

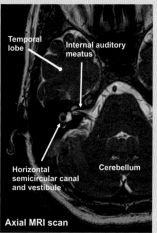

Axial MRI scan

Figure 21-14B. CT and MRI of Inner Ear Structures.

Recent developments in imaging resolution have made it possible to distinguish many of the anatomical features of the inner ear in human subjects. **Computed tomography (CT) imaging** of the temporal bones is helpful for evaluating bony anatomy, such as the middle ear ossicles and bony labyrinthine structures. CT is useful in cases of **trauma** to look for fractures and dislocations, **infection** and inflammatory processes to evaluate for bone erosion, and **congenital abnormalities** to explain hearing dysfunction. **Magnetic resonance imaging (MRI)** is most often performed to evaluate a patient with **sensorineural hearing loss.** It is used to exclude a **vestibular schwannoma** and, occasionally, to evaluate for infection. The brainstem, internal auditory canals, cranial nerves, and membranous labyrinthine structures (perilymph-filled cochlea, vestibule, and semicircular canals) are well evaluated on MRI. In the CT scan (*left*), bone is light and perilymph dark; these relations are reversed in the T2-weighted MRI (*right*).

SYNOPSIS 21-1 Pathologic and Clinical Terms for the Ear

■ *Sensorineural hearing loss:* Hearing loss that involves the loss of hair cells or neurons; accounts for about 90% of all hearing loss. Can occur after sound- or drug-induced damage to hair cells, disease-induced damage to neurons in the auditory system, and loss of hair cells with advancing age.

■ *Hydrops:* Excessive accumulation of clear, watery fluid in a tissue or cavity; **endolymphatic hydrops** refers to an accumulation of endolymph within the membranous labyrinth.

■ *Tinnitus:* Abnormal noise in the ear (e.g., ringing, whistling, hissing, roaring, chirping), ranging from "mild" to "extremely annoying"; inner ear trauma produced by loud noise is the leading cause; also occurs in Ménière disease. Advancing age is frequently accompanied by gradual loss of hair cells, producing sensorineural hearing impairment and tinnitus.

■ *Vertigo:* The illusory sensation of spinning or tilting most frequently caused by inner ear disturbances. Can last for minutes, days, or weeks and can be incapacitating; often accompanied by severe nausea.

■ *Conductive hearing loss:* Decrease in sound conduction to the inner ear. Possible causes include buildup of fluid pressure in the middle ear because of infection, blockage of external auditory meatus by wax, and disorders or traumatic damage of the ossicles.

■ *Erythema (erythematous):* Redness of a tissue as a result of inflammation.

■ *Otalgia:* Earache.

■ *Benign:* Description of a tumor that is nonmalignant, that is, does not invade surrounding tissues and does not metastasize to other locations in the body.

From Histology to Pathology

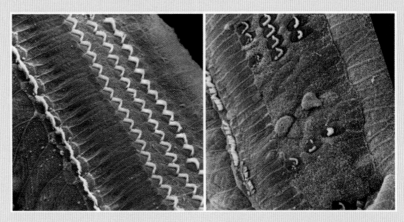

Figure 21-15.   Normal auditory hair cells and damaged auditory hair cells. SEM, ×376

Normal organ of Corti with three rows of outer hair cells and one row of inner hair cells from scanning electron micrographs (SEM) on the *left*, and **damaged auditory hair cells** on the *right*. The inner and outer hair cells have been damaged due to the prolonged noise. Durations of loud noise as short as a few minutes can produce detectable damage to stereocilia; longer duration exposure (as illustrated here) causes death of hair cells. Damaged hair cells are not replaced in mammals, although they are replaced in some birds and reptiles.

Clinical Vignette Questions

1. A 7-year-old boy complained about liquid discharge from his right ear for 3 weeks and a recent feeling of dizziness, imbalance, ear fullness, and hearing loss. History revealed the patient had two episodes of acute otitis media within the last 2 years. Otoscopic examination of the ears showed some epidermal debris in the external auditory canal and a white soft mass behind the right tympanic membrane within the middle ear space, which does not move with the tympanic membrane. A computed tomography scan showed minor erosion of the posterior wall of the external auditory canal and the mastoid bone. The mass and eroded structures were surgically removed within a week. Pathologic examination revealed desquamated squamous cells adjacent to stratified squamous epithelium. Which of the following is the most likely diagnosis in this case?

A. Adenocarcinoma
B. Cholesteatoma
C. Otitis externa
D. Otitis media
E. Otosclerosis

2. A 42-year-old man presented to the emergency department with chronic onset of headache, dizziness, tinnitus, and hearing loss in both ears. He was alert and oriented, without fever or hypertension. The patient had no history of previous hearing loss and no family history of dizziness. His blood tests were normal. CT scan of the brain revealed 3.2-cm and 4.5-cm masses in the cerebellopontine angles bilaterally. The lesions were well demarcated and extended into the internal auditory meatus. The patient underwent surgery, and the tumors were resected through a bilateral suboccipital craniotomy. Histologic examination of the tumors showed zones of alternately dense and sparse cellularity with no sign of atypia (a histopathologic term to describe atypical cells). Which of the following is the most likely diagnosis in this case?

A. Astrocytoma
B. Brain abscess
C. Glioma
D. Meningioma
E. Vestibular schwannoma

Appendix A

General Principles of Tissue Preparation and Staining

Introduction

The study of tissue structure relies on the preparation of tissue samples in ways that allow their structural details to be viewed at light or electron microscopic levels. First, there is the method of studying tissue using the light microscope. Second, there is the study of what is sometimes called the "ultrastructure" of tissue using the transmission electron microscope. There are numerous variations on these two general themes. Recognizing that a survey of all tissue preparation techniques is well beyond the scope of this atlas, the general features of the two methods mentioned are briefly summarized here.

Preservation Versus Fixation

Preservation and fixation of tissues, for subsequent treatments, share to varying degrees the common goals of minimizing any further tissue degradation and preserving the various components of the tissue in as lifelike a condition as possible. While the terms **preservation** and **fixation** are frequently used as interchangeable, they are, in fact, slightly different.

Preservation of tissue accomplishes the first goal stated above (prevents further degradation) but not necessarily the second. For example, a can of green peas contains preservatives; these may even be listed on the label. They protect the peas from further degradation. If you take a pea out of the can and look at it microscopically, its structure might be recognizable, but it is not very lifelike. Fish that are preserved in salt undergo significant changes that render the tissue useless for microscopic examination. Such structures are preserved but are not fixed. Many of the substances used to preserve tissues (animal and plant) can be ingested in moderation and cause absolutely no harm.

Fixation, on the other hand, protects against further degradation while preserving the internal components of the cell in a strikingly lifelike appearance. Fixation also hardens the tissue, making it possible to further manipulate the sample without damage. Tissue that is fixed will appear quite lifelike when viewed with a microscope. In this respect, a sample of tissue that is fixed is also preserved; however, a sample of tissue that is preserved is not necessarily fixed. Another important difference is the fact that most substances (except alcohol) used to fix tissue generally cannot be ingested; to do so, even in very moderate amounts, would cause significant harm or death.

Fixatives and Methods of Fixation

Fixatives

In addition to preventing tissue degradation, preserving components of the tissue, and hardening the tissue, proper fixation will also transform the contents of the cell from a semifluid to a semisolid and prepare the cell contents for visualization with stains, dyes, or metallic salts. There are numerous fixatives, many of which are designed for unique applications, which can be used separately or in combinations. Only representative examples are mentioned here.

Formalin (mixture of formaldehyde and alcohol), in solution of 5% to 10%, is one of the more commonly used general fixatives. It penetrates the tissue rapidly, leaves no residues, and requires little or no washing of the tissue to remove. It is used alone, in a solution buffered with sodium phosphate salts, or in other combinations. Buffered neutral formalin is usually preferred. Formalin acts through cross-linking between proteins.

Picric acid, in combination with formalin and glacial acetic acid (Bouin solution), is also used as a fixative. Its action of fixation is not fully understood, and it does not harden the tissue as much as formalin. Details of the nucleus are well demonstrated. However, picric acid in its dry form must be handled with care because it is an explosion hazard. Picric acid can also be used as a stain.

Aldehydes, such as glutaraldehyde and paraformaldehyde, are excellent fixatives for light microscopic applications and are also widely used in electron microscopy. Aldehydes act rapidly but tend to penetrate the tissue slowly. However, they provide excellent cellular detail regarding the contents of the cytoplasm and the nucleus. Osmium tetroxide, an oxidizing agent, is also used as a fixative for electron microscopy.

Alcohols, either methyl or ethyl alcohol, are also used as fixatives. Because they cause the tissue to become quite hard and, therefore, brittle, they are usually used in special applications such as smears of tissue or blood. Alcohol in various dilutions is also commonly used in tissue processing.

Mercuric chloride is used in combination with other substances in a variety of fixatives. Though the method of action at the cellular level is not well understood and fixatives containing this substance may penetrate the tissue slowly, they do provide excellent cellular detail.

Acetic acid, though rarely used as a fixative on its own, is used in combination with other agents in a variety of fixatives such as Bouin, Carnoy, and Clarke solutions. Although acetic acid may be used in concentrated form in certain applications, it is primarily used in combinations with other fixatives (and is thereby diluted); it is also commonly used by itself in dilutions of 1% to 5%.

Methods of Fixation

Fixation is usually accomplished in one of two ways. The first is by **immersion fixation**. The fixative is prepared, and a small piece of tissue removed and immersed in the fixative. It is common to suspend the tissue sample in the fixative; one method is to drape a delicate piece of cheesecloth in the fixative and place the sample in the sling thus created. This is advantageous because the fixative can penetrate from all sides of the tissue block. This method is useful when the tissue sample is small, and the fixative penetrates rapidly.

The second is **perfusion fixation**. In this method, the fixative is perfused through the intact vascular system of the organism. The fixative is preceded by a wash of physiological saline containing heparin and a substance that will paralyze the vessel walls, such as procaine hydrochloride, to ensure that the vascular bed will not contract in response to the fixative solution. This wash is followed immediately by the fixative. After perfusion, the tissue samples are removed and placed in more of the same fixative used in the perfusion. This method provides superior fixation of large pieces of tissue and is commonly used in many research applications.

FREEZING is also used as a method of fixation, especially in the clinical setting when a rapid diagnosis is needed during a medical procedure. A fresh tissue sample is retrieved from the patient or organism and immersed in liquid carbon dioxide or in a substance (such as isopentane) cooled extremely rapidly by dry ice. The best results are obtained with small tissue samples that are rapidly cooled to very low temperatures ($-40°C$ to $-60°C$). In general, rapid cooling causes very small ice crystals and minimal tissue disruption; slow cooling (like in your freezer) causes large ice crystals and maximum tissue disruption.

Processing of Fixed Tissue

Once the tissue sample is satisfactorily fixed, it must be taken through a series of steps that result in a thin slice of tissue mounted on a glass slide (for light microscopy) or an even thinner slice mounted on a copper grid (for electron microscopy). In general, this process requires three basic steps: (1) The water in the tissue needs to be removed; (2) the tissue must be passed through a solution that is miscible with water and with the substance in which the tissue will be embedded; and (3) the tissue must be passed through the embedding medium. Because the specific details of these steps may relate to the type of tissue being processed, only general comments are made here.

Dehydration: The goal of dehydration is to remove the water from the tissue. The most common method is to start with alcohol in a concentration of 75% to 80%. Recall that alcohol will mix with water; therefore, it can be used to remove water from the tissue. The tissue sample is passed, stepwise, through progressively higher concentrations (from 75% to 80% up to 100%) of alcohol; usually more than one step is used at 95% and 100%. Through this process, the water is completely removed from the tissue and replaced with alcohol.

Clearing: The clearing reagent is a substance that will mix both with alcohol and with the embedding medium. The most commonly used are xylene, toluene, and chloroform. The tissue is passed from 100% alcohol through changes of the clearing reagent. This stepwise process progressively removes the alcohol from the tissue and replaces it with the clearing reagent. This reagent is miscible with the embedding medium.

Impregnation and embedding: Because the clearing reagent will mix with the embedding medium, the tissue sample is taken from the last step in this reagent and placed in melted embedding medium (such as paraplast or bioloid—both are types of wax). The sample is then progressively passed through several changes of the embedding material. This stepwise process progressively removes the clearing reagent and replaces it with the embedding medium that will harden when cooled. Embedding is generally done in two steps. First, the tissue is removed from the last impregnation step and immediately placed in melted medium in a vacuum oven. The last traces of the clearing reagent and any minute bubbles are removed by vacuum. Second, the tissue sample is oriented in an embedding mold. The mold is then filled with melted medium and allowed to cool so the medium hardens. A similar set of steps are followed when a polymer is used as the embedding media for electron microscopy.

A comment on frozen sections: As noted above, rapid freezing can be used to fix tissue. Freezing can also be used to prepare tissues for sectioning. Small pieces can be rapidly frozen, mounted on a microtome, and sectioned. Larger pieces can be immersed in a sucrose solution until fully impregnated with the sucrose (the tissue initially floats and then sinks). The sucrose expedites the freezing process and renders minute ice crystals. The tissue is then mounted, frozen, and sectioned.

Sectioning and Mounting

Sectioning of prepared tissues is done on microtomes that are designed to accommodate sections mounted in paraplast (paraffin), frozen in ice, or embedded in plastic. The sections are cut using extremely sharp metal or glass knives, removed from the edge of the knife either as individual sections or as ribbons of sections, and floated in water (usually warmed) or in other fluids that are required by the unique features of the specific technique. For most applications in light microscopy, the sections range in thickness from about 5 to 12 μm (for paraffin embedded tissue) and from about 0.5 to 2.0 μm (for plastic embedded tissue). Special techniques may require sections up to 40 to 70 μm in thickness. At the opposite extreme of the microscopic continuum, glass or diamond knives are used to cut extremely thin sections for electron microscopy (EM, commonly called "TEM"). The thickness of sections for electron microscopy/transmission electron microscopy (EM/TEM) usually ranges from about 80 to 110 nm (10^{-9} m).

After the sections are cut, and before they are mounted, it is routine to make sure the glass slides are clean and to treat the slides so that the sections will not come off during the staining process. This may be accomplished by either spreading a drop of albumin on the slide or by adding a small amount of albumin (or gelatin) to the warm water bath in which the tissues are floated. Celloidin can also be used as an adhesive.

Staining

The goal of staining tissue slices is to use substances to impart color to various components of the section, making these components available for study. In many cases, the stain will visualize a specific component, such as fat, neurofibrils, or glycogen.

Stains are large molecules that are characterized by groups that absorb visible light (wavelengths between 380 and 760 nm) and groups that permit the attachment of the stain to the various chemical elements of the cell. The component of the stain that is responsible for light absorption is a system of conjugated double bonds known as the **chromophore**. The "combining" portion of the stain, which may also function as a solubilizing agent, is the **auxochrome**.

The simplest way that stains function is to exploit the electrostatic interactions between the stain molecules and components of the cell; positive charges on cellular structures attract negatively charged stain molecules and vice versa. **Basic dyes** carry positive charges and are, consequently, known as **cationic dyes**; they are attracted to negative charges within the tissue. Hematoxylin and toluidine blue are commonly used basic (cationic) dyes. They stain nuclear DNA, cytoplasmic RNA, sulfonated polysaccharides such as chondroitin sulfate, and polycarboxylic acids such as hyaluronic acid. **Acidic dyes** carry negative charges and are, consequently, known as **anionic dyes**; they are attracted to positive charges within the tissue. Eosin Y is a commonly used acidic (anionic) dye. It stains many proteins (and, therefore, stains many structures within the cell), and acid dyes also stain extracellular structures such as collagen.

There are literally hundreds of substances that are used as stains or dyes, or that may be used to impregnate tissues, and there are equally numerous methods or techniques that use these substances, in various combinations, to visualize the components of cells. Recognizing that even a brief survey of the broad range of methods is well beyond the scope of this atlas; the following focuses on the major stains used in this book.

Hematoxylin and eosin (H&E) is, by far, the most commonly used combination stain in basic sciences for general histological preparations and in clinical medicine for pathological specimens. This combination of cationic and anionic dyes results in most constituents of the cell (RNA, DNA, polysaccharides, and others) being stained various tones of either blue or pink. This method also stains extracellular collagen.

The **trichrome stains** are usually mixtures of acidic dyes, each having its own ionization constant. The Mallory trichrome stain, which is one of the more common, is a mixture of dyes used to demonstrate connective tissue (collagen stains blue) and other cellular constituents (nuclei and cytoplasm generally stain red), and blood cells (erythrocytes stain yellow). Trichrome stains are particularly useful for endocrine organs in which cells that produce different secretions can be stained different colors.

Wright stain is also a mixture of stains containing one acidic dye (methylene blue) and one basic dye (eosin). Wright stain is widely used for blood and bone marrow smears. Basophilic granules are deep purple, acidophilic (or eosinophilic) granules are reddish, and the cytoplasm is usually bluish gray, although it may appear pink to red (or mottled) if it contains acidophilic substances.

Elastic fiber stains are individual or combinations of dyes that stain cellular constituents but will also prominently stain elastic fibers. These exploit relatively nonspecific ionic and nonionic differences between collagen and elastin. Depending on the procedure used, elastic fibers may appear brown, deep purple, blue-black, or black.

Reticular fiber stains, as is the case for elastic stains, also exploit the relatively nonspecific differences in the amount of glycosylation of reticulin versus that of collagen. In general, reticular fibers are stained black, using silver as the chromophore, with the other cellular elements appearing as a monochromatic background of gray or various shades of light red. Whereas reticular fibers stand out in these special stains, other cellular detail does not.

Silver stains represent a large category of what are actually silver impregnation methods, not stains. In general, these methods use dilute solutions of silver nitrate (gold and mercury are also sometimes used) to impregnate blocks of nerve tissue and precipitate the metal ions on the cell membranes of neurons and glia. Tissue blocks, generally no more than 0.3 to 0.6 cm thick, are fixed in formalin, treated with a mordant solution such as potassium dichromate, suspended in a dilute silver nitrate solution for several days (with block cleaning and solution changing every day), and then encased in paraffin (not embedded). Sections are cut at thicknesses ranging from 40 to 70 µm and mounted on slides. Individual neurons and glia cells appear black on a light-yellow to off-white background. The mechanism of attachment of the silver ions to the cell membranes is not well understood.

The **periodic acid-Schiff** (**PAS**) reaction is a method that is more specific in its staining reaction than the anionic, cationic, or lipid soluble dyes. One such stain is the Schiff reagent (leucobasic fuchsin), which reacts specifically with free aldehydes. Pretreatment with periodic acid converts adjacent hydroxyl groups, such as those found in glycogen, into aldehydes. Treatment with the Schiff reagent stains the free aldehyde groups red; the sections are usually counterstained with H&E. The PAS reaction demonstrates sites of high concentrations of polysaccharide-containing components, such as glycogen and glycosaminoglycans.

Immunocytochemistry is a specialized method that can be used to precisely localize enzymes or large molecules (macromolecules) within the cell or on its membrane. The immune system of the body is able to defend itself against foreign molecules (antigens) by producing specific types of proteins (antibodies). Immunocytochemistry methods use this feature of cells to visualize specific molecules. For light microscopy, an antibody is produced (e.g., in rabbit tissue) against a specified protein or molecule, and the antibody is coupled with a dye, such as fluorescein or rhodamine B. When this labeled antibody attaches to a specific antigen and is exposed to ultraviolet light, it will fluoresce greenish yellow (fluorescein) or bright red (rhodamine B), thereby specifically identifying the location of that molecule. This is the direct method: An antibody is produced, coupled to a dye, attached to an antigen, and, thus, becomes visible. In the indirect method, unlabeled antibodies are produced in one animal (rabbit) against a specific antigen and then applied to a tissue to which they attach. The unlabeled antibodies are visualized by exposing them to labeled antibodies that are made in another species (goat) and that are directed against the immunoglobulins from the first species. One way to visualize this is as follows: An antibody is produced, not labeled, and attached to an antigen; a second antibody is produced, coupled with a dye, attached to the first unlabeled antibody, and, thus, then becomes visible.

Hematoxylin and eosin (H&E)

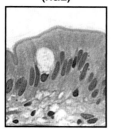

Mallory trichrome

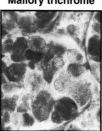

Wright stain

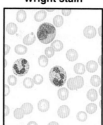

Elastic fiber stain

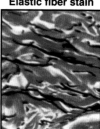

Reticular fiber stain

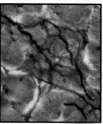

Silver stain

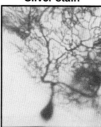

PAS reaction

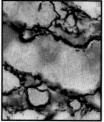

Immunohistochemistry

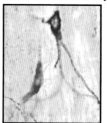

Transmission and Scanning Electron Microscopy

In slightly over 60 years, **TEM** has gone from a scientific curiosity to an essential tool in the study of tissue structure. The general steps used in TEM are conceptually similar to those used in light microscopy but customized to meet the unique needs of this technique. The tissue blocks are quite small, usually about 1 cubic millimeter, specially fixed to retain the fine integrity of the cellular constituents, and infiltrated with unpolymerized plastic rather than with wax or fluid. Sections usually in the range of 0.02 to 0.1 μm are cut using a knife fashioned from glass or diamond (steel cutting edges are not used in TEM). These tiny thin sections can be treated with solutions of heavy metal salts, such as lead citrate or uranyl acetate, to enhance contrast of the section. These salts become deposited on different structures within the cell making them electron dense, and they appear darker in electron micrographs. Once treated, the sections are mounted on perforated copper grids and the grids inserted into an electron microscope. A beam of electrons passes through the section, creating an image that can be viewed on a fluorescent plate and used to create a negative or digital image.

Scanning electron microscopy is similar, in many aspects, to TEM methods, except that small pieces of tissue are specially coated with a thin layer of gold or palladium. Sometimes, the tissue is frozen and then fractured to reveal internal structure before the metal-coating step. The electron beam passes over the surface of the specimen, and the metallic coating reflects some of these electrons. The reflected electrons are detected and are used to create a three-dimensional image of the surface of the specimen. Such images can be recorded as negatives or digital images.

Transmission electron microscopy (TEM)

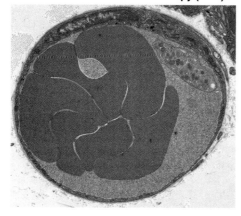

Scanning electron microscopy (SEM)

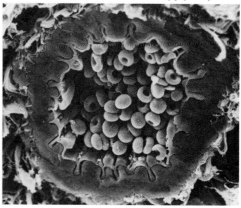

Appendix B

Answers and Explanations for Clinical Vignette Questions

Chapter 2 Cell Structure and Function

1. B. Competition with acetylcholine at nicotinic receptors

Explanation: Elapid snakes produce more neurotoxic poisons. Their venom acts on the neuromuscular junction, competing with acetylcholine at nicotinic receptors, inactivating acetylcholine, leading to muscular weakness of the legs and paralysis of the respiratory muscles (see Fig. 2-5B).

2. B. Mitochondria

Explanation: This patient has central core disease, which is a mitochondrion-associated disease. It causes predominantly proximal skeletal muscle weakness in infants. The muscle weakness may cause delays in milestones such as starting to walk. Often children with the disease have an abnormal gait and may appear to waddle. This weakness generally extends into adulthood but is not considered a severely progressive disease. Exercise and physical therapy can be of benefit. Muscle biopsies in affected patients reveal a central clearing of a portion or all of the myocytes under routine and special histologic stains. Ultrastructural examination of the central clearing reveals a marked reduction to a complete absence of mitochondria, the organelles responsible for cellular respiration and energy production. The disease is due to a mutation in the ryanodine receptor gene (*RYR1*). Some patients with central core myopathy are at risk for malignant hyperthermia, a severe reaction to certain anesthetics and depolarizing muscle relaxants (see Fig. 2-11B).

Chapter 3 Epithelium and Glands

1. E. Change from stratified squamous, nonkeratinized epithelium to mucus-secreting columnar epithelium

Explanation: This patient has Barrett esophagus, which is a complication of chronic gastroesophageal reflux disease (GERD) marked by metaplasia of the stratified squamous epithelium of the lower esophagus into a glandular epithelium with goblet cells as a response to prolonged reflux-induced injury. Patients with Barrett esophagus have an increased risk of developing adenocarcinoma (cancer of the esophagus) (see Fig. 3-16C).

2. D. IgG and/or C3 deposits in the basement membrane zone

Explanation: This patient had bullous pemphigoid (BP), which typically affects older individuals. In the bullous phase, tense fluid-filled blisters form, preferentially on the flexor forearms, inner thighs, and lower abdomen. The cause of BP is uncertain but appears to be related to radiation exposure, medications, and vaccinations in some cases. Immunofluorescence microscopy shows linear deposits of C3 and/or IgG in the basement membrane zone (see Fig. 3-20B).

3. D. Loss of normal villous architecture

Explanation: This 5-year-old boy has celiac disease, which is a disorder of the small intestine. Gluten, a substance found in wheat and barley, reacts with the lining of the small intestine (small bowel), leading to an attack by the immune system with damage to the microvilli and villi. Biopsies show increased T lymphocytes within the glandular epithelium, villous distortion and blunting, and increased chronic inflammation within the lamina propria. If left untreated, celiac disease can lead to malnutrition; anemia; bone disease; and, rarely, some forms of cancer (see Fig. 3-12C).

Chapter 4 Connective Tissue

1. C. Hydroxylation

Explanation: Although rare, vitamin C deficiency can be seen in individuals with inadequate diets and as a consequence of chronic alcohol abuse. Symptoms include swollen gums prone to bleeding, petechiae, particularly around hair follicles, scaly skin rash, bruising, coiled, fragile hairs, joint hemorrhage, and poor wound healing. Vitamin C is responsible for the hydroxylation of procollagen, and, in the deficient state, collagen produced by fibroblasts is weak and lacks tensile strength. Blood vessel fragility due to weak collagen predisposes to hemorrhage (see Fig. 4-6A).

2. C. *FBN1* genes

Explanation: This patient has Marfan syndrome, which is an autosomal-dominant disorder associated with fibrillin-1 (*FBN1*) gene mutations. This syndrome affects the formation of elastic fibers, particularly those found in the aorta, heart, eyes and skin. Signs and symptoms include tall stature with long limbs; long, thin fingers; and enlargement of the base of the aorta accompanied by aortic regurgitation and mitral valve prolapse (see Fig. 4-22C).

3. E. Actinic keratosis

Explanation: Actinic keratoses occur on sun-damaged skin and particularly affect fairer-skinned individuals. Clinically, these lesions appear scaly with a rough consistency and often appear on the face, hands, and arms. The histologic appearance shows hyperkeratosis (increased keratin in the stratum corneum), loss of the granular layer, and cellular atypia involving the keratinocytes within the lower layers of the epidermis. The dermis of sun-damaged skin shows solar elastosis, demonstrated histologically as blue-gray elastic fibers. Actinic keratoses, in time, may progress to squamous cell carcinoma. These lesions may be treated by surgical excision, cryotherapy, or topical chemotherapeutic medications (see Fig. 4-15C).

Chapter 5 Cartilage and Bone

1. B. Osteoarthritis

Explanation: This patient has osteoarthritis, or degenerative joint disease, the most common joint disorder in the United States. Osteoarthritis is typically a disease of older individuals, and it most often affects the knee and hip joints but may also affect the hands. Joint pain and stiffness are the most common symptoms, and, in contrast to the pain in rheumatoid arthritis that gets better with activity, the pain in osteoarthritis tends to get worse as the day progresses. Osteoarthritis is a noninflammatory type of arthritis treated with nonsteroidal anti-inflammatory drugs (NSAIDs) and, in cases of knee involvement, steroid injections. Imaging studies may reveal joint space narrowing and osteophytes. Pathologic examination of joints reveals changes in articular cartilage ranging from fibrillation to eburnation (wearing of the articular surface down to the bone) (see Fig. 5-4C).

2. B. Giant cell tumor

Explanation: This patient has a giant cell tumor, which is a benign bone tumor. Patients may present symptoms similar to that seen in arthritis, with local pain and swelling. Some patients experience a pathologic fracture due to the local destruction and weakening of the bone. The histologic appearance shows sheets of osteoclast-like giant cells and mononuclear cells, occasionally associated with necrosis and hemorrhage. The mononuclear cells are thought to be neoplastic primitive stromal cells that express the receptor activator of nuclear factor kappa-B ligand (RANKL), which stimulates the formation of the osteoclast-like giant cells (see Fig. 5-16).

3. E. Sheets of small, blue cells

Explanation: This patient has Ewing sarcoma, which is the second most common bone tumor in children, after osteosarcoma. This sarcoma has a predilection to arise in the diaphysis of long, tubular bones such as the femur. Patients may develop a local mass, pain, and occasional fever. Histologically, the tumor shows sheets of small, round blue cells. If neural differentiation is present, rosettes of cells may be seen. The t(11;22) chromosomal translocation is seen in the majority of Ewing sarcoma cases (see Fig. 5-14B).

Chapter 6 Muscle

1. A. Dermatomyositis

Explanation: This patient had dermatomyositis, which is a noninfectious inflammatory myopathy along with polymyositis and inclusion body myositis. Dermatomyositis, as the name suggests, is characterized by both skin and muscle findings. Patients with dermatomyositis appear to be at greater risk for the development of visceral cancers (cancers of the soft internal organs). The antinuclear antibody Jo-1 can be detected in some patients with inflammatory myopathies. Muscle biopsy findings include perifascicular atrophy of muscle fibers, a predominantly perivascular mononuclear inflammatory cell infiltrate, and necrosis of myocytes (see Fig. 6-4C).

2. B. Mutations in the dystrophin gene

Explanation: This patient has Duchenne muscular dystrophy (DMD), which is associated with early-onset muscle weakness, usually beginning between age 2 and 3 years. Most cases occur in males. In some cases, the onset of symptoms occurs later. Weakness selectively affects the proximal limb muscles first before the distal muscles and the lower extremities before the upper extremities. A child with DMD experiences difficulty running, jumping, and walking up steps. When rising from the floor, affected children may also use their hands to support and push themselves to an upright position, an action known as Gower sign. An unusual waddling gait, lumbar lordosis, and calf enlargement are usually observed. Growth delay and other motor signs and symptoms may also be present. Cardiomyopathy symptoms develop in the teenage years. Mutations in the dystrophin gene are responsible for the disease. Pathologic changes include large variation in muscle fiber diameter, muscle fiber necrosis, and centrally displaced nuclei. This disease is caused by mutations in the dystrophin gene. Skeletal muscle fibers are weakened and susceptible to mechanical injury. Regenerative capabilities are much lower than in normal muscle (see Fig. 6-7B and C).

Chapter 7 Nervous Tissue

1. A. Demyelination and perivascular infiltration of lymphocytes and macrophages

Explanation: This patient has multiple sclerosis, which is an autoimmune disease that attacks the myelin-producing oligodendrocytes of the central nervous system. T lymphocytes and macrophages play an important role in inflammation and destruction of the oligodendrocyte-myelin unit. Magnetic resonance imaging (MRI) is the test of choice in diagnosing multiple sclerosis. Lumbar puncture with oligoclonal bands in the cerebrospinal fluid also supports the diagnosis (see Fig. 7-6C).

2. C. Increase in amyloid plaques and intracellular neurofibrillary tangles

Explanation: This patient has Alzheimer disease, which is the most common form of dementia in the elderly. Patients show progressive memory loss, personality changes, and cognitive impairments. Pathologically, Alzheimer disease is characterized by extracellular deposition of amyloid-beta protein (plaques), intracellular neurofibrillary tangles, and loss of neurons and synapses in the cerebral cortex and some subcortical regions (see Fig. 7-12C).

3. A. Bacterial meningitis

Explanation: This patient has bacterial meningitis, which is an infectious inflammatory disease of the meninges. Patients with bacterial meningitis show more severe symptoms and more sudden onset than those caused by other infectious agents. Cerebrospinal fluid (CSF) findings help to differentiate causes of the meningitis. Patients with viral encephalitis show a slow onset and may have normal or slightly abnormal CSF findings. Pathologically, meningitis affects the pia-arachnoid and the CSF in the sub-arachnoid space and may extend into the cerebral ventricles. Characteristic findings include perivascular cuffs of acute and chronic inflammatory cells, which distend the arachnoid space. Lumbar puncture for CSF is an important diagnostic tool (see Fig. 7-14C).

Chapter 8 Blood and Hemopoiesis

1. B. t(9;22)

Explanation: This patient has chronic myelogenous leukemia (CML), which is a myeloproliferative disorder characterized by a chimeric *BCR-ABL* gene that comprises the *BCR* gene on chromosome 22 and the *ABL* gene on chromosome 9. In more than 90% of cases, this chimeric gene is due to a reciprocal translocation, t(9;22)(q34;q11), also known as the Philadelphia chromosome (see Fig. 8-8C).

2. D. Plasma cell myeloma

Explanation: This patient has a plasma cell myeloma (multiple myeloma), which is a malignant tumor that typically affects older individuals and is usually associated with the production of monoclonal proteins composed of intact immunoglobulin or immunoglobulin light chains. These monoclonal proteins can be detected electrophoretically in serum and urine. These light chains are rapidly filtered into the urine, where they are called "Bence-Jones proteins." Patients often present with bone pain and fatigue due to the infiltration of the bone marrow by malignant plasma cells, causing dissolution of the bone partly by the stimulation of osteoclasts. Bone marrow biopsy typically reveals sheets of plasma cells that may vary from histologically normal to bizarre (see Fig. 8-19).

3. A. Acute myeloid leukemia (AML)

Explanation: This patient has acute myeloid leukemia (AML), which is a heterogenous group of malignant myeloid neoplasms that occur due to genetic mutations leading to alterations in the normal maturation process. Many of the genetic defects are translocations, such as t(15;17) seen in acute promyelocytic leukemia (APL), one form of AML. As immature precursors accumulate in the marrow, normal hematopoietic cells are reduced, leading to anemia, thrombocytopenia, and a reduction in normal white blood cells. Patients often present with petechiae due to a decrease in platelets (thrombocytopenia). The peripheral white blood count is often markedly elevated due to the presence of the abnormal, immature cells. The cells of AML have the qualities of blasts with nucleoli and show different degrees of differentiation. One histologic hallmark of AML is the presence of rod-shaped cytoplasmic inclusions called Auer rods (see Fig. 8-1C).

Chapter 9 Circulatory System

1. B. Lymphocyte

Explanation: This patient has myocarditis, an inflammation of heart muscle due to a variety of causes including infectious agents, hypersensitivity reactions due to drugs, autoimmune diseases, transplant rejection, and sarcoidosis. Viral infection of the heart typically elicits an immune reaction with infiltration of myocardial tissue by lymphocytes (lymphocytic myocarditis) (see Fig. 9-2D).

2. B. Left atrium

Explanation: This patient has cardiac myxoma, a benign neoplasm that typically arises in the atria of the heart, particularly the left atrium in the region near the fossa ovalis. These neoplasms are often pedunculated (on a stalk) and may cause obstruction to blood flow through a valve. Myxomas may also cause valve damage in the long term. These lesions may become clinically apparent if a portion of the myxoma breaks apart from the main lesion causing systemic embolization. Treatment for cardiac myxoma involves surgical removal, which is usually curative. Approximately 10% of cardiac myxomas may be associated with a genetic syndrome known as the Carney complex, which is characterized by cardiac and extracardiac myxomas as well as pigmented skin lesions and endocrine overactivity. Grossly, myxomas appear soft and gelatinous. Histologically, myxomas exhibit myxoma cells arranged singly and in groups, often with an appearance of a blood vessel. The background is an amorphous and eosinophilic mucopolysaccharide ground substance, often showing hemorrhage and occasional mononuclear inflammatory cells (see Fig. 9-2C).

3. C. Acute coronary syndrome

Explanation: Acute coronary syndrome is a general term to describe conditions that may occur after a sudden reduction in blood flow to the heart. This patient has experienced stable angina over several months. Angina pectoris is chest pain due to myocardial ischemia—reduced blood flow to the heart. Stable angina is most often due to a fixed, critical stenosis in a coronary artery due to an atherosclerotic plaque. This type of angina is predictable in that it occurs on exertion and remits at rest. On the day she presented to the hospital, this patient was experiencing unstable angina. Unstable angina may occur at rest, and the chest pain tends to be severe and progressive. This type of angina is most often due to a change in an atherosclerotic plaque such as fissure or rupture, which causes a blood clot (thrombus) to form very quickly, thereby causing occlusion of the coronary artery lumen. The sudden onset of ischemia may cause sudden cardiac death, arrhythmia, or myocardial infarct, as seen in this case. The ECG changes and the characteristic rise of the marker of cardiac injury (high sensitivity troponin T) indicate a myocardial infarct. The troponin level will peak and slowly decline over a period of several days (see Fig. 9-13B).

Chapter 10 Lymphoid System

1. A. Decreased CD4 helper T cell numbers

Explanation: This patient has an HIV infection, which is associated with a progressive decline in CD4 helper T lymphocytes (T cells), resulting in immunosuppression. Patients with an acute HIV infection may experience fever, lymphadenopathy, pharyngitis (sore throat), rash, and myalgia (muscle ache). The chronic phase of HIV infection may last from months to years (see Figs. 10-5B and 10-12C).

2. D. Sarcoidosis

Explanation: This patient has sarcoidosis, which is a multisystem disease characterized by the presence of noncaseating (lacking necrosis) granulomatous inflammation. Patients often present with hypercalcemia and elevated angiotensin-converting enzyme (ACE) levels. Affected tissues show aggregates of epithelioid histiocytes called granulomas, often with multinucleated giant cells present. Necrosis is very unusual in sarcoidosis, but a variant does exist where necrosis is present (see Fig. 10-19).

3. A. Extramedullary hematopoiesis

Explanation: One of the many causes of pathologic extramedullary hematopoiesis is severe anemia, most often seen in the spleen and liver. This patient exhibits symptoms of anemia, including easy fatigability and tachycardia, which is usually seen only in severe anemia. Physical exam reveals pale conjunctivae, and laboratory studies confirm the anemia showing a markedly low hemoglobin level. Treatment includes red cell transfusion and vitamin supplements including B_{12} and folic acid (see Fig. 10-15B).

Chapter 11 Respiratory System

1. B. Hyaline membranes

Explanation: This patient has diffuse alveolar damage (DAD), which is acute lung injury, including acute respiratory distress syndrome (ARDS). Clinical features of ARDS include dyspnea and tachypnea followed by cyanosis, hypoxemia, and respiratory failure. ARDS may result from diverse conditions including those that cause direct lung injury like pneumonia, toxic inhalation, and lung contusion to indirect lung injury including sepsis, drug toxicity, massive transfusion, and trauma. Viral infections, including COVID-19, may lead to ARDS and diffuse alveolar damage. Endothelial activation and damage to type II pneumocytes lead to the accumulation of intra-alveolar fluid and ultimately the formation of hyaline membranes composed of protein and necrotic debris (see Fig. 11-12B).

2. D. *Pneumocystis jirovecii*

Explanation: This patient has pneumocystis pneumonia, also called *Pneumocystis jirovecii*. It is caused by fungal organism infection. Tissue diagnosis can be obtained from a variety of specimens including bronchial wash and bronchoalveolar lavage specimens, which tend to be higher yield in terms of demonstrating the organisms. The classic cytologic feature consists of foamy alveolar casts that contain the organisms (see Fig. 11-2C).

3. A. Adenocarcinoma

Explanation: This patient has adenocarcinoma of the lung, which is a primary malignant lung neoplasm commonly called "lung cancer." Adenocarcinomas tend to arise in the lung periphery, whereas small cell carcinoma and squamous cell carcinoma tend to arise more centrally. Although adenocarcinoma occurs more frequently in patients who smoke, it is less closely related to smoking than other forms of lung cancer. Other risk factors include exposure to environmental pollutants and radon gas. Histologically, these tumors range from well-differentiated, recapitulating, well-formed glandular structures to poorly differentiated structures in which sheets of malignant cells predominate with scarce evidence of glandular expression. Treatment includes surgery followed by chemotherapy and radiation, depending on the stage (extent of spread) of the tumor (see Fig. 11-19).

Chapter 12 Urinary System

1. A. Anti–glomerular basement membrane disease

Explanation: This patient has an anti–glomerular basement membrane disease (anti-GMB disease), also called Goodpasture syndrome. This syndrome involves the kidneys and lungs. It is rare and characterized by circulating antibodies to domains of type IV collagen in renal and alveolar basement membranes. It is more common in Caucasian populations, and it tends to show a bimodal distribution with individuals in the third and sixth decades of life. The etiology of the syndrome is uncertain, but it tends to occur more often in individuals with a genetic susceptibility and subsequent environmental triggers, such as smoking tobacco, hydrocarbon exposure, and infection (see Fig. 12-8B).

2. E. Urothelial cell carcinoma

Explanation: This patient has urothelial cell carcinoma, which is the most common urinary bladder carcinoma in adults. Urothelial carcinoma is most prevalent in older men, but it may occur at any age. Risk factors include cigarette smoking, exposure to arylamines and radiation, long-term use of cyclophosphamide, and infection by the parasite *Schistosoma haematobium*. Painless frank hematuria is the most common sign, and sometimes frequency, urgency, and dysuria may be present. The carcinomas typically display a papillary morphology, and they are subdivided into low and high grade depending on cytologic features and the amount of architectural disorder presents (see Fig. 12-15C).

3. D. Mesangial expansion, glomerular basement membrane thickening, and glomerulosclerosis

Explanation: This patient has diabetic nephropathy, which is a complication of both type 1 and type 2 diabetes mellitus. Hyperglycemia activates various inflammatory pathways, leading to podocyte injury, malfunction, apoptosis, and protein deposition in the extracellular matrix of the nephron, causing albumin to leak into the urine. Hypertension, obesity, high blood cholesterol levels, and genetic predisposition negatively impact disease progression. Glomerular and tubular basement membrane thickening and mesangial and interstitial expansion will be noticeable within 3 to 5 years of diabetes onset. As the disease progresses, glomerulosclerosis (Kimmelstiel-Wilson disease) will develop. Symptoms of diabetic nephropathy include edema, hypertension, foamy urine, fatigue, headache, nausea, and vomiting (see Fig. 12-5C).

Chapter 13 Integumentary System

1. D. Human herpesvirus type 8

Explanation: This patient has Kaposi sarcoma (KS), which is a vascular neoplasm. It affects older individuals in certain populations, including those of Mediterranean origin, Jews, and eastern Europeans, and is seen in patients with AIDS. KS is strongly associated with human herpesvirus type 8 (HHV-8) (see Fig. 13-8B).

2. E. Seborrheic keratosis

Explanation: This patient has seborrheic keratosis, which is the most common benign neoplasm of the skin, and it typically occurs in the mid to late adulthood. The histologic appearance is varied, and types include hyperkeratotic, clonal, and reticulated. These lesions may show signs of irritation with a pronounced inflammatory infiltrate. Invaginations of the surface produce horn cysts, which appear as cystic spaces containing keratin (see Fig. 13-15).

3. D. Merkel cell carcinoma

Explanation: This patient has Merkel cell carcinoma, which is an aggressive neuroendocrine carcinoma of the skin. It is thought to arise from Merkel cells that normally are scarce in the basal layer of the epidermis. These tumors typically show a high mitotic rate with occasional apoptotic cells. Merkel cell carcinoma typically expresses neuroendocrine markers and characteristic paranuclear dotlike positivity in cytokeratin 20 staining (see Fig. 13-2B).

Chapter 14 Oral Cavity

1. C. Dentinogenesis imperfecta

Explanation: This patient has dentinogenesis imperfecta, which is an autosomal-dominant genetic disorder of tooth development caused by mutations in the dentin sialophosphoprotein gene. Patients suffer frequent enamel fractures and enamel attrition. Full crowns will improve the appearance of the teeth and protect the teeth from damage. Histologically, dentinal tubules are irregular and are larger than normal in diameter, and an uncalcified matrix may be present (see Fig. 14-15C).

2. C. Enamel fluorosis

Explanation: This patient has an enamel fluorosis condition, which involves enamel changes caused by excessive fluoride intake during tooth development (generally children under 8 years old). These changes are characterized by diffuse, opaque, and white streaks that run horizontally across the enamel. Stains with rough, irregular enamel surfaces are common. A fluoride-induced toxic effect on ameloblasts during enamel formation is believed to be the mechanism of the condition (see Fig. 14-14C).

3. B. Nicotine stomatitis

Explanation: This patient has nicotine stomatitis, which is a nonprecancerous condition, characterized by a white lesion in the oral mucosa of the hard palate of the mouth. It is caused by long-term pipe smoking, cigarette smoking, and/or consumption of excessively hot beverages. Histologically, the squamous mucosa shows hyperkeratosis (thickening of the stratum corneum) and acanthosis (overgrowth of the stratum spinosum) (see Fig. 14-4C).

Chapter 15 Digestive Tract

1. D. Meckel diverticulum

Explanation: This patient has a Meckel diverticulum, which is a congenital abnormality characterized by an outpouching in the lower part of the small bowel due to failure of the vitelline duct to close. Most people with Meckel diverticulum are asymptomatic. Bleeding, inflammation, peptic ulceration, and perforation can occur, producing signs and symptoms similar to appendicitis (see Fig. 15-19C).

2. D. Crohn disease

Explanation: This patient has Crohn disease, which is a chronic autoimmune inflammatory disease of the gastrointestinal tract that may affect any location, from the oral cavity to the anus, but it mostly involves the distal small intestine and colon. Symptoms include abdominal pain, diarrhea, vomiting, and weight loss. Pathologic changes include mucosal neutrophil and mononuclear cell infiltration, ulceration, mucosal fissures, fistulae, serosal adhesions, abscesses, pseudopolyps, and noncaseating granulomas (see Fig. 15-21B).

3. A. Intraepithelial eosinophils in the proximal and distal esophagus

Explanation: This patient has eosinophilic esophagitis (EOE), which is an allergic inflammatory disease of the esophagus characterized by eosinophils within the stratified squamous epithelium (intraepithelial eosinophils). EOE affects children and adults, and presenting symptoms may include nausea, vomiting, pain, dysphagia (difficulty swallowing), and food impaction. Endoscopic examination of the esophagus may show esophageal rings, furrows, and edema. In severe cases, luminal stricture may occur. Histologic examination typically reveals basal cell hyperplasia; intraepithelial eosinophils (≥ 15 per high-power field); and occasional eosinophilic microabscesses in the upper, middle, and lower esophagus (see Fig. 15-1C).

Chapter 16 Digestive Glands and Associated Organs

1. B. CA19-9 antigen

Explanation: This patient has a pancreatic adenocarcinoma, also known as pancreatic cancer, which is a malignant neoplasm of the pancreas. It arises from the epithelium of pancreatic ducts. Pathologically, ductal adenocarcinomas show infiltrating small glands lined by low-columnar and mucin-containing cells. CA19-9 antigen is a tumor marker characteristically elevated in patients with pancreatic cancer (see Fig. 16-1C).

2. E. Warthin tumor

Explanation: This patient has Warthin tumor, also known as papillary cystadenoma lymphomatosum. It is a benign neoplasm of salivary glands, particularly the parotid gland. Clinically, Warthin tumors present as painless swellings in the area of the parotid gland, and they have a strong association with cigarette smoking. Grossly, the tumor is well-circumscribed and lobular, and it may be multifocal. Upon sectioning, the mass contains cystic spaces often filled with a dark brown mucoid material likened to used motor oil. The histologic appearance is striking and unique, with multiple cystic spaces and papillary formations set within a lymphoid stroma. The cysts and papillary areas consist of eosinophilic epithelial cells producing a two-layered epithelium. The basal layer is cuboidal and the luminal layer is columnar. These epithelial cells are described as "oncocytic" and upon ultrastructural examination reveal abundant mitochondria. Surgical excision with an adequate margin is considered curative (see Fig. 16-4C).

Chapter 17 Endocrine System

1. C. Parathyroid adenoma

Explanation: This patient has parathyroid adenoma, which is a benign neoplasm of the parathyroid gland, and it is the most common cause of primary hyperparathyroidism. Most cases of primary hyperparathyroidism are discovered incidentally when a patient is found to be hypercalcemic on routine laboratory studies. Other causes of primary hyperparathyroidism include parathyroid hyperplasia and parathyroid carcinoma. Parathyroid carcinoma can cause striking elevations in parathyroid hormone and calcium. Some cases of parathyroid adenoma are related to the multiple endocrine neoplasia syndromes MEN-1 and MEN-2. Parathyroid adenomas are well circumscribed and red-brown in color. They are invested within a thin fibrous capsule, and they often compress the adjacent normal parathyroid tissue (see Fig. 17-9C).

2. D. Medullary carcinoma

Explanation: This patient has medullary carcinoma, which is a malignant neuroendocrine neoplasm of the thyroid gland arising from the parafollicular, or C, cells that produce calcitonin. Most patients seek medical help due to an enlarging neck mass, but they may on occasion present with paraneoplastic symptoms due to the elaboration of polypeptide hormones like vasoactive intestinal peptide (CIP) and serotonin. The histologic appearance includes polygonal to spindle cells arranged in nests, cords, and follicles (see Fig. 17-17).

Chapter 18 Male Reproductive System

1. D. Testicular seminoma

Explanation: This patient has testicular seminoma, which is testicular cancer. Testicular seminoma arises from the germinal epithelium of the seminiferous tubules, and seminomatous components are the characteristic finding. Clinically, patients present with painless enlargement of the testis, which may also present with a hydrocele. Histologically, classic testicular seminoma consists of sheets of large cells with distinct cell borders and nucleoli, infiltrated with lymphocytes (see Fig. 18-15C).

2. B. Prostate adenocarcinoma

Explanation: This patient has prostate adenocarcinoma, which is the most common cancer in men and typically affects men over age 50 years. The majority of prostate cancers are adenocarcinomas arising from the glandular component of the prostate. Patients may present with urinary symptoms, such as difficulty initiating or stopping the urine stream, or dysuria (pain on urination). Patients may also present with bone pain due to advanced metastasis. Many patients are diagnosed through screening programs utilizing the digital rectal exam, the serum prostate-specific antigen (PSA) test, and transrectal needle biopsy if indicated. Histologically, the appearance of prostate cancer is highly varied, from well-formed tubular structures to individual infiltrating malignant cells (see Fig. 18-20C).

Chapter 19 Female Reproductive System

1. A. Ductal carcinoma *in situ*

Explanation: This patient has ductal carcinoma in situ (DCIS), which is a ductal adenocarcinoma of the breast. It has no transgression of the basement membrane or invasion of the adjacent fibrous stroma. Most DCIS results from changes in the ducts beginning as a proliferation of ductal cells. In time, these proliferating ductal cells may show signs of cellular atypia and eventually become DCIS, the precursor to infiltrating duct carcinoma (see Fig. 19-17C).

2. E. Papillary serous cystadenocarcinoma

Explanation: This patient has papillary serous adenocarcinoma, which is the most common malignant neoplasm of the ovary, and it arises from the ovarian surface epithelium. Symptoms include abdominal pain, gastrointestinal and urologic problems, and abdominal distension. Often, malignant ovarian tumors have already metastasized by the time of diagnosis. Histologically, papillary serous cystadeno-carcinomas show a papillary architecture and vary in the degree of differentiation (see Fig. 19-18).

3. A. Endometrial atrophy

Explanation: This patient has serous carcinoma of the endometrium, which is type II endometrial adenocarcinomas. Type II endometrial adenocarcinomas tend to occur in the setting of endometrial atrophy. They are often poorly differentiated and consist of the aggressive serous type. Treatment involves radical hysterectomy; lymph node dissection; and, in some cases, chemotherapy. The risk factors for type II adenocarcinoma include unopposed estrogen, obesity, diabetes, cigarette smoking, and infertility (see Fig. 19-11B).

Chapter 20 Eye

1. A. Acute angle-closure glaucoma

Explanation: This patient has acute angle-closure glaucoma, which is a form of glaucoma characterized by a sudden increase in intraocular pressure because the angle of the anterior chamber is blocked, and the aqueous humor cannot drain from the anterior chamber. It is usually unilateral, and excruciating pain may radiate to areas of trigeminal distribution. Atrophy of the optic nerve head ("cupping") along with peripheral vision defects is the common finding with acute angle-closure glaucoma. Treatment may involve surgery and medications to lower the intraocular pressure and reverse angle closure (see Fig. 20-12C).

2. E. Photoreceptor layer and pigment epithelium layer

Explanation: This patient has retinal detachment, which is an eye condition in which the sensory retina separates from the underlying retinal pigment epithelium. The retina covers the inner aspect of the posterior two thirds of the eyeball. The outer one third of the retina receives nutrients by diffusion from the choriocapillaris of the choroid, while the inner two thirds of the retina receive nutrients from retinal blood vessels. Direct impact and the shock wave from a deploying airbag can damage eye structures, resulting in retinal detachment (see Fig. 20-16B).

Chapter 21 Ear

1. B. Cholesteatoma

Explanation: This patient has a cholesteatoma, which is a mass of keratin-producing squamous epithelium that often grows from the tympanic membrane in the middle ear. As cholesteatoma progresses, it can cause damage to the ossicles, inner ear, mastoid air cells, and the external auditory canal leading to sepsis, meningitis, brain abscess, sensorineural hearing loss, vertigo, facial paralysis, and even death. Trauma and chronic inflammation of the tympanic membrane may increase the incidence of cholesteatoma. Surgery involving a tympanomastoidectomy remains the primary treatment for this condition (see Fig. 21-2C).

2. E. Vestibular schwannoma

Explanation: This patient has vestibular schwannoma, also known as neurilemmoma, which is a benign tumor mostly arising from Schwann cells of the vestibular branch of the eighth cranial nerve (vestibulocochlear nerve). Patients with vestibular schwannoma often present with headache, hearing loss, tinnitus, and vertigo. The cerebellopontine angle is a common site for vestibular schwannoma. The tumor is often well demarcated and extends into the internal auditory meatus. Histologic findings are characterized by alternately dense and sparse cellularity zones called Antoni A and Antoni B areas. Treatment options include surgery, radiation therapy, and observation, depending on the patient's health condition. Gamma knife surgery (GKS) is gradually becoming a standard treatment for vestibular schwannoma (see Fig. 21-14A).

Index